Time Perspective Theory; Review, Research and Application

Maciej Stolarski • Nicolas Fieulaine
Wessel van Beek
Editors

Time Perspective Theory; Review, Research and Application

Essays in Honor of Philip G. Zimbardo

Springer

Editors
Maciej Stolarski
Faculty of Psychology
University of Warsaw
Warsaw, Poland

Nicolas Fieulaine
Groupe de Recherche en Psychologie
Sociale, Institut de Psychologie
Université de Lyon
Bron, France

Wessel van Beek
GGZ Veenendaal
Veenendaal, The Netherlands

ISBN 978-3-319-07367-5 ISBN 978-3-319-07368-2 (eBook)
DOI 10.1007/978-3-319-07368-2
Springer Cham Heidelberg New York Dordrecht London

Library of Congress Control Number: 2014942519

Photo Credit goes to Linda A. Cicero/Stanford News Service, who kindly granted us the use of her picture on our cover.

Printed on acid-free paper

Springer is part of Springer Science+Business Media (www.springer.com)

To Phil Zimbardo,
our Teacher, our Mentor, our Friend

To all authors,
who promptly replied to our many requests
and patiently waited for ours

To our families and friends,
who supported and encouraged us
during this huge but exciting project

To our colleagues
from the TP international network and beyond

May the time be on your side!

Maciej, Nicolas, & Wessel

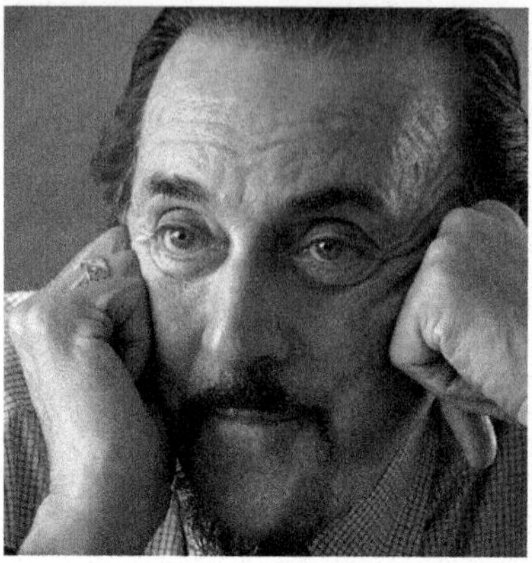

Philip Zimbardo *is internationally recognized as the "voice and face of contemporary psychology" through his widely viewed PBS-TV series, Discovering Psychology, his media appearances, best-selling trade books, and his classic research, The Stanford Prison Experiment.*

Zimbardo has been a Stanford University professor since 1968 (now emeritus), having taught previously at Yale, NYU, and Columbia University. He also continues to teach at the Naval Post Graduate School in Monterey (courses on the psychology of terrorism), and is professor at the Palo Alto University (teaching social psychology to clinical graduate students). Zimbardo has been given numerous awards and honors as an educator, researcher, writer, media contributor, and for service to the profession of psychology. He has been awarded the Vaclav Havel Foundation Prize for his lifetime of research on the human condition. Among his more than 400 professional publications, including 50 trade and textbooks, is the oldest current textbook in psychology, Psychology and Life, and Core Concepts in Psychology in its seventh edition. His popular book on shyness in adults was the first of its kind, as was the shyness clinic that he started in the community and continues as a treatment-research clinic at the Palo Alto University in Palo Alto.

His current research interests are in the domain of experimental social psychology, with a scattered emphasis on everything interesting to study from: time perspective, persuasion, madness, violence, political psychology, and terrorism. His current passion is The Heroic Imagination Project, exploring and encouraging the psychology of everyday heroes.

Noted for his personal and professional efforts to actually 'give psychology away to the public', Zimbardo has also been a social-political activist, challenging the Government's wars in Vietnam and Iraq, as well as the American Correctional System.

Zimbardo has been President of the American Psychological Association (2002), President of the Western Psychological Association (twice), Chair of the Council of Scientific Society Presidents (CSSP), and now Chair of the Western Psychological Foundation, as well as the Director of the Center for Interdisciplinary Policy, Education, and Research on Terrorism (CIPERT).

He is excited about his recent trade books, including: The Lucifer Effect *(Random House, 2007, paperback, 2008),* The Time Paradox *(with John Boyd, Free Press, 2008),* The Demise of Guys *(with Nikita Duncan, TED books, 2012), and* Time Cure *(with Richard and Rosemary Sword, Wiley, 2012).*

Foreword

Reflections on the Beginning of Time… Perspective

When Phil Zimbardo joined the Stanford faculty in the late 1960s, he came with prior training in hypnosis and experience in using it as a methodological tool (Zimbardo 1969). However, at Stanford he developed a new working relationship with the hypnosis laboratory run by his colleague, Jack Hilgard. Phil then organized a research team to use hypnosis methodology to study various cognitive and emotional processes. I was one of the members of that team, along with Gary Marshall and Greg White, and we conducted a number of different studies on such phenomena as unexplained arousal and control of physiological processes (see Maslach et al. 1979). The results of the unexplained arousal studies led Phil to do his later, innovative research on discontinuity theory and madness (Zimbardo 1999).

But the most exciting studies that our team conducted were those having to do with people's personal sense of time. Phil used both his own experiences and those of others to begin developing an idea that the way in which people understand and experience the flow of time as well as perceive distinctions between past, present, and future might provide great insights into various patterns of human behavior. He read all kinds of source materials with relevance to time, including historical, religious, economic, literary, and cross-cultural ones, and took his inspiration from these as well as from psychology, sociology, and anthropology. The discussions that we had about these new ideas, and about possible hypotheses, were truly fascinating.

Our first study focused on the notion of an expanded present, and we devised several behavioral measures to assess both the effectiveness of our hypnotic induction and of the hypothesized outcomes (Zimbardo et al. 1971). The research design compared the responses of twelve trained hypnotic subjects given the suggestion to "allow the present to expand and the past and future to become distant and insignificant" with those of eighteen other subjects distributed across three control conditions. In two of these conditions, the same expanded present time distortion instruction was given: half of these subjects were simulators, told to imagine how hypnotized subjects would respond and then to act in that way, while the other half were waking controls who merely received the expanded present instruction without any mention of hypnosis. The fourth group was a normal-time control, who did not receive any time distortion instructions (although they were asked to think about their own conception of time instead). All of the subjects engaged in three tasks. The first involved writing projective stories in response to two TAT pictures, one before and one after the time distortion manipulation. As predicted, the hypnotic subjects shifted to using more present tense verbs and making more references to present events and fewer to future ones. However, the simulators were able to figure out this response and did the same thing to an even greater degree. On the second task, the subjects were asked to listen to a tape recording of two comedians trying to make a radio commercial for their new film, and as these two made mistakes, they began to criticize and curse each other in increasingly obscene ways. While listening to this unexpected and socially inappropriate tape, subjects in the three control conditions were more restrained in their behavior and only smiled occasionally. But as predicted, the hypnotic "expanded present" subjects got totally caught up in the experience, laughed loudly, and expressed their comments in similarly humorous and obscene terms. The third task was designed to get the subjects involved in a sensory experience through the physical action of making something out of a large mound of sticky clay. All of the control subjects were upset about getting so messy and dirty while working with the clay, and they stopped the task as soon as they were told to. In vivid contrast, the hypnotic "expanded present" subjects were not at all concerned about the clay's messiness, but had more fun with it. Even more striking, when they were told to stop, they were so involved in the process that they just kept on playing with the clay for another five minutes (until the experimenter insisted that they stop and leave the room).

In addition to a subjective conceptualization of past, present, and future, people also develop a time sense of personal tempo. This involves both the estimation of the rate at which events are occurring and affective reactions to different rates of stimulus input. We designed a study in which this experienced tempo was altered through a hypnotic induction (Zimbardo et al. 1973). We assumed that if time is perceived as existing in a new relationship to the occurrence of certain events, then behavioral measures that are sensitive to the rate of responding should reveal this altered perception. All subjects in the study were taught to press a telegraph key at different rates in order to illuminate various target lights in an array of ten colored lights. They then participated in four trials, in which the first and third were baseline and the second and fourth were experimental. On one baseline trial, each subject was instructed to keep the red light illuminated (three presses per second), and on the other baseline trial, the subject was instructed to keep the blue light illuminated (six presses per second). Interspersed between these baseline trials were the instructions to modify personal tempo; on one trial, subjects were told to experience time as slowing down ("so that a second will seem like a minute, and a minute will seem like an hour"), while on the other trial, subjects were told to experience time as speeding up. Between these two tempo modification instructions (which were counterbalanced), subjects were told to normalize their experience of time. The 36 subjects were randomly assigned to one of three treatments: hypnosis, hypnotic simulation, and waking non-hypnotized control. Only the hypnotic subjects were reliably able to translate the verbal suggestion of asynchronicity between clock time and personal time into behavioral reality. This was shown in comparisons of mean rates of response, percentage of total time on and off target, mean deviation in individual response rates from baseline to experimental response levels, and even in the more subtle measure of displacement of the response distribution.

Although we were excited by these initial empirical findings on time, we did not follow up on them for quite a while, mainly for two reasons: in 1971 Phil conducted the Stanford Prison Experiment (which subsequently consumed a lot of his professional life), and I became an assistant professor at the University of California, Berkeley (where I had to start my own line of independent research). In addition, to be frank, there was not a lot of external interest in our time research at that point—the reactions were either dismissive of the hypnosis methodology or of the particular ideas.

Fortunately, many years later, Phil did return to his original fascination with time. With the collaboration of some graduate students, most notably John Boyd, Kelli Keough, Kent Harber, Alison Holman, and Alex Gonzalez, he did some new studies and developed a measure of time perspective, the Zimbardo Time Perspective Inventory (ZTPI). And then, to his great surprise and gratitude, the phenomenon of time perspective began to attract the attention of many researchers around the world. This global team of colleagues, many of whom have contributed to this volume, has done extraordinary work on time, with a remarkable level of collaboration and friendship.

All of this new work has brought great joy to Phil, and he continues to be in touch with this global team and to join them at various conferences. The fact that all of these colleagues have contributed their research to this book, in honor of Phil's 80th birthday, is absolutely the most wonderful gift they could give him, and I thank them all from the bottom of my heart!

References

Maslach, C., Zimbardo, P. G., & Marshall, G. (1979). Hypnosis as a means of studying cognitive and behavioral control. In E. Fromm, & R. Shor (Eds.), *Hypnosis: Developments in research and new perspectives* (2nd ed., pp. 649–683) Hawthorne: Aldine.

Zimbardo, P. G. (1969). *The cognitive control of motivation: The consequences of choice and dissonance.* Glenview: Scott Foresman.

Zimbardo, P. G. (1999). Discontinuity theory: Cognitive and social searches for rationality and normality – May lead to madness. *Advances in Experimental Social Psychology, 31,* 345–486.

Zimbardo, P. G., Marshall, G., & Maslach, C. (1971). Liberating behavior from time-bound control: Expanding the present through hypnosis. *Journal of Applied Psychology, 1,* 305–323.

Zimbardo, P. G., Marshall, G., White, G., & Maslach, C. (1973). Objective assessment of hypnotically induced time distortion. *Science, 181,* 282–284.

University of California
Berkeley, CA, USA

Christina Maslach

Laudation

The Life and Time of Philip Zimbardo

A Man of Consistent Extremes

I first met Phil in the spring of 1994. I had been admitted to Stanford for the fall term, and we were both excited to get to work early on time-related research. I had previously known him only through his publications and through *Discovering Psychology*, his PBS television series. I vividly remember being struck by contrasts as I walked into his office that beautiful spring Stanford day. My immediate sense was that Phil's public persona was inconsistent—some might say dissonant—with his true self. His office looked nothing like the staid, professional office that I had seen on TV. It instead looked like he had recently downsized from a much larger office and was still in the process of unpacking. Piles of papers, boxes of lecture material, and mail were strewn about. I was shocked. Over the years, however, I learned that Phil is not a man of inconsistencies, but a man of consistent extremes. His high future orientation does not conflict with his high present-hedonism. Phil is simply very high or very low on every dimension of time perspective, and most other individual difference measures as well. Back in 1994, I didn't realize this, and I remember thinking, just momentarily, "What have I gotten myself into?"

What I had gotten myself into, of course, was the adventure of a lifetime. I worked very closely with Phil over the next 5 years, and we continue to collaborate today. In the next few pages, I hope to provide some insight into what it was like to work closely with a man that is exceptional in more ways that anyone else that I've ever met. If you fail to be impressed, it's due to the limitation of my writing ability, not to my subject matter.

His Escape from Present-Fatalistic and Past-Negative Time Perspectives

Time had begun to shape Phil's life long before I showed up at his office door. In fact, it's no surprise that Phil ultimately studied time given the profound role that time—and his attitudes toward it—played in his life. Phil grew up in the Bronx, New York, which, like most of our hometowns, is a source both of great pride and modest insecurity. In Phil's eyes, the Bronx was a great place to be *from*. When he talks about it, he describes the neighborhood as a sea of poverty, ignorance, and hopelessness, which it undoubtedly was. Yet somehow the negativity and pessimism that permeated his youth never managed to stain Phil. His Present-Fatalism score is a remarkably low 1.1, and his Past-Negative score is an equally surprising 1.9. Through a combination of Past-Positive and a nascent Future time perspective, Phil was able to transcend the Present-Fatalism that could have defined his life.

His family—and his thick Sicilian blood, as he would say—was clearly a source of strength. Phil's father, the family bread winner, was relatively uneducated by current standards—he finished 8th grade—but he was extremely bright. He built the first TV in their neighborhood by hand, which would be quite an accomplishment even today. Phil's mother held the family together and insisted that Phil take care of his younger siblings. She was a saint, and she died in Phil's arms. Phil's brothers and sister were a constant source of playmates and support. Don, one of Phil's younger brothers, describes Phil alternately as a loving brother, the ring leader, the person that could hit the softball the farthest, the brother that could have played AAA baseball, and the brother that was blessed with a 160 IQ. Phil was obviously blessed in many ways: with great intellect, with great athletic skill, with great interpersonal skills, and with great drive. Perhaps his greatest gift, however, was his loving family that sheltered and protected him from the life that he could have had. Phil's Past-Positive time perspective is a remarkable 5.0.

An Education in Future Time Perspective

While Phil learned to embrace a Past-Positive and to ward off a Present-Fatalistic time perspective from his family, he began to learn a Future orientation from his teachers. He was very smart, and he quickly learned that, if he listen to what his teachers said now and did what they said later, he was rewarded. He passionately embraced a Future time perspective, and he never looked back. He worked extremely hard at whatever he did, and he was soon a track star and stellar student at James Monroe High School in the Bronx.

In retrospect, the social science curriculum at James Monroe is somewhat suspect. It seems highly coincidental that the two people most responsible for the creation of the morally responsible but occasionally bureaucratically impenetrable organization known as a Human Subject Committee would, by chance, be high school classmates. That's right. Phil Zimbardo and "little" Stanley Milgram were high school classmates. (Stan Getz, the famous jazz musician, whom Phil would befriend after moving to San Francisco, is also a James Monroe alumnus). By Phil's account, Stanley was the smartest guy in his high school class, and Phil was the most popular. I'm not sure about the first point, but I have no doubts about the second.

At some point during high school, Phil's family moved to Los Angeles. A relative had lined up a good job for Phil's dad. The time that Phil's family spent in LA was mostly unremarkable. The job was not as good as promised, and the family missed the Bronx. Phil felt stigmatized as a mafia family without the advantages of actually being a member. For the first time in his life, he developed asthma. After less than a year, they moved home.

What was remarkable about this episode was the journal that Phil kept during his family's road trip from New York to California. He found it while I was a graduate student with him. He showed it to me, because he was amazed by the younger version of himself. He was right to be impressed. It was, in essence, the most detailed lab journal that I have ever read. Each day started with the precise time that the family woke up, which was followed by what they had for breakfast, how much it cost, and the exact time that they began their journey. He covered the price of gas, the number of gallons purchased at each stop, and the number of miles driven. He then calculated the average miles per gallon. He noted the sights and scenes in such detail that his description could be used to rebuild the original Route 66.

The journal impressed me in multiple ways. First, and most personally, it was something that I would not have done. As much as I wanted to be like Phil, he is different than me, and, dare I say, he is likely different than you. Second, it reflected an attention to detail that I had not previously experienced. I have never met anyone else that would strive to capture life in such excruciating detail. It was a Jan Van Eyck painting in words. Finally, it reflected a future orientation that was clearly foreign to me when I was in high school. Who would read his treatise? It was either a future version of himself, which actually happened, or someone else. You might say that keeping a journal was a present-oriented way to pass the time. I would agree, if he only did it for a day or two. Phil kept it for the entire week-long journey.

As Phil would later document, future orientation is associated with academic success. He had to look no farther than his own life. His future orientation in high school led to academic success that led him to Brooklyn College, where he was the first person in his family to graduate from college. His future orientation at Brooklyn College led him to Yale, where he began his career as a behaviorist. That's right. The world's most famous social psychologist began his career running rats. His advisor suffered from depression and tragically committed suicide early during Phil's graduate career. Phil did what you would expect a brilliant, future-oriented grad student to do. He analyzed the remaining data, wrote the resulting papers, and got his advisor publications posthumously.

After the unfortunate death of his advisor, Phil gravitated to the work of Carl Hovland, whom Phil greatly admired. Phil recounted how Carl had acted at a multiday conference years before. Carl was the conference organizer, and, after the final presentation, Carl said that he thought that all of the presentations had been outstanding. Carl proceeded to summarize the best parts of each conference presentation without the benefit of notes so brilliantly that even if the original presentation was not outstanding, what Carl took from it was. According to Phil, Hovland was a brilliant, organized thinker, and from "good Midwestern stock," as was Ernest Hilgard with whom Phil would later collaborate on hypnosis research. For Phil, the term "good Midwestern stock" was a high compliment that signified the ability to work grueling hours in the pursuit of knowledge without showing visible signs of stress. Phil doesn't have the Midwestern genes, but he certainly has the trait, which is yet another case study suggesting that the situation matters.

A "Quantum Leap" in Future Orientation

In 1960, Phil moved to NYU in the Bronx, where he was an assistant professor. This was the most difficult stretch in Phil's professional career. He taught five courses each semester and was still expected to publish, which was a lot to ask even of Phil. He did manage to have some fun, such as the time he invited a young Muslim minister to speak to a largely Jewish class. The minister walked softly to the podium and quietly placed a Koran on it. He then humbly asked for the class's permission to begin with a prayer, which they of course granted. The lecture then began with a whisper. The tone of the minister's voice and the power of his words then grew to an impassioned crescendo. By the end, the entire class had joined the crusade for African American equality. Malcolm X was an even better speaker than you've been led to believe in movies.

During his seven years at NYU, Phil was invited to fill in for a year at Columbia University while Stanley Schachter was on sabbatical. Part of his responsibilities as an invited visitor was to act as host and tour guide for candidates for tenured positions that Phil coveted. This was an understandably awkward and embarrassing position for Phil, because he himself was obviously being overlooked in their search. At one point, an exasperated Phil asked the department chair what he needed to do to secure a tenured position. The department chair responded that Phil needed a "quantum leap in visibility," which only strengthened Phil's future orientation. As a result, hardworking Phil began to work even harder. As evidence of his hard work, there is a ten-year stretch from which Phil does not recognize any popular songs. Unfortunately for Phil, he picked a bad decade to miss, the 1960s.

Before you feel too sorry for future-oriented Phil, you should know how the NYU chapter ended. As Phil was toiling away for the benefit of NYU, he received an unexpected phone call. On the other end of the call was Albert Hastorf, chair of the Stanford Department of Psychology. Completely out of the blue, Al asked Phil what it would take for him to give up everything that he had going for him at NYU and to accept a position as a full, tenured professor at Stanford. Phil's answer: A bus ticket. Thus, Phil went from an assistant professorship at NYU to a full professorship at Stanford. There is some justice in this world.

Present-Hedonism Tempered by Future Time Perspective

It hasn't been all-work-and-no-play for Phil. While a Future time perspective has dominated his life, Phil, unlike many very successful people, has managed to maintain a healthy present-hedonism. He is a sucker for sweets and Macadamia nuts, and his 30-min meetings have been known to last hours. He loves physical contact, and he has the ability to be completely in the moment when he interacts, which is a trait that he greatly admires in others such as Bill Clinton. He loves parties, and he's a wonderful, gracious host. He likes to laugh. Phil's Present-Hedonistic time perspective is a high 3.5.

Despite his passion for life, Phil has managed to avoid the negative aspects of Present-Hedonism. He drinks alcohol, but I've never seen him drunk. He lived through the 1960s on college campuses, but, unlike Clinton, he didn't do drugs. You might find this somewhat surprising, given the enthusiasm with which he embraces deviance, but it makes perfect sense from the perspective of future orientation. The fact that Phil didn't try drugs wasn't a moral position. He just didn't have time. His Future time perspective interfered with his enjoyment of the music of the 1960s, but it also inoculated him against an aspect of the 1960s that, for many, was destructive.

Future Orientation as a Way of Life

Phil arrived at Stanford in 1968 feeling like his future orientation and hard work had finally paid off. They had. He had reached the top of the pyramid. He could now relax, kick back, and indulge his latent present-hedonism. But then he noticed something remarkable. Everyone else had gotten to Stanford because of their extreme Future time perspectives, too.[1] There was a new norm with which to compare himself, and, instead of changing, Phil became more of who he already was. Phil's Future time perspective is a very high 4.5. He doubled down on Future time perspective and soon produced what is undoubtedly his most important work, the Stanford Prison Experiment. He also wrote a book on shyness, conducted research on hypnosis with Hilgard, and became author of the longest continuously published introductory psychology textbook, *Psychology and Life*. He didn't let up. Over the next 40+ years, Phil became one of the most prolific, most influential, and most well-known psychologists of all time. Along the way, he produced the widely acclaimed *Discovering Psychology* series for public television, began work on his Discontinuity Theory of Madness, inspired heroes great and small, and, in the 1980s, turned his attention back to his roots with a renewed interest in time.

[1] The one bastion of present orientation at Stanford is the iconoclastic marching band. Somewhat ironically, the song that the band plays after the Stanford football team scores is Free's "All Right Now."

The Beginning of the Quantitative Investigation of Time

In 1985, Phil, Alex Gonzalez, and Robert Levine published articles in *Psychology Today* on how people's attitudes toward time affect their lives and how these attitudes differ across culture. Other brilliant thinkers had talked about time and its influence on our lives before them. Among them were such intellectual heavy hitters as Heraclitus and William James. These authors, however, had approached time from a philosophical and qualitative perspective that was largely foreign to American empirical psychology. Phil and Bob's work showed how attitudes toward time could be investigated using more rigorous and more modern quantitative methodologies. The 1985 *Psychology Today* publication marks the beginning of quantitative research on time perspective.

I read their work in the early 1990s and began to think about how their approach to studying time might be extended to explain what continues to be one of the most extreme human behaviors, suicide bombing. I added items to what was then the Stanford Time Perspective Inventory that I felt captured attitudes toward time after the imagined death of a person's physical body. I then administered the combined scale to several hundred people and factor analyzed the results. The items that I had added did indeed hold together as a distinct factor, which I called the post-Future time perspective. I wrote Phil a letter explaining my results, and, to my astonishment, I got a long letter in return. I was thrilled! I found the letter a couple of years into my graduate work at Stanford, and I showed it to Phil. His response was, "I should have been publishing." His extreme present orientation motivated him to write the letter. His extreme future orientation felt guilty for doing so. It was about this time that Phil renamed the "post-Future time perspective" the "transcendental-Future time perspective." Phil's score on the transcendental-future time perspective is a low 1.5.

What's Taken So Long?

It's been nearly 30 years since the publication of Phil's seminal article on time perspective and the publication of this work. A reasonable person might ask, "What's taken so long?" It's a good question, and there are a couple of reasonable answers.

One answer rests on the ephemeral, elusive nature of time itself. Much like gravity, which is not completely understood either, the fact that we live within time every second, minute, and hour of our lives makes research on time extremely challenging. Time controls us; we can't conduct controlled experiments on time.

A second answer relates to how completely our attitudes toward time color the way that we see the world. Our attitudes toward time shape our lives so that we are likely to be surrounded by others that share our time perspective. Phil's arrival at Stanford is a powerful example. He had indeed reached the top of the pyramid, but he found it populated only by other future-oriented people. All others had been left behind. In this world in which future orientation reigns supreme, it's taken people with unique experience and perspicacity to recognize the value and validity of competing time perspectives. Time is central to the human experience of the physical world, much like width, height, and depth. It is therefore not a stretch to claim that each individual's time perspective profile reflects an equally valid alternate conception of reality. The future-dominated world of academia has been slow to recognize this, and it's thus taken luminaries like Phil that possess experience with a diverse range of time perspectives to move the field forward. The fact that many of the chapters in this collected work are authored by people that have experience with more than just Future time perspective by virtue of culture and geography also supports this assertion.

When we first submitted our "Putting Time in Perspective" article to JPSP, the feedback was substantially less enthusiastic than we had hoped. It was as if a fish had proposed the study of water to a group of fish that didn't recognize the medium in which they lived. We persevered, as future-oriented people will, and the result is an article that has, in many ways, stood the test of time.

Thank You for the Time

I still have a key to Phil's psychology department office on my key chain. It is one of only five keys that I carry. I haven't used it in years, and I'm not sure that it would still work. Nonetheless, it's a way that I keep a part of him with me always, and it's a symbol of the doors that he unlocked for me. The time that Phil unselfishly gave to me changed the course of my life, and, if you're reading this, there's a good chance that he changed the course of yours as well. Phil, from all of us that you've touched over the years, thank you for the time.

Google Inc. John N. Boyd
San Francisco, CA, USA

Contents

Part II Evolutionary, Cultural, and Social Context of Time Perspective

Part III Cognitive, Emotional, and Motivational Processes in Time Perspective

Editors

Maciej Stolarski is currently an Assistant Professor at Faculty of Psychology, University of Warsaw, Poland, where he earned his MA and PhD degrees, both awarded with *summa cum laude* distinction. His scientific interests are very broad, including mutual influences between cognition and emotion, individual differences in temperament, IQ, and emotional intelligence, as well as analyses of aggregate psychological features of nations. He published in renowned peer-reviewed journals, including *Intelligence*, *Personality and Individual Differences*, *Journal of Happiness Studies*, and *PLOS One*, among others. His interest in Time Perspective phenomenon, as well as his collaboration with Phil Zimbardo began in 2010, after Phil's visit at University of Warsaw. Since that time Maciej conducted numerous studies investigating TP, mainly in its relation to emotional processes. He developed and validated the DBTP, an indicator of temporal balance, increasingly used in empirical research. Currently he conducts a research program investigating genetic, familial, and cultural bases of TP.

Nicolas Fieulaine is an Associate Professor of Social Psychology at the Institute of Psychology at the University of Lyon, France. He earned his BA, MA, and PhD from Provence University and works with Phil Zimbardo since 7 years to develop and structure time perspective research worldwide. He was awarded with several research grants for applied studies, and is the program director of the Master of Applied Social Psychology at the University of Lyon. His earliest research interests dealt with psychological correlates of socioeconomic precariousness which he studied using quantitative and qualitative methods. His findings rapidly bring him to be interested in the social roots and psychological implications of time perspective, mainly in the fields of inequalities related to health and access to rights. He is also interested in applying psychology to social issues through action-research, field experiments, or professional training. He is currently studying the role of psychological field properties on people's experiences, decisions, and behaviors.

Wessel van Beek studied clinical psychology at the University of Utrecht, the Netherlands, and earned his PhD from the Vrije Universiteit in Amsterdam. He has been working in clinical psychology and psychiatry for 20 years. Beside his work as a psychotherapist Wessel did research on the role of time perspective and Future thinking in suicidality, and he developed the Future Oriented Group Training for suicidal patients. As a clinician Wessel has special interest in how past, present, and future thinking are related and how they influence psychopathology. Wessel has been part of a core group of researchers working with Phil Zimbardo. He currently focuses on Prenatal Past, as a complementary time perspective, and is preparing a book on Time in Psychotherapy. Wessel is director of a small mental health care institute in The Netherlands.

Time Perspective Theory: The Introduction

Maciej Stolarski, Nicolas Fieulaine, and Wessel van Beek

In his numerous spirited lectures on Time Perspective, Professor Philip G. Zimbardo has often emphasized that time perspective remains one of the most powerful influences on human behavior (e.g., Zimbardo 2012). Quite an unusual claim, taking into account that it has been formulated by one of the most radical situationists (Zimbardo 2004) in contemporary psychology, with respect to construct which has a lot to do with individual differences. Since his early works on hypnotically induced focus on a particular time horizon (past, present or future Zimbardo et al. 1971; see also "Foreword" by Maslach, this volume), Zimbardo, has made an impressive contribution to psychology of time. His dissemination of Time Perspective Theory was initially presented to an enthusiastic group of young researchers, gathered originally through a seminar led at Moscow State University by Anna Sircova, and progressively structured into an International Research Network (see http://www.timeperspective.net) composed of more than 150 members from more than 40 countries. Dozens of articles published in high-impact, peer-reviewed journals confirmed the robustness of impact that Time Perspective Theory made on contemporary psychology. The impact that was perhaps most clearly visible was evident during the 1st International Conference on Time Perspective which took place in September 2012 in Coimbra, Portugal, with hundreds of

M. Stolarski (✉)
Faculty of Psychology, University of Warsaw,
Stawki Str. 5/7, 00-183 Warsaw, Poland
e-mail: mstolarski@psych.uw.edu.pl

N. Fieulaine
Groupe de Recherche en Psychologie Sociale, Institut de Psychologie,
Université de Lyon, 69600 Bron, France
e-mail: Nicolas.fieulaine@univ-lyon2.fr

W. van Beek
GGZ Veenendaal, Veenendaal, The Netherlands
e-mail: wessel.van.beek@gmail.com

M. Stolarski et al. (eds.), *Time Perspective Theory; Review, Research and Application: Essays in Honor of Philip G. Zimbardo*, DOI 10.1007/978-3-319-07368-2_1,

researchers from all around the world, presenting their research and discussing the nature and role of psychological time, as well as prominent keynotes, most of whom could be found among the authors of this book (Chapters "The Motivational Properties of Future Time Perspective Future Orientation: Different Approaches, Different Cultures" by Seginer and Lens; "Learning and Future Time Perspective: The Promise of the Future – Rewarding in the Present" by Husman et al.; "Time Perspective Therapy: Transforming Zimbardo's Temporal Theory into Clinical Practice" by Sword et al.; "Afterword" by Zimbardo; all in this volume).

We have decided to elaborate the present book for two equally important reasons: one personal and one scientific. First, to honor Professor Zimbardo, who celebrated his 80th birthday anniversary in March, 2013. Taking into account his outstanding contribution to both scientific psychology (from Stanford Prison Experiment to Time Perspective Theory) and practical psychology (from Shyness clinic to Heroic Imagination Project) this book summarizing his most recent area of research seemed natural and adequate for us, especially given that Phil Zimbardo has been a mentor, a friend, and an authority in our scientific careers. We all studied his classic handbook (Zimbardo 1992), we were all impressed and terrified with the results of the Prison Experiment (Haney et al. 1973), and we all anchored our research efforts and passion in Time Perspective Theory (Zimbardo and Boyd 1999, 2008). Our experience with Time Perspective theory and research led us to the conclusion that this area of temporal psychology definitely needs a holistic scientific review of the present state of art. Putting all the wonderful authors together, working with the most prominent authors in the field, as well as with young, albeit already experienced scientists, and developing our own research programs, has been a wonderful adventure for us, both at professional and personal level.

The Origins

Where in time do we start when giving an overview of the place of Zimbardo's Time Perspective Theory in social sciences? In this very limited overview we present some of the major publicists and researchers in the field of time science. We leave many people out, both from earlier times, and living in the very present.

Thinking about time is related to our frame of reference. Raju (2003) states it clearly: "time is where science meets religion. The interaction between science and culture is mediated by time beliefs". The presence or absence of God is one aspect we need to consider when we think about time (see chapter "Time Perspective and Transcendental Future Thinking" by van Beek and Kairys, this volume). The role of the interaction between mysticism or religion and time is clear when we regard time-telling artifacts, like Stonehenge, the Aztec calendar, and the Antikythera Mechanism. "We need to realize that these are not merely creations of the mind, but creations for the shaping of thought" (Birth 2013). We measure our time, the length of our lives, and try to relate our limited mortal presence to the infiniteness of God or eternity. Therefore, thinking about time and temporality might be as old as man is. In his 'Encyclopedia of Time' Birx (2009) mentions the ancient Greek Heraclitus, who proposed that the cosmos is endlessly changing, manifesting ongoing cyclical patterns, as one of the forefathers. After that, Plotinus and Saint Augustine were important contributors in this field.

In modern times we need to mention 'Being and Time' (1927/1996), by Martin Heidegger, a widely cited masterwork. But Heidegger's work 'On Time and Being' (1969/1972), in which he introduces the temporal character of Being itself, might be considered even more influential on his successors like Kurt Lewin. Heidegger was both personally and intellectually influenced by Edmund Husserl and his phenomenology. "If time finds its meaning in eternity, then it must be understood starting from eternity", as Heidegger (1927) pointed out.

In 1890, William James introduced a chapter on "The perception of Time" in his famous book "The Principles of psychology", and became one of the first researchers discussing the perception of time duration and the passage of time as a core concept in psychology. When stating that "*The knowledge of some other part of the stream, past or future, near or remote, is always mixed in with our knowledge of the present thing*" (p. 607) and that "*There is thus a sort of perspective projection of past objects upon present consciousness, similar to that of wide landscapes upon a camera-screen*" (p. 631), James introduced the foundations of conceptions that would become the time perspective theory, but also the concept itself ("*In hashish-intoxication there is a curious increase in the apparent time-perspective*", p. 631). At the same time, Henri Bergson in his thesis, "*Essai sur les données immédiates de la conscience*" (1889), discusses time as intuition of duration, felt through the stream of consciousness led by "*elan vital*" and stood internally in reference to the immediate experience. Subjective time is conceived by Bergson as a spatial degradation of "pure" time achieved by a symbolic representation constituted by the past, consisting of memory, and the future formed by expectations. In 1908, McTaggart also underlined the profound paradoxical status of time, in his "Unreality of time" paper, proposing a stimulating distinction between past/present and earlier/later positions in time (McTaggart 1908).

Other earlier psychologists studied the psychogenesis of time sense. The aim was to determine how time sensitivity is established in human psychology and to empirically explore the genesis of the idea of time (the earliest work in this perspective are those of Wundt 1897 and Guyau 1890). But the first and among the most disruptive exploration of the genesis and functioning of time in psychology is without any doubt the "psychology of time" published by Paul Fraisse in 1957. From an extensive review of psychological studies on time, he proposed a general model of the development of the sense and idea of time and tried to address the following question: If humans cannot objectively *perceive* the present, what perception of time is ? "*Time of things or duration of me? Duration from sensations, or duration from of our mind?*" (p. 79). Drawning from Gestalt Theory, he proposed that time perception comes from a "*bridge*" between the past, the present and the immediate future induced by the duration of perception. Then, "*as soon as we fix our attention, organization appears (…), distinguishing objects, isolating successive structures, which therefore are figures*" (p. 84). From this perception develops a "*time horizon, consisting of past and future time perspectives*" (p. 147), which then founded the abstract notion of time. This abstract notion is profoundly rooted in cultural and historical contexts, and a large body of research developed to explore and understand how societies create and maintain a specific relation to time (from the earliest studies of religious time by Hubert and Mauss 1905 or Durkheim in 1912, to the most recent works by Barbara Adams, e.g. Adams 1990).

But Time Perspective Theory finds its foundation in Kurt Lewin's work on time and future thinking. In his life-space model Lewin proposed to concentrate on 'what is' in the present. This includes the psychological past and the psychological future. He pinpoints the role of expectations, which tend to be 'affected by perception on the one hand and memory on the other' (Lewin 1943), and which affect current actions and emotions. His "*Time perspective and morale*" publication in 1942 is considered as the original reference for Time Perspective Theory, even if some authors also refer to the article by L.K. Franck in 1939. Hulett (1944), at the same period, published an influential article on Time Perspective and the Social Role, where he first emphasized the importance of cultural influences on time perspective.

But the contemporary research on time perspective was profoundly influenced by the publication of "*Future Time Perspective and Motivation*" by Joseph Nuttin and Willy Lens in 1980. Nuttin & Lens focused on the importance of future thinking as our primary motivational force. According to Nuttin we are driven by who we want to become. Our behavior is highly motivated by our thoughts about the future, or more precisely: "*the aggregate temporal distance to a person's self-listed goals*" (Nuttin and Lens 1985; see also Seginer 2009). One of us has in his hands the Phil Zimbardo's English copy of the Nuttin and Lens book. And annotations in the margins, dated 1985 (the year of Zimbardo's first publication on time perspective, Gonzales and Zimbardo 1985) are a testimony of the influence of this book on the future developments of time perspective theory and of the Zimbardo Time Perspective Inventory (Fig. 1).

To end with this short history of time psychology research, we have to mention three important contributions in the field, that have more or less influenced Phil Zimbardo's conception of time. First, the review "*Time and human interaction: Toward a social psychology of time*" by McGrath and Kelly (1986), a milestone in time perspective research and continues to illuminate students and academics in their studies and courses. J.T. Fraser, founder of the International Society for the Study of Time (ISST) also authored a famous series "*Time studies*" presenting interdisciplinary studies on time (see also Fraser 1989). Last, *but far from being the least*, there is one person that was also influential in Zimbardo's Time perspective Theory, namely Robert Levine. To use Phil's words, Levine wrote "the most fascinating book on time perspective." In "*A geography of Time*", Levine (1998) recounts his experiences as professor traveling through very different conceptions of time all over the world. Not only engaging and spirited, this book is the source of a great part of our actual knowledge of intercultural differences in time conceptions.

From this diverse background, the very performance of Phil Zimbardo and John Boyd was to develop an integrative approach, and to provide psychologists with a valid and reliable individual difference measure of time perspective. The 1999 paper in the "*Journal of Personality and Social Psychology*" was not only the presentation of a measure, but also a research program, and a call for re-launching research on

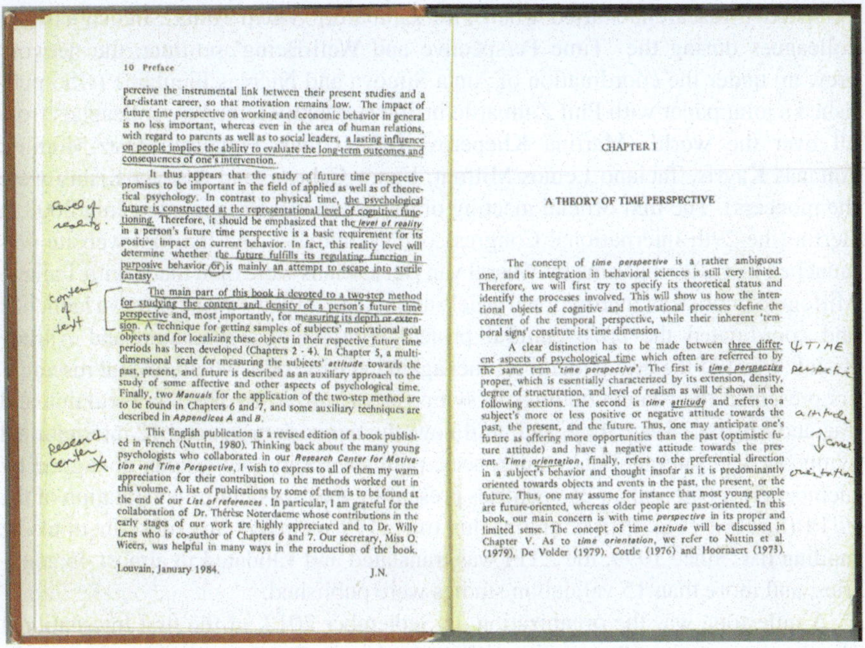

10 Preface

perceive the instrumental link between their present studies and a far-distant career, so that motivation remains low. The impact of future time perspective on working and economic behavior in general is no less important, whereas even in the area of human relations, with regard to parents as well as to social leaders, a lasting influence on people implies the ability to evaluate the long-term outcomes and consequences of one's intervention.

It thus appears that the study of future time perspective promises to be important in the field of applied as well as of theoretical psychology. In contrast to physical time, the psychological future is constructed at the representational level of cognitive functioning. Therefore, it should be emphasized that the *level of reality* in a person's future time perspective is a basic requirement for its positive impact on current behavior. In fact, this reality level will determine whether the future fulfills its regulating function in purposive behavior or is mainly an attempt to escape into sterile fantasy.

The main part of this book is devoted to a two-step method for studying the content and density of a person's future time perspective and, most importantly, for measuring its depth or extension. A technique for getting samples of subjects' motivational goal objects and for localizing these objects in their respective future time periods has been developed (Chapters 2 - 4). In Chapter 5, a multidimensional scale for measuring the subjects' *attitude* towards the past, present, and future is described as an auxiliary approach to the study of some affective and other aspects of psychological time. Finally, two *Manuals* for the application of the two-step method are to be found in Chapters 6 and 7, and some auxiliary techniques are described in *Appendices A* and *B*.

This English publication is a revised edition of a book published in French (Nuttin, 1980). Thinking back about the many young psychologists who collaborated in our *Research Center for Motivation and Time Perspective*, I wish to express to all of them my warm appreciation for their contribution to the methods worked out in this volume. A list of publications by some of them is to be found at the end of our *List of references*. In particular, I am grateful for the collaboration of Dr. Thérèse Noterdaeme whose contributions in the early stages of our work are highly appreciated and to Dr. Willy Lens who is co-author of Chapters 6 and 7. Our secretary, Miss O. Wieers, was helpful in many ways in the production of the book.

Louvain, January 1984. J.N.

CHAPTER I

A THEORY OF TIME PERSPECTIVE

The concept of *time perspective* is a rather ambiguous one, and its integration in behavioral sciences is still very limited. Therefore, we will first try to specify its theoretical status and identify the processes involved. This will show us how the intentional objects of cognitive and motivational processes define the content of the temporal perspective, while their inherent 'temporal signs' constitute its time dimension.

A clear distinction has to be made between three different aspects of psychological time which often are referred to by the same term '*time perspective*'. The first is *time perspective* proper, which is essentially characterized by its extension, density, degree of structuration, and level of realism as will be shown in the following sections. The second is *time attitude* and refers to a subject's more or less positive or negative attitude towards the past, the present, and the future. Thus, one may anticipate one's future as offering more opportunities than the past (optimistic future attitude) and have a negative attitude towards the present. *Time orientation*, finally, refers to the preferential direction in a subject's behavior and thought insofar as it is predominantly oriented towards objects and events in the past, the present, or the future. Thus, one may assume for instance that most young people are future-oriented, whereas older people are past-oriented. In this book, our main concern is with time *perspective* in its proper and limited sense. The concept of time *attitude* will be discussed in Chapter V. As to *time orientation*, we refer to Nuttin et al. (1979), De Volder (1979), Cottle (1976) and Hoornaert (1973).

Fig. 1 Phil's annotated version of Nuttin and Lens book on time perspective and motivation

time perspective. Phil and John then stated: "It is our hope that, as more researchers adopt the ZTPI as a measure of time perspective that is easy to administer and score, the empirical base of time perspective will be cumulatively solidified and its theoretical net stretched far and wide" (Zimbardo and Boyd 1999, p. 1284). It seems that their expectations are being met, and even beyond, due to Phil's power of conviction, and his mentoring role for a group of young scientist at different points around the globe. More basically, time perspective research was largely jeopardized by the heterogeneity of measures and definition, and thanks to the ZTPI's utility researchers were able to cumulate and compare findings, to collaborate and to build a scientific community all around the world.

The Time Perspective Network

Most of the contributors to this book were contacted on the behalf of the International Research Network on Time Perspective. Founded by Anna Sircova in 2007, this International Research Network gathered all the persons around the world interested in using, translating and validating the ZTPI. Originally established to facilitate the coordination of ZTPI translations, this research network became progressively a scientific community dedicated to the development and dissemination of Time

Perspective research. Started when Phil Zimbardo visited Anna Sircova and her colleagues during the 'Time Perspective and Well-Being' seminar, the network grew up under the coordination of Anna Sircova and Nicolas Fieulaine (who published a joint paper with Phil Zimbardo in 2007), rapidly joined by colleagues from all over the world (Martina Klicperova-Baker, Juan Francisco Diaz-Morales, Antanas Kayris, Taciano Lemos Milfont, Victor Cabrita, and Altinay Kislali were the pioneers). The first official meeting of the group was organized in July 2008 in Berlin (the 29th International Congress of Psychology), and the first website was launched just after that time by Wessel van Beek. Plans were then made with Taciano Milfont to publish an international article about the ZTPI and Anna Sircova launched and coordinated the cross-cultural project with Nicolas Fieulaine and Altinay Kislali. Most of the group members met again in Oslo 2009, where several researchers presented their latest findings in symposia organized by Nicolas Fieulaine and Taciano Milfont. Since then, and until now, the network organized 12 international symposia at 5 international conferences, published a journal article, co-signed by members from more than 25 countries presenting the cross-cultural validation of the ZTPI (Sircova et al. 2014), and at this time, 199 members are subscribers to the mailing list. Since 1999, the ZTPI was translated and validated in almost 45 countries, and more than 15 validation studies were published.

A milestone was the organization, in September 2012, of the first International Conference on Time Perspective (ICTP) by Victor Ortuño and his colleagues in Coimbra, Portugal, where 278 participants from 44 countries met each other in person. At this occasion, the editors presented the project of a book, the one you have in your hands now, Maciej Stolarski presented his plans to organize the second ICTP in Warsaw in July 2014, and Tomasz Rowiński announced a new website (see http://www.timeperspective.net/). Without this networking activity, animated by only a few persons under the caring and steady lead of Phil Zimbardo, this book, as the two ICTP, would be almost impossible, and it is our hope that the network will continue growing and find new ways and means to kindle warm relations, strong collaborations and diverse and innovative research on time perspective.

The Time Perspective Theory

Despite of the catchy character of Time Perspective Theory, especially in it simplified popular version ascribing individuals to particular "types" (e.g., "Present Hedonists"), it is actually not so easy to properly understand what time perspective really is. Zimbardo and Boyd (1999) define it as "the often nonconscious process whereby the continual flows of personal and social experiences are assigned to temporal categories, or time frames, that help to give order, coherence, and meaning to those events" (Zimbardo and Boyd 1999, p. 1271). The definition may sound a bit vague, as the "process" is definitely not intuitive (presumably because it is "often unconscious", thus we are less aware of it then, compared to our understanding of primary personality traits). In fact time perspective has a lot to do with cognitive processes. Before Kahneman (1973) emphasized a limitedness of our mental resources (particularly attention, but understood broadly, as a sort of "mental energy"), pointing out that they are continually "invested" into different activities, sources of information, or control processes. Thus, at one moment, only a tiny part of information is selected (Hunt and Lansman 1986), and becomes part of our conscious experience. Our past, present, and future permanently "fight" for resources, because focus on one of them usually pushes the remaining two outside of our field of attention.[1] In other words, if one becomes focused on her or his future, they will probably ignore their past, and leave only a small part of cognitive resources to control their present situation. Similarly, concentration on the present will reduce resources available for eventual considering future consequences of present behavior, and so on. Such momentary focus may have robust consequences for one's actual behavior (e.g., see studies reported by Maslach, as well as "Time and the Misfits: Temporal Framing and Priming in Persuasive Communications" by Martinez and Fieulaine, both in this volume). Naturally, albeit attention is often directed by properties of stimuli, it remains a subject of one's intentional control, thus we may choose to which time frame we want to refer to in a particular situation, for instance focusing our attention on considering possible future consequences of present behaviors.

Despite this central processing character of time perspective, through numerous learning processes (e.g., familial modeling, peer interactions, cultural influences etc.) individuals come to develop an habitual focus on one or more time zones and, as a consequence, tend to ignore the remaining ones. For example, training in gratification delay will probably enhance future focus and, to some degree, reduce Present-Hedonistic strivings. This habitual focus becomes so consolidated that it may be treated in a way similar to personality traits, or response styles. Zimbardo and Boyd (1999) distinguished five dimensions that can be used to describe one's time perspective, independently from the existence of the three natural time horizons (i.e., past, present, and future). Individuals may regard to each of them in different ways. For instance, a view of past may be positive, warm and nostalgic, as well as negative, full or regrets and traumas. What is worth emphasizing, these two ways of relating towards one's past are very weakly related (Zimbardo and Boyd 1999), thus an individual may reveal either a habitual focus on one of them, on both, or on neither. Analogically, one may perceive both present and future in different ways (see Table 1).

Moreover, numerous investigators of time perspective put a strong emphasis on a construct labeled Balanced Time Perspective (BTP, see chapter "Assessing Temporal Harmony: The Issue of a Balanced Time Perspective" by Stolarski et al., this volume). Balanced Time Perspective, understood as the optimal mix of time perspective, allowing an individual to optimize his or her functioning through flexible switching between adaptive views of each time zone, this remains a core of the Time Perspective theory (Boniwell and Zimbardo 2004).

---

[1] In some specific situations several temporal categories may coexist in consciousness; such situations usually regard meta-cognitive experiences of comparing two time zones, e.g., revising future plans under the influence of present events or reflections on recollections of own past.

Table 1 Time Perspectives distinguished by Zimbardo and Boyd (1999) in their Time Perspective Theory, and dimensions described in its extensions (Boyd and Zimbardo 1997; Carelli et al. 2011; Zimbardo et al. 2012)

Time perspective	Description	Sample correlates
Past-Negative (PN)	Relates to a generally negative, aversive view of the past, which may emerge as a result of actual experience of unpleasant or traumatic events, of a negative reconstruction of benign events, or of a mixture of both	Depression, aggression, low emotional stability, low self-esteem, trait anxiety
Past Positive (PP)	Reflects a warm, sentimental attitude toward the past	Friendliness, high self-esteem, low anxiety
Present-Hedonistic (PH)	Relates to a hedonistic, risk-taking and pleasure-oriented attitude towards life, with high impulsivity and little concern for future consequences of one's actions	Novelty and sensation seeking, low impulse control
Present-Fatalistic (PF)	"reveals a belief that the future is predestined and uninfluenced by individual action, whereas the present must be borne with resignation because humans are at the whimsical mercy of "fate"" (Zimbardo and Boyd 1999, p. 1278)	Depression, low consideration for future consequences, external locus of control
Future (F)	Relates to a general future orientation, with behavior dominated by striving for future goals and rewards	Conscientiousness, Consideration for future consequences
Future Transcendental (FT)[a]	Extends from the point of imagined death of the physical body to infinity; from this perspective behaviors often seen as irrational, such as suicide, extreme heroism, and excessive tithing, are transformed into rational behaviors expected to lead to fulfillment of transcendental-future goals	Religiosity, religious practices
Future Negative (FN)	Relates to a negative view of future, fulfilled with worry and future anxiety; with behavior dominated by avoidance of losses and suffering	Avoidant and dependent decision making styles
Future Positive (FP)	Reflects a positive view of future, with approach orientation; the dimension is in fact very similar to Zimbardo & Boyd F dimension (also at the measurement level)	Rational decision making style
Expanded Present (EP)	Reflects temporal coherence; future and past become balanced	Balanced Time perspective, mindfulness

[a]With a potential distinction into Positive and Negative Transcendental Future

The Impact

We already mentioned that Phil Zimbardo has always emphasized the robustness of the influence of time perspective on human behavior. Indeed, a body of empirical data based on the ZTPI confirms that time perspective dimensions predict numerous fundamental life outcomes, including health (see chapter "Time Perspective as a Predictor of Healthy Behaviors and Disease-Mediating States" by Hall et al., this volume), happiness (see chapter "Time Perspectives and Subjective Well-being: A Dual Pathway Framework" by Cunningham et al., this volume), financial (see chapter "Time Perspective in Consumer Behavior" by Klicperova et al., this volume) and pro-environmental behaviors (see chapter "Understanding Environmental Issues with Temporal Lenses: Issues of Temporality and Individual Differences" by Milfont and Demarque, this volume), among many others. The strength of these relationships, found in very diverse countries and cultures, is often indeed impressive. For instance, Zhang et al. (2013) shown that correlations between Balanced Time Perspective and well-being may reach the correlational level of .60, and time perspective dimensions are better predictors of well-being than are any of the famous Big Five personality traits (Zhang and Howell 2011). Numerous studies on time perspective revealed its fundamental role for different aspects of human functioning. To provide a reader with a brief review of the most important correlates of time perspective a nomological network was developed,[2] collecting a number of interesting results illustrating the role of each of the time perspective dimensions in different aspects of human functioning. The table is available as supplementary material at the end of the book. We are fully aware of the subjective nature of this selection – choices had to be made from the impressive number of highly important studies, and it could as well look completely different. We sincerely hope that authors of groundbreaking studies not mentioned here will forgive us our inadvertence.

Phil Zimbardo has always put an enormous effort to explore the paths linking academic psychology with real everyday life, and Time Perspective Theory is not an exception to the rule. Since the very beginning of his research on time perspective, he sought for ways to apply his theory to resolve fundamental social problems, including homelessness (Epel et al. 1999), substance abuse (Keough et al. 1999), and risky driving (Zimbardo et al. 1997). Probably the most famous application of his theory came as a result his cooperation with Hawaiian therapists, Richard and Rosemary Sword. Their innovative Time Perspective Therapy provided a novel approach for PTSD, revealing high effectiveness in a surprisingly short time (Zimbardo et al. 2012). Rick Sword recently passed away and Phil will always remember Rick's vitality, sense of humor, charming manner and his endless compassion for anyone in need of an act of kindness–his recent death at too young an age is a tragedy for humanity and all who loved him. Psychological practice based on Zimbardo & Boyd's theory proved useful also in other psychological disorders

[2] Originally presented as a supplementary material in Sircova et al. 2014, updated and presented for the present introduction after their authorization.

(see chapters "The Uncharted Territory: Time Perspective Research Meets Clinical Practice. Temporal Focus in Psychotherapy across Adulthood and Old Age" by Kazakina; "Friend or Foe? Escape from Death, or Death as an Escape?" by van Beek and Chistopolskaya, both this volume), as well as in positive interventions among healthy individuals (chapter "Time Perspective Coaching" by Boniwell and Osin, this volume).

The Book

The structure of the present book has been planned in a similar way as this opening chapter. The first part of the book provides a detailed review of Time Perspective Theory. It begins with its introduction in a reprint of the classic article by Philip Zimbardo and John Boyd (1999) from the "*Journal of Personality and Social Psychology*", which introduced the Zimbardo Time Perspective Inventory (ZTPI) to a broader audience, and remains the most cited paper in this area. In the first regular chapter, Maciej Stolarski with colleagues provide an analysis of the idea of Balanced Time Perspective, including both its theoretical background and empirical operationalizations. Further, a reader will find a detailed introduction into extensions of Time Perspective Theory in two chapters describing additional time perspective dimensions. Wessel van Beek and Antanas Kairys take a reader beyond the boundaries of earthly life, introducing the specificity of Future Transcendental Time Perspective, whereas Maria Grazia Carelli with her colleagues describes the "missing piece" of Time Perspective Theory, presenting the Future Negative dimension. Antanas Kairys and Audrone Liniauskaite analyze the complex issue of similarities and differences between time perspective and personality, while Zena Mello and Frank Worrell propose an alternative to original Time Perspective Theory, introducing a conceptual model of time perspective in adolescence. Jenefer Husman and her team take an in-depth look into the role of time perspective in learning processes, emphasizing the role of the connectedness between future and present horizons. Finally, Sam Magilo, Yacoov Trope and Nira Liberman provide an impressive, erudite analysis of Time Perspective Theory, framing it in a broader context of their theory of psychological distance.

The second part of the book puts time perspective into evolutionary, social and cultural contexts. It begins with an interesting text by Curtis Dunkel and Daniel Kruger, who view time perspective from an evolutionary perspective, reflecting on potential environmental pressures that may modify individual time perspective profiles. Their work is followed by a series of chapters focusing on cultural aspects of time perspective. The first presents a review of the huge cross-cultural project, aiming to establish time perspective profiles of cultures. A group of 61 scientists from 24 countries, led by Anna Sircova, present a valid, cross-cultural version of ZTPI, illustrating temporal features of each of the analyzed countries. Bob Levine takes the reader into a fascinating time travel, uncovering the mysteries of geography of temporality, whereas James Jones and Jordan Leitner describe the SANKOFA effect, comparing differences between views of time by Caucasians and Blacks.

Finally, Nicolas Fieulaine and Thémis Apostolidis analyze how poverty and social insecurity may interact to shape individual time perspectives.

In the third part, a reader will find a deepened analysis of various particular psychological processes in time perspective: cognition, emotion, and motivation. First, Maria Grazia Carelli and Carl Johan Olsson report their unprecedented study on neuropsychological correlates of particular time perspectives. Marcin Zajenkowski and colleagues discuss how is time perspective related to cognitive ability, Kathleen Arnold and Karl Szpunar show how time perspective predicts differences in future simulations, whereas Gerald Matthews and Maciej Stolarski provide deepened analyses of time perspective with respect to affective processes. Three following chapters focus directly on one of the time horizons – Future. Willy Lens and Rachel Seginer focus on motivational properties of future perspective. Juan Francisco Diaz-Morales and Joseph Ferrari take an in-depth look into the role which time perspectives play in procrastination, while Zbigniew Zaleski and Aneta Przepiórka provide an overview of the relationship between time perspective and future goals.

Part IV contains chapters describing some non-clinical applications of the Time Perspective Theory. It begins with an interesting analysis of the role of time perspective in health behavior performance, provided by Peter Hall and colleagues. Next, Martina Klicperova and Jaroslav Kostal report results shedding some light on the role of time perspective in financial behaviors, whereas Taciano Milfont and Christophe Demarque summarize research on Future time perspective's influence on pro-environmental attitudes and behaviors. The following chapter in this part by Frédéric Martinez and Nicolas Fieulaine raises a novel issue of the role of dispositional and situationally induced time perspective in the reception of persuasive communication in campaigns promoting sustainable behaviors. Healthy and wealthy life in a well maintained environment should lead to increased happiness, and this is why these chapters are succeeded with a final chapter on the fundamental role of time perspective in development of well-being by Kerry Cunningham and colleagues.

The fifth and last part of the present volume was organized around the new work of clinicians and practitioners to provide the first exhaustive set of texts pointing out the possible ways to apply Time Perspective Theory into clinical practice. Firstly, Pio Enrico Ricci Bitti and his collaborators focus on the role of time perspective in positive aging, whereas Ilona Boniwell with Evgeny Osin provide an impressive set of time perspective-focused techniques and exercises, which can be used to make coaching practice more effective. Then, Alison Holman argues that time perspective is an important cognitive process involved in adaptation to stressful life events, viewing it from a stress and coping perspective, whereas Wessel van Beek and Ksenia Chistopolskaya explore the relations of attitude towards death and time perspective in suicidal patients. The two last chapters, elaborated by Elena Kazakina, and Richard Sword and colleagues, provide useful guidelines for applying Time Perspective Theory in different types of psychotherapy.

The explicit intention of your editors was to provide the widest currently available compendium of knowledge on time perspective by bringing together a diversified set of authors, combining experience with passion, wisdom with youthfulness, science with practice. The task did initially seem daunting to us, however, when it comes to honoring Phil Zimbardo such concerns soon evaporate. Therefore, even if the present book is an effect of our joint, intensive work, it would never become real without Phil's indirect influence. By inspiring our ideas, by motivating us to develop a well grounded future orientation, by sharing his enthusiasm and irresistible youthfulness, Phil Zimbardo was in fact the one and true Editor of this book.

We hope that our work will become useful for all people who are or will become fascinated by the predominant influence of time on human life – and of the pervasive power of time in their own lives. May the best time be on our side!

References

Adam, B. E. (1990). *Time and social theory*. Cambridge: Polity Press.

Bergson, H. (1889/2007). *Essai sur les données immédiates de la conscience* [Time and free will]. Paris: Presses Universitaires de France.

Birth, K. (2013). Calendars: Representational homogeneity and heterogeneous time. *Time and Society, 22*, 216–236.

Birx, J. H. (Ed.). (2009). *Encyclopaedia of time*. London: Sage.

Boniwell, I., & Zimbardo, P. (2004). Balancing time perspective in pursuit of optimal functioning. In P. A. Linley & S. Joseph (Eds.), *Positive psychology in practice* (pp. 165–179). Hoboken: Wiley.

Boyd, J. N., & Zimbardo, P. G. (1997). Constructing time after death the transcendental-future time perspective. *Time & Society, 6*(1), 35–54.

Carelli, M. G., Wiberg, B., & Wiberg, M. (2011). Development and construct validation of the Swedish Zimbardo time perspective inventory. *European Journal of Psychological Assessment, 27*(4), 220–227.

Durkheim, E. (1912). *Les formes élémentaires de la vie religieuse*. Paris: PUF (ed. 1960).

Epel, S. E., Bandura, A., & Zimbardo, P. G. (1999). Escaping homelessness: The influences of self-efficacy and time perspective on coping with homelessness. *Journal of Applied Social Psychology, 29*(3), 575–596.

Fraisse, P. (1957/1963). *Psychologie du temps*. Paris: Presses Universitaires de France. English Translation: *The Psychology of time*. New York: Harper & Row.

Frank, L. K. (1939). Time perspectives. *Journal of Social Philosophy, 4*, 293–312.

Fraser, J. T. (1989). *Time and mind: Interdisciplinary issues*. Madison: International University Press.

Gonzales, A., & Zimbardo, P. G. (1985). Time in perspective: The sense we learn early affects how we do our jobs and enjoy our pleasures. *Psychology Today, 19*, 21–26.

Guyau, J. M. (1890). *La genèse de l'idée de temps* [The genesis of the idea of time]. Paris: Alcan.

Haney, C., Banks, W. C., & Zimbardo, P. G. (1973). Interpersonal dynamics in a simulated prison. *International Journal of Criminology and Penology, 1*, 69–97.

Heidegger, M. (1927/1996). *Being and time*. Albany: State University of New York Press.

Heidegger, M. (1969/1972). *On time and being* (Stambaugh, Trans.). New York: Harper & Row.

Hubert, H., & Mauss, M. (1905). *Mélanges d'histoire des religions*. Paris: Alcan (ed. 1929).

Hulett, J. E. (1944). The person's time perspective and the social role. *Social Forces, 23*, 155–159.

Hunt, E., & Lansman, M. (1986). Unified model of attention and problem solving. *Psychological Review, 93*, 446–461.

James, W. (1890). *The principles of psychology*. New York: Henry Holt.

Kahneman, D. (1973). *Attention and effort*. Englewood Cliffs: Prentice-Hall.

Keough, K. A., Zimbardo, P. G., & Boyd, J. N. (1999). Who's smoking, drinking, and using drugs? Time perspective as a predictor of substance use. *Basic and Applied Social Psychology, 21*, 149–164.

Levine, R. (1998). *A geography of time: The temporal misadventures of a social psychologist*. New York: Basic Books.
Lewin, K. (1942). Time perspective and morale. In G. Watson (Ed.), *Civilian morale* (pp. 48–70). Boston: Houghton Mifflin.
Lewin, K. (1943). Defining the "field at a given time". *Psychological Review, 50*, 292–310.
McGrath, J. E., & Kelly, J. R. (1986). *Time and human interaction: Towards a social psychology of time*. New York: Guilford Press.
McTaggart, J. E. (1908). The unreality of time. *Mind: A Quarterly Review of Psychology and Philosophy, 17*(68), 456–473.
Nuttin, J., & Lens, W. (1980/1985). *Motivation et perspectives d'avenir*. Louvain: Presses Universitaires de Louvain. English Translation: *Future time perspective and motivation*. Hillsdale: Lawrence Erlbaum.
Nuttin, J., & Lens, W. (1985). *Future time perspective and motivation: Theory and research method*. Leuven/Hillsdale: Leuven University Press/Erlbaum.
Raju, C. K. (2003). *The eleven pictures of time: The physics, philosophy, and politics of time beliefs*. New Delhi: Sage.
Seginer, R. (2009). *Future orientation: Developmental and ecological perspectives*. New York: Springer.
Sircova, A., Mitina, O. V., Boyd, J., Davydova, I. S., Zimbardo, P. G., Nepryakho, T. L., Nikitina, E. A., Semenova, N. S., Fieulaine, N., & Yasnaya, V. A. (2007). The phenomenon of time perspective in different cultures (based on research materials using ZTPI). *International Journal of Cultural-Historical Psychology, 4*, 18–35.
Sircova, A., Van De Vijver, F., Osin, E., Milfont, T. L., Fieulaine, N., Kislai-Erginbilgic, A., Zimbardo, P. G., & 50 Members of the International Time Perspective Research Project. (2014). *A global look at time: A 24-country study of the equivalence of the Zimbardo Time Perspective Inventory*. SageOpen 4(1), doi: 10.1177/2158244013515686
Wundt, W. (1897/1999). *Outlines of psychology*. Bristol: Thoemmes.
Zhang, J. W., & Howell, R. T. (2011). Do time perspectives predict unique variance in life satisfaction beyond personality traits? *Personality and Individual Differences, 50*(8), 1261–1266.
Zhang, J. W., Howell, R. T., & Stolarski, M. (2013). Comparing three methods to measure a balanced time perspective: The relationship between a balanced time perspective and subjective well-being. *Journal of Happiness Studies, 14*(1), 169–184.
Zimbardo, P. G. (1992). *Psychology and life* (13th ed.). New York: Harper Collins.
Zimbardo, P. G. (2004). A situationist perspective on the psychology of evil: Understanding how good people are transformed into perpetrators. In A. G. Miller (Ed.), *The social psychology of good and evil* (pp. 21–50). New York: Guilford Press.
Zimbardo, P. G. (2012, July). *The enormous silent power of time perspective in our lives and national destinies*. Keynote lecture at the 1st International conference of Time perspective, Coimbra, Portugal.
Zimbardo, P. G., & Boyd, J. N. (1999). Putting time in perspective: A valid, reliable individual-differences metric. *Journal of Personality and Social Psychology, 77*, 1271–1288.
Zimbardo, P. G., & Boyd, J. N. (2008). *The time paradox*. New York: Free Press/Simon & Schuster.
Zimbardo, P. G., Marshall, G., & Maslach, C. (1971). Liberating behavior from time-bound control: Expanding the present through hypnosis. *Journal of Applied Social Psychology, 1*, 305–323.
Zimbardo, P. G., Keough, K. A., & Boyd, J. N. (1997). Present time perspective as a predictor of risky driving. *Personality and Individual Differences, 23*, 1007–1023.
Zimbardo, P. G., Sword, R., & Sword, R. (2012). *The time cure: Overcoming PTSD with the new psychology of time perspective therapy*. San Francisco: Jossey-Bass.

Part I
Theory, Measurement, and Development of Time Perspective

Putting Time in Perspective: A Valid, Reliable Individual-Differences Metric

Philip G. Zimbardo and John N. Boyd

For us convinced physicists, the distinction between past, present, and future is an illusion, although a persistent one.

—Albert Einstein

Although Einstein's theory of relativity (1931) established the subjective nature of the physical phenomenon of time, the significance of the psychological interpretation of this relative phenomenon has been a source of controversy among philosophers, psychologists, and physical scientists. Monitoring time may be a basic function of human development that was vital in the evolution of human cognitive functioning (Suddendorf and Corballis 1997). Kant (1781/1965) believed time conception to be an "innate ability," arguing that it richly colored the way that people experience the world, and later existential philosophers and psychologists expounded on his notion of time (Heidegger 1927; Husserl 1964). William James (1950/1890) championed the concept of time as so central to psychology that he devoted an entire chapter to "time perception" in *The Principles of Psychology*. With the later behaviorist revolution came a restricted focus on the behavioral consequences of time-based experiences. This narrow view was rejected by Kurt Lewin (1942), whose views are more compatible with those of existential philosophers.

Lewin's life space model included the influence of both the past and the future on current behavior. Lewin (1951) defined time perspective (TP) as "the totality of the individual's views of his psychological future and psychological past existing at a given time" (p. 75). This integrative view of all temporal frames within the present moment is akin to Eastern Zen notions of time that are more circular (see Ornstein

Originally published in *Journal of Personality and Social Psychology, 77 (6), 1271–1288.*

P.G. Zimbardo (✉) • J.N. Boyd
Psychology Department, Stanford University,
Standard, CA 94305-2130, USA
e-mail: phil@heroicimagination.org; johnboyd@google.com

M. Stolarski et al. (eds.), *Time Perspective Theory; Review, Research and Application: Essays in Honor of Philip G. Zimbardo*, DOI 10.1007/978-3-319-07368-2_2,

1975), and it runs counter to the traditional Western view in which time flows at a constant, linear rate, never to be reclaimed. More recently, Joseph Nuttin (1964, 1985) supported the Lewinian time-filled life space, where "future and past events have an impact on present behavior to the extent that they are actually present on the cognitive level of behavioral functioning" (1985, p. 54). Contemporary social–cognitive thinking, as represented in Albert Bandura's (1997) self-efficacy theory, advances a tripartite temporal influence on behavioral self-regulation as generated by efficacy beliefs grounded in past experiences, current appraisals, and reflections on future options. Behavioral gerontologist Laura Carstensen and her colleagues (Carstensen et al. 1999) have proposed that the perception of time plays a fundamental role in the selection and pursuit of social goals, with important implications for emotion, cognition, and motivation.

Nevertheless, the study of psychological time in general, and of TP in particular, languishes off the shore of mainstream contemporary psychology. The goal of the research program reported here is to refocus efforts toward recognizing the centrality of TP in many domains of psychology as well as promoting the value of including TP in new research paradigms as an independent, dependent, or intervening variable.

Our General Conceptual Model of TP

The model guiding our thinking and research continues in, and extends, the Lewinian tradition by advancing a broad conceptualization of TP as a foundational process in both individual and societal functioning. TP is the often nonconscious process whereby the continual flows of personal and social experiences are assigned to temporal categories, or time frames, that help to give order, coherence, and meaning to those events. These cognitive frames may reflect cyclical, repetitive temporal patterns or unique, nonrecurring linear events in people's lives (Hall 1983). They are used in encoding, storing, and recalling experienced events, as well as in forming expectations, goals, contingencies, and imaginative scenarios. Between the abstract, psychological constructions of prior past and anticipated future events lies the concrete, empirically centered representation of the present.

We argue that these learned TPs exert a dynamic influence on many important judgments, decisions, and actions. For example, how might a decision to take an action be influenced by individual tendencies to emphasize a particular temporal frame? The dominant influence for some comes from the past, from recalling analogous prior situations, with memory of the costs and benefits that attended those decisions. Their recall may be nostalgic and positive or ruminative, traumatic, aversive, and negative, and they may remember accurately or distort the past. Such a focus on the past can significantly affect the interpretation of and response to the current decision situation, even dominating its intrinsic stimulus power. For others, the influential forces on this hypothetical decision come from anticipations and expectations constructed to embody an extension of the present into a future when the calculated costs of this current action will be paid or rewards will be reaped.

Their decision process may include creating alternative goal states, means–ends relationships, and probabilistic assessments of both desired components and reality-based potential impediments and challenges, as well as weighing predicted favorable consequences against longer-term estimated costs.

In both cases, the abstract cognitive processes of reconstructing the past and constructing the future function to influence current decision making, enabling the person to transcend compelling stimulus forces in the immediate life space and to delay apparent sources of gratification that might lead to undesirable consequences. In dramatic contrast to these, two "top-down" decision makers stand those whose decisions tend to be primarily "bottom-up," influenced by the sensory, biological, and social qualities associated with the salient elements of the present environment. Their actions are a product of the forces of situational press, the intensity or quality of the stimulus, the prevailing biological state, or the social aspects of the situation.

When a tendency develops to habitually overemphasize one of these three temporal frames when making decisions, it serves as a cognitive temporal "bias" toward being past, future, or present oriented. When chronically elicited, this bias becomes a dispositional style, or individual-differences variable, that is characteristic and predictive of how an individual will respond across a host of daily life choices. Of course, individuals use these temporal orientations to varying degrees, and each orientation may lead to an optimal decision in specific situations.[1] Temporal bias may include either habitual overuse or underuse of one or more of these temporal frames. Such limiting biases contrast with a "balanced time orientation," an idealized mental framework that allows individuals to flexibly switch temporal frames among past, future, and present depending on situational demands, resource assessments, or personal and social appraisals. The behavior of those with such a time orientation would, on average, be determined by a compromise, or balancing, among the contents of meta-schematic representations of past experiences, present desires, and future consequences.

Thus, we conceive of TP as situationally determined and as a relatively stable individual-differences process. Overreliance on particular temporal frames is multiply determined by many learned factors, with cultural, educational, religious, social class, and family modeling among the most prominent. Because the operation of TP is so pervasive in people's lives and is multiply determined, people are rarely aware of its subtle operation, influence, or biasing powers. It is our contention that this construct provides a foundation on which many more visible constructs are erected or embedded, such as achievement, goal setting, risk taking, sensation seeking, addiction, rumination, guilt, and more.

[1] At this point, we must acknowledge our theoretical and personal bias toward evaluating decisions from a future orientation. It is only from the perspective of future orientation that the decision to smoke can be seen to have a negative consequence: the future development of lung cancer. If judged solely through the lens of present orientation, smoking is just a pleasurable activity without articulated future consequences. In the context of present orientation, smoking may actually be the "right" decision, because it may lead to pleasure, however short lived.

State of Research on TP

Given the complexity of this construct, it is no wonder that TP has been measured and operationally defined in a variety of different ways by independent investigators. Most research has tried to relate either future or present orientation to other psychological constructs and to their effects on selected outcome behaviors, with relatively little attention to past orientation. In general, future orientation has been related to many positive consequences for individuals in Western society, such as higher socioeconomic status, superior academic achievement, less sensation seeking, and fewer health risk behaviors. The opposite holds for those with a dominant present orientation, who are seen as at risk for many negative life consequences, among them mental health problems, juvenile delinquency, crime, and addictions, when they function in a predominantly future-oriented society (e.g., see DeVolder and Lens 1982; Fraisse 1963; Levine 1997; Nuttin 1985; Strathman et al. 1994; Zaleski 1994).

We believe that the reason why this intriguing, seemingly central aspect of the human experience has not been incorporated into current domains of psychological science involves the disjointed, noncumulative nature of past research; the lack of adequate theory; and the absence of a standard, reliable, and valid measure for assessing TP. Previous attempts to capture the complexity of TP in a single index have used the Thematic Apperception Test (Wohlford 1966), the Experiential Inventory (Cottle 1968), the Circles Test (Cottle 1976), the motivational induction method (Nuttin 1985), questionnaires (Bond and Feather 1988; Roos and Albers 1965a, b), and time lines (Rappaport 1990), among others. However, none of these methods have been widely accepted because of their low reliability or scoring difficulties. Because the meaning of TP must be closely linked to the standardized operations used to assess it effectively, such disparate definitions and methods have hindered the fuller development of this domain of psychological inquiry.

Attempts at conceptual simplification have tended to focus on only a single dimension, such as the present or future, without the complicating influence of the other temporal dimensions; examples are a future anxiety scale (Zaleski 1996), the consideration of future consequences scale (Strathman et al. 1994), and a well-known sensation-seeking scale whose features emphasize present-oriented functioning (Zuckerman 1994). Although these scales are improvements over previous graphical or story-based attempts to measure TP, they are literally one dimensional. By focusing on but one dimension, they fail to provide assessments of the relative strengths of the other dimensions within individual temporal profiles. Moreover, they assume, incorrectly, that scoring low on a scale of future orientation is equivalent to scoring high on a scale of present orientation or that scoring low on a measure of the present is equivalent to being future oriented. (We present data later that challenge such reciprocal equivalencies.) Notably absent from these scales is any representation of the past. This shortcoming is especially troubling in light of the current debate in psychology and psychiatry concerning repressed memories versus "false memory syndromes," as well as the increased recognition of the ubiquity of posttraumatic stress disorders. These controversies suggest that the past, as personal reconstruction, plays a critical role in much individual and group behavior (Clark and Collins 1993).

We argue that the scale described in this article, the Zimbardo Time Perspective Inventory (ZTPI), addresses the shortcomings of previous scales. It is easy to administer and score, with a clear, replicable factor structure; reasonable subscale reliabilities; and demonstrated validity. It provides a quantifiable measure of multiple time frames as individual temporal profiles, assesses broad dimensions of TP, and is built on a theoretical foundation combining motivational, emotional, cognitive, and social processes that are assumed to contribute to—and are, in turn, influenced by—the operation of TP. Some of our research reveals the extent to which TP is related to a large, diverse constellation of well-known psychological constructs and personality scales. At a conceptual level, TP may unite or integrate diverse constructs in previously unrecognized ways, and use of the ZTPI, it is hoped, will serve as an impetus to bring order, coherence, and predictive power to the next generation of research on TP.

ZTPI Scale Construction

Overview

The process of developing the final version of the ZTPI presented in this article involved repeated iterations over many years. The scale is based on theoretical reflection and analyses, interviews, focus groups, repeated factor analyses, feedback from experiment participants, discriminant validity analyses, and specific attempts to increase factor loadings and internal consistencies by item analyses and revisions.

The initial impetus for developing this individual-differences measure came from early life experiences of Philip G. Zimbardo and his observations of the dramatic alterations in TP that occurred during the weeklong Stanford Prison Experiment (Zimbardo et al. 1973). One aspect of the power of the situation demonstrated by that study was the alteration in the subjective time sense of many of the participants from being relatively future-oriented college students to being totally immersed prisoners of the present moment, without concern for their shared past or any interest in the future after they were released. Growing up in poverty led Zimbardo to realize that his family and friends were prisoners of a fatalistic present. Education liberated him, and others, into a more future-oriented realm of existence.

Review of relevant research followed, along with conceptual analyses of the dynamic role that TP plays in everyday life decisions, goal setting, and actions. These early ventures were conducted with social psychologist Alex Gonzalez, who added a cultural dimension to our views of TP differences. We conducted interviews and focus groups with students, colleagues, and staff at Stanford University and Fresno State University, as well as with noncollege populations. We did so to elicit representative propositions that seemed to characterize their personal beliefs, preferences, and particular experiences concerning variations in subjective TPs. A first empirical demonstration of the utility of a scale to measure such differences came from a convenience sample of more than 12,000 respondents to a Psychology Today questionnaire that we had prepared on the basis of our exploratory investigations (Gonzalez and Zimbardo 1985; Zimbardo and Gonzalez 1984). Because of magazine space limitations and our primary interest at that time in differences between present-oriented and future-oriented individuals, we did not include items that might have tapped into a past orientation. However, factor analysis revealed a number of distinct temporal factors within the present and future domains, along with interesting correlations with many occupations and other lifestyle variables. That first scale became the core for the scale described in this article. It has been continually refined according to the results of many studies and has been used to preselect participants for experimental research projects and correlational studies.

Refinement of the ZTPI was empirically driven, based on repeated factor analyses of the pool of statements thought to characterize different TPs. These items, collected from many different sources, reliably produced five distinct factors when factor analyzed. There was no a priori theoretical prediction of the number or characteristics of the factors that we would obtain; their nature was determined solely by the pool of characteristic statements and repeated factor analyses of this pool. After the stability of the five-factor structure had been established, individual items were analyzed and revised to maximize factor loadings and increase the internal consistency of the subscales. The final factor analysis reported in this article thus represents the end product of a multipronged approach to the development of the ZTPI spanning more than a decade.

The scale items represent propositions about individuals' beliefs, preferences, and values regarding experiences that are temporally based but are not descriptive of time-related demographic information (e.g., "I have lived, now live, will live, in city X"). The scale's five-factor structure and relative loadings were replicated recently in an independent test with samples of respondents from three very different colleges ($N=612$; variance explained, 34 %), with only minimal changes found in factor loadings of specific items (Holman and Zimbardo 1999).

Exploratory Factor Analysis

The ZTPI asks respondents to indicate how characteristic a statement is of them on a 5-point Likert scale ranging from very uncharacteristic (1) to very characteristic (5). Students from the College of San Mateo and Stanford University ($N=606$) completed the 56 items of the ZTPI either for class credit or to be eligible to win a small cash prize. The Kaiser–Meyer–Olkin measure of sampling adequacy was .83 (see Table 1 for sample demographic characteristics).

Exploratory principal-components factor analysis (using varimax rotation and replacement of missing values with the mean) revealed five distinct TP factors that explained 36 % of the total variance (see Table 2). Inspection of both the scree plot and individual eigenvalues disclosed a precipitous drop in eigenvalues between the fifth and sixth factors. All items loaded above .30 on the first five factors, with an average loading of .45. The five latent constructs identified were theoretically viable

Table 1 Sample demographics

	Sample						
Characteristic	San Mateo[a]	Stanford[b]	Stanford[c]	Stanford[d]	SFSU[e]	Juvenile[f]	Interview[g]
n	205	79	224	99	361	38	28
Age range (years)	16–62	17–28	17–24	17–30	17–52	15–18	17–22
Main age (years)	23.6	19.1	18.8	19.2	19.4	16.5	18.6
Female (%)	65	57	57	52	61	24	56
Caucasian (%)	50	47	61	51	18	26	43
Asian American (%)	24	28	22	32	59	18	36
Hispanic (%)	14	11	9	1	11	32	7
African American (%)	2	8	4	11	5	18	7
Other ethnic background (%)	10	6	4	5	6	5	7

[a]College of San Mateo, introductory psychology classes, fall 1995
[b]Stanford University, introductory psychology class, winter 1996
[c]Stanford University, introductory psychology class, spring 1996
[d]Standford University, introductory psychology class, winter 1997
[e]San Francisco State University, introductory psychology class, spring 1996
[f]San Mateo County community schools, fall 1994
[g]Stanford University, introductory psychology students (18 from winter 1995 and 10 from fall 1995)

Table 2 Exploratory principal-components analysis: varimax-rotated factor matrix

ZTPI item	Past-Negative	Present-Hedonistic	Future	Past-Positive	Present-Fatalistic
1	.07	.42	−.02	.14	−.10
2	−.08	.18	.06	.62	.02
3	.24	.19	.09	.14	.44
4	.66	−.01	−.07	.05	.15
5	.41	.00	.02	.23	.13
6	.08	−.16	.46	.10	.02
7	−.25	.14	.01	.68	−.02
8	.03	.51	−.27	−.10	.05
9	−.09	.21	−.33	−.08	.12
10	−.16	.13	.56	−.03	−.09
11	−.41	.06	.03	.63	−.12
12	.09	.32	−.04	.13	.22

(continued)

Table 2 (continued)

ZTPI item	Past-Negative	Present-Hedonistic	Future	Past-Positive	Present-Fatalistic
13	–.08	–.17	.63	.04	.10
14	.10	.04	–.15	–.07	.64
15	.18	.09	.09	.63	.06
16	.69	.16	–.01	–.18	.06
17	–.20	.50	.19	.11	–.06
18	.11	.04	.48	–.06	–.04
19	.05	.38	.12	.10	.07
20	–.24	.24	.11	.64	–.03
21	–.12	.04	.46	.17	–.04
22	.49	.24	.07	–.20	–.04
23	.07	.51	–.25	–.12	.13
24	.06	.28	–.49	–.11	.20
25	.55	–.02	.02	–.52	.21
26	.05	.56	.05	.13	–.14
27	55	.03	–.18	.05	.02
23	.00	.36	–.30	.06	33
29	.04	.06	–.02	.64	.21
30	.00	.03	.37	.16	–.29
31	–.00	.70	–.02	–.00	.03
32	–.13	45	–.08	.08	.15
33	.43	.04	–.17	–.08	.29
34	.67	–.01	.05	–.25	.07
35	.20	.16	–.20	–.09	.42
36	47	.08	.06	.24	.21
37	.14	.17	–.12	–.04	.59
38	.17	–.02	.06	.02	.73
35	.04	–.02	–.01	–.10	.68
40	–.17	–.02	.61	–.01	.04
41	–.00	.00	–.00	–.45	.25
42	.00	.71	–.01	–.04	.08
43	–.05	.07	.45	.07	–.05
44	.18	.45	–.10	.07	.12
45	–.16	–.09	.61	–.06	–.06
46	.16	.44	–.22	.23	.10
47	.20	–.09	–.00	.09	.42
48	–.04	.45	–.16	–.10	.13
49	.10	–.06	.11	.47	–.03
50	.70	.06	.06	–.08	.05
51	.09	–.07	.53	.01	–.08
52	–.05	.28	–.18	–.04	.34
53	.08	.14	–.11	.02	.45
54	.63	–.07	–.13	.01	.21
55	.20	.44	–.00	.07	–.02
56	–.11	29	–.36	.09	.10

Note: ZTPI = Zimbardo Time Perspective Inventory

and were similar to those obtained in our earlier analyses. Two items, Items 11 and 25, loaded significantly on two factors but in opposite directions.[2] Both of these items were retained on the factor that was most theoretically justifiable.

Confirmatory Factor Analysis

Confirmatory factor analysis was performed (via maximum-likelihood estimation) on data from a new sample of San Francisco State University students ($N=361$). The model tested was based on the factor loadings of the exploratory analysis in which the items were driven by five latent TP constructs. All of the items had a significant relationship with the latent factor on which they were expected to load, and all but two items had a standardized loading above .30. Item 9 loaded at −.26, and Item 30 loaded at .29. We retained these two items because they added theoretical breadth to the factors and because deleting them did not significantly alter the factor structure. Because chi-square critical values are sensitive to degrees of freedom and the large number of degrees of freedom in our model (1,480), traditional goodness-of-fit indexes were not an appropriate test of our model's fit (see Pratte et al. 1994). Therefore, we resorted to an alternative method based on the relative chi-square value, which uses the ratio of χ^2/df (Carmines and McIver 1981).[3] Our χ^2/df ratio was 2.30 (3,398.73/1,480), which is within the acceptable ranges and suggests that the data are consistent with our model in which TP is represented by five latent factors.[4] (See the Appendix for the complete ZTPI scale.) The nature of each factor is described next.

The Five ZTPI Factors

Past-Negative

The first factor of the ZTPI, Past-Negative, reflects a generally negative, aversive view of the past (eigenvalue = 6.86; 12.3 % of variance explained; $n=10$; $M=2.98$, $SD=0.72$). Items that compose this factor include "I think about the bad things that have happened to me in the past," "I think about the good things that I have missed

[2] Both items loaded significantly on the Past-Negative and Past-Positive factors. They were retained on the Past-Positive scale on the basis of theoretical considerations, previous factor analyses of the scale, and a desire to increase the internal reliability of the scale.

[3] Although there are no clear criteria for interpreting this ratio, several researchers have proposed standards. Wheaton et al. (1977) suggested that a ratio of approximately 5 is acceptable when the sample size approaches 1,000 and that a ratio of 10 can be considered a good fit, and Carmines and McIver (1981) suggested that a ratio in the range of 2–3 is adequate.

[4] This was after allowing six pairs of factors to covary and freeing two off-diagonal elements of the theta–delta matrix. The items freed were 2 and 23, along with 31 and 42.

out on in my life," and "I often think of what I should have done differently in my life." Because of the reconstructive nature of the past, these negative attitudes may be due to actual experiences of unpleasant or traumatic events, to negative reconstruction of benign events, or to a mix of both. However, it seems reasonable to assume that the surprising prominence of this first strong factor is greater in the current United States cultural context in which the false memory syndrome–repressed memory controversy is publicized prominently and posttraumatic stress disorder is reported frequently in the media.

Significant ethnic differences were found, $F(4, 559) = 8.50$, $p < .01$, $\eta^2 = .06$. African Americans scored highest on the Past-Negative scale ($M = 3.20$, $SD = 0.75$), followed by Asians ($M = 3.10$, $SD = 0.69$), those of "other" ethnic backgrounds ($M = 3.10$, $SD = 0.73$), Hispanics ($M = 3.10$, $SD = 0.67$), and Caucasians ($M = 2.80$, $SD = 0.69$). Cronbach's alpha coefficient was .82.

Present-Hedonistic

The second factor, Present-Hedonistic, reflects a hedonistic, risk-taking, "devil may care" attitude toward time and life (eigenvalue = 5.01; 8.9 % of variance explained; $n = 15$; $M = 3.44$, $SD = 0.51$). It includes such diverse items as "Taking risks keeps my life from becoming boring," "I do things impulsively," "I often follow my heart more than my head," and "When listening to my favorite music, I often lose all track of time." It suggests an orientation toward present pleasure with little concern for future consequences. Cronbach's alpha coefficient was .79.

Future

The third factor reflects a general future orientation (eigenvalue = 3.54; 6.3 % of variance explained; $n = 13$; $M = 3.47$, $SD = 0.54$). Items typical of the Future factor include "I am able to resist temptations when I know that there is work to be done," "It upsets me to be late for appointments," "I complete projects on time by making steady progress," and (negatively) "I take each day as it is rather than try to plan it out." The Future scale suggests that behavior is dominated by a striving for future goals and rewards. Women scored significantly higher than men, $F(1, 585) = 16.20$, $p < .01$, $\eta^2 = .03$ (women, $M = 3.54$, $SD = 0.51$; men, $M = 3.36$, $SD = 0.51$). Cronbach's alpha coefficient was .77. (We were surprised that the Future factor did not decompose into several subfactors as had been found earlier (Gonzalez and Zimbardo 1985). However, that earlier sample included many older respondents in business and noncollege occupations whose future representations included their children, retirement, legacy, and other long-term factors not common in the thoughts of college students.)

Past-Positive

The fourth factor reflects an attitude toward the past that is very different from that captured by the first factor (eigenvalue = 2.50; 4.5 % of variance explained; $n=9$; $M=3.71$, $SD=0.64$). Whereas the first factor suggests trauma, pain, and regret, the Past-Positive factor reflects a warm, sentimental attitude toward the past. Items that load on the Past-Positive factor include “It gives me pleasure to think about the past,” “I get nostalgic about my childhood,” “I enjoy stories about how things used to be in the ‘good old times,’ ” and “I like family rituals and traditions that are regularly repeated.” Significant ethnic, $F(4, 559)=3.80$, $p<.01$, $\eta^2=.03$, and gender, $F(1, 585)=5.20$, $p<.05$, $\eta^2=.01$, differences were found on the Past-Positive scale. Caucasians scored highest ($M=3.80$, $SD=0.62$), followed by Hispanics ($M=3.80$, $SD=0.63$), African Americans ($M=3.70$, $SD=0.79$), Asians ($M=3.60$, $SD=0.59$), and those of other ethnic backgrounds ($M=3.40$, $SD=0.77$). Women ($M=3.70$, $SD=0.66$) scored higher than men ($M=3.60$, $SD=0.60$). Cronbach’s alpha coefficient was .80.

Present-Fatalistic

The fifth and final factor of the ZTPI reveals a fatalistic, helpless, and hopeless attitude toward the future and life (eigenvalue = 2.21; 3.9 % of variance explained; $n=9$; $M=2.37$, $SD=0.60$). Items that compose the Present-Fatalistic factor include “My life path is controlled by forces I cannot influence,” “You can’t really plan for the future because things change so much,” and “Often luck pays off better than hard work.” Significant ethnic differences were found, $F(4, 559)=4.46$, $p<.01$, $\eta^2=.03$. Asians scored highest ($M=2.60$, $SD=0.60$), followed by Hispanics ($M=2.50$, $SD=0.67$), those of other ethnic backgrounds ($M=2.40$, $SD=0.63$), Caucasians ($M=2.30$, $SD=0.55$), and African Americans ($M=2.20$, $SD=0.53$). Cronbach’s alpha coefficient was .74.

Test–Retest Reliability

Test–retest reliabilities of the five subscales of the ZTPI were established with 58 Stanford introductory psychology students over a 4-week period. Reliabilities ranged from .70 to .80. The Future scale demonstrated the best test–retest reliability (.80), followed by Present-Fatalistic (.76), Past-Positive (.76), Present-Hedonistic (.72), and Past-Negative (.70). All correlations were significant at $p<.01$ (see Table 3 for intercorrelations between the factors).

Table 3 Intercorrelations between Zimbardo Time Perspective Inventory factors: samples 1–4 ($n = 606$)

Factor	1	2	3	4	5
1. Past-Negative	–				
2. Present-Hedonistic	.16***	–			
3. Future	–.13**	–.29***	–		
4. Past-Positive	–.24***	.18***	.12**	–	
5. Present-Fatalistic	.38***	.32***	–.26***	–.09*	–

$*p<.05$; $**p<.01$; $***p<.001$

Convergent and Discriminant Validity

Having established the factor structure, test–retest reliability, and internal consistency of the ZTPI, we turn to issues of validity. As with the basic scale construction process, validation was complicated by the nature of this ephemeral but pervasive phenomenon. Time permeates and defines people's existence, so much so that it can be related to many diverse psychological constructs. Any attempt at validation, therefore, must include numerous psychological measures that conceptually might be related to any of our five TP factors. We next demonstrate the relationships of each of our scale factors with a network of traditional measures assumed to share some common variance with them. Our analyses reveal the unique contribution of our five temporal factors within the correlational structure existing between them and a dozen traditional measures.

Method

Evidence of convergent validity comes from support of hypotheses relating various established psychological constructs to each of the five subscales of the ZTPI. For evidence of divergent or discriminant validity, we hypothesized that subscales of the ZTPI would not be associated (or would be only weakly associated) with psychological constructs for which we did not make a prediction of convergent validity. After identifying relevant constructs from a literature review, we administered the appropriate scales along with the ZTPI to a subset of the participants in our first study. Space considerations do not allow us to detail all of the hypotheses we considered, so we focus on those we consider most important for the basic validation of our scale. It is important to note the wide range of diverse constructs that we believed were conceptually related to each of our TP factors. Moreover, it is equally interesting to highlight the many and varied constructs with which our TP factors overlap both empirically and conceptually.

Participants

Introductory psychology students from the College of San Mateo ($N=205$) participated in exchange for an opportunity to win cash prizes (see Table 1 for demographic characteristics). They completed a large set of 12 established scales, questionnaires and inventories, self-report items, and demographic measures, in addition to the ZTPI.

Materials

Aggression Questionnaire

The Buss and Perry Aggression Questionnaire (1992) contains four subscales that measure physical aggression, verbal aggression, anger, and hostility. The mean score for our sample was 2.63 ($SD=0.57$), men ($M=2.78$, $SD=0.59$) scoring significantly higher than women ($M=2.55$, $SD=0.56$), $t(196)=\eta^2.68$, $p<.01$. The alpha coefficient was .90.

Beck Depression Inventory

This scale (Beck et al. 1961) assesses the degree of negative cognitions associated with depression during the previous week. The average score in our sample was 5.77 ($SD=5.61$), and the alpha coefficient was .84.

Conscientiousness

The conscientiousness scale is a subscale of the Big Five Questionnaire (Caprara et al. 1993).[5] It has two facets: scrupulousness and perseverance. The scrupulousness facet measures dependability, orderliness, and precision, whereas the perseverance facet measures ability and motivation to fulfill one's tasks and commitments. The average score was 3.50 ($SD=0.42$), women ($M=3.55$, $SD=0.41$) scoring significantly higher than men ($M=3.40$, $SD=0.42$), $t(199)=2.29$, $p<.05$. The alpha coefficient was .79.

[5] Although specific predictions were made only for two of the Big Five Questionnaire factors, correlations with all five factors are presented in Table 4. TP correlations with the three factors for which predictions were not made suggest that TP, as measured by the ZTPI, is not strongly related to these factors. The strongest correlation between a ZTPI factor and one of these three factors for which no predictions were made was .30.

Consideration of Future Consequences Scale

This instrument (Strathman et al. 1994, p. 742) measures a "stable individual difference in the extent to which people consider distant versus immediate consequences of potential behaviors." The average score for this 12-item scale was 3.41 ($SD=0.57$), and the alpha coefficient was .78.

Ego-Control Scale (VI)

This scale (Block and Kremen 1996) has 38 items rated as to how true they are for the respondent. The scale is scored for undercontrol. The mean score was 2.57 ($SD=0.30$). The alpha coefficient was .80.

Impulse Control

The impulse control scale of the Big Five Questionnaire (Caprara et al. 1993) assesses one's ability to control irritation, discontent, and anger. The average score was 2.84 ($SD=0.52$), and the alpha coefficient was .72.

Novelty Seeking

This measure (Cloninger 1987) is a subscale of the Tridimensional Personality Questionnaire, which assesses three basic personality dimensions: novelty seeking, harm avoidance, and reward dependence. The novelty seeking scale measures "a tendency to be attracted to unfamiliar stimuli and is characterized by frequent exploratory activity and the avoidance of monotony" (Sher et al. 1995, p. 195). The average score (summing all of the true statements of the 34 that participants judged as true or false about themselves) was 17.93 ($SD=5.73$). The alpha coefficient was .79.

Preference for Consistency Scale

This scale (Cialdini et al. 1995; brief form) measures "a tendency to base one's responses to incoming stimuli on the implications of … previous expectancies, commitments, and choices" (p. 318). The average score was 5.61 ($SD=1.28$), and the alpha coefficient was .81.

Reward Dependence

This scale (Cloninger 1987) is a subscale of the Tridimensional Personality Questionnaire. Conceptually similar to delay of gratification, it measures "extreme sensitivity to reward cues, particularly social approval, and greater resistance to extinction of behavior" (Sher et al. 1995, p. 195). The personally relevant truth or falsity of each of 30 statements is rated. The average score in our sample (summing all of the true statements) was 19.94 ($SD=4.31$), women ($M=20.83$, $SD=3.98$) scoring significantly higher than men ($M=18.13$, $SD=4.38$), $t(200)=4.45$, $p<.01$. The alpha coefficient was .71.

Rosenberg Self-Esteem Scale

The 10 items of this scale (Rosenberg 1965) assess the degree of one's perceived self-esteem. The average score was 4.0 ($SD=.74$). Men ($M=4.2$, $SD=0.68$) scored significantly higher than women ($M=3.9$, $SD=0.76$), $F(1, 301)=7.0$, $p<.01$, $\eta^2=.02$. The alpha coefficient was .90.

Sensation-Seeking Scale

The 40 items of this scale (Zuckerman 1994; Zuckerman et al. 1978) describe individuals' preferences regarding seeking sensation and excitement. The average score in our sample was 59.2 ($SD=6.4$), men ($M=60.3$, $SD=6.2$) scoring marginally higher than women ($M=58.6$, $SD=6.4$), $F(1, 200)=3.1$, $p=.08$; $\eta^2=.01$. The alpha coefficient was .79.

State-Trait Anxiety Inventory

The 20 items of this instrument (Spielberger et al. 1970) measure either state or trait anxiety. We used the trait version, which measures relatively stable individual differences between people in their tendency to respond with anxiety to situations perceived as threatening. The average score was 2.12 ($SD=0.47$), and the alpha coefficient was .89.

Self-Report and Demographic Questions

Several self-report and demographic items were also included in the surveys: grade point average (GPA), hours studied per week, creativity, happiness, lying, and shyness. These single self-report items obviously do not have the reliability of the other established scales. Nevertheless, we expected them to be related to our ZTPI factors, and, if so, they could provide useful information for future research.

Results

Support for the validity of the ZTPI comes from the general pattern of results, which is quite consistent with our theory and hypotheses. Predictions involving specific constructs and facets of TP are discussed subsequently. Correlations were corrected for attenuation (taking account of the reliability of each scale; for a complete set of correlations, see Tables 4 and 5).

Table 4 Convergent and discriminant validity: Zimbardo Time Perspective Inventory correlations ($n = 205$)

Scale	Past-Negative	Present-Hedonistic	Future	Past-Positive	Present-Fatalistic
Aggression	.49***	.29***	–.31***	–.16***	.39***
Depression	.59***	.20**	–.19**	–.17*	.37***
Energy	–.18**	.27***	.30***	.15**	–.21***
Friendliness	–.11*	.05	.04	.22***	–.08
Conscientiousness	–.11*	–.20***	.57***	.04	–.22***
Emotional stability	–.45***	–.19***	.06	.08	–.19***
Openness	–.10	.05	.11*	–.01	–.19***
Consideration of future consequences	–.19**	–.31***	.52***	.02	–.55**
Ego control	.26***	.60***	–.39***	–.04	.29***
Impulse control	–.34***	–.25***	.29***	–.01	.23**
Novelty seeking	.29***	.57***	–.41***	–.03	.28***
Preference for consistency	–.10	–.41***	.47***	.09	–.16*
Reward dependence	.01	–.01	.37***	.18*	–.13
Self-esteem[a]	–.48***	.11	.13*	.28***	–.28***
Sensation seeking	.05	.57***	–.31***	–.05	.17*
Trait anxiety	.62***	.07	–.14*	–.25***	.38***

[a]Samples 4 and 5 ($n = 312$)
*$p<.05$; **$p<.01$; ***$p<.001$

Table 5 Zimbardo Time Perspective Inventory and Single Self-Report Item correlations: College of San Mateo and San Francisco State University data ($n = 566$)

Characteristic	Past-Negative	Present-Hedonistic	Future	Past-Positive	Present-Fatalistic
Age	–.08	–.10*	.23***	.01	–.08*
Grade point average	–.05	–.07	.21***	.07	–.08*
Hours of studying per week	.06	–.15**	.28***	.01	.02
Level of creativity	–.06	.28***	.09*	.13***	–.11*
Level of happiness	–.41***	.16***	.01	.36***	–.23***
Frequency of stealing	.12*	.16**	–.02	.04	.13*
Frequency of lying	.18***	.16***	–.20***	.03	.17***
Level of shyness	.20***	–.16**	.00	–.13**	.13**
Temper	.18***	.05	–.08	–.06	.18***

*$p<.05$; **$p<.01$; ***$p<.001$

Past-Negative

This factor embodies a pessimistic, negative, or aversive attitude toward the past. Previous research has shown that negative rumination is associated with depression (Lyubomirsky and Nolen-Hoeksema 1995; Nolen-Hoeksema and Morrow 1993). Therefore, Past-Negative scores were predicted to be associated with depression, anxiety, unhappiness, and low self-esteem. As predicted, Past-Negative score was significantly associated with depression, $r(203)=.69$, $p<.01$; anxiety, $r(205)=.73$, $p<.02$; self-reported unhappiness, $r(205)=-.41$, $p<.01$; and low self-esteem, $r(312)=-.56$, $p<.01$.[6] An additional, unexpected finding was the strong relationship between Past-Negative scores and aggression, $r(200)=.57$, $p<.01$.

Evidence for discriminant validity was provided by null relationships with reward dependence and sensation seeking. Reward dependence was predicted—and found—to be strongly associated with scores on the Future scale, and sensation seeking was associated with scores on the Present-Hedonistic scale.

Present-Hedonistic

This factor is characterized by an orientation toward present enjoyment, pleasure, and excitement, without sacrifices today for rewards tomorrow. Accordingly, we hypothesized that high scores on this scale would be associated with a lack of consideration of future consequences, a low preference for consistency, a low ego or impulse control, and an emphasis on novelty and sensation seeking. These predictions were validated; robust correlations emerged with ego undercontrol, $r(205)=.75$, $p<.01$; novelty seeking, $r(204)=.72$, $p<.01$; sensation seeking, $r(205)=.72$, $p<.01$; and (negatively) preference for consistency, $r(205)=-.51$, $p<.01$. In contrast to these predicted strong correlations, the scale did not correlate significantly with any of the past-oriented or future-oriented constructs, such as reward dependence and anxiety, and negatively with the self-report shyness item.[7]

Future

This factor is characterized by planning for and achievement of future goals. Predicted relations were thus expected with consideration of future consequences, conscientiousness, preference for consistency, and reward dependence, along with low levels of novelty and sensation seeking. We also expected Future scores to be negatively associated with behaviors that might jeopardize future goals, such as aggression, ego undercontrol, impulsivity, and risk taking. Indeed, as predicted, the Future factor correlated significantly with conscientiousness, $r(205)=.73$, $p<.01$; consideration of future consequences, $r(205)=.67$, $p<.01$; preference for consistency, $r(205)=.59$, $p<.01$; and the self-report item regarding hours spent studying per week, $r(205)=.28$, $p<.01$. As expected, it also correlated negatively with novelty seeking, $r(204)=-.53$, $p<.01$, and sensation seeking, $r(205)=-.40$, $p<.01$, and it correlated weakly with anxiety, $r(205)=-.17$, $p<.05$, and depression, $r(203)=-.24$, $p<.01$. It was unrelated to aggression.

---

[6] Self-esteem data are from Samples 4 and 5 (see Table 1).

[7] The sample size was smaller because participants who reported that they were "not shy" in preceding questions did not respond to the "how shy" question.

Past-Positive

This factor is characterized by a glowing, nostalgic, positive construction of the past. Its opposition to the Past-Negative factor should lead to negative associations with all of the behaviors typical of those high on the Past-Negative factor. High scorers on this factor were predicted to be low in depression and anxiety but high in self-esteem and happiness. This factor taps a healthy outlook on life, in contrast with the potentially pathological focus of high scorers on the Present-Fatalistic and Past-Negative scales. As expected, it correlated significantly and negatively with aggression, $r(200)=-.19$, $p<.05$; depression, $r(203)=-.20$, $p<.05$; and anxiety, $r(205)=-.30$, $p<.01$. Each of these correlations was opposite to that found for the Past-Negative factor. The factor also correlated significantly with self-esteem, $r(315)=.33$, $p<.01$ (see Table 1, sample Stanford[c]). It did not correlate significantly with present-oriented or future-oriented constructs such as novelty seeking, sensation seeking, and preference for consistency.

Present-Fatalistic

This factor reflects the absence of a focused TP. It lacks the goal focus of future-oriented individuals, the emphasis on excitement of hedonists, and the nostalgia or bitterness of those high on the two past factors. Instead, it reveals a belief that the future is predestined and uninfluenced by individual actions, whereas the present must be borne with resignation because humans are at the whimsical mercy of "fate." Such individuals should score high on measures of depression and anxiety. In addition, their perceived lack of control over future events should show up in a negative relationship with consideration of future consequences. As predicted, this factor correlated significantly and strongly with aggression, $r(200)=.48$, $p<.01$; anxiety, $r(205)=.47$, $p<.01$; and depression, $r(203)=.45$, $p<.01$. It correlated negatively with consideration of future consequences, $r(205)=-.72$, $p<.01$. It did not correlate significantly with future-oriented constructs such as reward dependence.

Supporting External Validation Studies

Next, we report an additional study by independent investigators, which used the ZTPI with other constructs, that provides further external validation. We also include here some relevant research from our own TP research program.

The Big Five Questionnaire

A recent study by independent investigators found discriminating patterns of correlation between our ZTPI factors and the five dimensions of the Big Five Questionnaire (Goldberg and Maslach 1996). For example, the Present-Hedonistic factor correlated positively and significantly with energy but negatively with conscientiousness and emotional stability. The Future factor correlated very strongly with conscientiousness as well as energy. The Present-Fatalistic factor correlated negatively with energy, conscientiousness, openness, and emotional stability. The Past-Positive factor correlated positively with energy and agreeableness, whereas the Past-Negative factor was related significantly but negatively to emotional stability, energy, conscientiousness, and agreeableness (see Table 4 for a complete list of correlations).

Risk Taking and Substance Use

In two large-scale companion studies (*N* = >2,600), present TP was highly related to risky driving (Zimbardo et al. 1997) and also to more frequent smoking, consumption of alcohol, and drug use (Keough et al. 1999). Risky driving included driving fast, driving under the influence of alcohol, riding bikes without mandatory helmets, and taking risks that might result in crashes and accidents. Substance use included heavy drinking as well as smoking and taking drugs. These socially significant results were obtained across 15 diverse samples (college and high school students and driving school adults), with several independent replications. TP remained an independent predictor of risk and substance use even after controlling for the effects of many of the personality measures previously reported as associated with these classes of outcome measures. In addition, the strongly positive correlations between present TP and each of the risk and substance use variables contrast with their weakly negative associations to Future TP. That contrast speaks to the relative independence of these temporal factors and to the caution against assuming that low values of one of these factors imply high values of the other factor. In a later section, we present additional research showing the predictive utility of the ZTPI for other health risk behaviors.

Additional Tests of Discriminant Validity

A potential criticism of the ZTPI is that it does nothing more than serve as "a new bottle for old wines." That damaging view would be supported if there was evidence that the strong correlations obtained between our time scale and traditional psychological constructs are tapping the same underlying psychological dimensions with little added value provided by the ZTPI. To assess this hypothesis, we examined in depth two very robust correlations between different ZTPI factors and established psychological constructs: depression and conscientiousness. Our data were subjected to a special statistical evaluation to determine whether these variables and the relevant ZTPI factors, Past-Negative and Future, were tapping into a common shared dimension or whether the ZTPI maintained conceptual and empirical independence despite the surface correlations.

The Past-Negative subscale of the ZTPI correlated (disattenuated for measurement error) highly with the depression scale at .69, whereas our Future subscale correlated with the Big Five Questionnaire conscientiousness scale at a solid .73. We used these relationships as a test case for the discriminant validity of the ZTPI by separately factor analyzing each of our scales with the relevant personality scale.

As a means of investigating the possibility that the first pairing was measuring the same construct, first all ZTPI items and then the items from the depression scale were factor analyzed together via varimax rotation (replacing missing values with the mean). The solution was constrained to six factors, which explained 36 % of the variance. Factor 1 (13 % of the variance) appeared to be the "depression" factor. All of the items from the depression scale loaded on this factor at greater than .30 (average loading of .55). None of the depression items loaded above .3 on any other factor. Seven items from the ZTPI Past-Negative subscale also loaded above .3 on this first factor (average loading of .31). Five of these seven items, however, loaded higher on Factor 6. The two items from the ZTPI Past-Negative subscale that loaded more highly on the "depression" factor were "It's hard for me to forget unpleasant images of my youth" and "I think about the good things that I have missed out on in my life." Both suggest depressive rumination. Factor 6, which accounted for 3 % of the variance, appeared to be the "Past-Negative" factor, because 8 of the 12 items from the ZTPI Past-Negative subscale loaded above .3 on this factor (average loading of .38). None of the depression scale items loaded above .3 on Factor 6 (average loading of .09).

Factor loadings were standardized, and then mean factor loadings for Factors 1 and 6 were compared with the scale from which the items were taken. Analysis of variance revealed that there was a significant interaction between the scale from which an item was taken and its factor loading, $F(1, 48) = 84.5$, $p < .01$. Items from the ZTPI Past-Negative scale loaded significantly higher on Factor 6, whereas depression items loaded significantly higher on Factor 1. It seems reasonable to conclude, then, that although the Past-Negative subscale of the ZTPI and depression are strongly correlated, they remain distinct and not entirely overlapping constructs.

As a means of investigating the possibility that the ZTPI Future subscale might be isomorphic with the content of the conscientiousness scale, items from the latter were factor analyzed with all items from the ZTPI. The varimax rotation (missing values replaced with the mean) constrained the solution to six factors (34 % of the variance). Factor 1 appeared to be the "Future" factor, and it accounted for 12 % of the variance. Of the 15 items of the ZTPI Future subscale, 12 had loadings above .30 on this first factor (average loading, .40). Thirteen of the 24 items of the conscientiousness scale also loaded above .30 on the first factor, with an average loading of .15. However, no clear "conscientiousness" factor emerged, making comparison of mean factor loadings less meaningful. Eight conscientiousness items loaded above .3 on Factor 1, six loaded above .3 on Factor 4, and seven loaded above .3 on Factor 6. Three of the 24 conscientiousness scale items failed to load above .3 on any factor. Items from the Future subscale that loaded above .30 on factors other than Factor 1 and Factor 6 were reversals of their earlier loading direction that made sense in this setting. The item that loaded (.34) on Factor 3, the "Present-Hedonistic" factor, was "I feel that it's more important to enjoy what you're doing than to get work done on time." This item had previously loaded negatively on the Future subscale of the ZTPI. The item that loaded on Factor 4 (at .47), the "Present-Fatalistic" factor, was "It takes the joy out of the process and flow of my activities, if I have to think about goals, outcomes, and products." Again, this item had previously loaded negatively on our Future subscale. The items that loaded on Factor 6 (at .36), the "conscientiousness-mixed" factor, was "I believe that a person's day should be planned ahead each morning." This item had previously loaded positively on the Future subscale.

These results were interpreted as providing evidence of discriminant validity for the Past-Negative and Future subscales of the ZTPI. Past-negative TP and the depression scale were highly correlated with depression, a highly consistent construct that explains a larger portion of the variance. However, Past-Negative remained a distinct factor, with items from the depression scale loading significantly higher on the "depression" factor than Past-Negative items. The reverse was true for items from the Past-Negative subscale, which loaded significantly higher on the "Past-Negative" factor than did the depression items.

In the case of Future TP and conscientiousness, the evidence more strongly supports the discriminant validity of the ZTPI. Although the items from the conscientiousness scale do not form a coherent factor, the items from the Future subscale of the ZTPI do. The Future factor appears more coherent and explains more variance than does the conscientiousness scale.

This overall pattern of results is clearly consistent with our theory that TP is a fundamental psychological dimension from which more complex psychological constructs may emerge and to which more complex psychological constructs may be related. We arbitrarily selected two of the more robust correlations between our new scale and established scales as test cases for the assertion that the ZTPI is but a new instrument for replaying old tunes. That is not the case here, nor do we believe it would be so with similar analyses applied to the other time factors. Thus, we can assert with greater confidence that although the subscales of the ZTPI correlate with a variety of predicted psychological constructs, they maintain their conceptual independence and coherence as explanatory constructs. And, as shown next, they also have predictive utility of considerable value.

Discussion

The results of our validation study, supplemented by independent investigations, give us confidence in the ZTPI as an individual-differences metric that assesses fundamental dimensions of the human condition. We have shown that it is related in significant ways to many established psychological concepts, as we had predicted, with an encouraging breadth and robustness of the obtained relationships. Because each of our subscales correlated with diverse measures that do not appear to assess identical concepts, we may begin to uncover commonalities among these important psychological constructs using TP as an integrating and analytic process. Doing so may help explain the temporal basis of some of these relationships, such as that between anxiety and depression, and may also guide the development of future psychological constructs.

Studies of Predictive Validity

The final step in evaluating the usefulness of this new psychological measure is to demonstrate its predictive validity. Does it enable predictions of a range of significant outcomes based on predictor scores on each of the subscales, in addition to their simultaneous correlations? The main study presented next as an affirmative answer to that question used in-depth case study interviews and observations of participants selected as high on each one of the five ZTPI factors. Further supportive evidence of the predictive utility of the ZTPI is then presented through brief reports on several health-relevant experiments involving college students and cancer survivors, on high-risk sexual behaviors of female prisoners, on sleep and dreaming disorders, and on the influence of roles and status on TP among classes of military academy personnel. Included is an interesting study showing that students' decisions as to when during the school term to sign up for participation in experiments are predicted by whether they are present or future oriented. These results suggest a systematic, unrecognized potential biasing effect on experimental data collected at different points of the school term. Finally, predictive utility is shown further in a recent study relating TP to coping strategies of homeless people.

Time Perspective Case Studies

This validation of the ZTPI is by means of intensive case study research. The predictive validity of the ZTPI is demonstrated across a wide range of behaviors that were assessed through in-depth interviews with individuals who had previously scored high on one of the five factors of our measure.

Method

Participants

Introductory psychology students at Stanford University who scored above the 95th percentile on one of the ZTPI factors, but below the 95th percentile on the other four factors ($N = 31$), were individually invited (and paid) to participate in a research project involving a personal interview. Participants were selected to represent nearly equal numbers of each TP factor, and they were randomly and individually assigned to each of 31 separate interviewers who remained unaware of the TP bias of their interviewee until after submitting their case reports.

TP Semistructured Interview

A semistructured interview was designed to associate a wide range of specific behaviors with specific TPs (in collaboration with a TP research group consisting of graduate and honor students). The interview was formulated to generate a behavioral profile predictive of a "typical" high scorer on each subscale. The interview included sections on general background, friendships, romantic relationships, personal items, risk taking, significant life events, academics, typical day, stress, money, expected longevity, life goals, spirituality, health, and sexuality. (Copies of the interview are available on request.)

Procedure

Thirty-one trained interviewers, members of the TP research group and undergraduates in a TP seminar, interviewed the 31 preselected students individually during a long session that averaged 87 min. The interviews were conducted in students' dormitory rooms to facilitate their being at ease and to enable the interviewer to record aspects of the room. All interviews were typed, according to a prearranged scoring format, and then scored independently by two trained judges and reviewed by a third. Only data on which there was agreement between two of the three raters were included. The results of the 31 case studies are pooled here, and only significant results are presented. These individual interviews were gathered about 2 months after the ZTPI scale had been administered in a large-group setting.

Results

Although unaware of the TP factor bias of the participants, 14 of 31 interviewers correctly identified the TP for which their interviewee had been selected, $\chi^2\,(1) = 12.3$, $p < .01$. This is particularly impressive given that our Stanford student population probably had a more restricted range of TP than the general population and that some participants were also relatively high on some of the other four factors (but less than 95 %). In general, the characteristics of these participants were as we had predicted. For brevity, we summarize the major results in terms of a characteristic profile for each of the ZTPI factor "types." Because of the relatively small sample size for each subscale, we are taking the liberty of reporting statistical findings in predicted directions that exceed traditional significance values.

Past-Negative

Those scoring high on this factor present a potentially disturbing portrait. In general, their interpersonal relationships are minimal and unsatisfactory, and they are not motivated to work for future rewards. They reported having fewer close friends both at Stanford, $r(30) = -.40$, $p < .05$, and elsewhere, $r(30) = -.38$, $p < .05$. When asked whether their significant life events involved people, experiences, or both people and experiences, those who reported "people" most frequently were likely to be the high-scoring Past-Negative respondents $F(2, 27) = 5.00$, $p < .05$, $\eta^2 = .27$. They also exercised less but liked gambling more than did those in the other TP groups: exercising regularly, $F(3, 23) = 2.80$, $p < .10$, $\eta^2 = .27$, and feelings toward gambling, $F(2, 27) = 2.70$, $p < .10$, $\eta^2 = .17$. Past-negative TP individuals were less likely to have had sex than their peers in the other TP groupings. The 60 % of this total sample who had not had sex scored higher on the Past-Negative scale, $F(1, 26) = 3.90$, $p < .10$, $\eta^2 = .13$. In general, there were few aspects of their current life in which they reported taking pleasure.

Present-Hedonistic

The picture of highly Present-Hedonistic students was well predicted by our earlier-reported data and TP theory. Interviewers clearly believed that these respondents were living for pleasure today with little regard for tomorrow. They used alcohol more, had unclear future goals, were not religious, and did not wear wristwatches, and more of them had parents who had divorced; however, they communicated with their families more often than students in the other TP categories. Specifically, those who used alcohol more often scored higher on the Present-Hedonistic scale than those who used alcohol less often, $F(2, 25) = 2.60$, $p < .10$, $\eta^2 = .18$. Individuals with less clearly defined future goals scored higher on this factor as well, $F(3, 26) = 3.30$, $p < .05$, $\eta^2 = .28$. The same was true for not being religious, $F(1, 26) = 3.10$, $p < .10$, $\eta^2 = .23$; not wearing a wristwatch, $F(1, 26) = 4.10$, $p < .10$, $\eta^2 = .14$; having divorced parents, $F(3, 25) = 2.50$, $p < .10$, $\eta^2 = .23$; and communicating with family more often, $r(29) = .40$, $p < .05$. These individuals also tended to be highly energetic, engaging in many activities and a wide variety of sports.

Future

Our interviews revealed that future-oriented TP students were highly organized, ambitious goal seekers who felt pressed for time but were willing to sacrifice present enjoyment to achieve their career objectives. They stood out from their peers on most dimensions of organizational planning and efficiency. Those scoring high on the Future scale were most likely to make "to-do" lists, $F(1, 27) = 8.30$, $p < .01$,

$\eta^2=.23$; use a day planner, $F(1, 28)=9.20$, $p<.01$, $\eta^2=.25$; wear a watch, $F(1, 27)=3.90$, $p<.10$, $\eta^2=.36$; and balance their checkbook, $F(3, 23)=9.75$, $p<.01$, $\eta^2=.56$. Similarly, those students reporting that they had more order and structure in their lives also scored higher on the Future subscale, $F(4, 26)=5.80$, $p<.01$, $\eta^2=.48$, and they had more clearly defined future goals, $F(3, 27)=5.50$, $p<.01$, $\eta^2=.38$.

This focus on organization in their lives may arise from a sense of "time crunch" and a need to use time wisely to fulfill the many tasks they engage in and to reach their high standards. Those highest on the Future factor were most likely to report the presence of stress, $F(1, 27)=8.80$, $p<.01$, $\eta^2=.25$, as well as a high degree of stress, $F(4, 26)=3.30$, $p<.05$, $\eta^2=.34$. They also reported pressure to use time efficiently, $F(1, 28)=7.40$, $p<.05$, $\eta^2=.21$, while simultaneously noting that they had little "free time" available in their current lives, $F(4, 26)=6.20$, $p<.01$, $\eta^2=.49$. However, the trade-offs for dealing with this pressured lifestyle derive from its rewarding consequences, because ambition, organization, striving, and stress result in higher GPAs, $r(27)=.40$, $p<.05$, and fewer course "incompletes," $r(30)=-.39$, $p<.05$, relative to classmates.

Another aspect of their eye on living for tomorrow and their self-centeredness was evident in reports about wanting to live to be older, $r(28)=.36$, $p<.10$; preferring nutrition over taste in selecting foods, $F(2, 25)=3.20$, $p=.06$, $\eta^2=.20$; and planning to have fewer children, $r(29)=-.41$, $p<.05$. But a significant cost that is packaged with this ambitious goal seeking for future-oriented individuals is the social deficit that is created by having no time to "waste" hanging out with friends or even making them in the first place. However, they imagine that it would be good to be able to do so, as shown by the result that those wishing they had more time to spend with their friends scored significantly higher on the Future scale, $F(1, 28)=6.00$, $p<.05$, $\eta^2=.18$.

Past-Positive

These high scorers who focus nostalgically on good times from the past are somewhat introverted, yet they get involved in relationships with friends and, in general, tend to act in ways that their parents would support as "better safe than sorry." High scorers on the Past-Positive scale were more likely to be shy, $F(1, 25)=7.60$, $p<.05$, $\eta^2=.23$; involved in a current relationship, $F(1, 28)=6.59$, $p<.05$, $\eta^2=.19$; and spiritual, $F(1, 27)=4.30$, $p<.05$, $\eta^2=.14$. They were also more likely to have married parents, $F(3, 26)=2.80$, $p<.10$, $\eta^2=.24$. Their cautious behavioral style stood in dramatic contrast with those scoring high on the Present-Hedonistic scale. They reported having had less sex, $F(1, 26)=6.50$, $p<.05$, $\eta^2=.20$, and those who had engaged in sex had fewer partners, $r(28)=-.42$, $p<.05$. Moreover, they consumed alcohol less often, $F(2, 26)=3.10$, $p<.10$, $\eta^2=.19$, and took fewer risks, $F(3, 27)=3.40$, $p<.05$, $\eta^2=.27$. Interviewers noted that these students were more likely to keep a clock prominently on their desks, $F(1, 28)=3.50$, $p<.10$, $\eta^2=.12$.

Present-Fatalistic

These students present a puzzling problem because they are intelligent young men and women living in a generally optimistic environment that encourages a sense of personal efficacy, yet they do not believe that anything they do, or will do, is likely to make a difference in their lives. More than any other group, they tended to be dissatisfied with their present life and did not think that it would improve. One manifest aspect of this negativity was their lower GPA, $r(27) = -.37$, $p < .10$. They did not wish that they had more time to spend with their friends, $F(1, 28) = 5.50$, $p < .05$, $\eta^2 = .16$. Perhaps most telling about the depth of the fatalism embraced by these students is the fact that they wanted to live shorter lives than did the other students we interviewed, $r(28) = -.46$, $p < .05$. They were also likely to have many sexual partners, with high Present-Fatalistic scores positively correlated with number of different sexual partners, $r(28) = .36$, $p < .10$. (Other data indicated that they were not likely to practice safe sex, and, with this promiscuity, one can predict that they will be overrepresented among those who contract sexually transmitted diseases and are at risk for HIV.)

Discussion

These interview results bolster our earlier validity findings while extending the vast array of behaviors that are influenced by the operation of TP biases. TP was related to such diverse behaviors and dispositions as wearing a watch, choice of food based on taste or nutrition, how long individuals want to live, sexual experiences, parental marital state, desire to spend more or less time with friends, risk taking, goal focus, grades, stress, perceived time pressures, shyness, and spirituality. Of course, we recognize that the small sample sizes in each of the cells of this case study limit the generalizability of our conclusions. Nevertheless, taken in aggregate with the earlier-reported data from large-scale studies, these results add breadth and depth to the emerging portrait of how major differences in temporal perspective may come to shape the thoughts, feelings, actions, and dispositional tendencies of many individuals. We next present research relating TP to important areas such as health and coping, sleep and dreaming, roles and status, and when during a school term students sign up to participate in experiments.

Health-Relevant Research

Several studies have examined health-related consequences of various TP biases, some from our laboratory and others conducted by independent investigators. A study of childhood cancer survivors ($N = 40$) randomly assigned participants to write about selected events in the past, present, or future over a 2-week period (Mann et al. 1999). Future TP was positively correlated with optimism ($r = .35$, $p < .05$; Life Orientation Test; Scheier and Carver 1985). Optimists scored higher on future orientation ($M = 3.80$) than did pessimists ($M = 3.40$), $t(37) = 2.91$, $p < .01$. Writing about the future led to significant increases in optimism ($M = 10.6$ %, $z = 2.08$, $p < .05$), writing about the present had no effect, and writing about the past decreased optimism, although not significantly so ($M = -2.7$ %). Pessimists were most helped by writing about the future; their optimism increased by 17 % relative to 3 % for the optimists, $t(13) = 2.14$, $p < .05$.

An Italian study using our TP scale produced important health data regarding women who seek breast cancer screening and those who do not (Guarino et al. 1999). A group of 150 women was given an Italian translation of the ZTPI in the waiting room of a breast cancer clinic in a public hospital in Rome. An equal number of matched control women who did not participate in regular breast cancer screening were tested at their homes. Preliminary findings indicated that, as expected, women seeking breast cancer screening scored higher on the Future scale than the no screening controls, who in turn scored higher on the Present-Hedonistic scale.

Rothspan and Read (1996) used our ZTPI with a sample of 188 heterosexual college students to investigate HIV risk and TP. They predicted and found that those high in present orientation (both hedonists and fatalists) were more sexually active and had more sexual partners than those high in future orientation, but the latter were more likely to use alternate methods of reducing HIV exposure.

Because rates of HIV risk behavior and HIV infection are high among female prisoners, an interdisciplinary team of health researchers investigated the relationships between ZTPI scores and HIV risk behaviors among 177 incarcerated women in the Maryland Correctional Institution for Women (Hutton et al. 1999). The study sample was comparable to the general population ($N = 978$) at that institution in regard to most demographic characteristics. As a group, these female prisoners scored a standard deviation higher on present TP than did female students. These findings indicate that “a future time perspective may reduce the likelihood of practicing HIV risk behavior” (Hutton et al. 1999, p. 14). Female prisoners who scored high on the Future subscale were less likely to have had an intravenous-drug-using sex partner, to have had large numbers of sex partners, or to have been “high” on drugs or alcohol during sex than peers who scored low on this scale. They were also less likely to have had a lifetime psychiatric dependency on cocaine or heroin. All of these associations were unconfounded by age, HIV infection, education, or race factors. Prisoners who scored high on the Present-Fatalistic scale were significantly more likely to engage in high-risk HIV behaviors by having sex when high on drugs or alcohol and to share needles or syringes (but these results were not significant when adjusted for sociodemographic variables). Finally, higher Present-Hedonistic scores were associated with prostitution (but also not when adjusted for sociodemographic variables).

Holman and Zimbardo (1999) investigated relationships among TP, coping with trauma, and social support issues in several college student samples. There was a negative association between how much students spoke with family members about their stressful experiences and Past-Negative ($r(124) = -.26$, $p < .01$) and Present-Fatalistic ($r(124) = -.18$, $p < .05$) TP, but a positive association between how much students spoke with friends about their stress and degree of Present-Hedonism, $r(124) = .21$, $p < .05$. After students experienced stress, Past-Positive TP was positively associated with the degree of social support they received, $r(164) = .27$, $p < .001$, whereas Past-Negative TP was associated with the degree of social conflict they reported in the aftermath of stress, $r(159) = .16$, $p < .05$. In regard to coping activities used to deal with stress, Future TP was strongly associated with active problem-solving coping, $r(125) = .41$, $p < .001$, and emotional growth coping, $r(125) = .27$, $p < .01$. Present-Fatalistic TP was negatively associated with active problem-solving coping, $r(125) = -.21$, $p < .05$. Past-Positive TP was associated with positive emotional growth coping, $r(125) = .29$, $p < .001$, and Past-Negative TP was negatively associated with emotional growth coping, $r(125) = -.24$, $p < .01$. Present-hedonistic TP was associated with avoidance coping, $r(125) = .22$, $p < .05$.

The predictive value of the ZTPI was evident in correlations with measures taken 3 months later. In the aftermath of stress reported in the pretest–posttest assessment interval, the degree of social conflict reported was positive for Past-Negative TP, $r(63) = .28$, $p < .05$, but negative for Past-Positive TP, $r(63) = -.28$, $p < .05$, as well as Future TP, $r(63) = -.25$, $p < .05$. This data set supports the notion that the ZTPI may play a useful role in focusing attention on various stress reactions and coping strategies of specific groups of clients varying in their TPs.

Sleep and Dreaming Problems

In a study from the sleep laboratory of Robert Hicks, dreaming was related to ZTPI scores (Marquez et al. 1999). Posttraumatic dream reports correlated with scores on the Past-Negative scale, $r(294) = .19$, $p < .05$; the Present-Fatalistic scale, $r(294) = .13$, $p < .05$; and the Present-Hedonistic scale, $r(294) = .12$, $p < .05$. However, they did not correlate with Future or Past-Positive scale scores. Given that the frequent use of drugs, alcohol, or tobacco has detrimental effects on sleep and TP has been related to these behaviors (Keough et al. 1999), Hicks's research team reasoned that TP should relate to sleep problems. They found highly significant correlations ($p < .001$) between each of the three sleep problem scales and each of the five subscales of the ZTPI. These results suggest that "the ZTPI has implications for health-related behaviors in addition to the frequent use of certain substances" (Vranesh et al. 1999, p. 24).

Influence of Roles and Status

A demonstration of the influence that situational factors can have on TP comes from a recent study examining changes in dominant ZTPI factors across 4 years of cadet experience at the US Air Force Academy, as students progress from freshmen to seniors and then on to officer status (Samuels 1997). The ZTPI was administered to 136 cadets and officers, about an equal number from each of the four classes, as well as officers at the academy. Officers were much lower than cadets of any level on Present-Fatalistic, Past-Negative, and Present-Hedonistic TP. On the Future factor, officers were highest (3.8), seniors were lower (3.5), and freshmen were lowest (3.3). Past-Positive scores showed a systematic increase over each of the 4 years of military training, from 3.7 in the freshman year up to 4.0 in the senior year. These data are in line with expectations based on the type of students recruited, the goals of military training, and officer job demands and reward contingencies (S. Samuels, personal communication, December 23, 1998). This cross-sectional study is being replicated with a longitudinal design to examine changes within individuals over time.

Research Participation Timing

Scores on the ZTPI predict the timing during a school term when college students sign up for participation in required research (Harber et al. 1999). The goal-directed, efficient work style of future-oriented students should encourage them to dispatch this requirement as early as possible, whereas their present-oriented peers should delay initiating this new demand on their time, procrastinate, become distracted, and thus begin their research commitment later and require more time to complete it. They should also be more tardy in meeting research obligations and more likely to be "no-shows" for experiments they signed up for than future-oriented students. Each of these predictions was confirmed.

Dates of research participation were monitored for 167 students in the initial study and for 287 students in a replication. As predicted, future-oriented students began participating sooner than present-oriented peers by 7.2 days ($p < .05$), a substantial disparity in a quarter system of only 9 weeks. By midterm, that discrepancy was maintained with a 7.1-day gap ($p < .05$), and completion of the quota took 8.5 days longer for present-oriented students ($p < .05$). This pattern was replicated the next year, with future-oriented students starting their participation earlier than present-oriented students ($p < .06$) and increasing it to a school week sooner both by midterm ($p < .01$) and by completion ($p < .05$). The Big Five Questionnaire trait of conscientiousness was evaluated as the possible mediating variable in this relationship, because it correlated positively with Future TP ($r = .38$) and negatively with present TP ($r = -.27$). Conscientiousness had no effect on any of the three research times, and when it was covaried out of the data, results remained significant for future-oriented students completing the requirement sooner than present-oriented students.

In addition, present-oriented students were three times as likely as future-oriented students to be "no-shows" even after they had signed up for given studies ($p < .05$). We also found that they were significantly more likely to be tardy than future-oriented students in submitting self-report data in a study colleagues were doing that involved emotion diary reports being submitted regularly over a 4-week period. Despite the researchers' repeated emphasis that late data could not be used, present-oriented participants more frequently missed self-report submission deadlines than did their future-oriented peers, $t(31)=3.12$, $p<.01$, being tardy an average of 3.4 times to only once for future-oriented participants. Thus, this differential failure to meet contractual obligations could bias the results of the study if TP were related to the phenomenon under investigation. Similarly, the data on TP variations in research participation sign-ups could be a source of unrecognized error variance in many studies. Research conducted primarily early in a term will involve an overrepresentation of future-oriented participants, whereas present-oriented participants should predominate in research conducted near the end of a term, thereby yielding failures to replicate or other distortions in research conclusions depending on the relationship of TP to the processes being studied.

Coping With Homelessness

Finally, we present a field study that extends the range of applicability of the TP construct beyond college student samples to reveal its functioning among homeless people living in city shelters (Epel et al. 1999). On arrival at a temporary family shelter, homeless adults ($N=82$) completed our TP scale along with self-efficacy measures. When they were leaving 1–3 months later, they completed a report on their interim activities and their job and housing situations. Those higher on Future TP had shorter durations of homelessness, were more likely to enroll in school, and were more likely to report learning from and gaining positive benefits from their predicament. In contrast, those higher on present TP used more avoidant coping strategies, spending more time watching TV and eating, working less, and not saving money. Efficacy predicted time spent searching for housing and employment, but neither TP nor efficacy predicted obtaining stable housing, a social–economic–political issue beyond the realm of individual-differences effects. However, it is evident that the personal construction of psychological time has a significant impact on whether homeless people use their time in shelters constructively or "waste time" in indulgent, unproductive activities that reduce their likelihood of obtaining jobs or housing.

Conclusion and General Discussion

The overall pattern of data emerging from the array of research presented here provides strong evidence for the value of the ZTPI as an index of the fundamental and vital psychological construct of TP. The robust pattern of diverse, yet significant, relationships with a host of traditional personality measures and behavioral indexes reveals that the ZTPI is a reliable and valid measure of TP. Our scale also has demonstrated predictive utility in experimental, correlational, and case study research.

It promises to offer conceptual integration of many seemingly unrelated psychological concepts as long as they have a temporal underpinning. The reasonableness of that strong claim comes from acknowledging that humans exist in time, that every human life is time bound, and that time is ubiquitous in every known culture. Many basic psychological processes rely on some aspect of time, such as habituation, conditioning, memory, reinforcement contingencies, self-efficacy, anticipation, violations of expectation, evolutionary adaptiveness, guilt, depression, and anxiety, to name but a few. Even fundamental distinctions between cognitions and emotions are reconcilable within the framework provided by a temporally based theory in which emotions are cast as being evolutionarily more primal for immediate responding, whereas cognitions are cast as later adaptations for planning and reflective responding (Boyd 1999).

Our decades-long research and personal involvement with aspects of temporal perspective have convinced us that there are few other psychological variables capable of exerting such a powerful and pervasive impact on the behavior of individuals and the activities of societies. It is our hope that, as more researchers adopt the ZTPI as a measure of TP that is easy to administer and score, the empirical base of TP will be cumulatively solidified and its theoretical net stretched far and wide.

Limits and Extensions of the ZTPI

Although the development of the ZTPI emerged from the earlier scale designed by Gonzalez and Zimbardo (1985) and administered to a large, diverse population, its psychometric properties in the current research program were established with a variety of college student samples. Perhaps the greater range of ages, backgrounds, and career diversity of that normative sample contributed to the resulting four subfactors of the Future factor (Future-Work Motivation–Perseverance, Future-Goal Seeking–Long-Term Planning, Future-Specific Daily Planning, and Future-Pragmatic Action for Later Gain). By contrast, the ZTPI has but one Future TP. Perhaps further factor analyses of our scale with a variety of noncollege populations will again show a more complex set of future subfactors.

A further limitation of the generalizability of our scale may lie in its cultural relevance to individualist societies and their ambitions, tasks, and demands rather than to more collectivist, interdependent societies in which time is differently valued and conceptualized (Levine 1997). Obvious cross-cultural adaptations of the ZTPI are called for.

ZTPI and Personality Processes

Evident from much of the research reported here is the considerable overlap between the ZTPI and traditional personality measures, notably the five-factor model of personality. Some of our TP factors may be manifestations of inherent temperament characteristics; if so, exploring how temporal dimensions relate to temperament may add new understandings of some of the Big Five dimensions. But recall that we have shown that, despite this overlap, there remains a uniquely independent contribution of our time factors, many of which relate to a greater range of behaviors than do the personality measures with which they correlate highly. In addition, future research may profit from the use of combined "profile patterns" of the five ZTPI factors instead of independent examination of ZTPI subscales. In this sense, we are allied to personality psychologists, who "explore the mechanisms that mediate person-environment transactions and the ways in which these psychological mechanisms give rise to the uniqueness of each person" (Caprara 1999, p. 127). As social psychologists, we also acknowledge the power of situations to modify even stable individual differences. As demonstrated, TP can be influenced by situational forces such as status change, trauma, or altered states of consciousness, as seen in the Stanford Prison Experiment (Zimbardo et al. 1973), or by hypnotic alteration of time orientation (Zimbardo et al. 1971).

Transcendental Future TP

For many people, the focus on the future does not terminate with the death of the body, because they believe in some form of existence after death. We recently developed a separate scale to assess individual differences in this postdeath dimension of TP among a large sample of 1,235 respondents (Boyd and Zimbardo 1996). Respondents who score high on the Transcendental Future scale believe that they will be rewarded or punished for their present behavior, just as those high on the traditional Future scale do, but for the former reinforcement comes only after their death. This time factor was higher for women than men and higher for those more than 50 years old than those in their 20s. It was highest for those high in religiosity and religious practices, for African Americans and Hispanics, and for Protestants and Catholics and lowest for Buddhists and Jews. It was related to both past ZTPI factors and to the Present-Fatalistic factor but not to the traditional Future and Present-Hedonistic factors. Moreover, when factor analyzed with the 132 items of the Big Five Questionnaire, Transcendental Future remained a distinct factor, suggesting that it is an individual-differences dimension unaccounted for by traditional personality analyses.

Power of Past TP

We were surprised to find that the Past-Negative scale occupied such a prominent place in the factor structure of the ZTPI. Recently, the important role of past temporal orientation and the psychological distress of trauma victims was documented in a longitudinal, cross-sectional study conducted by Holman and Silver (1998). These researchers found that a past orientation focusing cognitively and emotionally on a prior trauma is associated with prolonged elevated levels of distress. In addition, those most traumatized by their experience often exhibit "temporal disintegration," in which the present is isolated from the past and future. This time zone discontinuity was found to contribute to greater suffering among these already-distressed victims.

Quite the opposite was found among college students in a study that examined how a Past-Positive TP might build functional bridges to the future (Goldberg and Maslach 1996). Nearly 300 participants completed the ZTPI, the Big Five Questionnaire, and a detailed report of their past and present familial experiences. Past-positive TP was positively correlated with practicing traditions, planning to practice family traditions, including more generations in describing important family events, seeing family members for everyday events or for no particular reason, and writing about routine family events. In contrast, Past-Negative TP was negatively correlated with practicing traditions and writing about routine family events but positively correlated with writing about rare family events. The authors made a strong case for the importance of the positive past temporal orientation as contributing to developing a sense of personal continuity over time and thus feeding into a richer Future perspective (see also Kamiol and Ross 1996).

The Present-Oriented Child in a Future-Oriented Educational Environment

We have reported at length about the syndrome of behaviors and traits that are associated with a present TP and how they combine to predispose such individuals to greater likelihood of failure when faced with situations demanding delay of gratification, planning, goal setting, and resisting temptations and distractions when there is work to be done. We have come to believe that high dropout rates among students of low socioeconomic status at all levels of schooling are more a consequence of "TP discordance" than deficits in intelligence or intellectual abilities. Those high on present TP may be "speaking a present-oriented dialect" in a setting that recognizes only the meaning and value of future-oriented language. Children from families and communities where present fatalism and hedonism predominate will not be as prepared as their peers to think in terms of causalities, probabilities, and if–then sequences or to tolerate boring lessons even if they may reap a payoff later. We advocate novel interventions that would teach these children the "language" of Future TP and how to use whatever TP is most appropriate to the school, work, home, or community setting in which they find themselves.

A second practical consequence of altering Present-Hedonistic and Present-Fatalistic TP is the increased likelihood that those with these TP biases will be seduced into substance abuse, dangerous sexual activities, and failure to use relevant health maintenance or illness-prevention strategies. Educational messages that encourage primary prevention strategies are most instrumental in changing behavior in desired directions (Sundberg 1985), but they will be effective primarily for those who are already future oriented and rarely for those who are present oriented and need to practice them most (see Alvos et al. 1993). Individuals without a well-developed Future TP may not have the cognitive scaffolding on which to hang mental scenarios of the negative future consequences of their present behavior. New persuasive appeals are called for that are tailored in style and content to the present orientation of adolescents and adults.

Our investigation into the dynamics of TP has made us aware of a completely neglected area of psychological research, that of the psychology of temptation. The classical biblical situation of acting now to get immediate pleasures of the flesh while failing to recognize the "wages of sin" that will lead to damnation has not been studied by psychological researchers. It is quite different from the research protocol of delay of gratification studies (Mischel et al. 1988), in which a person chooses between a small immediate reward and a bigger delayed one, because in temptation the choice is certain pleasure now and probable pain later. This important psychological phenomenon (that should trap present-oriented individuals most often) deserves to be explored experimentally, with the blessings of human subjects research committees.

At the other end of the spectrum, we are concerned for those excessively future-oriented people who cannot "waste" time relating to family or friends, in community activities, or enjoying any personal indulgence. Such a "time press" fuels high stress levels, especially in today's global economy in which excessive workloads seep over into personal time through the availability of technology to work anywhere, anytime (Levine 1997). Driven by the curse of having their ambitious goals realized by endless work agendas, these people—successful in careers but unsuccessful in life—may need "time therapy" to develop a broader temporal perspective in which to integrate work, play, and social responsibility.

A Balanced TP

This conjecture leads us to promote the ideal of a "balanced TP" as most psychologically and physically healthy for individuals and optimal for societal functioning. Balance is defined as the mental ability to switch flexibly among TPs depending on task features, situational considerations, and personal resources rather than be biased toward a specific TP that is not adaptive across situations. The future focus gives people wings to soar to new heights of achievement, the past (positive) focus establishes their roots with tradition and grounds their sense of personal identity, and the present (hedonistic) focus nourishes their daily lives with the playfulness of youth and the joys of sensuality. People need all of them harmoniously operating to realize fully their human potential.

Annexes A

Zimbardo Time Perspective Inventory Items

1. I believe that getting together with one's friends to party is one of life's important pleasures.
2. Familiar childhood sights, sounds, and smells often bring back a flood of wonderful memories.
3. Fate determines much in my life.
4. I often think of what I should have done differently in my life.
5. My decisions are mostly influenced by people and things around me.
6. I believe that a person's day should be planned ahead each morning.
7. It gives me pleasure to think about my past.
8. I do things impulsively.
9. If things don't get done on time, I don't worry about it.
10. When I want to achieve something, I set goals and consider specific means for reaching those goals.
11. On balance, there is much more good to recall than bad in my past.
12. When listening to my favorite music, I often lose all track of time.
13. Meeting tomorrow's deadlines and doing other necessary work comes before tonight's play.
14. Since whatever will be will be, it doesn't really matter what I do.
15. I enjoy stories about how things used to be in the "good old times."
16. Painful past experiences keep being replayed in my mind.
17. I try to live my life as fully as possible, one day at a time.
18. It upsets me to be late for appointments.
19. Ideally, I would live each day as if it were my last.
20. Happy memories of good times spring readily to mind.
21. I meet my obligations to friends and authorities on time.
22. I've taken my share of abuse and rejection in the past.
23. I make decisions on the spur of the moment.
24. I take each day as it is rather than try to plan it out.
25. The past has too many unpleasant memories that I prefer not to think about.
26. It is important to put excitement in my life.
27. I've made mistakes in the past that I wish I could undo.
28. I feel that it's more important to enjoy what you're doing than to get work done on time.
29. I get nostalgic about my childhood.
30. Before making a decision, I weigh the costs against the benefits.
31. Taking risks keeps my life from becoming boring.
32. It is more important for me to enjoy life's journey than to focus only on the destination.
33. Things rarely work out as I expected.
34. It's hard for me to forget unpleasant images of my youth.

35. It takes joy out of the process and flow of my activities, if I have to think about goals, outcomes, and products.
36. Even when I am enjoying the present, I am drawn back to comparisons with similar past experiences.
37. You can't really plan for the future because things change so much.
38. My life path is controlled by forces I cannot influence.
39. It doesn't make sense to worry about the future, since there is nothing that I can do about it anyway.
40. I complete projects on time by making steady progress.
41. I find myself tuning out when family members talk about the way things used to be.
42. I take risks to put excitement in my life.
43. I make lists of things to do.
44. I often follow my heart more than my head.
45. I am able to resist temptations when I know that there is work to be done.
46. I find myself getting swept up in the excitement of the moment.
47. Life today is too complicated; I would prefer the simpler life of the past.
48. I prefer friends who are spontaneous rather than predictable.
49. I like family rituals and traditions that are regularly repeated.
50. I think about the bad things that have happened to me in the past.
51. I keep working at difficult, uninteresting tasks if they will help me get ahead.
52. Spending what I earn on pleasures today is better than saving for tomorrow's security.
53. Often luck pays off better than hard work.
54. I think about the good things that I have missed out on in my life.
55. I like my close relationships to be passionate.
56. There will always be time to catch up on my work.

Note: Respondents are asked to read each item and, as honestly as they can, answer the following question: "How characteristic or true is this of you?" (1 = very uncharacteristic, 2 = uncharacteristic, 3 = neutral, 4 = characteristic, 5 = very characteristic).

References

Alvos, L., Gregson, R. A., & Ross, M. W. (1993). Future time perspective in current and previous injecting drug users. *Drug and Alcohol Dependence, 31*, 193–197.

Bandura, A. (1997). *Self-efficacy: The exercise of control*. New York: Freeman.

Beck, A. T., Ward, C. H., Mendelson, M., Mock, J., & Erbaugh, J. (1961). An inventory for measuring depression. *Archives of General Psychiatry, 4*, 561–571.

Block, J., & Kremen, A. M. (1996). IQ and ego-resiliency: Conceptual and empirical connections and separations. *Journal of Personality and Social Psychology, 70*, 349–361.

Bond, M., & Feather, N. T. (1988). Some correlates of structure and purpose in the use of time. *Journal of Personality and Social Psychology, 55*, 321–329.

Boyd, J. N. (1999). *The interaction of affect and cognition: It's about time.* Manuscript submitted for publication.

Boyd, J. N., & Zimbardo, P. G. (1996). Constructing time after death: The transcendental-future time perspective. *Time & Society, 6*, 35–54.

Buss, A. H., & Perry, M. (1992). The Aggression Questionnaire. *Journal of Personality and Social Psychology, 63*, 452–459.

Caprara, G. V. (1999). The notion of personality: Historical and recent perspectives. *European Review, 7*, 127–137.

Caprara, G. V., Barbaranelli, C., Borgogni, L., & Perugini, M. (1993). The "Big Five Questionnaire:" A new questionnaire to assess the five factor model. *Personality and Individual Differences, 15*, 281–288.

Carmines, E. G., & McIver, J. D. (1981). Analyzing models with unobserved variables: Analysis of covariance structures. In G. W. Bohinstedt & E. F. Borgatta (Eds.), *Social measurement: Current issues* (pp. 65–115). Beverly Hills: Sage.

Carstensen, L. L., Isaacowitz, D. M., & Charles, S. T. (1999). Taking time seriously: A theory of socioemotional selectivity. *American Psychologist, 54*, 165–181.

Cialdini, R. B., Trost, M. R., & Newsom, J. T. (1995). Preference for consistency: The development of a valid measure and the discovery of surprising behavioral implications. *Journal of Personality and Social Psychology, 69*, 318–328.

Clark, L. F., & Collins, J. E. (1993). Remembering old flames: How the past affects assessments of the present. *Personality and Social Psychology Bulletin, 19*, 399–408.

Cloninger, R. (1987). A systematic method for clinical description and classification of personality variants. *Archives of General Psychiatry, 44*, 573–588.

Cottle, T. J. (1968). *The location of experience: A manifest time orientation*. Cambridge, MA: Harvard University Press.

Cottle, T. J. (1976). *Perceiving time: A psychological investigation with men and women*. New York: Wiley.

DeVolder, M., & Lens, W. (1982). Academic achievement and future time perspective as a cognitive-motivational concept. *Journal of Personality and Social Psychology, 42*, 566–571.

Einstein, A. (1931). *Relativity: The special and general theory* (R. W. Lawson, Trans.). New York: Crown.

Epel, E. S., Bandura, A., & Zimbardo, P. G. (1999). Escaping homelessness: The influences of self-efficacy and time perspective on coping with homelessness. *Journal of Applied Social Psychology, 29*, 575–596.

Fraisse, P. (1963). *The psychology of time* (J. Leith, Trans.). Westport, CT: Greenwood Press.

Goldberg, J., & Maslach, C. (1996, April). *Understanding time: Connections between the past and future.* Paper presented at the annual convention of the Western Psychological Association, San Jose, CA.

Gonzalez, A, & Zimbardo, P. G. (1985, May). Time in perspective: A *Psychology Today* survey report. *Psychology Today,* pp. 21–26.

Guarino, A., DePascalis, V., & DiChiacchio, C. (1999). *Breast cancer prevention, time perspective, and trait anxiety.* Unpublished manuscript, University of Rome.

Hall, E. T. (1983). *The dance of life: The other dimension of life*. Garden City: Anchor Press.

Harber, K. D., Zimbardo, P. G., & Boyd, J. N. (1999). *Participant self selection biases as a function of individual differences in time perspective.* Manuscript submitted for publication.

Heidegger, M. (1927). *Being and time*. Halle: Niemeyer.

Holman, E. A., & Silver, R. C. (1998). Getting "stuck" in the past: Temporal orientation and coping with trauma. *Journal of Personality and Social Psychology, 74*, 1146–1163.

Holman, E. A., & Zimbardo, P. G. (1999). *The time of our lives: Time perspective and social relations in young adulthood.* Unpublished manuscript, Stanford University.

Husserl, E. (1964). *Phenomenology of internal time consciousness* (J. Churchill, Trans.). Bloomington: Indiana University Press.

Hutton, H. H., Lyketsos, C. G., Hunt, W. R., Bendit, G., Harrison, R. B., Swetz, A, & Treisman, G. J. (1999). *Personality characteristics and their relationship to HIV risk behaviors among women prisoners.* Manuscript submitted for publication.

James, W. (1950). *The principles of psychology* (Vol. I). New York: Dover. (Original work published 1890).
Kamiol, R., & Ross, M. (1996). The motivational impact of temporal focus: Thinking about the future and the past. *Annual Review of Psychology, 47*, 593–620.
Kant, I. (1965). *Critique of pure reason* (N. Smith, Trans.). New York: St. Martin's Press. (Original work published 1781).
Keough, K. A., Zimbardo, P. G., & Boyd, J. N. (1999). Who's smoking, drinking, and using drugs? Time perspective as a predictor of substance use. *Journal of Basic and Applied Social Psychology, 21*, 149–164.
Levine, R. (1997). *A geography of time: The temporal misadventures of a social psychologist, or how every culture keeps time just a little bit differently*. New York: Basic Books.
Lewin, K. (1942). Time perspective and morale. In G. Lewin (Ed.), *Resolving social conflicts* (pp. 103–124). New York: Harper.
Lewin, K. (1951). *Field theory in the social sciences: Selected theoretical papers*. New York: Harper.
Lyubomirsky, S., & Nolen-Hoeksema, S. (1995). Effects of self-focused rumination on negative thinking and interpersonal problem solving. *Journal of Personality and Social Psychology, 69*, 176–190.
Mann, T., Kato, P. M., Figdor, E. J., & Zimbardo, P. G. (1999). *How to make a pessimist behave like an optimist: Future writing, optimism, and health behaviors in cancer survivors and HIV patients*. Manuscript submitted for publication.
Marquez, H. B., Madrid, S. D., Nguyen, T. T., & Hicks, R. A (1999, April). *College students' time perspective and dreams*. Paper presented at the annual convention of the Western Psychological Association, Irvine, CA.
Mischel, W., Shoda, Y., & Peake, P. K. (1988). The nature of adolescent competencies predicted by preschool delay of gratification. *Journal of Personality and Social Psychology, 54*, 687–696.
Nolen-Hoeksema, S., & Morrow, J. (1993). Effects of rumination and distraction on naturally occurring depressed mood. *Cognition & Emotion, 7*, 561–570.
Nuttin, J. R. (1964). The future time perspective in human motivation and learning. *Acta Psychologica, 23*, 60–83.
Nuttin, J. R. (1985). *Future time perspective and motivation: Theory and research method*. Hillsdale: Erlbaum.
Ornstein, R. (1975). *On the experience of time*. Baltimore: Penguin.
Pratte, F., Sidanius, J., Stallworth, L. M., & Malle, B. F. (1994). Social dominance orientation: A personality variable predicting social and political attitudes. *Journal of Personality and Social Psychology, 67*, 741–763.
Rappaport, H. (1990). *Marking time*. New York: Simon & Schuster.
Roos, P., & Albers, R. (1965a). Performance of retardates and normals on a measure of temporal orientation. *American Journal of Mental Deficiency, 69*, 835–838.
Roos, P., & Albers, R. (1965b). Performance of alcoholics and normals on a measure of temporal orientation. *Journal of Clinical Psychology, 21*, 34–36.
Rosenberg, M. (1965). *Society and the adolescent self- image*. Princeton: Princeton University Press.
Rothspan, S., & Read, S. J. (1996). Present versus future time perspective and HIV risk among heterosexual college students. *Health Psychology, 15*, 131–134.
Samuels, S. M. (1997). *Time perspective in the military: Cadets versus officers*. Unpublished manuscript, U.S. Air Force Academy, Colorado Springs, CO.
Scheier, M. F., & Carver, C. S. (1985). Optimism, coping, and health: Assessment and implications of generalized outcome expectancies. *Health Psychology, 4*, 219–247.
Sher, K. J., Wood, M. D., Crews, T. M., & Vandiver, P. A. (1995). The Tridimensional Personality Questionnaire: Reliability and validity studies and derivation of a short form. *Psychological Assessment, 7*, 195–208.

Spielberger, C. D., Gorsuch, R. L., & Lushene, R. E. (1970). *The State Trait Anxiety Inventory*. Palo Alto: Consulting Psychologists Press.

Strathman, A., Gleicher, F., Beninger, D., & Edwards, C. (1994). The consideration of future consequences: Weighing immediate and distant outcomes of behavior. *Journal of Personality and Social Psychology, 66*, 742–752.

Suddendorf, T., & Corballis, M. C. (1997). *Mental time travel and the evolution of the human mind*. New York: Basic Books.

Sundberg, N. D. (1985). The use of future studies in training for prevention and promotion in mental health. *Journal of Primary Prevention, 15*, 131–134.

Vranesh, J. G., Madrid, G., Bautista, J., Ching, P., & Hicks, R. A. (1999). Time perspective and sleep problems. *Perceptual and Motor Skills, 88*, 23–24.

Wheaton, B., Muthen, B., Alwin, D. F., & Summers, G. F. (1977). Assessing the reliability and stability in panel models. In D. R. Heise (Ed.), *Sociological methodology* (pp. 84–136). San Francisco: Jossey-Bass.

Wohlford, P. (1966). Extension of personal time, affective states, and expectation of personal death. *Journal of Personality and Social Psychology, 3*, 559–566.

Zaleski, Z. (1994). *Psychology of future orientation*. Lublin: Towarzystwo Naukowe KUL.

Zaleski, Z. (1996). Future anxiety: Concept measurement and preliminary research. *Personality and Individual Differences, 21*, 165–174.

Zimbardo, P. G., & Gonzalez, A. (1984, February). A *Psychology Today* reader survey. *Psychology Today*, pp. 53–54.

Zimbardo, P., Marshall, G., & Maslach, C. (1971). Liberating behavior from time-bound control: Expanding the present through hypnosis. *Journal of Applied Social Psychology, 1*, 305–323.

Zimbardo, P. G., Haney, C., Banks, W. C., & Jaffe, D. (1973, April 8). The mind is a formidable jailer: A Pirandellian prison. *New York Times Magazine*. p. 36ff.

Zimbardo, P. G., Keough, K. A., & Boyd, J. N. (1997). Present time perspective as a predictor of risky driving. *Personality and Individual Differences, 23*, 1007–1023.

Zuckerman, M. (1994). *Behavioral expressions and biosocial bases of sensation seeking*. New York: Cambridge University Press.

Zuckerman, M., Eysenck, S. B. G., & Eysenck, H. J. (1978). Sensation seeking in England and America: Cross-cultural, age, and sex comparisons. *Journal of Consulting and Clinical Psychology, 39*, 308–321.

Assessing Temporal Harmony: The Issue of a Balanced Time Perspective

Maciej Stolarski, Britt Wiberg, and Evgeny Osin

Introduction

The issue of time perspective's (TP) balance has been the essential point of most of the discussions and research which concerned human's temporality understood in the way proposed by Philip G. Zimbardo (Zimbardo and Boyd 1999, 2008). TP is defined as "the often nonconscious process whereby the continual flows of personal and social experiences are assigned to temporal categories, or time frames, that help to give order, coherence, and meaning to those events" (Zimbardo and Boyd 1999, p. 1271). Such a perceptual process is dynamic; however, particular individuals usually put a relative emphasis or develop a habitual focus on one of the time frames,[1] which results in emergence of relatively stable bias (Boniwell and Zimbardo 2003), reflected in individual TP profile. Our time is limited, and overusing one temporal category naturally leads to underusing others. For instance, one may remain permanently focused on their future, achieving impressive career successes, but could in parallel fail to achieve happiness, due to developed inability of living in their present.

[1] Zimbardo and Boyd (1999) empirically distinguished five dimensions (or TPs), on which human's temporality can be described: Past Negative (PN), Past Positive (PP), Present Fatalistic (PF), Present Hedonistic (PH) and Future (F). A particular description of each may be found in Zimbardo and Boyd's "Putting Time in Perspective", this volume.

M. Stolarski (✉)
Faculty of Psychology, University of Warsaw,
Stawki Str. 5/7, 00-183 Warsaw, Poland
e-mail: mstolarski@psych.uw.edu.pl

B. Wiberg
Department of Psychology, Umeå University, SE-901 87 Umeå, Sweden
e-mail: Britt.Wiberg@psy.umu.se

E. Osin
Department of Psychology, National Research University
Higher School of Economics, Moscow, Russia
e-mail: eosin@hse.ru

M. Stolarski et al. (eds.), *Time Perspective Theory; Review, Research and Application: Essays in Honor of Philip G. Zimbardo*, DOI 10.1007/978-3-319-07368-2_3,

Such temporal bias could be a consequence of a number of factors, including culture, religion, social class, education (Zimbardo and Boyd 2008), personality (Dunkel and Weber 2010), individual experiences (Kruger et al. 2008), and traumas (Zimbardo et al. 2012). In cases of a seriously maladaptive TP profile, one may require a “time perspective therapy” (Zimbardo and Boyd 1999; Sword et al. 2014) or other ways of intervention (Boniwell 2005), focused on enhancing neglected time categories. Such psychological interventions generally facilitate a formation of an ideal, perfectly harmonized combination of time horizons which allows an individual to effectively adapt to environment (Kruger et al. 2008), which in turn results in higher levels of happiness (Boniwell and Zimbardo 2003). The most adaptive manner of temporal framing has been labeled balanced time perspective (BTP; Zimbardo and Boyd 1999). The authors initially defined balance as “the mental ability to switch effectively among TPs depending on task features, situational considerations, and personal resources, rather than be biased towards a specific TP that is not adaptive across situations” (Zimbardo and Boyd 1999, p. 1285).

From the very beginning, TP was considered as a basic aspect of individual subjective experience, influencing individual and social choices and actions. After the 9/11 terrorist attacks, Zimbardo emphasized the role of balancing individual (and, in consequence, national) time perspective in order to reinvent a “stronger nation, one with renewed civic engagement, and an awareness of the fragility and preciousness of every human life” (Zimbardo 2002, p. 62). The vital construct of BTP has been further theoretically developed within the scope of positive psychology (Boniwell and Zimbardo 2003, 2004; Boniwell and Osin, chapter “Time Perspective Coaching,” this volume).

The importance of the issue of balance was emphasized by Kazakina (1999), who probably first attempted to empirically operationalize BTP. The authoress, basing on Cottle’s (1976) work, suggested that psychological time integration manifests both in time relatedness and in temporal balance. According to Kazakina, “Time orientations are ‘in balance’ when individual’s thoughts and feeling are relatively equally allocated to past, present and future. In other words, balance involves a degree of variability in the assessment of one’s past, present, and future” (1999, p. 107). She claims that the more consistent an individual is in their evaluation of personal past, present, and future, the more balanced past, present, and future are in their TP. Her operational definition of balance simply involved standard deviation as a measure. Kazakina took three items from Time Opinion Survey (Kuhlen and Monge 1968), assessing an individual’s relative focus on their past, present, and future. Using a 5-point Likert-type scale, respondents were required to assess how much their thoughts focus on each of the time zones. Such procedure provides three estimates for an individual: estimate of their focus on the past, present, and future. Balance is estimated via standard deviation, which is a measure of variability of a sample of scores from their mean (e.g., one individual scoring 3, 4, and 3, respectively, on past, present, and future items reveals more balanced temporal profile than another scoring 1, 5, and 3). Kazakina broadened the spectrum of balance estimates adding two other balance estimates: Index of Balanced Density and Indices of Balanced Emotional Valence. Likert-type scales and standard deviations were applied to these measures.

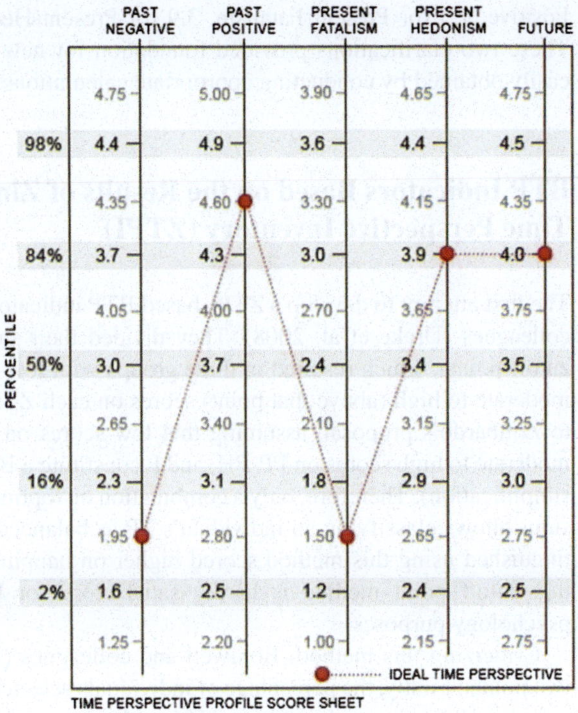

Fig. 1 The graph illustrates the BTP profile and is taken from the Time Paradox webpage (www.timeparadox.com/surveys/)

Although it seemed promising, the balance measure proposed by Kazakina (1999) has not been widely accepted and applied. Presumably, this was due to a lack of direct reference to other well-established frameworks for research on human temporality (e.g., Nuttin and Lens 1985) or to time perspective theory, proposed by Zimbardo and Boyd (1999). TP researchers widely accepted the Zimbardo Time Perspective Inventory (ZTPI) as a measure of temporal orientation, and thus it was obvious that to conduct research in this paradigm, a BTP estimate based on ZTPI scores had to be created.

Although Zimbardo and Boyd (2008) did not develop any direct indicator of BTP, they proposed an interesting starting point for its empirical operationalizations by formulating a description of an optimal mix of time perspectives. Basing on their research, the authors propose that the optimal TP profile consists of:

- High scores on Past Positive TP
- Moderately high scores on Future TP
- Moderately high scores on Present Hedonistic TP
- Low scores on Past Negative TP
- Low scores on Present Fatalistic TP

Although Zimbardo is aware of possible bias, resulting from subjective assessment and functioning in the Western cultural context (Zimbardo and Boyd 1999), he proposes an even more precise definition of BTP on Time Paradox webpage (www.timeparadox.com/surveys/). The graph presented (Fig. 1) here nearby illustrates this profile, locating "optimal" ZTPI raw scores at 1.95 for Past Negative, 4.6 for Past

Positive, 1.5 for Present Fatalism, 3.9 for Present Hedonism, and 4.0 for Future. These two clarifications provided foundation for new BTP indicators that can be easily obtained by conducting appropriate calculations on ZTPI scale scores.

BTP Indicators Based on the Results of Zimbardo Time Perspective Inventory (ZTPI)

The first attempt to develop a ZTPI-based BTP indicator came from Lisa Drake and colleagues (Drake et al. 2008). They divided their sample using 33rd percentile cutoff points, which resulted in three groups with low (below 33rd percentile) and moderate to high (above that point) scores on each ZTPI dimension. They referred to Zimbardo's proposal, assuming that low scores on PN and PF combined with moderate to high scores on PP, PH, and F constitute a BTP (which is certainly some simplification). Therefore, only a combination of "optimal" scores on all five dimensions allows classifying an individual's TP as balanced. Although participants distinguished using this method scored higher on happiness and mindfulness scales, this cutoff point method is hardly satisfactory for both clinical and scientific psychology purposes.

Criticizing this method, Boniwell and colleagues (Boniwell et al. 2010) make two points: Firstly, the percentage of individuals selected as having a BTP using this criterion depends on the extent ZTPI scales are correlated in a specific sample, rather than on real psychological differences between individuals. Usually, this approach results in selecting about 5 % respondents with a balanced TP (13 of 260 participants in the study reported by Drake et al. (2008); 12 of 179 participants in the case of Boniwell et al. 2010). Thus, an individual classified as balanced in a specific sample could be labeled as not balanced in another sample with a higher percentage of respondents having a BTP. Secondly, and perhaps most important, is that there is no evidence that these arbitrarily chosen cutoff points are optimal. Boniwell and colleagues (2010) show that using 50th percentile (rather than 33rd percentile) as a cutoff point criterion results in selecting another subsample of individuals as having a BTP. The groups of BTP individuals selected using these two arbitrary approaches overlap by only 50 % but have similar effect sizes on well-being scales, suggesting that the real percentage of BTP respondents is higher that 5–7 % selected using this criterion.

Taking into account these weaknesses of Drake's method, Boniwell and colleagues (2010) proposed cluster analysis approach as a more adequate method to operationalize BTP. It is based on person-oriented approach (Magnusson 1999, 2003), which aims to identify subgroups of individuals exhibiting similar score patterns (using simultaneous measurement of a number of different constructs) or developmental change trends (using longitudinal data). Technically, the procedure used by Boniwell and colleagues involves applying cluster analysis (Ward's method based on Squared Euclidean metric calculated using standardized scores for the 5 scales of the ZTPI) and comparing models with different number of clusters in order to choose one that is both comprehensive (in terms of describing different ZTPI score patterns peculiar to specific sample) and parsimonious (in terms of having a limited number of interpretable clusters, usually 4–6). The cluster models can also be evaluated by the proportion of variance of the ZTPI scales they explain, using an elbow criterion similar to the Cattell scree test (Everitt et al. 2001). One of the clusters that emerges usually shows a pattern similar to BTP (relatively high or above average scores on F, PH, and PP combined with relatively low or below average scores on PN and PF). This approach has been applied by the authors to British and Russian samples, resulting in a larger proportion of respondents selected as having a BTP (10–23 %) with similar or larger effect sizes for the differences between BTP and non-BTP groups on well-being measures, compared to the percentile cutoff criteria. Boniwell and her colleagues' (2010) person-oriented approach was certainly a milestone in the research on exploring the BTP construct.

However, Zhang et al. (2013) noted that also this method does have certain drawbacks. The technique endorsed by Boniwell and colleagues (2010) also resulted in a rather small number of people being categorized as having a BTP. Moreover, both methods are sample dependent. Both cluster and cutoff approaches may categorize individuals as having a "balanced" time perspective whose time perspective profile is different from the way Zimbardo and Boyd (1999) originally defined BTP, and it is difficult to compare results from BTP studies done in different samples. In addition, the cluster analysis procedure used may introduce its artifacts, for instance, Ward's method tends to create clusters of roughly equal size (Everitt et al. 2001), which may not always be appropriate for the study of BTP. Finally, and most important is that cluster analysis provides a binomial measure of BTP (classifying each individual either into BTP or into not-BTP subgroup). It may be useful to measure BTP as a relative, rather than absolute construct, although more advanced clustering techniques, such as fuzzy or "soft" clustering, overcome this limitation (Everitt et al. 2001).

Addressing the abovementioned concerns, Stolarski et al. (2011) developed a new indicator of BTP: the Deviation from Balanced Time Perspective (DBTP). It is a measure of difference between individuals' time perceptions and the optimal time perspective profile as stated by Zimbardo and Boyd (2008) which indicates how ill-balanced the time perspective of each person is. At the root of the DBTP is the assumption that there is an "optimal" point on each of the time perspective scales. The main determinant of a BTP is how close an individual is to these optimal points. Following the abovementioned "optimal" points on each TP dimension, proposed by Zimbardo and Boyd (2008), the following formula is then applied in calculating the DBTP:

$$\mathrm{DBTP} = \sqrt{(\mathrm{oPN} - \mathrm{ePN})^2 + (\mathrm{oPP} - \mathrm{ePP})^2 + (\mathrm{oPF} - \mathrm{ePF})^2 + (\mathrm{oPH} - \mathrm{ePH})^2 + (\mathrm{oF} - \mathrm{eF})^2}$$

where oPN – ePN is (optimal Past Negative) – (an individual's empirical Past Negative); this procedure is repeated for each time perspective dimension. Thus, the root of the sum of squared deviations of individual's scores from the optimal points on each ZTPI dimension is calculated. DBTP values close to zero indicate almost perfectly balanced time perspective (the theoretical ideal), whereas large positive values indicate individual time perspective that is out of balance (and is expected to be maladaptive).

One may argue that the applied procedure is overcomplicated and simple sum of absolute values of the optimal and empirical scale scores would reveal analogical results. Although it may seem redundant, this "complication" was intentional. Each scale deviation is squared to capture the nature of maladaptive influence of the deviation from each of the time perspective dimensions (which we believe to be parabolic rather than linear). This effect may be best illustrated with an example. An individual who differs from the "optimal" by .20 point on every time perspective dimension is in fact closer to BTP than an individual who obtained a perfect fit on four of the five time perspectives and differs by 1 point on the fifth time perspective (see Zimbardo and Boyd 2008). If we simply add the absolute deviations for each person, the obtained value is the same for both. However, if we apply the above formula for the DBTP assuming that maladaptive influence of the deviations from the optimal scores increases nonlinearly as the deviations increase, the former person obtains a DBTP score of .45, while the latter person obtains a score of 1.0. This difference reflects the more maladaptive time perspective profile of the second individual.

Also, the square root of the sum of squares is applied in order to maximize the possibility of obtaining a normal distribution. This is because squaring each of the differences between optimal and obtained scores naturally results in right-skewed distribution. This effect remains also after summing the differences for all TP dimensions. Therefore, calculating a square root allows to reverse this skewing effect and restore normal distribution of the variable (see Ferguson and Takane 1989 for a review of "normalizing" procedures).

In a study by Zhang et al. (2013), the DBTP proved to have significantly better predictive validity with regard to well-being than both of the other existing approaches to balanced time perspective's: a cutoff point approach (Drake et al. 2008) and a cluster analysis (Boniwell et al. 2010). The DBTP provides a linear variable and allows avoiding dichotomize people into "balanced" and "not balanced." Following this point of view, balanced TP is a complex personality characteristic and a normally distributed trait. It does not determine whether one's TP is balanced or not; it shows how far is an individual from developing the most adaptive (according to Zimbardo and Boyd) TP profile.

However, also this method is not free from drawbacks. Firstly, the contribution of the three temporal domains is not equal: ZTPI has two Present and two Past scales and only one Future scale. Secondly, the optimal scores used to calculate a DBTP was based on the arbitrary recommendation from Zimbardo and Boyd (2008). Whether these are true optimal scores should be explicitly tested. An attempt to develop an optimal BTP profile (using criteria measures, such as subjective well-being scores) is currently being undertaken by Mitina and Osin. Thirdly, this approach still does not "catch" the ability to flexibly switch between particular time zones, which is considered essential to BTP (Zimbardo and Boyd 1999). Therefore, besides verifying reasonability of distinguishing these and not others, "optimal" points on each TP, perhaps enriching ZTPI with a few new items, making up a new dimension of temporal flexibility, could also be considered.

There are also other approaches to BTP based on the ZTPI that have been suggested but received more limited research attention (e.g., Sircova and Mitina 2008).

A fourth, combined approach to BTP has been developed by Wiberg et al. (2012a). According to Zimbardo and Boyd (1999), BTP individual's actions are shaped by a consideration of all three temporal zones (past, present, future). The basic assumption in their study is based on the theoretical model by Zimbardo (2002, p. 62), who wrote that "in an optimally BTP, the past, present and future components blend and flexibly engage, depending on a situation's demands and our needs and values." In that sense, an individual with BTP is assumed to operate within temporal frames which are more appropriate than an individual with less BTP or biased TP. The aims of their study were to examine and compare earlier operationalizations of BTP (Boniwell 2005; Boniwell et al. 2010; Drake et al. 2008; Sircova and Mitina 2008) and also to present an alternative proposal in order to give a sample independent operationalization of BTP, in which BTP is measured as a multidimensional, rather than a binary construct. Two versions of Zimbardo Time Perspective Inventory were administered to a Swedish sample of 502 individuals: the original ZTPI with the five TP dimensions (PN, PP, PF, PH, and F (Zimbardo and Boyd 1999)) and the Swedish version of ZTPI (S-ZTPI; Carelli et al. 2011), where the Future temporal dimension is extended and divided in both a Future Positive and a Future Negative scale[2] and therefore consists of six dimensions (or TPs) (PN, PP, PF, PH, FP, and FN). Wiberg and colleagues (2012b) proposed an operationalization of BTP, based on the theoretical model initially proposed by Boniwell and Zimbardo (2004) that a person with a BTP, when assessed with ZTPI, should score low on PN and PF, moderate on PH and F, and high on PP, but Zimbardo (2006) later changed opinion toward scoring moderately high on F. For the ZTPI and S-ZTPI instruments, this means that a person with a BTP, in the stringent case, should score:

- Low (scoring 1 or 2 on most items) on PN, PF, and FN
- Moderate (scoring 3 on most items) on PH
- Moderately high (scoring 3 or 4 on most items) on F and FP
- High (scoring 4 or 5 on most items) on PP

The levels of balance (see Table 1) may appear overlapping, but this is not a problem since they were comparing each individual within a TP dimension, which means that whether the individual fulfilled the definition for that dimension or not. A person's level of balance depended on how many parts of the BTP definition were

[2] Carelli et al. (2011) empirically distinguished six temporal dimensions (or TPs), on which human's temporality can be described: Past Negative (PN), Past Positive (PP), Present Fatalistic (PF), Present Hedonistic (PH), Future Positive (FP) and Future Negative (FN). A particular description of each dimension may be found in their works, as well as in the chapter by Carelli et al. (chapter "Broadening the TP Profile: Future Negative Time Perspective", this volume).

Table 1 Proposed BTP operationalization for the subscales in ZTPI and S-ZTPI (Wiberg et al. 2012a, b)

TP dimensions ZTPI and S-ZTPI	Number of items	Level of balance	Limit scores
PN	10	Low	1.00–2.50
PP	9	High	3.50–5.00
PF	9	Low	1.00–2.50
PH	15	Moderate	2.70–3.30
F[a]	13	Moderately high	3.00–4.00
FP[b]	11	Moderately high	3.00–4.00
FN[b]	10	Low	1.00–2.50

[a]Only included in ZTPI
[b]Only included in S-ZTPI

Table 2 Levels of balance for the ZTPI and S-ZTPI in the proposed operationalization ($n=502$) (Wiberg et al. 2012a, b)

	ZTPI participants		S-ZTPI participants	
Level of balance	Number	Percentage	Number	Percentage
0	21	4.2	17	3.4
1	66	13.1	55	11.0
2	114	22.7	98	19.5
3	150	29.9	125	24.9
4	113	22.5	107	21.3
5	38	7.6	76	15.1
6	–	–	24	4.8

fulfilled. One has to bear in mind that they did not consider an individual to be either balanced or not balanced, but considered that an individual may be more or less balanced, depending on their level of BTP.

Every person was classified on each TP dimension (PN, PP, PF, PH, FP, FN) as whether or not fulfilling the BTP definition for that particular scale, and the researchers classified the individuals' level of balance (range 0–5 for ZTPI and range 0–6 for S-ZTPI) due to how many parts of the BTP definition were fulfilled. Applying this BTP operationalization for the 502 Swedish participants on ZTPI and S-ZTPI, they obtained respectively 38 (7.6 %) and 24 (4.8 %) fully balanced individuals (see Table 2). The highest percentage is at the middle level of BTP (level 3), which seemed to be the most common pattern in their Swedish sample. The latter result seems to be perfectly in line with the Stolarski and colleagues' (2011) assumption that BTP is a normally distributed trait.

A limitation of the study by Wiberg and her colleagues (2012a) was that the proposed BTP operationalization was not completely validated. The BTP construct was based on a theoretical model in the literature, and the definition of the underlying concepts that constitutes BTP, i.e., the different temporal dimensions (or TP's) and their interrelationships, was used. Their proposal of a new operationalization of

BTP can be used independently of obtained samples and is also concerning the ecological validity. Their BTP model is also closer to the everyday complexity of the construct and defines levels of balance in line with the idea that a person is seldom balanced or not balanced.

Alternative Ways to Assess Balance

In parallel to the endeavors for the most optimal BTP indicator based on ZTPI, other researchers seek alternative ways to assess temporal harmony. First such effort came from Webster (2011) who developed the Balanced Time Perspective Scale (BTPS). The measure comprises of two subscales (Past and Future) due to the author who assumed that for developing BTP, an individual should counterbalance one time zone with the other. Basing on the scores of the two subscales and median cutoff splits, Webster distinguished four types of individuals: time restrictive (low scores on both Past and Future), futurists (low score on Past and high on Future), reminiscers (high score on Past and low on Future), and time expansive (i.e., balanced; scoring high on both Past and Future). Although the author provided some evidence for the validity of BTPS, its predictive value is not convincing. First, time expansive individuals did not score higher than futurists on any of applied criterion variables (well-being, self-esteem, and happiness). Thus, there is no evidence that BTPS time expansive individuals are better adapted than futurists (however, they did score higher than time restrictive, and, in some cases, than reminiscers). Moreover, once again, a typological approach has been proposed, resulting in loss of significant amount of information. Substituting this cutoff point approach with linear indicators of balance based on the two subscales Past and Future (e.g., a square root of the product of these two scores) could provide a joint indicator of temporal expansion and balance.

Although the author shows some BTPS' advantage over analogical procedure conducted using Past Positive and Future scales of the ZTPI, the BTPS scores do not take into account the other ZTPI dimensions. It is highly probable that the five scales of Zimbardo's TP inventory would have explained much higher amount of criterion variables' variance. Moreover, the Webster's BTPS measure does not take into account negative aspects of time perspective despite the fact that it is now broadly accepted that negative affective states are not opposite to positive affective states (e.g., Tomkins 1980). One more weakness of the scale is that it does not cover the present time zone. One may balance her/his Past and Future, but at the same time could be unable to live in the moment, to enjoy immediate pleasures of her/his life, and to experience satisfying social relationships. Thus, to effectively measure balance, BTPS needs to be significantly improved.

Another approach to the BTP construct has been explored in Sweden as a case study with combinations of qualitative and quantitative methods (Wiberg et al. 2012b). The aim of this study was to get a deeper understanding of the BTP concept by studying people with BTP with both deep interviews (combined with Cottle's

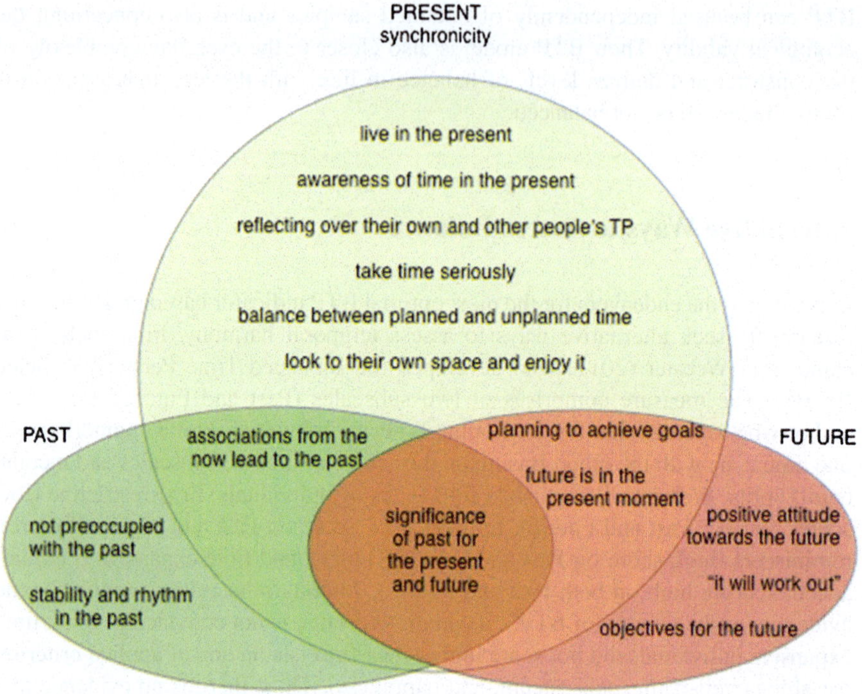

Fig. 2 Overarching themes categorized into Past, Present, and Future, illustrating the synchronicity (Lindvall 2011)

test, 1976) and several self-rating instruments, such as SCL-90, Life Events scale, Scales of Psychological Well-Being (C. Ryff), and Satisfaction with Life Scale (E. Diener). Seven people with balanced time perspective (BTP) according to Swedish Zimbardo Time Perspective Inventory (S-ZTPI; Carelli et al. 2011) have been studied at two occasions. S-ZTPI was administered in order to study the stability and change in BTP level at two occasions with about 18 months in between. The results of the S-ZTPI showed a great stability in the BTP level among the seven participants, although a small change was observed, and the results will be presented in a forthcoming publication by Wiberg and colleagues at Umeå University.

The 14 interviews were analyzed according to Interpretative Phenomenological Analysis (IPA; Smith et al. 2009). The preliminary analysis of the interviews shows a consciousness about the "now" among these seven people with a BTP profile. They expressed a synchronicity between the present and the past in the theme "associations from the now lead to the past," and they also expressed a synchronicity between the present and the future in the themes "planning to achieve goals" and "future is in the present moment" (see Fig. 2).

The preliminary results from this case study give strength to a holistic present scale (Zimbardo and Boyd 2008) and an "extended now" according to the overarching theme "significance of past for the present and future" (Fig. 2). This study may be helpful to get a deeper understanding of the BTP construct and also gives opportunity to formulate further research questions. In that sense, the results from a case study may give some ideas for the future directions in the research on BTP with both quantitative and qualitative methods.

Future Directions in Research on BTP

In theory, balanced time perspective is characterized by flexible switching between a person's past, present, and future time orientations, depending on situational demands, personal resources, or personal and social evaluations. Thus, BTP is considered to be associated with most psychological and physical health for individuals and optimal societal functioning. The construct of balanced time perspective (BTP) was initially proposed by Zimbardo and Boyd (1999) along with introducing the final version of Zimbardo Time Perspective Inventory (ZTPI). Since then, several attempts have been made to operationalize the BTP construct (Drake et al. 2008; Boniwell et al. 2010; Stolarski et al. 2011; Zhang et al. 2013; Wiberg et al. 2012a, b). The results of the proposed operationalizations are that there are both strong sides and drawbacks of each approach and that the BTP construct is not yet totally explored and clarified. A great amount of work has to be done in the future to get a clearer and more complete picture of the BTP construct from empirical studies in order to get an opportunity to theorize about balanced time perspective.

Possible options for future research are, firstly, to conduct more empirical studies in order to establish relationships between the BTP construct and other psychological constructs, e.g., psychological well-being, quality of life, and other aspects of positive functioning and also with different cognitive, clinical, and life satisfaction measures. By using multidimensional instruments with high validity and reliability, one may get a clearer and more complete picture of what BTP is and not is. This suggestion is in line with, for example, Wiberg and colleagues' (2012a, b) research directions. Also, usage of a wide range of psychological well-being indicators could help to answer the question of the "optimal" BTP profile based on ZTPI (e.g., one on which the DBTP is based).

Secondly, longitudinal studies might be very useful to answer the research question about the change or stability of BTP over time, and such empirical data should be connected to demographical aspects such as age, gender, marital status, occupational, and ethno-cultural aspects as well as positive and negative/stressful life events. This suggestion was also proposed by Boniwell and Zimbardo (2004) and aims to investigate the role of the level of balance in practice and also to clarify the "moderately high on Future TP" discussion. As Wiberg and colleagues (2012a, b) comment, there is no research available on the negative effects of being too high on the Future dimension.

Thirdly, a combination of qualitative and quantitative methods may be used in, e.g., single case study and multiple case studies in exploring the individual BTP profiles with a combination of deep interviews and self-report instruments.

This may be done in order to answer research questions about the way an individual's own view of her/his time orientation influences her/his daily life and also in order to arrive at new research questions and hypotheses concerning the BTP construct.

Fourthly, it may perhaps also be meaningful and useful to conduct more research around the new idea of viewing BTP as an ordinal-level variable or even a continuous trait instead of an either-or typology. Such operationalizations make sense from a psychological perspective and are adjustable for studying country differences.

Fifthly, future research should take into account a possible interplay between particular TP dimensions. This suggestion first of all applies to Present Hedonistic and Future orientations. Already Zimbardo and Boyd (2008) emphasized that excessive development of one of these TPs results in numerous threats (e.g., addictions in Present Hedonists and workaholic tendencies in Future-oriented individuals) if it is not counterbalanced with an appropriate level of the other. Recently, it was empirically demonstrated that the two dimensions should not be analyzed separately, as significant effects of interaction and suppression between these variables were obtained for such outcomes as well-being (Stolarski et al. 2012) or mood (Stolarski et al. 2013).

Finally, the dynamic nature of TP needs to be acknowledged. If TP is indeed "dynamic, perceptual flow," as Boniwell and Zimbardo (2003) claimed, then balancing one's TP is a flexible process, leading to immediate adaptive responses to changing environmental contexts. There are a few existing self-report approaches in psychology that allow the study of dynamic processes and could be used to investigate the extent to which different temporal dimensions are integrated into individual life and to assess BTP. For instance, an approach similar to Day Reconstruction Method (DRM; Kahneman et al. 2004) could be applied to assess retrospectively the extent to which individual's subjective experience during the previous day was affected by past, present, or future events. A variant of Experience Sampling Method (ESM; Larson and Csikszentmihalyi 1983) could be used to study the influence of the past, present, and future within the context of daily life. However, the assessment of dynamic processes using traditional self-report questionnaire techniques still has its limitations.

As an alternative, a dynamic assessment that has been developed within the scope of dynamic social psychology (Nowak and Vallacher 1998) could be applied to BTP-focused research programs. Mouse paradigm (Vallacher and Nowak 1994) is probably the most promising of the available methods. This innovative technique was initially developed to investigate moment-to-moment evaluations of social stimuli, basing on the assumption that attitude is an implicit approach-avoid response (Hovland et al. 1953). In further studies, it has been modified to investigate other robust psychological outcomes (e.g., depression; Johnson and Nowak 2002). Mouse paradigm is great in its simplicity. In its initial version, an individual was asked to think of themselves and move the mouse cursor toward the red circle in the center of a computer screen when their thoughts are positive. If the thoughts become negative, the cursor should be moved toward the edge of a screen. Dynamics of the cursor are being registered throughout all the procedure. Analyses of datasets obtained in such way allow for calculating not only average self-esteem during this period but also its variability and allocation and strength of points of stability, labeled attractors. The empirical studies revealed that temporal dynamics of self-esteem or mood are often even more important than average scores (Johnson and Nowak 2002).

The dynamic nature of measurement, characteristic for this method, and its effectiveness in the diagnose of psychological dynamisms suggest that mouse paradigm could become an interesting alternative for more traditional methods of estimating balance, described in the present chapter. Studies aimed at development of special computer software measuring temporal dynamics of focus on particular time zones and their emotional loadings, are currently being conducted at the University of Warsaw.

The method seems promising especially due to the fact that conditions provided in mouse paradigm investigation are analogous to the trade-off between particular time zones we inevitably deal with in real life. While responding to the ZTPI or BTPS items, one can easily describe themselves as equally highly past, present, and future oriented. However, the reality is completely different: we incessantly have to manage our attention resources allocating them to one of the time zones. In the mouse paradigm, the experimental situation is similar: our time is limited, and only one time zone could remain in attention focus in a particular moment. Flexibility in switching the temporal attention and ability to develop stable but not immobilizing positive temporal attractors may prove to be the most effective and theoretically anchored BTP estimate.

Conclusions

In theory, balanced time perspective is characterized by flexible switching between a person's past, present, and future time orientations, depending on situational demands, personal resources, or personal and social evaluations. Thus, BTP is considered to be associated with psychological and physical health in individuals and optimal societal functioning. The construct of balanced time perspective (BTP) was initially proposed by Zimbardo and Boyd (1999) along with introduction of the final version of Zimbardo Time Perspective Inventory (ZTPI). Since then, several attempts have been made to operationalize the BTP construct (Boniwell et al. 2010; Drake et al. 2008; Stolarski et al. 2011; Wiberg et al. 2012a, b; Zhang et al. 2013). The results of the proposed operationalizations suggest that each approach has specific strengths and drawbacks, and that the BTP construct is not yet totally explored and clarified. A great amount of work has to be done in the future to get a clearer and more complete picture of the BTP construct from empirical studies in order to theorize about balanced time perspective.

References

Boniwell, I. (2005). Beyond time management: How the latest research on time perspective and perceived time use can assist clients with time-related concerns. *International Journal of Evidence Based Coaching and Mentoring, 3*(2), 61–74.

Boniwell, I., & Zimbardo, P. G. (2003). Time to find the right balance. *The Psychologist, 16*(3), 129–131.

Boniwell, I., & Zimbardo, P. G. (2004). Balancing time perspective in pursuit of optimal functioning. In P. A. Linley & S. Joseph (Eds.), *Positive psychology in practice* (pp. 165–178). Hoboken: Wiley.

Boniwell, I., Osin, E., Linley, P. A., & Ivanchenko, G. V. (2010). A question of balance: Time perspective and well-being in British and Russian samples. *The Journal of Positive Psychology, 5*(1), 24–40.

Carelli, M. G., Wiberg, B., & Wiberg, M. (2011). Development and construct validation of the Swedish Zimbardo time perspective inventory. *European Journal of Psychological Assessment, 27*(4), 220–227.

Cottle, T. J. (1976). *Perceiving time*. New York: Wiley.

Drake, L., Duncan, E., Sutherland, F., Abernethy, C., & Henry, C. (2008). Time perspective and correlates of wellbeing. *Time and Society, 17*(1), 47–61.

Dunkel, C. S., & Weber, J. L. (2010). Using three levels of personality to predict time perspective. *Current Psychology, 29*(2), 95–103.

Everitt, B. S., Landau, S., & Leese, M. (2001). *Cluster analysis*. London: Edward Arnold.

Ferguson, G. A., & Takane, Y. (1989). *Statistical analysis in psychology and education*. New York: McGraw-Hill.

Hovland, C. I., Janis, I. L., & Kelley, H. H. (1953). *Communication and persuasion; psychological studies of opinion change*. New Haven: Yale University Press.

Johnson, S. L., & Nowak, A. (2002). Dynamical patterns in bipolar depression. *Personality and Social Psychology Review, 6*(4), 380–387.

Kahneman, D., Krueger, A. B., Schkade, D. A., Schwarz, N., & Stone, A. A. (2004). A survey method for characterizing daily life experience: The day reconstruction method. *Science, 306*(5702), 1776–1780.

Kazakina, E. (1999). *Time perspective of older adults: Relationships to attachment style, psychological well-being and psychological distress*. Unpublished doctoral dissertation, Columbia University.

Kruger, D. J., Reischl, T., & Zimmerman, M. A. (2008). Time perspective as a mechanism for functional developmental adaptation. *Journal of Social, Evolutionary, and Cultural Psychology,* 2(1), 1–22.

Kuhlen, R. G., & Monge, R. H. (1968). Correlates of estimated rate of time passage in the adult years. *Journal of Gerontology, 23*(4), 427–433.

Larson, R., & Csikszentmihalyi, M. (1983). The experience sampling method. *New Directions for Methodology of Social & Behavioral Science, 15*, 41–56.

Lindvall, M. (2011). *Förändring och förhållande till tiden ur ett balanserat tidsperspektiv.* Psykologexamensuppsats, 30 hp, Institutionen för psykologi, Umeå universitet, Umeå.

Magnusson, D. (1999). On the individual: A person-oriented approach to developmental research. *European Psychologist, 4*, 205–218.

Magnusson, D. (2003). The person approach: Concepts, measurement models and research strategy. *New Directions for Child and Adolescent Development, 101*, 3–23.

Nowak, A., & Vallacher, R. R. (1998). *Dynamical social psychology*. New York: Guilford Press.

Nuttin, J. R., & Lens, W. (1985). *Future time perspective and motivation: Theory and research method.* Leuven: Leuven University Press/Lawrence Erlbaum.

Sircova, A., & Mitina, O. (2008). *Balanced time perspective (BTP) as a resource of person's optimal functioning.* Paper presented at the 4th European conference on positive psychology, Opatija, Croatia.

Smith, J. A., Flowers, P., & Larkin, M. (2009). *Interpretative phenomenological analysis, theory, method and research*. London: SAGE Publications Ltd.
Stolarski, M., Bitner, J., & Zimbardo, P. G. (2011). Time perspective, emotional intelligence and discounting of delayed awards. *Time and Society, 20*(3), 346–363.
Stolarski, M., Zimbardo, P. G., Howell, R. T., & Zhang, J. W. (2012). *Looking for the bright side of life: How to shape your time perspective to become happier?* Paper presented at the 1st international conference on time perspective, Coimbra, Portugal.
Stolarski, M., Matthews, G., Postek, S., Zimbardo, P. G., & Bitner, J. (2013). How we feel is a matter of time: Relationships between time perspectives and mood. *Journal of Happiness Studies*. Advanced online publication. doi:10.1007/s10902-013-9450-y.
Sword, R. M., Sword, R. K. M., Brunskill, S. R., & Zimbardo, P. G. (2014). Time perspective therapy: A new time-based metaphor therapy for PTSD. *Journal of Loss and Trauma, 19*(3), 197–201. doi:10.1080/15325024.2013.763632.
Tomkins, S. S. (1980). Affect as amplification: Some modifications in theory. In R. Plutchik & H. Kellerman (Eds.), *Emotion: Theory, research, and experience* (Vol. 1, pp. 141–164). London: Academic.
Vallacher, R. R., & Nowak, A. (1994). The stream of social judgment. In R. R. Vallacher & A. Nowak (Eds.), *Dynamical systems in social psychology* (pp. 251–255). London: Academic.
Webster, J. D. (2011). A new measure of balance time perspective: Initial psychometric findings from the balanced time perspective scale (BTPS). *Canadian Journal of Behavioural Science, 43*(2), 111–118.
Wiberg, M., Sircova, A., Wiberg, B., & Carelli, M. G. (2012a). Operationalizing balanced time perspective in a Swedish sample. *The International Journal of Educational and Psychological Assessment, 12*(1), 95–107.
Wiberg, B., Wiberg, M., Carelli, M. G., & Sircova, A. (2012b). *A qualitative and quantitative study of seven persons with balanced time perspective (BTP) according to S-ZTPI*. Poster presented at the Ist international conference on time perspective and research: Converging paths in psychology time theory and research (pp. 120–120). ESPACOBRANCO.
Zhang, J. W., Howell, R. T., & Stolarski, M. (2013). Comparing three methods to measure a balanced time perspective: The relationship between a balanced time perspective and subjective well-being. *Journal of Happiness Studies, 14*(1), 169–184.
Zimbardo, P. G. (2002). Just think about it: Time to take our time. *Psychology Today, 35*, 62.
Zimbardo, P. G. (2006, October). *The secret power of time: Influencing personal decisions and national destinies*. Paper presented at the Department of Psychology, Lomonosov Moscow State University, Moscow, Russia.
Zimbardo, P. G., & Boyd, J. N. (1999). Putting time in perspective: A valid, reliable individual-difference metric. *Journal of Personality and Social Psychology, 77*(6), 1271–1288.
Zimbardo, P. G., & Boyd, J. N. (2008). *The time paradox. The new psychology of time that will change your life*. New York: Free Press.
Zimbardo, P. G., Sword, R. M., & Sword, R. K. (2012). *The time cure: Overcoming PTSD with the new psychology of time perspective therapy*. San Francisco: Jossey-Bass.

Time Perspective and Transcendental Future Thinking

Wessel van Beek and Antanas Kairys

Introduction

In 1997, Boyd and Zimbardo published their article "Constructing Time After Death: The Transcendental-Future Time Perspective." In this manuscript, the authors present their ideas about partitioning the psychological future into a pre- and post-death time frame, the latter transcending life and living. When human behavior is at least partly motivated by thoughts about the past, the present, and the future, it seems obvious that thoughts about the afterlife need to be integrated in time-related models in psychology. As we will see, this is not as self-evident as it may seem.

Let us present few core definitions we are going to follow in this chapter. Religion is "a particular system of faith and worship" (Stevenson 2013); the differences between religion and spirituality will be discussed later. Transcendence is defined as "existence or experience beyond the normal or physical level" (Stevenson 2013). We shall elaborate on the concept of transcendent time perspective in the following chapter. It is worth mentioning however that "'transcendental-future' time perspective, postulated to be distinct and separate from the traditional future, encompasses the period of time from the imagined death of the physical body to infinity. The transcendental-future may contain goals such as reunion with deceased loved ones, eternal life, reincarnation, the avoidance of eternal damnation, and the elimination of current poverty, pain, suffering and shame" (Boyd and Zimbardo 1997, p. 36).

In this chapter, we shall discuss the relationship between spirituality, religion, and time perspective theory. We shall focus on the role of thinking about death in

W. van Beek (✉)
GGZ Veenendaal, Veenendaal, The Netherlands
e-mail: wessel.van.beek@gmail.com

A. Kairys
Department of General Psychology, Vilnius University, Vilnius, Lithuania

M. Stolarski et al. (eds.), *Time Perspective Theory; Review, Research and Application: Essays in Honor of Philip G. Zimbardo*, DOI 10.1007/978-3-319-07368-2_4,

psychology, and how it can be measured. Some empirical data on transcendental Future time perspective will be presented and discussed. However, first of all, we shall present and discuss the transcendental future thinking in religion.

Transcendental Future Thinking, Spirituality, and Religion

Life after death, or the absence of it, is regarded to be an important motivational factor by Boyd and Zimbardo (1997). It encompasses the time from the imagined death of the physical body to infinity (Boyd and Zimbardo 1997). This predicted eternal reward or punishment in the afterlife can be of utmost significance for an individual and, by such, substantially affect one's present life.

Transcendental future thinking is related to religion and spirituality, as it stands for the belief in something larger than life, an energy or an entity that transcends the present or the immediate future. In religion, this is referred to as "God"; in spirituality, it is sometimes addressed as a "Higher Power." Spirituality and religion have overlapping but different meanings. Cook et al. (2009) define spirituality as "a distinctive, potentially creative and universal dimension of human experience arising both within the inner subjective awareness of individuals and within communities, social groups and traditions. It may be experienced as relationship with that which is intimately 'inner', immanent and personal, within the self and others, and/or as relationship with that which is wholly 'other', transcendent and beyond the self" (p. 4). According to these authors, most studies are concerned with religion, because it has been impossible to separate spirituality and religion in research. Although we know that there is a high correlation with religiosity (Boyd and Zimbardo 1997), we can assume that transcendental future thinking defines a separate factor, because if focuses on the distinct aspect of thoughts about life after death, whereas spirituality and religion encompass related traditions and rituals.

Nelson (2009) describes two implications of religion. It is defined as a worldview, consisting of historical, cultural, and personal elements, providing meaning for the individual. All major religions have a view of transcendence: the divine surpassing the material world and a concept of what is beyond life. The second implication Nelson mentions is that of the behavioral consequences: religion as human activity, to look at it in terms of its functions, instead of its contents and specific beliefs. Ostow (2007) defines religion as "a social system in which the spiritual drive is channeled into a set of modes of worship, a set of beliefs, and a set of behavioral imperatives and prohibitions, all within a social structure" (p. 61). An essential feature of spirituality is that experiences essentially reach out to an imagined transcendent presence that seems so compellingly inviting that it challenges our notion of reality.

There has been a shift in Western society from institutionalized religion, toward a broader sense of spiritual awareness. "Spirituality [...] is a way of being and experiencing that comes through awareness of a transcendental dimension and that is characterized by certain identifiable values in regard to self, others, nature, life and whatever one considers to be ultimate" (Elkins et al., 1988, cited in Swinton 2001, p. 20).

When we have a closer look on thoughts about life after death, we know that women are more afraid of death than men and younger people more than older people (Thorson et al. 1988). In their study among cancer patients, McClain-Jacobson et al. (2004) come to the conclusion that spirituality has a much more powerful effect than actual beliefs in life after death. Other research has shown that religion is a protective factor from and in illness but also may have negative effects (Koenig et al. 2001), particularly regarding mental health problems. Some studies stress the contribution of religion in providing hope and meaning. A minimal claim would be that the evidence presented within this chapter suggests that spirituality is an important dimension of human experience which can significantly affect the process of mental health care (Swinton 2001).

A recent study by Ellis et al. (2012) reveals that Muslims are more anxious about death than Christians, possibly due to a vindictive versus forgiving image of God. Less death anxiety was found in Christian believers and people who expressed not to be religious. We know that firmness and consistency of beliefs and practices, rather than religiousness per se, buffer against death anxiety in old age (Wink and Scott 2005). According to a study among bereaved people (Smith et al. 1992), the feeling of recovery following bereavement is enhanced by high belief in afterlife and diminished by losing the loved one via suicide or accident. Some studies suggest that religious beliefs are an important factor in providing meaning and thereby protecting against mental health problems (Flannelly et al. 2006). And unpleasant beliefs about life after death are strongly associated with poorer mental health (Flannelly et al. 2008).

The awareness of death is a unique human characteristic. Believing that death is not the end of one's individual existence, an afterlife, is found in almost every religious and spiritual approach. But there are differences as well. Whereas in Western religions the individual transcends the limitation of life to live an extension in some kind of afterlife, Eastern religions are mostly nonpersonalistic (Obayashi 1992). This simple notion has huge psychological and sociological effects, which we will discuss later on.

We first evaluate the ideas about life after death in the major denominations. Our choice of these five religions is based upon the scale of followers, not on personal or other considerations. The descriptions we provide are based upon traditional religious beliefs, for it is impossible to include the many interpretations within each of these religions. The overview is in alphabetical order.

Buddhism

According to Buddhism, death is part of an ongoing process of life, death, and rebirth. Although the recognition of phenomenological reality may eventually lead to so-called release from the power of death, for the majority of followers, release from this ongoing process of birth and dying is out of the question. Rebirth may lead to life in a more advantageous position in the human world but also to life in one of the many Buddhist hells. In short, one way of affecting this process is moderating desires in one's current life, learning from to Buddha's teachings (c.f. Thompson 2008).

Christianity

The apocalyptical conceived Christianity is based upon the idea of rebirth. In its origins, it was envisioned that the Final Judgment would lead to a sudden end of the world, followed by the second coming of Jesus. Rebirth would lead to a second, eternal spiritual life. In the history of the Christian tradition, a shift took place, from an announced end of the world to the individual soul who enters heaven through God's judgment and admission. "Human beings are mortal, and only by faith in God's power of resurrection, conquering death, can they hope to be raised into a new life" (Obayashi 1992, p. 111). No longer a sinning world coming to an end, but individuals who will be personally judged. Human life can be seen as a preparation for death, a preparation for eternal life (Tiso 2008).

Judaism

Contrary to most other religions, Judaism focuses more on traditions and rituals than on a uniform cosmological understanding, and there is room for personal opinions. The central view on life after death is not clearly defined, for it is considered a matter of the Divine. Ancient Judaism did not entertain thoughts of personal resurrection, nor a judgment after death (Casey 2009); but in common Jewish tradition, the souls pass into the next realm after death. There is a transition from the physical body, and the soul returns to its divine source. The body and the soul are separated, and the physical body returns to the soil. The soul, with its memories and its individuality, is held accountable for God. Death is another step in the metaphysical journey to the World to Come, a process that starts in the living world.

Kabbalistic tradition teaches that the soul consists of five levels. These levels, and sublevels, provide direction and structure for the individual in life before death. There is no concept of hell or eternal damnation in Judaism. Although reincarnation is debated among Jewish mystics, it is considered to be an ancient, mainstream belief in Judaism.

Some Jewish texts mention a complex process of post-death interaction between the body and the soul; but according to the Zohar, "once the Angel of Death removes the soul from a person's body, death occurs instantaneously. At that point, the person's spirit comes out and sits on the tip of the nose until the body begins to decay" (Seltzer 2008, p. 10).

Hinduism

Hinduism is not a monotheistic model. There is not one God, nor one uniform set of beliefs about death and the afterlife. Hinduism does not endorse a dichotomous difference between life and not-life, but worldly life and afterlife are on a continuum.

According to this perspective, people die and are reborn, and to be freed from this endless cycle, the person must follow the path of ritual action and the path of knowledge. The afterlife in Hinduism may be reached through a ritual cremation tradition, through which a person may or may not enter the World of the Fathers. This ceremony, and therefore afterlife, depends on one's descendants to establish and sustain it. Death of the individual is only a transition point in a system of duties according to class and stage of life, which will take many cycles of birth and death.

Islam

The Koran tells people that all things have come from God and return to him. Muslims believe in resurrection of the body and the existence of heaven and hell. After death, Islam distinguishes three major stages of becoming after death. In the "interworld," from death to until the day of resurrection, or "the end of the world," the soul is imaginal. This soul does not enter heaven or hell until the day of resurrection, based upon the deeds performed in this world. Islam teaches that believers should not long for death or look forward to dying, although life is regarded as the believer's current prison he parts with once he passes away (Timani 2008).

We can conclude that spirituality and religion play important role in transcendental future thinking as well as we can see that major religions can provide the frame for individual thoughts about the life after death. In the next paragraph, we will shortly discuss some psychological conceptions about transcendental future thinking.

Transcendental Future Thinking in Psychology: Current Models and Ideas

The research on transcendental future is one of the emerging trends in psychology. The issues of death and dying which are near to Time Perspective Theory have been the subject of the investigation for several decades. We start our short overview with some words about Freud's notions on religion. Freud (1968) stated that religion can be understood as a projection of one's inner needs and desires. That people are, at least partly, driven by needs that have not been met in childhood, and desires and hopes and expectations are projected on a transcendental state (life after death) or an omnipotent fatherly figure (God). What can't be gotten, can't be reached, or can't be fulfilled in this life might be in the afterlife. Freud (1959) referred to religion as a "universal obsessional neurosis," a collaborate defense against the awareness of death.

Neither the matters of death and dying nor the ones of the transcendental future are popular and widely researched comparing to other areas of psychology. This may be due to the subject matter being complex, mysterious, and uncanny or to the propensity of human nature to avoid going deep into phenomena which are beyond the grasp by direct experience and accompanied by emotional pain and negative feelings. Most probably it is the combination of these factors.

After decades of philosophical contemplation, the research in the psychology of death was boosted with the attempts to give a psychological evaluation of death and dying. Hood and Morris (1983) identify three main research areas on death in psychology. Those are the research on death as a process, the experience of death, and the attitudes toward the death. The greater part of research on death as a process started with the work by Kübler-Ross (1969), who was interested in the process of dying and grief. Later, the research evolved to such topics as near terminal experiences and death attitudes. In the mean time, the transcendental future time perspective as well as any other relatively new phenomena cannot boast a broad research field. Currently, there are several research trends which represent somewhat different theories and models in the transcendental future time perspective paradigm. Those are death transcendence theory, terror management theory, and of course the transcendental Time Perspective Theory. They are by no means the only conceptual models which try to integrate transcendental future thinking. The meaning maintenance model (Heine et al. 2006) is also worth mentioning as it emphasizes the importance of symbolic immortality. We will however pay more attention to the three theories mentioned above as they are currently the most influential in the field of transcendental time perspective.

Death transcendence theory stems from R. J. Lifton's (1979) ideas about individuals' awareness of their inevitable death and the attempts to seek immortality using symbolic means. Lifton distinguishes five modes of symbolic immortality. Later, the abovementioned Hood and Morris (1983) elaborated Lifton's ideas and created an instrument to evaluate them (the Death Transcendence Scale). Lifton (1979) and Hood and Morris (1983) claim that the five modes of symbolic immortality are as follows:

1. Biological (biosocial) mode. By using this mode, individuals believe they remain immortal in their offspring despite actual death. This mode also involves remaining in the memory of the social group.
2. Creative mode – remaining through the works of science or art that individuals create throughout their lives and which remain after the death of their authors. Recollections of the close and significant relationships (i.e., patient–doctor) also belong to this mode.
3. Religious or theological mode related to the life after the death postulate of most religions. This postulate also means transition to the other, a higher quality existential level.
4. Naturalistic mode means understanding that the nature surrounding us is illimitable and will continue even after our death. Unity with nature also belongs to this mode of symbolic immortality.
5. Experiential (mystical) transcendence encompasses the unity with something that stretches beyond the individual, also mystical and ecstatic experience (Lifton 1979; Hood and Morris 1983).

Lifton (1979) and Hood and Morris (1983) distinguish between the first four and the last mode of symbolic immortality. While the former modes stem from the cognitive awareness, the latter one, the mystical mode cannot be explained by cognitive beliefs only.

Terror management theory is without a doubt the most elaborated theory among others mentioned in this chapter. It stems from Ernest Becker's ideas on individuals' relationship with death. The basic assumptions of the theory claim that individuals have biological self-preservation and reproduction predispositions. In the process of evolution, people gained consciousness which led to the awareness about being mortal. This awareness of death creates the possibility for experiencing the paralyzing terror. It becomes vital to protect ourselves from this terror experience. Certain cultural worldviews create the perception of the world being meaningful, human existence has its significance or state that immortality can be achieved through the immortal soul either through symbolic means described by Lifton (1979) in his work on transcendence, help to fight the terror feeling. The culture also brings certain requirement, the fulfillment of which boosts self-esteem. The higher levels of self-esteem buffer the death anxiety (Pyszczynski et al. 1997; Solomon et al. 2000).

The transcendental future time perspective concept was offered by Zimbardo and Boyd (Boyd and Zimbardo 1997; Zimbardo and Boyd 2008) as a logical extension to five mundane time perspectives. The authors suggest that people divide the psychological future to pre- and post-death time frames. The transcendental future time perspective involves individuals' goals, expectations, and beliefs related to the time frame from physical death of the body to eternity. Boyd and Zimbardo (1997) point out five possible goals of transcendental future: "reunion with deceased loved ones, eternal life, reincarnation, the avoidance of eternal damnation, and the elimination of current poverty, pain, suffering and shame" (Boyd and Zimbardo 1997, p. 36). This kind of time perspective operates in the same mode as the other five mundane time perspectives; however, because of the orientation to the indefinite future, it can be a very powerful source of motivation. According to Zimbardo and Boyd, the transcendental future time perspective can take part in understanding such extreme behavior as suicide explosions, ritual suicides, etc.

Boyd and Zimbardo (1997) brought some insight about the differences between the three theories mentioned in this chapter on transcendental future thinking in psychology. According to them, Becker's ideas (terror management theory) were "narrow and unidimensional and sought to demonstrate that people expect to transcend death in multiple ways, not just through denial" (Boyd and Zimbardo 1997, p. 38). One should bear in mind that within the context of terror management theory which got the most of the empirical support comparing to other theories, some research has been carried out that broadened its limits. There are some studies which try to emphasize the ways by which individuals assume to be able to seek immortality. The example of those could be the studies which suggest that individuals react in a different way to the mortality salient situations if their thoughts about the possibility of the life after death were aroused comparing to those who were not (Dechesne et al. 2003; Wojtkowiak and Rutjens 2011). Florian and Mikulincer (1998) related

Lifton's ideas on death transcendence and terror management theory. They concluded that "the findings of our series of studies seem to corroborate Lifton's (1979) theoretical assumptions and to provide systematic empirical support to the hypothesis that a sense of symbolic immortality can serve as a shield against the fear of death" (Florian and Mikulincer 1998, p. 731). So it seems like terror management theory could significantly benefit from incorporating the constructs from death transcendence and transcendental future time perspective theories.

Commenting on death transcendence theory ideas, Boyd and Zimbardo state that research on transcendental future time perspective differs from the others that primarily address death beliefs as they seek to "stress not the plausibility of these beliefs, but their possible impact on present behavior" (Boyd and Zimbardo 1997, p. 38). We agree to this critique but only partly and want to draw attention to the essential distinction between death transcendence and transcendental future time perspective concepts which lies in the viewpoint of weather the individuals' goals and beliefs concerning life after death are of single dimensions, or if we can distinguish several different ways of death transcendence.

Despite the fact that the three theories mentioned above differs in views on individuals' relationship with the time after the death of their physical body, we find it meaningful to look for the commonalities and to attempt to integrate them. Studies that incorporate the ideas of several concepts and of various research methods would serve this goal. We suggest that the transcendental future time perspective concept provides suitable grounds for the integration as it also involves mundane time perspectives which were repeatedly proven to be significant in predicting human behavior. The merger of mundane time and transcendental time perspectives would expand the life space of human existence.

Less scientific but more popular theories about life after death are based upon near-death experiences. Due to the lack of scientific research on near death experiences, we decided to leave it out.

Research and Measurement

Before moving on to the research on transcendental future time perspective, we will provide a brief summary of the studies carried out within the framework of the other two mentioned concepts and their importance in terms of a transcendent future time perspective.

Based on Lifton's ideas, several scales were created: Death Transcendence Scale (Hood and Morris 1983; Vandecreek and Nye 1993) and Sense of Symbolic Immortality Scale (Drolet 1990). The studies using those scales proved the possibility of symbolic immortality beliefs, and the five modes of death transcendence were confirmed by the factor analysis. However, those studies gained greater significance only in the context of terror management theory.

A great body of research was promoted by the terror management theory (Burke et al. 2010; Arndt and Vess 2008). The results of the research confirm death- and afterlife-related thoughts to be important psychological constructs. Recent research shows that mortality salience supports, for instance, teleological beliefs (Davis et al. 2011) and preferences for law and justice TV programs (Taylor 2012). The detailed survey of the research made in the framework of terror management theory is not the subject this chapter, and the readers interested in more detailed analysis should refer to the works of Burke et al. (2010), Arndt and Vess (2008), and some others. As already mentioned in paragraph 3, the interaction between symbolic immortality and the mortality salience is the research direction which is currently relevant in the field of terror management theory. The results suggest the symbolic immortality feeling can buffer against the fear of death (Florian and Mikulincer 1998).

Unfortunately, the research on transcendental future perspective is scarce indeed. The first to mention is the research made by Boyd and Zimbardo (1997) that laid the grounds for the research area and offered an instrument – the Transcendental Future Time Perspective Scale. This study also established and theoretically justified the links between the transcendental time perspective, values, personality traits, and religious affiliation. In summary, this particular study confirmed the value of transcendental future time perspective as an independent and significant construct. Regrettably, not much research followed. Transcendental Future Time Perspective Scale was adapted to use in Portugal (Ortuño et al. 2011a, 2012); this instrument was applied to evaluate the links between time perspective and religiousness (Ortuño et al. 2011b); a study of development of transcendental future time perspective was carried out (Ortuño et al. 2011c). Although the adaptations of Transcendental Future Time Perspective Scale in Lithuania and the Netherlands have not been published yet, meaningful results of preliminary researches were reported (Kairys and Liniauskaite 2012; Van Beek et al. 2011). Chistopolskaya and Enikolopov (2012a) studied the terror management patterns of individuals attempted to commit suicide (see van Beek and Chistopolskaya, chapter "Friend or Foe? Escape from Death, or Death as an Escape?," this volume). The authors assumed mundane time perspectives can serve as defense mechanism against the fear of death. The authors however did not include the transcendental future time perspective in their research.

The role of transcendental future thinking in depressed non-suicidal and suicidal patients was investigated by Van Beek, Beekman, and Kerkhof (submitted). The main research question was whether stronger beliefs in an afterlife would protect from having suicidal thoughts. Using the Transcendental Future Time Perspective Scale, these researchers found no differences between suicidal patients and non-suicidal patients. This can be explained by the diversity of attitudes of suicidal patients toward death. For some it is a relief, while others believe that they will be called to account and punished if they should commit suicide. For others who believe in rebirth, the prospect of life after suicide might be negative as well.

During the first conference on time perspective in Coimbra, Portugal, in 2012, several communications were presented on the subject matter. The symposium called "Transcendental future time perspective: how life after death motivates us?" raised several questions as well as future research directions. Ortuño et al. (2012) presented some evidence of construct validity of Portuguese version of Transcendental Future Time Perspective Scale; however, Seema et al. (2012a, b) argued that validity of TFTPS is questionable. In their opinion TFTPS measures beliefs instead of time perspective. Kairys and Liniauskaite (2012) presented interrelations between transcendental Future time perspective and values and also showed that transcendental Future time perspective alongside with mundane time perspectives helps to find meaningful clusters in the sample. Chistopolskaya and Enikolopov (2012b) as well as Van Beek (2012a, b) discussed role of time perspective in suicidal process. In his presentation of Van Beek (2012b) raised the idea of a prenatal time perspective. He stated that what is complementary interesting is how the role of the time before the actual conception can be taken into account. Where and who was the child before it was born, and how does this affect one's current life? This "before-birth" time zone is part of the context the person is born in, sometimes implicit and maybe even unconscious, but in some religious traditions manifest and of utmost importance. As we have seen, mostly in non-Western religions and from other than linear time perspectives, people can be motivated by transindividual aspects, like forefathers or rebirth. The cyclic nature of this way of looking upon time and temporality makes a specific afterlife time zone even redundant. But even from a Western perspective, the ideas, dreams, beliefs, wishes, and anxieties of the parents and environment affect the development of the infant, and it would enrich time perspective theory to address this as well. If anywhere the traditional science of psychology pays attention to prenatal period, the time immediately before conception is looked through (Van Beek 2012b). We can conclude that this symposium could be considered as the first signs of increasing interest to this particular research area.

Positive and Negative Transcendental Future

Following the distinction between positive and negative aspects of the past (Zimbardo and Boyd 1999 and Carelli and Ollson (chapter "Neural Correlates of Time Perspective," this volume) and Van Beek and Chistopolskaya (chapter "Friend or Foe? Escape from Death, or Death as an Escape?," this volume) regarding the future, the distinction between positive and negative aspects of the transcendental future might provide additional information as well. Transcendental future may not be the mono-dimensional construct as it is considered in the TFTPS. While some people hold a positive view of the afterlife, as an end to the suffering and sinfulness of mortal man, others are scared of what is to come after death. Death as the end of pain in religious worldviews or death as the end of simply everything among atheists. Or, for people who consider God to be punishing, the possibility of hell and eternal suffering after Final Judgment. While others believe to live another life and get another chance after rebirth. Depending of the prior life or not.

Figure 1 depicts a very basic overview of suggested aspects of a more elaborate view of transcendental future. Both positive and negative, many people may have a neutral or obscure outlook on the transcendental future.

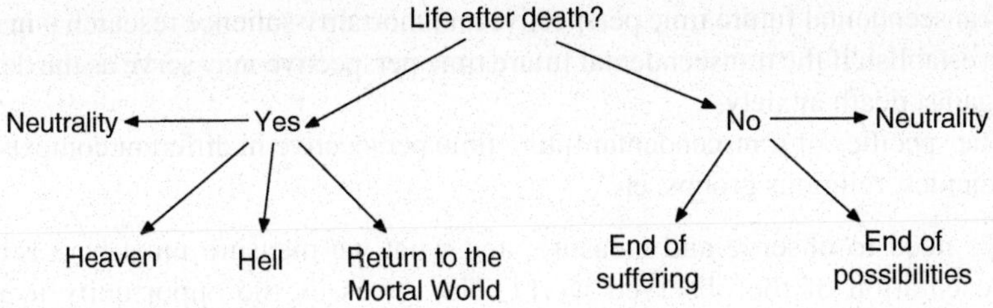

Fig. 1 Aspects of life after death

What is the meaning a person gives to life after death or the absence of life after death? And what is the role of this meaning in human motivation? We feel that a more comprehensive view of transcendental future theory could add to time perspective theory in general.

Discussion

The commonality in the findings on the role of thoughts about life after death in health care, and particularly in mental health care, makes sense. The assumption that something better awaits you when the current suffering is over is likely to be comforting. The findings regarding suicidal patients might indicate that things are not that simple though. Life after death, when you struggle with thoughts about ending your own life, is not something to cling onto. Some preliminary findings in the other research areas seem to confirm importance of transcendental future time perspective in human functioning.

In their pioneering work Boyd and Zimbardo (1997) tried to integrate their notions about the role of the afterlife in time perspective theory, but not much has happened since their 1997 manuscript. One of the problems that we are facing when it comes to transcendental future thinking is the dominance of positivism and empiricism in current research paradigms. We can state that we need to expand the research in various areas related to transcendental future thinking. We hope numerous and diverse research in the area of transcendent future time perspective will emerge in the nearest future. In our opinion, the most important guidelines for the future research are as follows:

- Qualitative research in the field of transcendental future thinking.
- The adaptation of the Future Time Perspective Scale to a larger number of countries due to lack of research in different cultures. It is very likely that the transcendent future time perspective may be culturally sensitive. The studies on construct, convergent, and divergent validity of the scale, since there are doubts about its validity.

- Transcendental future time perspective and mortality salience research – in order to establish if the transcendental future time perspective may serve as the defense against death anxiety.
- The specifics of transcendental future time perspective in different contexts, i.e., suicides, religious groups, etc.

We need to observe and measure, and what we measure must be a reliable representation of the observed world. This gives us the opportunity to place transcendental future thinking in a broader context. And we need to continue to integrate transcendental time perspective or even prenatal time perspective in to the mainstream research.

References

Arndt, J., & Vess, M. (2008). Tales from existential oceans: Terror management theory and how the awareness of our mortality affects us all. *Social and Personality Psychology Compass, 2*(2), 909–928.

Boyd, J. N., & Zimbardo, P. G. (1997). Constructing time after death: The transcendental-future time perspective. *Time and Society, 6*, 35–54.

Burke, B. L., Martens, A., & Faucher, E. H. (2010). Two decades of terror, management theory: A meta-analysis of mortality salience research. *Personality and Social Psychology Review, 14*(2), 155–195.

Casey, J. (2009). *After lives: A guide to heaven, hell, and purgatory*. New York: Oxford University Press.

Chistopolskaya, K. A., & Enikolopov, S. N. (2012a). Terror management after a recent suicide attempt. *Psychology in Russia: State of the Art, 5*, 142–156.

Chistopolskaya, K. A., & Enikolopov, S. N. (2012b). To forget, to embrace, to fear: Death attitudes and time perspectives after recent unsuccessful suicidal attempt. In M. P. Paixão, V. E. C. Ortuño, P. Cordeiro, & R. David (Eds.), *First international conference on time perspective: Converging paths in psychology time theory and research. Book of abstracts* (p. 88). Coimbra: University of Coimbra.

Cook, C. C. H., Powell, A., & Sims, A. (2009). *Spirituality and psychiatry*. London: RCPsych Publications.

Davis, W. E., Juhl, J., & Routledge, C. (2011). Death and design: The terror management function of teleological beliefs. *Motivation and Emotion, 35*, 98–104.

Dechesne, M., Pyszczynski, T., Arndt, J., Ransom, S., Sheldon, K. M., van Knippenberg, A., & Janssen, J. (2003). Literal and symbolic immortality: The effect of evidence of literal immortality on self-esteem striving in response to mortality salience. *Journal of Personality and Social Psychology, 84*(4), 722–737.

Drolet, J. L. (1990). Transcending death during early adulthood: Symbolic immortality, death anxiety, and purpose in life. *Journal of Clinical Psychology, 46*(2), 148–160.

Ellis, L., Wahab, E., & Ratnasingan, M. (2012). Religiosity and fear of death: A three-nation comparison. *Mental Health, Religion & Culture, 16*(2), 1–21.

Flannelly, K. J., Koenig, H. G., Ellison, C. G., Galek, K., & Krause, N. (2006). Belief in life after death and mental health: Findings from a national survey. *The Journal of Nervous and Mental Disease, 194*, 524–529.

Flannelly, K. J., Ellison, C. G., Galek, K., & Koenig, H. G. (2008). Beliefs about life after death, psychiatric symptomology and cognitive theories of psychopathology. *Journal of Psychology and Theology, 36*, 94–103.

Florian, V., & Mikulincer, M. (1998). Symbolic immortality and the management of the terror of death: The moderating role of attachment style. *Journal of Personality and Social Psychology, 74*(3), 725–734.

Freud, S. (1959). The defense neuro-psychoses. In E. Jones (Ed.), & J. Riviere (Trans.), *Collected papers* (Vol. 1, pp. 59–75). New York: Basic Books. (Original work published in 1894.)

Freud, S. (1968). *The future of an illusion. The standard edition of the complete psychological works of Sigmund Freud* (Vol. 21, J. Strachey, Trans.). London: Hogarth Press. (Original work published in 1927.)

Heine, S. J., Proloux, T., & Vohs, K. D. (2006). The meaning maintenance model: On the coherence of social motivations. *Personality and Social Psychology Review, 10*(2), 88–110.

Hood, R. W., & Morris, R. J. (1983). Toward a theory of death transcendence. *Journal for the Scientific Study of Religion, 22*(4), 353–365.

Kairys, A., & Liniauskaite, A. (2012). Transcendental future time perspective and values. In M. P. Paixão, V. E. C. Ortuño, P. Cordeiro, & R. David (Eds.), *First international conference on time perspective: Converging paths in psychology time theory and research. Book of abstracts* (p. 88). Coimbra: University of Coimbra.

Koenig, H. G., McCullough, M. E., & Larson, D. B. (2001). *Handbook of religion and health*. London: Oxford University Press.

Kübler-Ross, E. (1969). *On death and dying*. New York: Macmillan.

Lifton, R. J. (1979). *The broken connection: On the death and the continuity of life*. New York: Basic Books.

McClain-Jacobson, C., et al. (2004). Belief in an afterlife, spiritual well-being and end-of-life despair in patients with advanced cancer. *General Hospital Psychiatry, 26*, 484–486.

Nelson, J. M. N. (2009). *Psychology, religion and spirituality*. New York: Springer.

Obayashi, H. (Ed.). (1992). *Death and the afterlife: Perspectives of world religions*. Westport: Praeger Publishers.

Ortuño, V., Paixão, M. P., & Janeiro, I. (2011a). *Exploratory study of the Portuguese transcendental – Future time perspective scale*. Poster presentation. Retrieved from: http://victortuno.netii.net

Ortuño, V., Paixão, M. P., & Janeiro, I. (2011b). *Diferenças na Perspectiva Temporal entre estudantes religiosos e não religiosos*. Actas do VIII Congresso Iberoamericano de Avaliação Psicologica. Lisboa: Universidade de Lisboa.

Ortuño, V., Paixão, M. P., & Janeiro, I. (2011c). Tempo e Universidade: A Evolução da Perspectiva Temporal ao Longo do Percurso Universitário. In L. Faria, A. Araújo, F. Morais, E. Sá, J. Pinto, & A. Silva (Eds.), *Carreira, Criatividade e Empreendedorismo* (pp. 217–225). Braga: APDC Edições.

Ortuño, V., Paixão, M. P., & Janeiro, I. (2012). The nature of transcendental future. In M. P. Paixão, V. E. C. Ortuño, P. Cordeiro, & R. David (Eds.), *First international conference on time perspective: Converging paths in psychology time theory and research. Book of abstracts* (pp. 87–88). Coimbra: University of Coimbra.

Ostow, M. (2007). *Spirit, mind, and brain: A psychoanalytic examination of spirituality and religion*. New York: Columbia University Press.

Pyszczynski, T., Greenberg, J., & Solomon, S. (1997). Why do we need what we need? A terror management perspective on the roots of human social motivation. *Psychological Inquiry, 8*(1), 1–20.

Seema, R., Sircova, A., Baltin, A., & Pork, M. (2012a). Transcendental future – Is it a healthy belief or time perspective? Time Perspective Inventory (TTPI) (Boyd & Zimbardo, 2006) in Estonians. In M. P. Paixão, V. E. C. Ortuño, P. Cordeiro, & R. David (Eds.), *First international conference on time perspective: Converging paths in psychology time theory and research. Book of abstracts* (p. 88). Coimbra: University of Coimbra.

Seema, R., Sircova, A., Baltin, A., & Pork, M. (2012b). *Transcendental future – Is it a healthy belief or time perspective? Time Perspective Inventory (TTPI) (Boyd & Zimbardo, 2006) in Estonians*. Oral presentation presented on First International Conference on Time Perspective, Coimbra, Portugal.

Seltzer, A. (2008). Judaism: The journey of the soul. In S. J. Rosen (Ed.), *Ultimate journey: Death and dying in the world's major religions* (pp. 1–20). London: Praeger.

Smith, P. C., Range, L. M., & Ulmer, A. (1992). Belief in afterlife as a buffer in suicidal and other bereavement. *OMEGA–Journal of Death and Dying, 24*(3), 217–225.

Solomon, S., Greenberg, J., & Pyszczynski, T. (2000). Pride and prejudice: Fear of death and social behavior. *Current Directions in Psychological Science, 9*(6), 200–204.

Stevenson, A. (Ed.). (2013). *Oxford dictionary of English*. Retrieved January 14, 2014, from Oxford Reference website: http://www.oxfordreference.com/view/10.1093/acref/9780199571123.001.0001/m_en_gb0699400?rskey=vuPeb1&result=70906

Swinton, J. (2001). *Spirituality and mental health: Rediscovering a forgotten dimension*. London: Jessica Kingsley.

Taylor, L. D. (2012). Death and television: Terror management theory and themes of law and justice on television. *Death Studies, 36*, 340–359.

Thompson, J. M. (2008). Awakening to mortality: Buddhist views of death and dying. In S. J. Rosen (Ed.), *Ultimate journey: Death and dying in the world's major religions* (pp. 83–114). Westport: Praeger Publishers.

Thorson, J. A., Powell, F. C., Kara, G., & Uhl, H. S. M. (1988, May 4). *Personality correlates and changes in medical students' attitudes toward old people and death anxiety*. A paper presented at the 45th annual scientific meeting of the American Geriatrics Society, Anaheim, CA.

Timani, H. S. (2008). Death and dying in Islam. In S. J. Rosen (Ed.), *Ultimate journey: Death and dying in the world's major religions* (pp. 59–82). Westport: Praeger Publishers.

Tiso, F. V. (2008). Preparation of eternal life: Christian teaching on death and dying. In S. J. Rosen (Ed.), *Ultimate journey: Death and dying in the world's major religions* (pp. 21–58). Westport: Praeger Publishers.

Van Beek, W. (2012a). When there's life after death, suicide is useless. In M. P. Paixão, V. E. C. Ortuño, P. Cordeiro, & R. David (Eds.), *First international conference on time perspective: Converging paths in psychology time theory and research. Book of abstracts* (p. 89). Coimbra: University of Coimbra.

Van Beek, W. (2012b). *When there's life after death, suicide is useless*. Oral presentation presented on first international conference on time perspective, Coimbra, Portugal.

Van Beek, W., Berghuis, H., Kerkhof, A. J. F. M., & Beekman, A. T. F. (2011). Time perspective, personality and psychopathology: Zimbardo's time perspective inventory in psychiatry. *Time and Society, 20*(3), 364–374.

Vandecreek, L., & Nye, C. (1993). Testing the death transcendence scale. *Journal for the Scientific Study of Religion, 32*(3), 279–283.

Wink, P., & Scott, J. (2005). Does religiousness buffer against the fear of death and dying in late adulthood? Findings from a longitudinal study. *Journal of Gerontology: Psychological Sciences, 60B*(4), 207–214.

Wojtkowiak, J., & Rutjens, B. T. (2011). The postself and terror management theory: Reflecting on after death identity buffers existential threat. *The International Journal for the Psychology of Religion, 21*, 137–144.

Zimbardo, P. G., & Boyd, J. N. (1999). Putting time in perspective: A valid, reliable individual-differences metric. *Journal of Personality and Social Psychology, 77*(6), 1271–1288.

Zimbardo, P. G., & Boyd, J. N. (2008). *The time paradox: The new psychology of time that will change your life*. New York: Free Press.

Broadening the TP Profile: Future Negative Time Perspective

Maria Grazia Carelli, Britt Wiberg, and Elisabeth Åström

Introduction

How we perceive time is part of the human experience and essential for everyday behavior and for the survival of the individual (Pöppel 1997; Wittmann 2009). Particularly intriguing in the last years has been the study of how people differ in their perceptions of the present, past and future, despite the unidirectional progression of time (Bluedorn 2002).

This overall orientation to time is often referred as Time Perspective (TP; Lewin 1951; Zimbardo and Boyd 1999). Within the area of time perspective research a variety of studies have established that there are reliable individual differences in whether people are predominantly focused on the past, present, or future. These differences, in turn, have been linked to a number of important behaviors and outcomes, such as achievement (Kahana et al. 2005) learning and self-regulation (Sanna et al. 2003) and adaptation to life events (Holman and Silver 1998).

However, the philosophical perspective asserting that *the future* dominates human consciousness (Heidegger 1992) has influenced much of the psychological research on time perspective, and as result the Future time perspective has received much attention in scientific terms, in comparisons with the present or past time perspectives.

Researchers have been referring to *future perspective* using different conceptualizations, including *future-oriented thinking* and Future time perspective. The former refers to our plans, expectations, and various scenarios through which these potential outcomes may or may not be realized (see e.g., Aspinwall 2005,

M.G. Carelli (✉) • B. Wiberg • E. Åström
Department of Psychology, Umeå University, SE-901 87 Umeå, Sweden
e-mail: grazia.carelli@psy.umu.se; Britt.Wiberg@psy.umu.se; elisabeth.astrom@psy.umu.se

M. Stolarski et al. (eds.), *Time Perspective Theory; Review, Research and Application: Essays in Honor of Philip G. Zimbardo*, DOI 10.1007/978-3-319-07368-2_5,

for a review), whereas the latter is defined as the present anticipation of future goals and refers to an individual's beliefs or perspective toward the future concerning temporally distant goals (Bembenutty and Karabenick 2004; Nuttin and Lens 1985). Thinking about the future has also been defined in terms of *episodic future thinking* (Atance and O'Neill 2001; see also Tulving 2001), a projection of the self into the future in order to pre-experience an event. Related to this term, *temporal foresight* and *mental time travel* in the future (Suddendorf and Corballis 1997) have been conceptualized as the human capacity to imagine, plan for, and shape the future. Further, thinking about the future, conceived as the ability of planning, has been considered as "*The capacity that have long been of major importance to our survival and may have been a prime mover in human cognitive evolution*" (Suddendorf 2006, p. 1006).

Psychologists have stressed the benefits of future-oriented thinking, arguing that it is motivational for health behaviors and well-being (see e.g., Boyd and Zimbardo 2005 for a review), influences the nature of social relationships (Lang and Carstensen 2002), and can promote goal setting, motivation and achievement strivings (Shipp et al. 2009).

Nonetheless, to focus on the future perspective as a single unipolar construct (e.g., Zimbardo and Boyd 1999), while ignoring negative effects of thinking about future events and actions is a too simplistic view of the future. Research on Future time perspective has focused much less attention on how a "negative" Future perspective may impact overall well-being. Loss of control and fear of future threat have been found to be strong predictors of Post-Traumatic Stress Disorder (PTSD) and depressive symptomatology among survivors of the war in the former Yugoslavia (Basoğlu et al. 2005). Furthermore, the concept of "future anxiety" (FA: Zaleski 1996) – a state of uncertainty, apprehension, fear and worry of unfavorable changes in a more remote personal future – has also been associated with high levels of stress among young adults (Otrar et al. 2002). Together, these findings suggest that the Future time perspective may have a double valence: when it is positive and motivational for achieving goals, it may benefit wellbeing, but when it involves a predominantly negative vision of the future, it may destabilize mental and/or physical health.

Assessment of Future Time Perspective

Healthy adults appear to differ in their ability to think about the future. While some consider the future as a challenge full of striving and achievements, for others the future represents uncertainty and preoccupation. Several measures have been developed to assess this temporal dimension, trying to capture its many aspects. These measures consist mainly of self-report instruments that either focus solely on the future dimension or utilize the future as a reference point to which the past and the present are compared.

Unidimensional Measurements of Future Time Perspective

Unidimensional measurement techniques such as the Future Time Perspective Instrument (FTP; Daltrey 1982), the Future Time perspective Orientation (FTO; Husman and Shell 2008), the Consideration of Future Consequences Scale (CFC; Strathman et al. 1994), the Future Anxiety Scale (FAS; Zaleski 1996), and the Future Time Perspective Scale (FTPS; Husman and Shell 2008) represent earnest attempts to overcome low psychometric properties of previous story based or projective tests (e.g. Future Event Test (Kasterbaum 1961, see also Lasane and O'Donnel 2005, for a review).

In the CFC (Strathman et al. 1994) the future dimension is conceived as the "*extent to which individuals consider the potential distant outcomes of their current behaviors and the extent to which they are influenced by these potential outcomes*" (Strathman et al. 1994, p. 743). The CFC construct refers to a stable individual difference variable representing the extent to which people consider distant versus immediate consequences of potential behavior. Strathman and colleagues (1994) suggested that this variable reflects an intrapersonal struggle between present behavior and immediate outcomes versus future outcomes. The CFC construct seems to be related to individual differences in health and environmental attitudes and behaviors (Atance and O'Neill 2001) and may play a regulatory role in the affective responses to negative events (Boninger et al. 1994).

Zaleski (1996) emphasized the negative side of the future by introducing the concept of Future Anxiety (FA). In the 29-item measurement scale (FAS) the author describes the FA concept as a personality characteristic where a negative Future time perspective functions as the basis for FA. Individuals scoring high on the FAS scale demonstrate some specific cognitive and behavioral patterns. They tend to use harder power strategies to influence others in the superior-subordinate situation, are more pessimistic regarding future solution to global problems and on an interpersonal level they use others to secure their own future. Moreover, they treat future matters with less humor and have more somatic symptoms when thinking about the future (Zaleski 1996, 2005).

The Future Time Perspective Scale (FTPS; Husman and Shell 2008; Shell and Husman 2001) was devised to measure future perspective as a set of stable beliefs and expectations about the future. The FTPS scale is composed by 27 items with four subscales representing distinct temporal dimensions: *speed*, *connectedness*, *value* and *extension*. The concept of *speed* refers to the speed at which individuals feel time is passing (e.g. "I always seem to be doing things at the last moment") whereas *connectedness* is the tendency to make connections between present activities and future goals, as well as a general concern for future consequences (e.g. "What will happen in the future is an important consideration in deciding what action to take now"). Interestingly, this aspect of the FTPS seems to be present in other measures of future orientation, including the CFC (Strathman et al 1994, e.g. "I consider how things might be in the future, and try to influence those things with my day to day behavior"). *Value* is operationalized as the importance individuals place on goals attainable in the future and more specifically, the willingness to make sacrifices in the present to support the future (e.g. "It is more important to save for the future than to buy what one wants today"). Finally, the fourth dimension of the FTPS, *extension*, refers to the amount of future time that a person can conceptualize, defined by Daltrey and Langer (1984) as "How far ahead a person projects one's thoughts" (p. 719). Goals that are within a person's projected future "time space" generally appear closer and more attainable, in comparison to goals that temporally extend outside this time space.

Even though a series of studies have shown a good construct validity of the FTPS, further research remains on its predictive and divergent validity before it can be concluded that the FTPS reliably measures a persons' future time perspective.

Multidimensional Measures of Time Perspective: Comparing the Future with the Past and the Present

Several approaches ranging from the Time Attitude Scale (TAS; Nuttin 1972), the Time Orientation Questionnaire (TOQ; Shirai 1997), to the Zimbardo Time Perspective Inventory (ZPTI; Zimbardo and Boyd 1999) try to capture the complexity of future dimension in one instrument by considering – and comparing – the temporal dimensions of past, present and future.

Nuttin (1972) developed the Time Attitude Scale (TAS), a multidimensional scale used to measure a person's affective attitudes towards multiple time periods. Nuttin's research was particularly important in setting the basis for the initial development of time perspective instruments described in the current set of studies. In the TAS subjects were asked to rate their attitudes towards the past, the present and future on a 7-point scale with two bipolar adjectives, such as "pleasant" and "unpleasant" as anchors (Nuttin and Lens 1985). Research indicates that attitudes towards time have meaningful relationships with several other variables, including educational outcomes and psychological well-being (Calster et al. 1987).

The Time Orientation Questionnaire (TOQ; Shirai 1997) was created in order to measure Time orientation. Following Nuttin's distinction between time perspective, time attitude, and time orientation, the latter is considered as the preferred or predominant direction of the individual's behavior and thoughts toward objects or events in the past, the present, or the future (Nuttin and Lens 1985). TOQ consists of five predominant time orientations: Positive Future Orientation (PFO), Positive Present Orientation (PPO), Negative Future Orientation (NFO), Negative Present Orientation (NPO), and Past Orientation (PNO). Each of these temporal profiles are obtained by combining two dimensions, namely the most important time frame and the connection of the present with the future. More specifically, subjects' degree of time integration among the three temporal dimensions are based on the explanation for their preference in response to the following open-ended question "Which is the most important time for you, the future, the present, or the past? Please write down why you prefer this and do not prefer the others" (Shirai et al. 2012, p. 277). The

Positive future orientation (e.g. "I prefer the future because the present is a step to attain future goals") of TOQ seems to emphasize both the importance individuals place on goals or *valence* (de Volder and Lens 1982), as well as *connectedeness*, the tendency to make connections between present activities and future goals (Strathman et al. 1994). Some aspect of the Negative future orientation (e.g. "I prefer the future since my present is unpleasant but my future is unknown") is also present in other measures of future orientation/perspective, including Zaleski's concept of future anxiety (FA).

Yet, despite the TOQ showing psychometrically sound properties (e.g. test-retest reliability at 0.80, and content analysis reliability is 81.1 %), additional research is required to shed more light on the role and connection of the past with the other time frames.

Since 1999 the dominant approach to time perspective has been the Zimbardo Time Perspective Inventory (ZPTI; Zimbardo and Boyd 1999). The ZTPI seeks to address the shortcomings of the previous scales, represents a step forward in multi-dimensional assessment of TP, and finally takes into account the dimension of emotional valence (Boniwell et al. 2010).

According to Boyd and Zimbardo (2005), individuals with a more future oriented perspective are more optimistic and able to anticipate positive outcomes, engage in risky behavior less often than individuals high in present time perspective and are able to cope with negative life situations more effectively. To have a more future-oriented outlook is therefore regarded as the more constructive TP in terms of engaging in positive health behaviors.

Developing and Extending the Future Dimension of the ZTPI: The Future Negative Scale

Although the ZTPI has been used and validated extensively in past research, the future dimension needs to be extended and specified better. Specifically, the future dimension includes a mixture of negative and positive items, whereas the past-orientation dimension is based on separate scales. In the original article, Zimbardo and Boyd (1999) were aware of the necessity to include a future subfactor: "*By contrast, the ZTPI has but one future TP. Perhaps further factor analyses of our scale with a variety of non-college populations will again show a more complex set of future subfactors*" (Zimbardo and Boyd 1999, p. 1284). Also, Worrell and Mello (2007) suggested the possibility of a six-factor structure.

In a recent study, Carelli et al. (2011) extended and revised the ZTPI by decomposing its Future (F) scale into to the Future Negative (FN) and Future Positive (FP) scales, respectively. Specifically, two of the original F-items (#9: "If things don't get done on time, I don't worry about it", and #20: "It upsets me to be late for appointments", reversed coded item) were defined as FN-items and the remaining 11 items as FP-items. The final FN scale was then developed by including eight new items (see items I-VIII in Table 1).

Table 1 Future Negative (FN) scale (S-ZTPI, Carelli et al. 2011)

Future negative time perspective scale	
(I)	I often think that I do not have time for everything I have planned to do in one day
(II)	Usually, I do not know how I will be able to fulfill my goals in life
(III)	At night I often reflect on tomorrow's challenges
(IV)	I often feel that I cannot fulfil my obligations to friends and authorities
(V)	If I have to take a quick decision I am often worried that it was wrong
(VI)	I feel pressure not to be finished with different projects on time
(VII)	To think about my future makes me sad
(VIII)	The future contains too many boring decisions that I do not want to think about
(IX)	If things don't get done on time, I don't worry about it. (R)*
(X)	It upsets me to be late for appointments

*(R)** reversed coded item

Following the line of reasoning outlined above, the main argument was that the assessment of TP should not be limited to Positive Future evaluations. Instead the ZTPI should also include a negative dimension which involves thinking about the future with worry, anticipating negative outcomes, in a similar way as the Past Negative time perspective is described in the original scale. Zaleski's (1996) and Nurmi's (2005) research on the relationship between future and affective aspects support this argument. Both authors point out that the Future TP is often described in positive terms. This bias seems reasonable as we usually associate the concept of future with hope, success and related attributes. However, there are other kind of associations, such as fear, anxiety, preoccupation and uncertainty. These negative aspects of the Future TP are often neglected. The individual personal future must be conceived evoking emotional and cognitive attitudes that range from positive (e.g., hope, joy, success) to negative attributes (e.g., concerns, anxiety). Moreover, the Future Negative dimension can be very effective in facing dangerous situations, discomfort or pain. Individuals who are future oriented may be more likely to think of strategies that they can engage in to reduce the discomfort/pain. They can plan more effectively in order to anticipate negative future outcomes, and may be more able to cope with discomfort or pain (Andersson and Wood 2005; Higgins 1997).

Reviews of adults' future orientation (Nurmi 2005) showed that fears and worries about the future are also an important part of peoples' future perspective. As Nurmi (1991, 2005) suggests, negative aspects of the future differ from one stage of life to another. Young people, for example, report concern related to dealing with normative developmental tasks (e.g., unemployment, low level of school achievement), and facing a divorce in the future (Solantaus 1987). Young people seem also concerned about possible negative life events that might happen to their parents and family members (e.g., divorce, health problems), as well as events on the society level such as environmental problems (Poole and Cooney 1987). Beginning in middle adulthood, health related fears became more frequent in adults' future concerns and worries. Fears related to societal problems, such as war, were found to increase in the later years of middle adulthood (Nurmi 2005).

Research suggests that people's future orientation changes again when they move from middle to late adulthood. Relatively few studies have analyzed the Future-Negative perspective or outcomes in later life. Lang and Carstensen (2002) suggested that, as people grow older, they increasingly perceive their future as limited. This constricted time perspective leads older people to value personal goals related to the task of finding out about one's role in the society (e.g., receiving social acceptance), and to vocational or career interests (e.g., become financially independent).

In summary, we suggest the relationship between Future time perspective, well-being and long-term adjustment is more complex than originally thought. Thinking about the future in negative terms may ultimately have an unfavorable impact on overall mental and physical health over time. As Holman and Silver (2005) pointed out: "*Both positively and negatively valenced future thinking contributed independently to different indices of adjustment, suggesting that focusing on future goals can help us to adapt life's main changes, but having fears about an ambiguous future may also take a toll on our enjoyment of life and render us vulnerable to the negative impact of chronic stress*" (Holman and Silver 2005, p. 407).

The Future Negative Scale and Anxiety: A New Perspective

We have argued throughout the chapter for the double emotional valence of the Future time perspective and its differential relationship with well-being on one hand and distress on the other hand. In a recent study, we investigated time perspective in relation to anxiety and we were specifically interested in the relationship between the FN scale and anxiety symptoms. Theoretical conceptualizations and empirical research on anxiety suggest that anxiety is associated with a temporal bias towards thinking about the future in negative terms (Barlow 2002; Beck and Emery 2005). Worry, which is present to a significant degree in all the anxiety disorders, is described as being temporally oriented towards the future, with anticipation of future threat or harm (Barlow 1988). However, Zimbardo and Boyd (1999), when investigating time perspective in anxiety using the ZTPI, found only a weak correlation between anxiety and the Future scale. Anxiety was more strongly correlated with both the Past Negative (PN) and the Present Fatalistic (PF) scale. This result may sound puzzling at first, but considering that the Future scale in the original version of the ZTPI does not include a negative perspective of the future, this result is less surprising. We argued that to get a full comprehension of time perspective profiles in persons with anxiety, feelings and attitudes towards the future including worry and anticipation of negative outcomes also need to be comprehended. To test this assumption, we conducted two studies with a total of 120 adults with varying degrees of anxiety (Wiberg and Carelli 2014). In both studies we used the S-ZTPI (described in the previous section of the paper) for assessing time perspective. Both studies showed that anxiety was associated with higher scores on the FN scale, but also on the PN scale. Although conceptualizations of anxiety focus on the future negative perspective, our studies also demonstrate the link between anxiety and the PN time perspective. This further stresses the importance of the PN time perspective in relation to mental distress, which has been suggested by previous research in psychiatric populations (Van Beek et al. 2011), and in traumatized individuals (Holman and Silver 1998).

Our study provide support for the application and usefulness of the S-ZTPI and its added FN scale for a more comprehensive view of time perspective and anxiety. Its application may however be broader than this particular study. The FN scale is constructed to assess a wider concept than worry covering both negative anticipation as well as a negative attitude towards the future. This implies that the FN time perspective may play a role in other clinical conditions as well. For instance, a recent study on ADHD population suggest a clear ADHD-related biases in time perspective as measured by the S-ZTPI (Carelli and Wiberg 2012). In this study, the future perspective of the participants in the ADHD group was more negative than that of the participants in the control group. ADHD was associated with the lowest scores (agreement) with the future-oriented (positive) statements of the S-ZTPI that involve planning, organization, and timekeeping.

Moreover, past research has revealed that depressive symptoms may be associated with less anticipation of future positive experiences (MacLeod and Byrne 1996) and negative future thinking (Lavender and Watkins 2004). Together, these findings support our argument that both the negative and positive aspects of future-directed thinking should be simultaneously considered.

Directions for Future Work

Our research suggests that the FN scale contributes to a fuller understanding of time perspective in persons with anxiety. The question remains however, whether the FN orientation precedes the anxiety, rendering "Future Negative" individuals vulnerable to anxiety, or if their time perspective is colored by anxious emotion. Zaleski's (1996) related concept of Future Anxiety proposes that a Negative Future time perspective precedes the affect. Zimbardo's (Zimbardo and Boyd 1999; Boyd and Zimbardo 2005) view of time perspective as a stable individual differences variable may also suggest that it is the FN time perspective that precedes the affect. This would mean that time perspective is an important variable to consider in preventive measures of mental health problems. But there is much need for longitudinal research on the stability of TP-profiles over time, both in normal and in clinical populations.

Conclusions

In the field of clinical psychology, greater attention to time perspective and future thinking can provide a basis for distinguishing between different types of psychopathology, and a more refined understanding of one hallmark feature of anxiety, namely, *a negative outlook with respect to the future*.

We have suggested that positive and negative aspects of the future represent two important and separate dimensions of temporal experience. The distinction of positive and negative aspects of experience into two, at least partly, independent dimensions represents a line of thought that runs through different levels of analysis, including clinical aspects, motivational, as well as cognitive.

Future research might reveal not only quantitative but also qualitative differences in the types of *positive and negative future outcomes* individuals anticipate and shed more light on how people conceptualize their unique way to think, feel and plan for the future.

References

Andersson, K. B., & Wood, M. D. (2005). Considering the future consequences of aggressive acts: Established and potential effects in the context of the general aggression model. In A. Strathman & J. Joireman (Eds.), *Understanding behavior in the context of time* (pp. 85–107). Mahwah: Lawrence Erlbaum Associates.

Aspinwall, L. G. (2005). The psychology of future-oriented thinking: From achievement to proactive coping, adaptation, and aging. *Motivation and Emotion, 29*(4), 203–235. doi:10.1007/s11031-006-9013-1.

Atance, C. M., & O'Neill, D. K. (2001). Episodic future thinking. *Trends in Cognitive Sciences, 5*(12), 533–539.

Barlow, D. H. (1988). *Anxiety and its disorders: The nature and treatment of anxiety and panic*. New York: The Guilford Press.

Barlow, D. H. (2002). *Anxiety and its disorders: The nature and treatment of anxiety and panic* (2nd ed.). New York: The Guilford Press.

Basoğlu, M., Livanou, M., Crnobarić, C., Frančišković, T., Suljić, E., Durić, D., & Vranešić, M. (2005). Psychiatric and cognitive effects of war in former Yugoslavia. *JAMA, 294*, 580–590.

Beck, A. T., & Emery, G. (2005). *Anxiety disorders and phobias*. New York: Basic Books.

Bembenutty, H., & Karabenick, S. A. (2004). Inherent association between academic delay of gratification, future time perspective, and self-regulated learning. *Educational Psychology Review, 16*(1), 35–57.

Bluedorn, A. C. (2002). *The human organization of time: Temporal realities and experience*. Stanford: Stanford University Press.

Boninger, D. S., Gleicher, F., & Strathman, A. (1994). Counterfactual thinking: From what might have been to what may be. *Journal of Personality and Social Psychology, 67*, 297–307.

Boniwell, I., Osin, E., Linley, P. A., & Ivanchenko, G. V. (2010). A question of balance: Time perspective and well-being in British and Russian samples. *The Journal of Positive Psychology, 5*(1), 24–40.

Boyd, J. N., & Zimbardo, P. G. (2005). Time perspective, health, and risk taking. In A. Strathman & J. Joireman (Eds.), *Understanding behavior in the context of time* (pp. 85–107). Mahwah: Lawrence Erlbaum Associates.

Calster, K. V., Lens, W., & Nuttin, J. R. (1987). Affective attitude toward the personal future: Impact on motivation in high school boys. *American Journal of Psychology, 100*(1), 1–13.

Carelli, M. G., & Wiberg, B. (2012). Time out of mind: Temporal perspective in adults with ADHD. *Journal of Attention Disorders, 16*(6), 460–466.

Carelli, M. G., Wiberg, B., & Wiberg, M. (2011). Development and construct validation of the Swedish Zimbardo Time Perspective Inventory. *European Journal of Psychological Assessment, 27*(4), 220–227.

Daltrey, M. H. (1982). *The development and evaluation of a future time perspective instrument.* Doctoral dissertation, University of Colorado, Boulder.

Daltrey, M. H., & Langer, P. (1984). Development and evaluation of a measure of future time perspective. *Perceptual and Motor Skills, 58*(3), 719–725.

de Volder, M. L., & Lens, W. (1982). Academic achievement and future time perspective as a cognitive-motivational concept. *Journal of Personality and Social Psychology, 42*(3), 566–571.

Heidegger, M. (1992). *The history of the concept of time: Prolegomena.* Oxford: Blackwell Publishers.

Higgins, E. T. (1997). Beyond pleasure and pain. *American Psychologist, 52*(12), 1280–1300.

Holman, E. A., & Silver, R. C. (1998). Getting "stuck" in the past: Temporal orientation and coping with trauma. *Journal of Personality and Social Psychology, 74*, 1146–1163.

Holman, E. A., & Silver, R. C. (2005). Future-oriented thinking and adjustment in a nationwide longitudinal study following the September 11th terrorist attacks. *Motivation and Emotion, 29*, 389–410.

Husman, J., & Shell, D. F. (2008). Beliefs and perceptions about the future: A measurement of future time perspective. *Learning and Individual Differences, 18*, 166–175.

Kahana, E., Kahana, B., & Zhang, J. (2005). Motivational antecedents of preventive proactivity in late life: Linking future orientation and exercise. *Motivation and Emotion, 29*(4), 443–464.

Kasterbaum, R. (1961). The dimension of future time perspective, an experimental analysis. *Journal of Genetic Psychology, 65*, 203–218.

Lang, F. R., & Carstensen, L. L. (2002). Time counts: Future time perspective, goals, and social relationships. Stanford University. *Psychology and Aging, 17*(1), 125–139.

Lasane, T. P., & O'Donnell, D. A. (2005). Time orientation measurement: A conceptual approach. In A. Strathman & J. Joireman (Eds.), *Understanding behavior in the context of time* (pp. 11–30). Mahwah: Lawrence Erlbaum Associates.

Lavender, A., & Watkins, E. R. (2004). Rumination and future thinking in depression. *British Journal of Clinical Psychology, 43*, 129–142.

Lewin, K. (1951). *Field theory in the social sciences: Selected theoretical papers*. Oxford: Harpers.

MacLeod, A. K., & Byrne, A. (1996). Anxiety, depression, and the anticipation of future positive and negative experiences. *Journal of Abnormal Psychology, 105*(2), 286–289.

Nurmi, J.-E. (1991). How do adolescents see their future: A review of the development of future orientation and planning. *Developmental Review, 11*, 1–59.

Nurmi, J.-E. (2005). Thinking about and acting upon the future. Development of future orientation across the lifespan. In A. Strathman & J. Joireman (Eds.), *Understanding behavior in the context of time* (pp. 31–58). Mahwah: Lawrence Associates Publishers.

Nuttin, J. (1972). *Time Attitude Scale (TAS).* Unpublished manual, Louvain, Research Center for Motivation and Time Perspective.

Nuttin, J. R., & Lens, W. (1985). *Future time perspective and motivation: Theory and research method.* Leuven/Hillsdale: Leuven University Press/Lawrence Erlbaum Associates.

Otrar, M., Eksi, H., Dilmac, B., & Sikin, A. (2002). The sources of stress, coping, and psychological well- being among Turkic and relative societies' students in Turkey. *EDAM Egitim Danismanligi Ve Arastirmalari Merkezi, 2*, 473–506.

Poole, M. E., & Cooney, G. H. (1987). Orientations to the future: A comparison of adolescents in Australia and Singapore. *Journal of Youth and Adolescence, 16*(2), 124–151.

Pöppel, E. (1997). A hierarchical model of temporal perception. *Trends in Cognitive Sciences, 1*, 56–61.

Sanna, L. J., Stocker, S. L., & Clarke, J. A. (2003). Rumination, imagination, and personality: Specters of the past and future in the present. In E. C. Chang & L. J. Sanna (Eds.), *Virtue, vice, and personality: The complexity of behavior* (pp. 105–124). Washington, DC: American Psychological Association.

Shell, D. F., & Husman, J. (2001). The multivariate dimensionality of personal control and future time perspective in achievement and studying. *Contemporary Educational Psychology, 26*, 481–506.

Shipp, A. J., Edwards, J. R., & Lambert, L. S. (2009). Conceptualization and measurement of temporal focus: The subjective experience of the past, present, and future. *Organizational Behavior and Human Decision Processes, 110*, 1–22.

Shirai, T. (1997). Time orientation and identifying adolescence and middle age. *Memoires of Osaka Kyouku University, Ser. IV, Education, Psychology, Special Education, and Physical education, 45*(2), 207–226.

Shirai, T., Nakamura, T., & Katsuma, K. (2012). Time orientation and identity formation: Long-term longitudinal dynamics in emerging adulthood. *Japanese Psychological Research, 54*(3), 274–284.

Solantaus, T. (1987). Hopes and worries of young people in three European countries. *Health Promotion, 2*, 19–27.

Strathman, A., Gleicher, F., Boniger, D. S., & Edwards, C. S. (1994). The consideration of future consequences: Weighing immediate and distant outcome behavior. *Journal of Personality and Social Psychology, 66*(4), 742–752.

Suddendorf, T. (2006). Foresight and the evolution of the human mind. *Science, 312*, 1006–1007.

Suddendorf, T., & Corballis, M. C. (1997). Mental time travel and the evolution of the human mind. *Genetic, Social, and General Psychology Monographs, 123*, 133–167.

Tulving, E. (2001). Origin of autonoesis in episodic memory. In H. L. Roedediger et al. (Eds.), *The nature of remembering: Essays in honor of Robert G. Crowder* (pp. 17–34). Washington, DC: American Psychological Association.

Van Beek, W., Berghuis, H., Kerkhof, A., & Beekman, A. (2011). Time perspective, personality and psychopathology: Zimbardo's Time Perspective Inventory in psychiatry. *Time and Society, 20*(3), 364–374.

Wiberg, M., & Carelli, M. G. (2014). Insights into features of anxiety through multiple aspects of psychological time. *Journal of Integrative Psychology and Therapeutics, 2*, 3. doi:10.7243/2054-4723-2-3.

Wittmann, M. (2009). The inner experience of time. *Philosophical Transactions of the Royal Society B, 364*, 1955–1967.

Worrell, F. C., & Mello, Z. R. (2007). The reliability and validity of Zimbardo Time Perspective Inventory scores in academically talented adolescents. *Educational and Psychological Measurement, 67*, 487–504.

Zaleski, Z. (1996). Future anxiety: Concept, measurement, and preliminary research. *Personality and Individual Differences, 20*(2), 165–174.

Zaleski, Z. (2005). Future orientation and anxiety. In A. Strathman & J. Joireman (Eds.), *Understanding behavior in the context of time: Theory, research, and application* (pp. 125–141). Mahwah: Lawrence Erlbaum Associates.

Zimbardo, P. G., & Boyd, J. N. (1999). Putting time in perspective: A valid, reliable individual-differences metric. *Journal of Personality and Social Psychology, 77*(6), 1271–1288.

Time Perspective and Personality

Antanas Kairys and Audrone Liniauskaite

While trying to define psychological phenomena there is also an attempt to answer the question about their place in the structure of personality. Therefore, any other psychological variable, including time perspective, has to find its place in the context of personality. Most of authors who do research in the field of time perspective tend to refer to the time perspective as to attitudes or cognitive – motivational phenomena (Lens and Moreas 1994; Zimbardo and Boyd 2008). Nevertheless, some studies and theoretical assumptions (Harber et al. 2003; Kairys 2010a, b) imply that individuals' attachment to specific time zones is relatively stable and that prompts further search of time perspective's place among structural parts of personality. We believe there are two important issues addressing this problem: (1) in a great variety of personality theories the ways of integrating various constructs to the personality field depend on the paradigm; (2) human behaviour in a given situation is a result of interaction between situational circumstances and personality.

Currently there is a great range of personality concepts however regardless of authors' position explaining the personality it is commonly agreed that in general personality is one of the most fundamental mechanisms, regulating person's functioning in the environment. According to Funder (2001), several theories compete for the prevalence (classic psychoanalytic, trait, behaviourist evolved to social-cognitive, and the humanistic paradigms; biological and evolutionary theory have also attained the status of new paradigms for personality), suggesting slightly differing concept of personality as well as research methods. The trait theory is one that gains popularity and support among researchers. It develops rapidly and offers few

A. Kairys (✉)
Department of General Psychology, Vilnius University, Vilnius, Lithuania
e-mail: kairys.antanas@gmail.com

A. Liniauskaite
Department of Psychology, Klaipeda University, Klaipeda, Lithuania
e-mail: audrone.liniauskaite@gmail.com

M. Stolarski et al. (eds.), *Time Perspective Theory; Review, Research and Application: Essays in Honor of Philip G. Zimbardo*, DOI 10.1007/978-3-319-07368-2_6,

relevant theoretical models (Eysenck, Cloninger, Zuckerman, Strelau, Gray theories, HEXACO model, etc.), the Big Five/Five Factor model being one of the most popular (Matthews et al. 2003). The main representatives of this model define traits as "dimensions of individual differences in tendencies to show consistent patterns of thoughts, feelings, and actions" (McCrae and Costa 2003, p. 25), whereas personality is characterized as the totality of traits (McCrae 2005). Due to its' popularity, development, and great amount of empirical studies this model became the basis of the Chapter.

As already mentioned the position of time perspective in the context of personality structure is determined not only by the chosen theoretical paradigm, but also by the principle endorsed in psychology by Lewin (1936) who is also the father of idea of time perspective. He stated that the person's behaviour depends on both the personality and the characteristics of the situation (B = f (P; E), where B stands for behaviour, P – personality and E – environment). Cattel (1965/2008) elaborated further on the principle and expanded the Lewin's formula emphasizing that behaviour depends on various personality and situational factors, which are present at a given moment. The interaction between environment and personality retains its relevance nowadays (see Bond 2013; Kihlstrom 2013; Snyder 2013). Moreover, this issue of interactions between situation and personality becomes essential in the context of personality traits and time perspective associations, since the nature of time perspective is still being debated.

This chapter will present theoretical assumptions as well as the analysis of empirical studies, allowing us to associate personality traits with time perspective and also discuss the possible position of time perspective in the context of personality traits.

Time Perspective in the Personality Space: Theoretical Predispositions

In contemporary psychology the concept of time perspective and its position in the system of psychological phenomena is not unequivocal or established. There are several different ways of defining the time perspective. The time perspective can be viewed as (1) perceived task characteristic (Gjesme 1983; Lens and Moreas 1994); (2) motivational – cognitive process, commonly emphasizing planning, goal setting and similar processes, however other processes like autobiographic memory are also mentioned (Andriessen et al. 2006; Lens and Moreas 1994; Seijts 1998); (3) attitude or viewpoint (Zimbardo and Boyd 2008); (4) construct, similar to personality traits, highlighting individual differences and stability of time perspective (Harber et al. 2003; Kairys 2010b). Despite the ongoing discussion about the nature of time perspective, most agree that time perspective regulates individual's relationship with time and also with memories, plans, objectives, relationships with others, etc. Various authors state that "time perspective can become a dispositional characteristic which influences individual choices, actions, and decisions" (Luyckx et al. 2010, p. 240), it is a "fundamental psychological process" (Luyckx et al. 2010, p. 243), "basic aspect of individual subjective experience" (Boniwell and Zimbardo 2004, p. 8), etc. All these are the functions of the personality construct. Therefore, it can be considered that time perspective might be a construct similar to a personality trait.

The general principle that the behaviour is the result of the interaction between situation and personality should not be forgotten or disregarded however. Therefore even if time perspective is considered as a stable dispositional construct, it has to be recognised that time perspective can be greatly affected by the situation. For example, we are more present-oriented when playing a game, compared to discussing investment options (Zimbardo and Boyd 2008). This is most likely associated with the duality of time perspective, since on the one hand it is the process of attributing the constant flow of experiences to certain time frames (Zimbardo and Boyd 1999), and on the other – a more stable dispositional attachment to time frames.

Quite a few similarities were discovered while analysing and comparing descriptions and correlates of time perspective (Zimbardo and Boyd 1999, 2008, etc.) along with descriptions of traits in the Five Factor model (Costa and McCrae 1992; McCrae 2005, etc.). These similarities are presented in Table 1. These similarities further support the assumption that at least to some degree, time perspective is a stable dispositional characteristic.

Thus, theoretically, personality traits and time perspective are similar constructs to a certain degree. But is this supported by empirical research?

Empirical Research of Links Between Time Perspective and Personality Variables

Few researchers attempted to relate time perspective and personality traits or other personality dispositions empirically. Six studies were found in which both Five Factor personality traits and time perspective were researched: Zimbardo and Boyd (1999) performed validation of Zimbardo time perspective inventory (ZTPI) with 566 USA college students, the Big Five Questionnaire was used as well. Dunkel and Weber (2010) did a research with 196 USA college students using ZTPI and Big Five Personality Inventory. Adams and Nettle (2009) with ZTPI Future TP scale and 50-item five-factor scale from the international personality item pool did a research in order to evaluate how those variables predict smoking, body mass, and physical activity. 423 participants from USA urban areas were recruited for that research. There are two studies by Kairys (2010b) in which both ZTPI and personality was evaluated. In the larger scale research 636 participants from general Lithuanian population were recruited and NEO-FFI as personality measure was used, in the other research 153 participants from general Lithuanian population took part and NEO PI-R as more thorough personality measure was used. Zhang and Howell (2011) did a research with USA undergraduate college students (N=754) in which ZTPI and Sausier's mini-markers were used. Correlations between Time

Table 1 Similarities between descriptions of personality traits and time perspective

Trait and its descriptions	Time perspective and its description
Neuroticism – "general tendency to experience negative affects such as fear, sadness, embarrassment, anger, guilt, and disgust is the core of the N domain" (Costa and McCrae 1992, p. 14). Neuroticism includes facets like anxiety, depression, etc. (Costa and McCrae 1992; Matthews et al. 2003)	**Past Negative TP** includes "a pessimistic, negative, or aversive attitude toward the past" (Zimbardo and Boyd 1999, p. 1277). It is associated with anxiety, depressiveness, unhappiness, low self-esteem (Zimbardo and Boyd 1999, 2008)
	Present Fatalistic TP – a fatalistic and helpless attitude toward future and life. It is associated with increased levels of depression and anxiety (Zimbardo and Boyd 1999, 2008)
	Past Positive TP. This TP is the opposite of the Past Negative TP, therefore positively past-oriented individuals are characterized by low levels of depression and anxiety (Zimbardo and Boyd 1999)
Extraversion: "extraverts are friendly, sociable, […], assertive, active, and talkative" (Costa and McCrae 1992, p. 15). Stimulation seeking is typical for extraverts (McCrae 2005)	**Present Hedonistic TP** is described as orientation towards present pleasures, entertainment, excitement. Individuals with Present Hedonistic orientation are open to meeting new people (Zimbardo and Boyd 1999)
	Future TP is associated with less need for social interaction (Boniwell and Zimbardo 2004)
	Past Positive TP is associated with maintaining long-term relationships with friends (Boniwell and Zimbardo 2004)
Openness to experience: related to preference for variety, attentiveness to feelings, active experience seeking for the sake of sheer experience, openness to ideas, values. Individuals who are closed to experience tend to be conservative (Costa and McCrae 1992; Matthews et al. 2003; McCrae 2005)	People who have strongly expressed **Present Hedonistic TP** are prone to novelty-seeking, sensation-seeking (Zimbardo and Boyd 1999).
	People with **Past Negative TP** orientation are conservative, avoiding change, novel cultures or experiences (Boniwell and Zimbardo 2004).
	Future TP is associated with low novelty-seeking and low sensation-seeking (Zimbardo and Boyd 1999)
Agreeableness. Agreeable person is altruistic, sympathetic, while disagreeable individual, in contrast, is egocentric, adverse, competitive, antagonistic (Costa and McCrae 1992; McCrae 2005)	Individuals who have expressed **Past Negative TP** tend to be aggressive (Zimbardo and Boyd 1999, 2008).
	Individuals with **Past Positive TP** orientation are less aggressive, are good at maintaining long-term relationships with friends (Boniwell and Zimbardo 2004; Zimbardo and Boyd 1999, 2008)

(continued)

Table 1 (continued)

Trait and its descriptions	Time perspective and its description
Conscientiousness. Conscientious individuals are persistent, purposeful, determined. They have better self-control and are able to resist the impulses. Individuals with low conscientiousness are indifferent to pursuit of objectives, careless, more hedonistic and more interested in sex. Conscientiousness is associated with academic and occupational achievements (Costa and McCrae 1992; McCrae 2005)	**Future TP** is associated with planning, purposefulness. Individuals who are strongly future-oriented are usually successful in academic field and career (Boniwell and Zimbardo 2004; Zimbardo and Boyd 1999, 2008) Individuals with **Present Hedonistic TP** orientation do not sacrifice present comforts for the sake of the future, they do not consider future consequences, have poor ego or impulse control. They tend to have more sexual relationships (Boniwell and Zimbardo 2004; Zimbardo and Boyd 1999) **Present Fatalistic TP** reflects carelessness toward future, assumption that consequences are not controlled by actions (Zimbardo and Boyd 1999, 2008)

Adapted with permission from Kairys (2010b)

perspective and Five factor personality traits, which were obtained in these 6 studies, as well as weighted averages of correlations, calculated using Hunter and Schmidt (2004) formula $\overline{r} = \frac{\sum_{i=1}^{k} n_i r_i}{\sum_{i=1}^{k} n_i}$, are presented in Table 2.

Table 2 presents the findings of six studies (Adams and Nettle 2009; Dunkel and Weber 2010; Kairys 2010b; Zhang and Howell 2011; Zimbardo and Boyd 1999), which give the clear view of connection patterns between time perspective and Five Factor personality traits. There is a strong positive connection between Future time perspective and conscientiousness ($\overline{r} = 0.60$). Present Fatalistic time perspective is not only negatively associated with conscientiousness, but also has a positive relation with neuroticism; this relation wasn't established only in one study (Dunkel and Weber 2010), what might be due to the characteristics of the sample and the research tools. Present Hedonistic time perspective is positively associated with extraversion and negatively associated with conscientiousness. The results of four out of five studies suggest that Present Hedonistic time perspective and openness are related ($\overline{r} = 0.23$). Past Positive time perspective has a positive correlation with extraversion and agreeableness; Past Negative time perspective is positively related to neuroticism ($\overline{r} = 0.48$), this being the second strongest weighted mean correlation coefficient, and negatively – to extraversion and conscientiousness; three studies also revealed negative association with agreeableness. Other identified correlations between personality traits and time perspective are weaker, inconsistent

Table 2 The association between time perspective and five factor personality traits

	Neuroticism/emotional stability[a]	Extraversion/energy	Openness	Agreeableness/friendliness	Conscientiousness
Future TP	$\bar{r}$ **=−0.07**	$\bar{r}$ **=0.10**	$\bar{r}$ **=0.03**	$\bar{r}$ **=0.14**	$\bar{r}$ **=0.60**
	−0.06 ZB	0.30*** ZB	0.11* ZB	0.04 ZB	0.57*** ZB
	0.19** DW	0.02 DW	−0.04 DW	0.19** DW	0.67*** DW
	−0.08 AN	0.01 AN	0.06 AN	0.03 AN	0.57*** AN
	−0.15*** K1	0.05 K1	−0.12** K1	0.19*** K1	0.66*** K1
	−0.05 K2	−0.05 K2	−0.15 K2	−0.01 K2	0.67*** K2
	−0.07* ZH	0.11** ZH	0.15*** ZH	0.24*** ZH	0.54*** ZH
Present fatalistic TP	$\bar{r}$ **=0.26**	$\bar{r}$ **=−0.10**	$\bar{r}$ **=−0.15**	$\bar{r}$ **=−0.07**	$\bar{r}$ **=−0.25**
	0.19*** ZB	−0.21*** ZB	−0.19*** ZB	−0.08 ZB	−0.22*** ZB
	0.13 DW	0.09 DW	0.13 DW	0.00 DW	−0.33*** DW
	0.32*** K1	0.06 K1	−0.11** K1	0.09* K1	−0.14** K1
	0.44*** K2	−0.22** K2	−0.13 K2	0.26** K2	−0.47*** K2
	0.25*** ZH	−0.19*** ZH	−0.22*** ZH	−0.27*** ZH	−0.29*** ZH
Present hedonistic TP	$\bar{r}$ **=0.08**	$\bar{r}$ **=0.30**	$\bar{r}$ **=0.23**	$\bar{r}$ **=0.02**	$\bar{r}$ **=−0.18**
	0.19*** ZB	0.27*** ZB	0.05 ZB	0.05 ZB	−0.20*** ZB
	−0.16* DW	0.31** DW	0.25*** DW	0.18** DW	−0.15* DW
	0.08 K1	0.38*** K1	0.34*** K1	−0.13** K1	−0.19*** K1
	0.06 K2	0.53*** K2	0.43*** K2	−0.13 K2	−0.26** K2
	0.07 ZH	0.22*** ZH	0.23*** ZH	0.12*** ZH	−0.14*** ZH
Past positive TP	$\bar{r}$ **=−0.08**	$\bar{r}$ **=0.18**	$\bar{r}$ **=0.09**	$\bar{r}$ **=0.24**	$\bar{r}$ **=0.13**
	−0.08 ZB	0.15** ZB	−0.01 ZB	0.22*** ZB	0.04 ZB
	−0.14* DW	0.17* DW	0.06 DW	0.29*** DW	0.02 DW
	0.03 K1	0.22*** K1	0.05 K1	0.24*** K1	0.20*** K1
	−0.01 K2	0.16* K2	0.2* K2	0.16* K2	−0.03 K2
	−0.17*** ZH	0.17*** ZH	0.19*** ZH	0.25*** ZH	0.19*** ZH

Past negative TP	$\bar{r}$ =**0.48**	$\bar{r}$ =**−0.24**	$\bar{r}$ =**−0.07**	$\bar{r}$ =**−0.12**	$\bar{r}$ =**−0.19**
	0.45*** ZB	−0.18** ZB	−0.1 ZB	−0.11* ZB	−0.11* ZB
	0.47*** DW	−0.34*** DW	0.03 DW	−0.26*** DW	−0.19** DW
	0.46*** K1	−0.19*** K1	−0.05 K1	−0.11** K1	−0.16*** K1
	0.61*** K2	−0.32*** K2	−0.18* K2	0.11 K2	−0.29*** K2
	0.49*** ZH	−0.30*** ZH	−0.07* ZH	−0.15*** ZH	−0.25*** ZH

Note. Weighted averages of correlations are presented in *bold*.
ZB – Zimbardo and Boyd (1999). DW – Dunkel and Weber (2010). AN – Adams and Nettle (2009). K1 – Kairys (2010b), ZTPI and NEO-FFI were used; K2 – Kairys (2010b); ZTPI and NEO PI-R were used. ZH – Zhang and Howell (2011)
*p<005; **p<0.01; ***p<0.001
[a]Zimbardo and Boyd (1999) used Big Five Questionnaire with higher scale scores representing low neuroticism, thus correlations were reversed

and do not allow establishing any clear tendencies and might be related to the specific characteristics of the sample and the research tools.

It may be assumed that some associations between time perspective and personality traits are determined by cultural differences – correlations between Present Fatalistic time perspective and neuroticism are significant ($p<0.001$) and relatively strong (0.32–0.44; Kairys 2010b) in Lithuanian sample, while in the USA those are weaker or insignificant (Dunkel and Weber 2010; Zhang and Howell 2011; Zimbardo and Boyd 1999), either way such an assumption needs further studying.

To examine the associations between time perspective and facets of the personality traits, Kairys (2010b) used NEO PI-R, which evaluates not only five personality traits, but also subordinate dimensions (i.e. facets) of each of the five personality factors. Correlations between time perspective and facets of the personality traits are presented in Table 3.

The results presented in Table 3 suggest each time perspective is related to personality facets.

Future time perspective is related to all conscientiousness trait facets correlations with achievement striving ($r=0.64$) and self-discipline (0.60) being particularly strong. Past positive time perspective scale positively correlates with warmth and altruism, and they are of average effect size. This time perspective has the least correlations with personality traits. Present fatalistic time perspective is related to higher values of neuroticism facets, the strongest correlation being with vulnerability to stress ($r=0.47$), also with lower values of conscientiousness facets, especially with competence ($r=-0.5$) and achievement striving ($r=-0.49$). Present hedonistic time perspective correlates with all extraversion facets establishing a clear trend of higher Present Hedonistic time perspective's values related to greater excitement seeking ($r=0.56$), tendency to engage in new actions ($r=0.45$), impulsiveness ($r=0.41$) and lower deliberation ($r=-0.45$). Past negative time perspective has the similar trend of correlations to the facets as Present Fatalistic time perspective: there are positive correlations with the facets of neuroticism and negative with the facets of conscientiousness, correlations with depression ($r=0.63$) and vulnerability to stress ($r=0.52$) being particularly strong. This pattern of correlations between time perspective and personality facets not only confirms the time perspective concept by Zimbardo and Boyd (1999, 2008) but allows to better understanding of the peculiarities of different time perspectives as well. The strong links between time perspective and some lower lever personality traits are obvious and allow the assumption about the similarities of discussed phenomena.

Some published studies link personality traits with various psychological time variables. Rammsayer (2002) studied associations between perception of short intervals and Big Three personality traits (extraversion, neuroticism, psychoticism). Associations were found only with psychoticism – individuals having high scores for psychoticism showed better temporal processing in the range of seconds. Kelly and Johnson (2005) found that perceived time use effectiveness relates to conscientiousness, though there were no connections established with other personality traits. Gomez et al. (2009) investigated interaction between personality traits and evaluation of life events (which could be a measure of time perspective) and

Table 3 Correlations between time perspective and facets of personality traits

	Future TP (N=148)	Past positive TP (N=151)	Present fatalistic TP (N=151)	Present hedonistic TP (N=147)	Past negative TP (N=148)
N1 anxiety	0.01	0.04	**0.38*****	−0.07	**0.48*****
N2 hostility	0.08	0.00	0.24**	**0.24****	**0.35*****
N3 depression	−0.07	−0.1	**0.38*****	−0.08	**0.63*****
N4 self-consciousness	0.11	0.00	**0.32*****	−0.16	**0.49*****
N5 impulsiveness	−0.19*	0.01	0.10	**0.41*****	0.14
N6 vulnerability to stress	−0.17*	0.00	**0.47*****	0.02	**0.52*****
E1 warmth	−0.03	**0.37*****	0.05	**0.39*****	−0.01
E2 gregariousness	−0.18*	0.07	−0.10	**0.39*****	−0.17*
E3 assertiveness	0.05	0.00	**−0.35*****	**0.29*****	**−0.30*****
E4 activity	0.13	0.03	**−0.24****	**0.35*****	**−0.28****
E5 excitement seeking	−0.16*	0.13	−0.15	**0.56*****	−0.20*
E6 positive emotion	−0.03	0.17*	**−0.26****	**0.32*****	**−0.40*****
O1 fantasy	**−0.39*****	0.13	0.05	**0.31*****	−0.05
O2 aesthetics	−0.07	0.20*	0.10	**0.24****	0.04
O3 feelings	−0.01	0.12	−0.05	**0.31****	−0.04
O4 actions	−0.10	0.13	−0.17*	**0.45*****	**−0.28****
O5 ideas	0.18*	0.09	**−0.34*****	0.10	−0.19*
A1 trust	0.09	0.22**	−0.01	0.12	−0.12
A2 straightforwardness	0.02	0.02	0.11	−0.23**	0.01
A3 altruism	−0.08	**0.29*****	0.24**	0.11	0.09
A4 compliance	−0.04	−0.02	0.14	**−0.33*****	0.06
A5 modesty	−0.01	−0.04	0.21**	**−0.28****	0.20*
A6 tendermindedness	−0.01	0.19*	**0.31*****	0.21**	0.18*
C1 competence	**0.31*****	0.04	**−0.50*****	−0.07	**−0.39*****
C2 order	**0.42*****	−0.02	**−0.30*****	−0.19*	**−0.25*****
C3 dutifulness	**0.48*****	0.02	−0.17*	−0.10	−0.04
C4 achievement striving	**0.64*****	0.02	**−0.49*****	−0.10	−0.24**
C5 self-discipline	**0.60*****	−0.06	**−0.41*****	−0.22**	**−0.28****
C6 deliberation	**0.51*****	−0.11	−0.24**	**−0.45*****	−0.11

Adapted with permission from Kairys (2010b)

Note: Correlations exceeding least medium effect size (r=0.24) according to Cohen (as cited in Volker 2006) are presented in *bold*; O6 Values scale was omitted due to low Cronbrach's alpha coefficient

***$p<0.001$; **$p<0.01$; *$p<0.05$

used both variables to predict subjective well-being. Results of the research showed that neuroticism is associated with negative evaluation of life events, while positive evaluation of life events was linked to openness.

Few studies investigated relations between time perspective and other personality variables. Connections between **time perspective and locus of control** were explored and it was established that internality positively correlated with future-orientation and negatively – with Past Negative and Present Fatalistic time perspective (Kolesovs 2002). Brannigan et al. (1992) found that people with strong expression of externality tend to engage in daydreaming related to past events, meanwhile Muzdybajev (Муздыбаев 1983) found that individuals with strong manifestation of either externality or internality, are more satisfied with their present than past, but have different opinions regarding the future: external individuals are more optimistic about future and are less likely to fill past, present and future time zones.

Time perspective and self-efficacy are substantially related: positive associations were established between self-efficacy and Future time perspective (Epel et al. 1999; Luszczynska et al. 2004). Epel et al. (1999) found that stronger expression of present time perspective among homeless was related to lower self-efficacy.

There also are associations between **time perspective and sensation seeking** behaviour: it was found that Present Hedonistic and Fatalistic time perspective is related to higher level of sensation seeking (Zimbardo and Boyd 1999), while Future time perspective is related to lower level of excitement seeking (Robbins and Bryzan 2004; Zimbardo and Boyd 1999).

There are few time perspective connections to other personality characteristics: MacKillop et al. (2003) established that impulsiveness of pathological gamblers is positively associated with Past Negative, Present Fatalistic and Hedonistic and also negatively with Future time perspective; risky and reckless behaviour is related to Present Hedonistic time perspective; empathy is positively associated with Past Positive and Future time perspective.

Discussion

We came down to what we began with – time perspective can be attributed to various phenomena: dynamic cognitive-motivational processes (Nuttin 1985; Gjesme 1983; Lens and Moreas 1994; Seijts 1998; Vazquez and Rapetti 2006), more stable dispositions (Boniwell and Zimbardo 2004; Lens and Moreas 1994; Gjesme 1983; Zaleski 1994) or less stable phenomena – attitudes (Zimbardo and Boyd 1999, 2008). The answer to "what is the nature of time perspective?" would also give us the understanding of what is the place of time perspective in the context of personality. The final answer however is yet to be found.

Lets' try and attend two essential questions: (1) if time perspective is an independent construct or is it the set of personality traits? (2) is time perspective is stable enough and has other features typical of a stable personality disposition?

Considering constructs which correlate strongly with personality traits (and it was shown that time perspective has rather strong correlations) the question arises if the construct in question has additional prognostic value and having the personality traits is not enough to explain the behaviour. There is some research that shows time perspective has additional prognostic value even controlling for personality traits.

There is ample of research (see Boniwell et al. 2010; Zhang et al. 2013) relating time perspective to personal well – being and being satisfied with life. There are also a lot of studies (see DeNeve and Cooper 1998; Lucas and Diener 2008; Schmutte and Ryff 1997) proving personality traits being valid predictor of well – being. Zhang and Howell (2011) on the basis of performed regression analysis concluded that "relations between personality traits and life satisfaction can, quite significantly, be explained by individual differences in time perspective – specifically, the past time perspectives. As a result, while personality traits are strongly associated with life satisfaction (Diener and Lucas 1999) we suggest that at least some, if not most, of the association between an individual's disposition and their life satisfaction may be due to how they relate their personal and social experiences to time." (p. 1265). Bagdonas et al. (2013), while analysing the data of Lithuanian representative sample found that time perspective is as valid as Five Factor personality traits in predicting well – being and has more potential in predicting well – being than clinical MMPI – 2 scales. It should be mentioned however that in both of the cases the common method bias was not controlled for which can explain the great predictive value (Podsakoff et al. 2012). Kairys (2010b) presents evidence of time perspective remaining important predictor of health, alcohol consumption and faith even after controlling for personality traits. Summarizing, time perspective is an important and independent construct and the links found with other variables (such as well-being) in various research cannot be explained by mere correlations with personality traits.

While considering second question about the stability and independent features of time perspective it is worth noticing that personality trait has to satisfy a large number of conditions that are described in the works of contemporary trait theory researchers (Matthews et al. 2003; McAdams and Pals 2006; McCrae and Costa 1995; McCrae 2005, etc.). Summarizing these conditions, we have to admit that if a construct is claimed to be a trait, it has to be a dimension of individual differences related to "consistent patterns of thoughts, feelings, and actions" (McCrae and Costa 2003, p. 25). What is more, these stable features must be found in a broad spectrum of psychological phenomena, like wishes, motives, attitudes, behaviour, etc. That is what separates traits from other mental phenomena that are classified as characteristic adaptations, e.g. values, attitudes, habits (McCrae and Costa 1995; McCrae 2005). So if time perspective indeed possesses similarities with personality traits (is stable enough and covers vide range of phenomena) it can be considered a relatively stable personality disposition.

Time perspective research on development and stability is particularly lacking. However, there are some cross-sectional (i.e. Cate and John 2007; Fingerman and Perlamutter 1993; Lang and Carstensen 2002; Zacher and Frese 2009 etc.), and longitudinal studies (Cate and John 2007; Holman and Silver 1998; Luyckx et al. 2010; Nurmi 1989), but the authors are usually focused only on one age group or one time perspective (future). Kairys (2010a, b) simultaneously studied time perspective and five personality traits in three age groups. Research results show that correlations between time perspective and stable personality traits are similar in all the age groups. The relatively stable correlations with personality traits allow for the assumption that time perspective can be stable as well (Kairys 2010a, b). However in order to give the definite answer to the question whether time perspective is more stable or more changing long-term longitudinal studies incorporating all time perspectives are needed.

Time perspective can be noticed in a broad spectrum of mental phenomena and this gives it even more reason that time perspective is similar to personality disposition. According to Zimbardo model, clear differences are seen amongst people having different combination of time perspective. These differences can be observed in emotions (e.g., past negative oriented person's depressiveness), anticipations, goal setting (e.g. future oriented person tends to plan ahead, present hedonistic oriented person – lives in the moment), behaviour (reckless driving, choice of leisure activities, alcohol use, etc.) (Apostolidis et al. 2006; Keough et al. 1999; Wills et al. 2001; Zimbardo and Boyd 1999, 2008, etc.). Although, time perspective wasn't as vastly researched as Five Factor model, there are enough arguments to state that time perspective covers a broad pattern of behavioural, emotional, attitudinal and other psychological phenomena. Moreover, the research with the most common time perspective instrument – ZTPI – is being done in various cultures and this is another point in the discussion that time perspective is at least partly culturally universal. However broader cross cultural research is needed especially using emic research strategy.

A trait is considered to have evolutionary and biological basis, and to be at least partially innate (Matthews et al. 2003; McCrae and Costa 1995; McCrae 2005). However, very little is known about the nature of time perspective. Time perspective is considered to be a fundamental process of psyche (Zimbardo and Boyd 1999), it is often stated that its development is influenced by sociocultural context: family, social groups or other circumstances (Luyckx et al. 2010; Zimbardo and Boyd 2008). The research proving this is still scarce. It is obvious, that further studies, that could evaluate if time perspective is determined by social context or people who are biologically predisposed to one or another time perspective are more susceptible to sociocultural influences, are needed.

Summarizing, there are sufficient research findings speaking in favour of time perspective being an independent construct that has additional prognostic value even after controlling for personality traits. It is also evident that time perspective has likeliness to personality trait – is stable, broad and therefore can be considered as relatively stable dispositional characteristic. Referring to the mentioned in the introductory part interaction between personality and environment as well as to time perspective being defined both as a process during which the flow of experience is attributed to time frame and stable attachments to those frames, it can be assumed that the nature of the time perspective is twofold. The core of the time perspective is relatively stable and similar to the trait and the shell of it is dynamic and subjective to situational changes.

References

Adams, J., & Nettle, D. (2009). Time perspective, personality and smoking, body mass, and physical activity: An empirical study. *British Journal of Health Psychology, 14*, 83–105.

Andriessen, I., Phalet, K., & Lens, W. (2006). Future goal setting, task motivation and learning of minority and non-minority students in Dutch schools. *British Journal of Educational Psychology, 76*, 827–850.

Apostolidis, T., Fieulaine, N., Simonin, L., & Rolland, G. (2006). Cannabis use, time perspective and risk perception: Evidence of a moderating effect. *Psychology and Health, 21*(5), 571–592.

Bagdonas, A., Kairys, A., Liniauskaite, A., & Pakalniskiene, A. (2013). *Lietuvos gyventojų psichologinė gerovė ir jos veiksniai [Psychological well-being of residents of Lithuania and its factors]*. Vilnius: Vilniaus universiteto leidykla.

Bond, M. H. (2013). Refining Lewin's formula: A general model for explaining situational influence on individual social behaviour. *Asian Journal of Social Psychology, 16*, 1–15.

Boniwell, I., & Zimbardo, P. G. (2004). Balancing one's time perspective in pursuit of optimal functioning. In P. A. Linley & S. Joseph (Eds.), *Positive psychology in practice* (pp. 165–181). Hoboken: Wiley.

Boniwell, I., Osin, E., Linley, P. A., & Ivanchenko, G. V. (2010). A question of balance: Time perspective and well-being in British and Russian samples. *The Journal of Positive Psychology, 5*(1), 24–40.

Brannigan, G. G., Shahon, A. J., & Schaller, J. A. (1992). Locus of control and time orientation in daydreaming: Implications for therapy. *Journal of Genetic Psychology, 153*(3), 359–361.

Cate, R. A., & John, O. P. (2007). Testing models of the structure and development of future time perspective: Maintaining a focus on opportunities in middle age. *Psychology and Aging, 22*(1), 186–201.

Cattell, R. B. (1965/2008). *The scientific analysis of personality*. New Brunswick: Aldine Transaction.

Costa, P. T., & McCrae, R. R. (1992). *Revised NEO Personality Inventory (NEO PI - R™) and NEO Five – Factor Inventory (NEO-FFI)*. Lutz: PAR.

DeNeve, K. M., & Cooper, H. (1998). The happy personality: Traits and a meta-analysis of 137 personality subjective well-being. *Psychological Bulletin, 124*(2), 197–229.

Dunkel, C. S., & Weber, J. L. (2010). Using three levels of personality to predict time perspective. *Current Psychology, 29*(2), 95–103.

Epel, E., Bandura, A., & Zimbardo, P. G. (1999). Escaping homelessness, the influences of self-efficacy and time perspective on coping with homelessness. *Journal of Applied Social Psychology, 29*(3), 575–596.

Fingerman, K. L., & Perlamutter, M. (1993). Future time perspective and life events across adulthood. *The Journal of General Psychology, 122*(1), 95–111.

Funder, D. C. (2001). Personality. *Annual Review of Psychology, 52*, 197–221.

Gjesme, T. (1983). On the concept of future time orientation: Considerations and some functions' and measurements' implications. *International Journal of Psychology, 18*, 443–461.

Gomez, V., Krings, F., Bangerter, A., & Grob, A. (2009). The influence of personality and life events on subjective well-being from a life span perspective. *Journal of Research in Personality, 43*, 345–354.

Harber, K. D., Zimbardo, P. G., & Boyd, J. N. (2003). Participant self-selection biases as a function of individual differences in time perspective. *Basic and Applied Social Psychology, 25*(3), 255–264.

Holman, E. A., & Silver, R. C. (1998). Getting "stuck" in the past: Temporal orientation and coping with trauma. *Journal of Personality and Social Psychology, 74*, 1146–1163.

Hunter, J. E., & Schmidt, F. L. (2004). *Methods of meta-analysis: Correcting error and bias in research findings*. Thousand Oaks: Sage.

Kairys, A. (2010a). Correlations between time perspective and personality traits in different age groups. *Tiltai, 2*, 159–173.

Kairys, A. (2010b). *Laiko perspektyva: sąsajos su asmenybės bruožais, amžiumi ir lytimi (daktaro disertacija)* [Time perspective: Its link to personality traits, age, and gender (Doctoral dissertation)], Vilnius University, Vilnius.

Kelly, W. E., & Johnson, J. L. (2005). Time use efficiency and the five-factor model of personality. *Education, 125*(3), 511–515.

Keough, K. A., Zimbardo, P. G., & Boyd, J. N. (1999). Who's smoking, drinking, and using drags? Time perspective as a predictor of substance use. *Basic and Applied Social Psychology, 21*(2), 149–164.

Kihlstrom, J. F. (2013). The person–situation interaction. In P. E. Nathan (Ed.), *The Oxford handbook of social cognition* (pp. 786–806). Oxford: Oxford University Press.

Kolesovs, A. (2002). The relation between time perspective and locus of control in high school students. *Baltic Journal of Psychology, 3*(2), 7–19.

Lang, F. R., & Carstensen, L. L. (2002). Time counts: Future time perspective, goals, and social relationships. *Psychology and Aging, 17*(1), 125–139.

Lens, W., & Moreas, M. A. (1994). Future time perspective: An individual and a societal approach. In Z. Zalesky (Ed.), *Psychology of future orientation* (pp. 23–28). Lublin: Towarzystwo Naukowe.

Lewin, K. (1936). *Principles of topological psychology*. New York: McGraw Hill Book Company.

Lucas, R. E., & Diener, E. (2008). Personality and subjective well-being. In O. P. John, R. W. Robins, & L. A. Perwin (Eds.), *Handbook of personality. Theory and research* (pp. 795–814). New York: The Guilford Press.

Luszczynska, A., Gibbons, F., Piko, B. F., & Tekozel, M. (2004). Self-regulatory cognitions, social comparison, and perceived peers' behaviors as predictors of nutrition and physical activity: A comparison among adolescents in Hungary, Poland, Turkey, and USA. *Psychology and Health, 19*(5), 577–593.

Luyckx, K., Lens, W., Smits, I., & Goossens, L. (2010). Time perspective and identity formation: Short-term longitudinal dynamics in college students. *International Journal of Behavioral Development, 34*(3), 238–247.

MacKillop, J., Anderson, A. J., Castelda, B. A., Mattson, R. A., & Donovick, P. J. (2003). Convergent validity of measures of cognitive distortions, impulsivity, and time perspective with pathological gambling. *Psychology of Addictive Behaviors, 20*(1), 75–79.

Matthews, G., Deary, I. J., & Whiteman, M. C. (2003). *Personality traits*. Cambridge: Cambridge University Press.

McAdams, D. P., & Pals, J. L. (2006). A new big five: Fundamental principles for an integrative science of personality. *American Psychologist, 61*(3), 204–217.

McCrae, R. R. (2005). Personality structure. In V. J. Derlega, B. A. Winstead, & W. H. Jones (Eds.), *Personality. Contemporary theory and research* (pp. 192–217). Belmont: Wadsworth Publishing.

McCrae, R. R., & Costa, P. T. (1995). Trait explanations in personality psychology. *European Journal of Personality, 9*, 231–252.

McCrae, R. R., & Costa, P. T. (2003). *Personality in adulthood*. New York: The Guilford Press.

Муздыбаев, К. [Muzdybajev, K.]. (1983). *Психология ответственности* [The psychology of responsibility]. Ленинград [Leningrad]: Наука [Nauka].

Nurmi, J. E. (1989). Development of orientation to the future during early adolescence: A four-year longitudinal study and two cross-sectional comparisons. *International Journal of Psychology, 24*, 195–214.

Nuttin, J. (1985). *Future time perspective and motivation*. Leuven: Leuven University Press.

Podsakoff, P. M., MacKenzie, S. B., & Podsakoff, N. P. (2012). Sources of method bias in social science research and recommendations on how to control it. *Annual Review of Psychology, 65*, 539–569.

Rammsayer, T. H. (2002). Temporal information processing and basic dimensions of personality: Differential effects of psychoticism. *Personality and Individual Differences, 32*, 827–838.

Robbins, R. N., & Bryzan, A. (2004). Relationships between future orientation, impulsive sensation seeking, and risk behavior among adjudicated adolescents. *Journal of Adolescent Research, 19*, 428–445.

Schmutte, P. S., & Ryff, C. D. (1997). Personality and well-being: reexamining methods and meanings. *Journal of Personality and Social Psychology, 73*(3), 549–559.

Seijts, G. H. (1998). The importance of future time perspective in theories of work motivation. *The Journal of Psychology, 132*(3), 154–168.

Snyder, M. (2013). *B=f (P, S)*: Perspectives on persons and situations, from Lewin to Bond and beyond. *Asian Journal of Social Psychology, 16*, 16–18.

Vazquez, S. M., & Rapetti, M. V. (2006). Future time perspective and motivational categories in Argentinean adolescents. *Adolescence, 41*(163), 511–532.

Volker, M. A. (2006). Reporting effect size estimates in school psychology research. *Psychology in the Schools, 43*(6), 653–672.

Wills, T. A., Sandy, J. M., & Yaeger, A. M. (2001). Time perspective and early – Onset substance use: A model based on stress – Coping theory. *Psychology of Addictive Behaviors, 15*(2), 118–125.

Zacher, H., & Frese, M. (2009). Remaining time and opportunities at work: Relationships between age, work characteristics, and occupational future time perspective. *Psychology and Aging, 24*, 487–493.

Zaleski, Z. (1994). Towards a psychology of the personal future. In Z. Zaleski (Ed.), *2* (pp. 23–38). Lublin: Towarzystwo Naukowe.

Zhang, J. W., & Howell, R. T. (2011). Do time perspectives predict unique variance in life satisfaction beyond personality traits? *Personality and Individual Differences, 50*, 1261–1266.

Zhang, J. W., Howell, R. T., & Stolarski, M. (2013). Comparing three methods to measure a balanced time perspective: The relationship between a balanced time perspective and subjective well-being. *Journal of Happiness Study, 14*, 169–184.

Zimbardo, P. G, & Boyd, J. N. (1999). Putting time in perspective. A valid, reliable individual-difference metric. *Journal of Personality and Social Psychology, 77*, 1271–1288.

Zimbardo, P. G., & Boyd, J. N. (2008). *The time paradox*. New York: Free Press.

The Past, the Present, and the Future: A Conceptual Model of Time Perspective in Adolescence

Zena R. Mello and Frank C. Worrell

"Perhaps no area is more in need of exploration since all human conduct…is conditioned by the time perspectives of the individual" (Frank 1939, p. 294). Almost 75 years later, this statement is still relevant. This paper seeks to promote research on time perspective in adolescence by presenting a new multidimensional conceptual model. Scholars have provided compelling evidence showing that how individuals feel about the past, the present, and the future predicts important developmental outcomes, such as academic achievement (Mello and Worrell 2006; Zimbardo and Boyd 1999), risky behavior (Zimbardo et al. 1997), substance use (Keough 1999), and physical activity (Henson et al. 2006). To complement this research, this paper proposes (a) additional dimensions of time perspective that may illuminate its relationships with human behavior, (b) a focus on adolescence as a developmental period that is particularly salient for the expression of time perspective, and (c) potential implications for incorporating time perspective into interventions.

Time Perspective

Time perspective is conceptualized as a cognitive and motivational construct that is individually varying (see Fig. 1 for a conceptual model), and this conceptualization is based on four premises. First, time perspective is cognitive because it originates in the thoughts of individuals and it is motivational because thoughts about time

Z.R. Mello (✉)
San Francisco State University, San Francisco, California
e-mail: zmello@sfsu.edu

F.C. Worrell
University of California, Berkeley, CA, USA
e-mail: frankc@berkeley.edu

M. Stolarski et al. (eds.), *Time Perspective Theory; Review, Research and Application: Essays in Honor of Philip G. Zimbardo*, DOI 10.1007/978-3-319-07368-2_7,

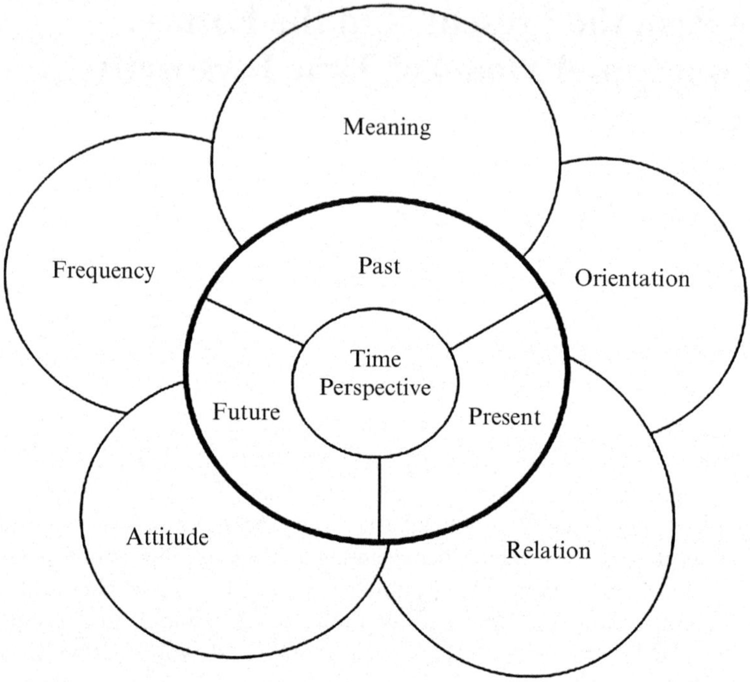

Fig. 1 A conceptual model of time perspective dimensions

lead individuals to make particular decisions and engage in specific behaviors. Second, time perspective encompasses three temporal periods—namely the past, the present, and the future—and each period contributes uniquely to an individual's time perspective. Moreover, individual functioning may vary in relationship with each time period. For example, academic outcomes may be more closely tied to individuals' perspective toward the future than the past, whereas risk taking may be more closely tied to an orientation to the present. Further, to understand completely an individual's time perspective, all three time periods must be considered. Thus, an individual's perspective toward the present will not necessarily convey their perspective toward the past or the future.

Third, time perspective differs among individuals as a result of learning and experiences in various contexts, such as family, school, and community. For example, Mello and Swanson (2007) showed how adolescents' expectations for the future varied by neighborhood socioeconomic status. Lastly, time perspective is multidimensional and may be conceptualized in terms of (a) attitude, (b) orientation, (c) relation, (d) frequency, and (e) meaning, with each dimension yielding a distinct and meaningful part of the construct. In the subsequent sections, I define each dimension with research on adolescents, outline age-related changes of these dimensions in adolescence, and provide examples of interventions that have included time perspective.

Time Attitudes

Time attitudes are defined as positive and negative feelings toward the past, the present, and the future and are the most commonly studied element of time perspective. As early as 1953, Lewin stated, "The behavior of an individual does not depend entirely on his present situation. His mood is deeply affected by his hopes and wishes and by his views of his own past" (p. 75). Although named differently, time attitudes have been studied most frequently with the Zimbardo Time Perspective Inventory (ZTPI; Zimbardo and Boyd 1999). The ZTPI measures individual-variation in college-aged populations and is comprised of five subscales: Past Positive, Past Negative, Present Hedonism, Present Fatalism, and Future. ZPTI scores are related to a variety of constructs in adolescent and adult samples (Apostolidis et al. 2006; Henson et al. 2006; Keough et al. 1999; Mello and Worrell 2006; Rothspan and Read 1996; Shores and Scott 2007; Wills et al. 2001; Zimbardo and Boyd 1999).

The most recent addition to measuring time attitudes is a new instrument developed to assess time attitudes in adolescents, given prior research indicating that the ZTPI may have limited utility with adolescents (Worrell and Mello 2007). Mello and Worrell (2010) created the Adolescent Time Inventory (ATI). The time attitude dimension of time perspective on the ATI is represented by the Adolescent Time Attitude Scale (ATAS; Mello and Worrell 2007), which assesses positive and negative attitudes toward the past, the present, and the future. The ATAS includes six subscales that comprise five items each: Past Positive, Past Negative, Present Positive, Present Negative, Future Positive, and Future Negative. In studies with American and German adolescents, the ATAS has yielded valid and reliable scores, which have theoretically consistent relationships with a variety of constructs, including academic self-concept, global self-esteem, hope, optimism, and perceived stress (Worrell and Mello 2009; Worrell et al. 2013). Clusters based on ATAS scores indicate that adolescents in several countries have meaningful time attitude profiles, which also predict differences on academic constructs (Alansari et al. 2012; Andretta et al. 2014; Buhl and Lindner 2009).

Studies using other instruments have indicated that time attitudes are associated with developmental outcomes in adolescents, such as delinquency, substance use, and academic achievement (Jew and Green 1998; Landau 1976; Lennings et al. 1998; Robbins and Bryan 2004). As is evident, time attitudes are related to many important developmental outcomes, and are certainly worthy of greater systematic research scrutiny. For example, unlike the ZPTI, ATAS scores are focused only on time without additional constructs, such as hedonism. The ATAS will allow us to examine questions, such as if present attitudes are related to risk taking and depression independently of constructs such as hedonism and fatalism, respectively.

Time Orientation

Time orientation refers to the emphasis one places on the past, the present, and/or the future. Lewin (1935, 1939, 1942) described how varying thoughts about time periods could predict human behavior, and time orientation research shows that individuals vary in how they much they emphasize the past, the present, and the future (e.g., Cottle 1967b). Zimbardo and Boyd (1999, p. 1272) argued that a "balanced" orientation, with an equal emphasis on the past, the present, and the future, would be associated with the healthiest behaviors. Using a variety of instruments, research has shown that individuals are most interested in the future or the present and least interested in the past. For example, delinquent adolescent males preferred the future over the present or the past (Landau 1976). Studies with adults indicate that the present is the most important, followed by the future and the past (Cottle 1967b; Israeli 1932) or that the future is valued the most, followed by the present, and the past (Carreras et al. 2008; Jason et al. 1989). In a study with children and late adult participants, Gonzalez and Zimbardo (1985) reported that more than half selected a phrase including the present and the future, followed by a third who selected a phrase with the future, a smaller group who selected a phrase with the present, and a very small group who selected a phrase with only the past.

Studies using various measures have shown relationships between time orientation and developmental outcomes. Researchers have found that future orientation is positively associated with achievement in adolescent males (Haldeman 1992; Tehan 1957) and with academic behaviors in college students (Lasane and Jones 1999). In an experimental study, Brock and Giudice (1963) showed that participants who stole were three times more likely than non-stealers to select the word "yesterday" and no difference was observed with the word "tomorrow." Regarding psychological outcomes, optimism was positively related to an orientation toward the future in adolescents (Haldeman 1992) and was inversely related to the past in adults (Shipp et al. 2002).

Extant research is limited because most available instruments do not enable researchers to assess an orientation towards one, two, or three time periods. To address this limitation, the ATI's Time Orientation section (ATI-TO) was developed to assess adolescents' orientation towards the past, the present, and the future (Mello and Worrell 2010). The ATI-TO includes circles of varying sizes labeled the past, the present, and the future. Respondents choose from one of seven configurations (e.g., Past emphasis, Present and Future emphasis) to indicate which time period or periods are most important to them. It is possible that different relationships may emerge among individuals who are oriented towards a single time period, multiple time periods, or specific time periods. Results from a recent study using a previous version of the ATI-TO (Mello et al. 2013) showed that participants who were oriented towards *only* the present or *only* the future had lower self-esteem and academic achievement and reported engaging in more risky-behavior than those oriented towards two or three time periods.

Time Relation

Time relation reflects the degree to which individuals perceive that the past, the present, and the future are related to one another. This concept is premised on an understanding of potential causal relations between what has occurred (the past) and what is occurring (the present), between the present, and what might occur (the future), and among the past, present and future. Indeed, some scholars have argued that perceiving a connection among time periods is beneficial for health (Cottle 1967b; Lennings et al. 1998). Thus, adolescents who conceive of time periods as related may better understand that today's actions will have an influence on tomorrow's outcomes, and such thinking may lead to healthier decisions. Zimbardo and Boyd (2008) have referred to a Holistic Present, which is a focus on the present time period, where the present contains both the past and the future. They liken this notion to mindfulness practices and suggest this conceptualization leads to healthier individuals. Time relation may be a way to operationalize the construct.

Researchers have employed various instruments to examine time relation. In a study of late adolescents, Cottle (1967a) asked participants to draw circles indicating the relationship among the past, the present, and the future. Results indicated that the most common configuration included a set of circles overlapping in a linear pattern (i.e., past overlapping present, and present overlapping future), followed by unrelated circles. In other studies using participant drawn circles, the overlapping time period pattern was positively associated with valuing achievement (Cottle 1969) and intelligence (Getsinger 1975) and inversely associated with anxiety (Cottle 1969; Getsinger 1975). In another study of the interrelationship among time periods, college students who perceived a connection between current and future goal-related behaviors also reported higher academic achievement (Shell and Husman 2001). Lastly, qualitative research has illustrated that some adolescents think the time periods are interconnected: "Well, I think it's kind of like steps, the past can influence the future, but you have to think about the past in the present to influence the future" (Mello et al. 2009a, p. 547).

As with time orientation, our knowledge of time relation has been restricted due to the absence of a standardized measure. To address this gap, the ATI (Mello and Worrell 2010) has a Time Relation section, the ATI-TR, comprised of configurations of circles labeled the past, the present, and the future. Configurations vary in overlap among time periods to indicate the degrees to which individuals perceive that time periods are related to one another, and include four options: unconnected time periods, past alone/present and future connected, linearly connected, and interconnected (i.e., a Venn diagram). Using an earlier three-option version of the ATI-TR, Mello et al. (2013) reported that 50 % perceived time as interconnected, 35 % perceived the time periods as linearly related and 10 % reported no relationship. In the second part of the study, with the four-option ATI-TR, 38 % of adolescents perceived the time periods as interconnected, 33 % chose present/future connected, 20 % selected the linear relationship, and 10 % chose no connection. Adolescents who selected the interconnected and linearly connected options had higher grade point averages, higher scores on goal setting and self-esteem, and lower risky behaviors, such as stealing or running away from home than those who selected unrelated circle configurations. It will be important for these findings to be replicated and extended to other areas including clinical depression, delinquency, and physical activity, for example.

Time Frequency

Time frequency refers to the rate with which individuals report thinking about the past, the present, and the future. This concept is similar to scope and extension. Lewin (1939, 1942) described scope when he contended that from childhood to adolescence, individuals increase their perspective from days and weeks to months and years. Extension is a similar construct and refers to the distance one thinks into the future (Nuttin 1985). Time frequency (ATI-TF) has been measured with items that assess how often individuals think about the past, the present, and the future, such as daily, weekly, monthly, and never (Mello and Worrell 2010). In a recent study of adolescents, Mello et al. (2009b) found that two-thirds of the sample thought about the present and the future on a daily basis, whereas only about half thought about the past on a daily basis. Results also indicated that participants who thought about the past on a daily or weekly basis had higher academic achievement than their counterparts who reported thinking about the past on a monthly basis or never. In another study, findings showed that most adolescents thought about the past on a weekly basis (Finan 2012); however, no comparison with the other two time periods was available in this study. Future research should examine time frequency with psychological and behavioral outcomes, as it is possible that such relationships may vary by time periods.

Time Meaning

Time meaning (ATI-TM) refers to how individuals *define* the past, the present, and the future (Mello and Worrell 2010). In a focus-group study of academically talented adolescents, participants reported tremendous variation in how they conceptualized time periods (Mello et al. 2009a). For example, participants defined the past as "when I was younger, my family's past, or what already happened in history." Results also revealed that participants' definitions included analogies, affect, or relationships among the time periods. In another focus-group study of adolescents (McKay et al. 2012), participants used different time periods to define time, such as short-term, medium-term, and long-term. Participants in this sample also mentioned domains, such as school, work, and family in their reports on the meaning of the time periods. Similar to Mello et al. (2009a), results indicated that participants used personal, familial, and large-scale definitions for the past and that genders did not vary in time meanings.

Time meaning may also reveal important cross-cultural variation by illuminating how cultures vary in their understanding of time. For example, Nunez and Sweetser (2006) conducted research with the Aymaran community, which resides in areas of Bolivia, Chile, and Peru. In this community, the temporal arrangement of the past, the present, and the future differs from other peoples. Specifically, in this group, time is ordered with the future first, followed by the present and then the past. Alternately, what constitutes time may vary across cultures. In some Native American tribes, time is considered to be cyclical and is intrinsically tied to the earth, with seasons used to mark changes from one period to the next (Lake 1991). Seginer (2009) has also presented a conceptual model of future orientation, a topic similar to time perspective that incorporates culture. She highlights how educational and occupational opportunities vary both between and within cultures, and contends that the perceptions of such opportunities shape adolescents orientation toward the future.

Summary

As highlighted in the preceding discussion, there are multiple dimensions of time perspective, and the ATI (Mello and Worrell 2010) assesses five of these: attitudes, orientation, relation, frequency, and meaning. Time meaning has the potential to be useful in illustrating cross-national variation in how individuals define time (Lake 1991; Nunez and Sweetser 2006), and extant findings have revealed substantial individual variation in adolescent samples (McKay et al. 2012; Mello et al. 2009a). In keeping with other research, a study using the ATI (Mello et al. (2009b) indicated that adolescents think more often about the present and the future than the past and that the past time frequency. Time attitudes have received the most attention, given the frequent use of the ZPTI (Zimbardo and Boyd 1999), although data suggest that in adolescents, the ATAS (Alansari et al. 2013; Buhl and Lindner 2009; Worrell and Mello 2007; Worrell et al. 2013) yields more reliable and valid scores. Generally, extant research indicates that time attitudes are related to outcomes in the academic, psychological, and physical health domains (e.g., Apostolidis et al. 2006; Henson et al. 2006; Shores and Scott 2007). Although time attitudes are generally interpreted as indicative of time orientation (e.g., Zimbardo and Boyd 1999, 2008), time orientation and time relation have received limited consideration since Cottle (1967b) published a projective measure to assess these constructs. By providing another way to assess these time orientation and time relation, the ATI may be useful in clarifying their relationships with time attitudes, time frequency, and important developmental outcomes.

Time Perspective Research and Development in Adolescence

Adolescence is an important period of the lifespan to investigate time perspective, given developmental changes that occur at this age. Adolescents mature in cognitive capacities (Piaget 1955, 1975) and engage in the process of identity formation (Erikson 1968), which enable them to think about time in a new way when compared to childhood. Scholars describing time perspective have posited that age-related changes may occur across the life-span including the transition from childhood to adolescence (Frank 1939; Lewin 1935, 1946).

Research on cognitive abilities indicates that adolescents are capable of abstract thinking and considering the hypothetical (Piaget 1955, 1975), advances that enable the consideration of time perspective. Piaget (1955) postulated that the capacity for individuals to understand time was an indicator of intellectual development. To demonstrate the emergence of time concepts, Piaget developed studies to show how children come to understand movement, sequence, and velocity (Flavell 1963). Abstract thinking is necessary to consider the past, the present, and the future at the same time, as it permits individuals to place themselves hypothetically in varying time periods of their life. Piaget (1955) described time as a logical concept containing order and duration and argued that the understanding of time would follow the same sequence as general cognitive development. In adolescence, individuals are able to think about the order or sequence of the past, the present, and the future, as well as the duration of events in the stream of time.

The seminal work by Erikson (1968) on identity formation also provides support for the relevance of time perspective during adolescence. Erikson described identity formation as the primary developmental task of adolescence with an identity achieved through the integration of one's past, present, and future selves. Erikson's description of identity formation alludes to the presence of time perspective. He wrote about the importance of integrating the time periods when forming a personal identity: "Identity contains a complementarity of past and future…it links the actuality of a living past with that of a promising future" (Erikson 1968, p. 310). Erikson also discussed how individuals may have the inability to integrate their past, present, and future. As he stated, "every adolescent… knows at least fleeting moments of being thus at odds with time itself" (Erikson 1968, p. 181). Erikson proposed that adolescents could recognize the complexity of time and would express a preference for an orientation toward the future.

In 1935, Lewin argued that, in childhood, individuals are focused on the present, and in adolescence, individuals learn that life includes both a past and a future. Frank (1939) discussed how children will have a time perspective of limited range and that older individuals will show more extensive ranges in thinking about time. Lewin (1946) also noted how adolescence results in an increased focus on the future and in future-related planning. Extant studies on time perspective in adolescent samples have focused on time attitude, time orientation, and time relation.

Time Attitudes in Adolescence

In a study of high school students (*M* age = 16.5) and college students (*M* age = 19.4), Lennings et al. (1998) did not observe age differences in negative attitudes toward time. Mello and Worrell (2006) showed how Present Hedonism scores increased with age in a cross-sectional study of individuals aged 11–18, although the effect size for this result was small. In this study, age was positively related to Future Positive scores, although also with a small effect size, in a study of academically talented participants aged 12–19 (Worrell and Mello 2009).

Time Orientation in Adolescence

Research on time orientation and adolescents has generally focused on single time periods. Cross-sectional research focusing on the future indicates that adolescence is associated with an increase in thinking about this time period. In a study of adolescents aged 9–15, an emphasis on the future was shown to become greater with age (Lessing 1972). Researchers have examined extension, the distance one thinks into the future, and have concluded that adolescence is characterized by an increase in future thinking compared to childhood (Wessman and Gorman 1977). Greene (1986) examined the future thinking of individuals aged 15, 17, and 19 years old with a measure of future extension. Results indicated that older participants reported thinking farther into the future than their younger counterparts. However, Lennings et al. (1998; see also Lenning 1994) did not find differences on past or future time extension between high schoolers with an average age of 16 and college students with an average age of 19. In a review of neuroscience research examining structural changes in the brain, Steinberg (2008) reported that future orientation increases from early to mid-adolescence. In a subsequent study of individuals aged 10–30, Steinberg et al. (2009) found that adolescents aged 16 and older were more oriented towards the future compared to their younger counterparts. In this study, future orientation was defined by a concern for the future, anticipation of consequences, and delay discounting. This latter study's results may explain the lack of differences in the Lennings study.

In contrast with the studies reported in the previous paragraph, some researchers have found that adolescence is characterized by an increased emphasis on the present. Klineberg (1967) showed that adolescents were oriented toward the present and then the future, compared to children who were predominantly oriented toward the future. Tismar (1987) reported similar results in a study of adolescents ($M=14$ years old), late adolescents ($M=18$ years old), and young adults ($M=23$ years old). This author found that present orientation increased and future orientation decreased from mid- to late adolescence, and that young adults reported more emphasis on the past compared to adolescents. In a study of adolescents aged 12–17, Bowles (1999) reported that older adolescents emphasized the present, followed by the past, and the future, and younger adolescents emphasized the present and the future more than older adolescents. However, in contrast to these results, Cottle (1967b) showed that younger adolescents generally drew circle configurations indicating a present orientation compared to their older counterparts, with age groups comprised of individuals under and over age 15 and ranging from 12 to 18.

Additional cross-sectional research employing various instruments has also shown an increase in present orientation in adolescence. Webb and Mayers (1974) conducted a study with children and adolescents aged 9–10, 12–13, 15–16, and 18–19, and used a sentence-completion task to discern orientation toward the past, the present, and the future. Results indicated a larger emphasis on the present in adolescents aged 15–16 compared to other age groups. In a study of individuals ranging in age from 8 to over 90 years old, Gonzalez and Zimbardo (1985) found that younger participants were more likely to focus on the present than their older counterparts, and in a study of elementary and secondary school students, Anderssen et al. (1992) reported that older participants had higher scores in fatalistic orientation, defined as a present focus and an inability to consider the future, compared to their younger counterparts.

Time Relation in Adolescence

Very little research has been conducted on time relation and adolescence. Lewin (1939) argued that the awareness of the influence of present behavior on the future emerges in this age period. Cottle and Klineberg (1974) also argued that the recognition of the relatedness of the past, present, and future time period would manifest in adolescence. Some support for this notion came from a prior study. Specifically, Cottle (1967a) administered a projective test involving drawn circle configurations to adolescents and reported that more 15–18 year olds indicated the time periods were interrelated than 12–15 year olds. In contrast, Lennings et al. (1998) found that high schoolers obtained significantly higher scores than university students on two measures of time relation. However, the effect sizes for both comparisons were small (i.e., $d < .26$), suggesting that the differences were not meaningful.

Summary

Developmental theory provides some support for the notion that with the transition from childhood to adolescence (Erikson 1968; Piaget 1955), individuals' time perspectives will change. However, the specific ways in which age-related change may occur is difficult to discern, given the scarcity of research and inconsistency in results. Some studies indicate an increase in positive attitudes toward the present (Mello and Worrell 2006) and the future (Worrell and Mello 2009), although other studies have not replicated these results (Lennings 1994; Lennings et al. 1998). Findings on time orientation and time relation are also mixed, suggesting a great need for research in this area. Research on the relationship of age to time frequency and time meaning has yet to be conducted.

Time Perspective Intervention Implications

Time perspective has implications for promoting positive developmental outcomes in various domains such as education (Phalet et al. 2004) and physical health (Rakowski 1985). Zimbardo and Boyd (1999) described how researchers might conceive of programs to alter time perspectives so that individuals with a present orientation might learn how to think in a more future-oriented manner. Some scholars have described how time perspective can contribute to the prevention of and intervention with health problems (Rakowski 1985).

Extant intervention programs serve as examples of the potential for time perspective research to foster healthy adolescent development. Results from the *Going for the Goal* program (Danish 1997) suggest that teaching adolescents to identify positive future goals resulted in better school attendance compared to non-participants. Similarly, Oyserman et al. (2002) reported that an intervention program that taught adolescents to construct plans and goals for adulthood resulted in participants reporting more strategies to attain goals and better school attendance than non-participants. Hall and Fong (2003) designed an intervention to promote future-oriented thinking in decisions regarding physical fitness by encouraging college-aged participants to consider the consequences of present actions. Results from a 10-week follow-up indicated that participants in the time perspective condition reported increased levels of physical activity compared to the remaining groups, a finding that was replicated in a second study with college students.

Directions for Further Research

As this brief review has highlighted, despite the interest in the time perspective construct over the past 75 years, there is still a limited understanding of the complexity of the construct and the role that the various time perspective dimensions play in adolescent functioning. The majority of research studies have been on time attitudes, but even in that domain, strong conclusions are limited by problematic operationalizations and inconsistency of findings. In addition to examining time perspective dimensions *in* adolescence, there are several directions for additional research on time perspective, including studies that focus on differences by age and cultural group membership. Although we have argued that adolescence is a particularly salient period to examine time perspective, the topic may be meaningful in other periods of the life-span or in transitions into and out of adolescence. Examining the stability of scores by age over the time perspective dimensions and how these scores change across the life-span is a fruitful direction to pursue.

On a related topic, longitudinal research designs are greatly needed for facilitating a comprehensive understanding of age-related variation in the time perspective dimensions and across the three time periods. The majority of research has used cross-sectional designs that limit our ability to understand changes in time perspective dimensions across developmental periods. Longitudinal research designs will also help to disentangle age-related changes from changes related to social phenomena or levels of education.

Additional areas of study include cross-cultural and cross-national research. Time perspective may vary substantially across cultural communities. Indeed, the limited research on this topic suggests that how individuals think about time may be related to their cultural contexts (e.g., Alansari et al. 2013; Andretta et al. 2013;

Lake 1991; Nunez and Sweetser 2006; Seginer 2009). It will be important for further research to explore the ways in which time perspective differs across ethnicities and nations.

Lastly, in this paper, we described dimensions of time perspective that might be useful in predicting developmental outcomes in adolescents including attitudes, orientation, relation, frequency, and meaning. An important direction for future research is the examination of the interrelationships among these dimensions. For example, time orientation and time frequency should be positively related, given that they both assess focus on specific time periods. It is also possible that interactions among the dimensions may be meaningfully associated with outcomes, such that individuals who have *both* positive attitudes toward the future and think about that time period frequently are healthier than their counterparts who do not think as favorably or as often about the future.

Conclusion

This paper presented a conceptual model of time perspective that is multidimensional and developmental. It was argued that time perspective is an individually varying cognitive-motivational construct that has a particular salience in the period of adolescence. Using early and contemporary research on time perspective to provide a foundation, we have argued for a new and broader conceptualization of time perspective that includes three time periods and several dimensions. We also argued that these dimensions apply to each of the three time periods and may vary in relationship with specific areas of human functioning, such as academic or psychological outcomes. Extant studies were reviewed that showed age-related changes in some time perspective dimensions, although the findings are inconsistent. Some studies also suggest that time perspective can be the foundation for interventions intended to facilitate positive developmental outcomes. In closing, we contend that time perspective has the potential to contribute much to our understanding of adolescents specifically and of human behavior more generally.

References

Alansari, M., Worrell, F. C., Rubie-Davies, C., & Webber, M. (2013). Adolescent Time Attitude Scale (ATAS) scores and academic outcomes in secondary school females in New Zealand. *International Journal of Quantitative Research in Education, 1*, 251–274.

Anderssen, E. C., Myburgh, C. P. H., van Zyl, M. A., & Wiid, A. J. B. (1992). A differential analysis of time-use attitudes of high school students. *Adolescence, 27*, 64–72.

Andretta, J. R., Worrell, F. C., & Mello, Z. R. (2014). Predicting educational outcomes and psychological wellbeing in adolescents using time attitude profiles. *Psychology in the Schools, 51*, 434–451. doi:10.1002/pits.21762.

Andretta, J. R., Worrell, F. C., Mello, Z. R., Dixson, D. D., & Baik, S. H. (2013). Demographic group differences in adolescents' time attitudes. *Journal of Adolescence, 36*, 289–301. doi:10.1016/j.adolescence.2012.11.005.

Apostolidis, T., Fieulaine, N., & Soule, F. (2006). Future time perspective as a predictor of cannabis use: Exploring the role of substance perception among French adolescents. *Addictive Behaviors, 31*, 2339–2343. doi:10.1016/j.addbeh.2006.03.008.

Bowles, T. (1999). Focusing on time orientation to explain adolescent self-concept and academic achievement: Part II testing a model. *Journal of Applied Health Behavior, 1*, 1–8.

Brock, T. C., & Giudice, C. D. (1963). Stealing and time orientation. *Journal of Abnormal and Social Psychology, 66*, 91–94. doi:10.1037/h0042834.

Buhl, M., & Linder, D. (2009). Time perspectives in adolescence: Measurement, profiles, and links with personality characteristics and scholastic experience. *Diskurs Kindheits und Jugendforschung* [Research on Child and Adolescent Development], *2*, 197–216.

Carreras, O., Lemercier, C., & Valax, M. F. (2008). Knowing which day of the week it is: Temporal structure and dynamics of memory. *Psychological Reports, 102*, 893–902. doi:10.2466/pr0.102.3.893-902.

Cottle, J. T. (1967a). Adolescent perceptions of time: The effect of age, sex, and social class. *Journal of Personality, 37*, 636–650. doi:10.1111/j.1467-6494.1969.tb01770.x.

Cottle, T. J. (1967b). The circles test: An investigation of perceptions of temporal relatedness and dominance. *Journal of Projective Techniques & Personality Assessment, 31*, 58–71. doi:10.1080/0091651X.1967.10120417.

Cottle, T. J. (1969). Future orientation and avoidance: Speculations on the time of achievement and social roles. *The Sociological Quarterly, 10*(4), 419–437.

Cottle, T. J., & Klineberg, S. L. (1974). *The present of things future*. New York: Macmillan.

Danish, S. J. (1997). Going for the goal: A life skills program for adolescents. In G. W. Albee & T. P. Gullotta (Eds.), *Primary prevention works* (Vol. 6, pp. 291–312). Thousand Oaks: Sage.

Erikson, E. (1968). *Identity: Youth and crisis* (1st ed.). New York: Norton.

Finan, L. J. (2012). *Daydreaming or distraught? Past time perspective and perceived stress among adolescents*. Unpublished master's thesis, The University of Colorado, Colorado Springs, CO.

Flavell, J. H. (1963). *The developmental psychology of Jean Piaget*. Princeton: D. Van Nostrand Company.

Frank, L. K. (1939). Time perspectives. *Journal of Social Philosophy, 4*, 293–312.

Getsinger, S. H. (1975). Temporal relatedness: Personality and behavioral correlates. *Journal of Personality Assessment, 39*, 405–408. doi:10.1207/s15327752jpa3904_14.

Gonzalez, A., & Zimbardo, P. (1985). Time in perspective: A Psychology Today survey report. *Psychology Today, 19*, 21–26.

Greene, A. L. (1986). Future-time perspective in adolescence: The present of things future revisited. *Journal of Youth and Adolescence, 15*(2), 99–113.

Haldeman, D. H. (1992). *The Cottle circle test: Its validity for identifying adolescent time perspective*. Unpublished doctoral dissertation, The Pennsylvania State University, State College.

Hall, P. A., & Fong, G. T. (2003). The effects of a brief time perspective intervention for increasing physical activity among young adults. *Psychology and Health, 18*, 685–706. doi:10.1080/0887044031000110447.

Henson, J. M., Carey, M. P., Carey, K. P., & Maisto, S. A. (2006). Associations among health behaviors and time perspective in young adults: Model testing with boot-strapping replication. *Journal of Behavioral Medicine, 29*, 127–137. doi:10.1007/s10865-005-9027-2.

Israeli, N. (1932). The social psychology of time: Comparative rating of and emotional reactions to the past, present, and future. *Journal of Abnormal and Social Psychology, 27*, 209–213.

Jason, L. A., Schade, J., Furo, L., Reichler, A., & Brickman, C. (1989). Time orientation: Past, present, and future perceptions. *Psychological Reports, 64*, 1199–1205. doi:10.2466/pr0.1989.64.3c.1199.

Jew, C. L., & Green, K. E. (1998). Effects of risk factors on adolescents' resiliency and coping. *Psychological Reports, 82*, 675–678.

Keough, K. A., Zimbardo, P. G., & Boyd, J. N. (1999). Who's smoking, drinking, and using drugs?: Time perspective as a predictor of substance use. *Basic and Applied Social Psychology, 21*(2), 149–164.

Klineberg, S. L. (1967). Changes in outlook on the future between childhood and adolescence. *Journal of Personality and Social Psychology, 7*, 185–193. doi:10.1037/h0024988.

Lake, R. A. (1991). Between myth and history: Enacting time in Native American protest rhetoric. *Quarterly Journal of Speech, 77*, 123–151. doi:10.1080/00335639109383949.

Landau, S. F. (1976). Delinquency, institutionalization, and time orientation. *Journal of Consulting and Clinical Psychology, 44*, 745–759.

Lasane, T. P., & Jones, J. M. (1999). Temporal orientation and goal-setting: The mediating properties of a motivational self. *Journal of Social Behavior and Personality, 14*, 31–44.

Lennings, C. J. (1994). An investigation of the effects of agency and time perspective variables on career maturity. *The Journal of Psychology, 128*, 243–253. doi:10.1080/00223989809599294.

Lennings, C. L., Burns, A. M., & Cooney, G. (1998). The profiles of time perspective and personality: Developmental considerations. *The Journal of Psychology, 132*, 629–641.

Lessing, E. E. (1972). Extensions of personal future time perspective, age, and life satisfaction of children and adolescents. *Developmental Psychology, 6*, 457–468. doi:10.1037/h0032576.

Lewin, K. (1935). *A dynamic theory of personality*. New York: McGraw-Hill.

Lewin, K. (1939). Field theory and experiment in social psychology: Concepts and methods. *The American Journal of Sociology, 44*, 868–897.

Lewin, K. (1942). Time perspective and morale. In K. Lewin (Ed.), *Resolving social conflicts and field theory in social science* (pp. 80–93). Washington, DC: American Psychological Association.

Lewin, K. (1946). Behavior and development as a function of the total situation. In L. Carmichael (Ed.), *Manual of child psychology* (2nd ed., pp. 918–970). New York: Wiley.

McKay, M. T., Cole, J. C., Sumnall, H. R., & Goudie, A. J. (2012). Framing health messages for adolescents: Should we use objective time periods, temporal benchmarks, or both? *Journal of Youth Studies*, 1–18. doi:10.1080/13676261.2012.663897.

Mello, Z. R., & Swanson, D. P. (2007). Gender differences in African American adolescents' personal, educational, and occupational expectations and perceptions of neighborhood quality. *Journal of Black Psychology, 33*, 150–168. doi:10.1177/0095798407299514.

Mello, Z. R., & Worrell, F. C. (2006). The relationship of time perspective to age, gender, and academic achievement among academically talented adolescents. *Journal for the Education of the Gifted, 29*, 271–289.

Mello, Z. R., & Worrell, F. C. (2007). *The Adolescent Time Perspective Inventory-English*. Unpublished scale: University of California, Berkeley.

Mello, Z. R., & Worrell, F. C. (2010). *The adolescent time inventory: Preliminary technical manual*. Berkeley: Colorado Springs, CO.

Mello, Z. R., Bhadare, D., Fearn, E. J., Galaviz, M. M., Hartmann, E. S., & Worrell, F. C. (2009a). The window, the river, and the novel: Examining adolescents' conceptions of the past, the present, and the future. *Adolescence, 44*, 539–556.

Mello, Z. R., Worrell, F. C., & Andretta, J. R. (2009b). Variation in how frequently adolescents think about the past, the present, and the future in relation to academic achievement. *Research on Child and Adolescent Development* [Diskurs Kindheits-und Jugendforschung], *2*, 173–183.

Mello, Z. R., Finan, L. J., & Worrell, F. C. (2013). Introducing an instrument to assess time orientation and time relation in adolescents. *Journal of Adolescence, 36*, 551–563. doi:10.1016/j.adolescence.2013.03.005.

Nunez, R. E., & Sweetser, E. (2006). With the future behind them: Convergent evidence from Aymara language and gesture in the crosslinguistic comparison of spatial construals of time. *Cognitive Science, 30*, 1–49.

Nuttin, J. (1985). *Future time perspective and motivation: Theory and research method*. Hillsdale: Lawrence Erlbaum.

Oyserman, D., Terry, K., & Bybee, D. (2002). A possible selves intervention to enhance school involvement. *Journal of Adolescence, 25*, 313–326.

Phalet, K., Andriessen, I., & Lens, W. (2004). How future goals enhance motivation and learning in multicultural classrooms. *Educational Psychology Review, 16*, 59–89.

Piaget, J. (1955). The development of time concepts in the child. In P. H. Hoch & J. Zubin (Eds.), *Psychopathology of childhood* (pp. 34–44). New York: Grube & Stratton.

Piaget, J. (1975). The intellectual development of the adolescent. In A. H. Esman (Ed.), *The psychology of the adolescent?: Essential readings* (pp. 104–108). New York: International Universities Press.

Rakowski, W. (1985). Future time perspective: Application to the health context of later adulthood. *American Behavioral Scientist, 29*, 730–745. doi:10.1177/000276486029006007.

Robbins, R. N., & Bryan, A. (2004). Relationships between future orientation, impulsive sensations seeking, and risk behavior among adjudicated adolescents. *Journal of Adolescent Research, 1*, 428–445. doi:10.1177/0743558403258860.

Rothspan, S., & Read, S. J. (1996). Present versus future time perspective and HIV risk among heterosexual college students. *Healthy Psychology, 15*, 131–134. doi:10.1037/0278-6133.15.2.131.

Seginer, R. (2009). *Future orientation: Developmental and ecological perspectives*. New York: Springer.

Shell, D. F., & Husman, J. (2001). The multivariate dimensionality of personal control and future time perspective beliefs in achievement and self-regulation. *Contemporary Educational Psychology, 26*, 481–506. doi:10.1006/ceps.2000.1073.

Shipp, A. J., Edwards, J. R., & Lambert, L. S. (2002). Conceptualization and measurement of temporal focus: The subjective experience of the past, present, and future. *Organizational Behavior and Human Decision Processes, 110*, 1–22. http://dx.doi.org/10.1006/obhd.2001.2988.

Shores, K., & Scott, D. (2007). The relationship of individual time perspective and recreation experience preferences. *Journal of Leisure Research, 1*, 28–59.

Steinberg, L. (2008). A social neuroscience perspective on adolescent risk-taking. *Developmental Review, 28*, 78–106. doi:10.1016/j.dr.2007.08.002.

Steinberg, L., Graham, S., O'Brien, L., Woolard, J., Cauffman, E., & Banich, M. (2009). Age differences in future orientation and delay discounting. *Child Development, 1*, 28–44. doi:10.1111/j.1467-8624.2008.01244.x.

Tehan, J. E. (1957). Future time perspective, optimism, and academic achievement. *Journal of Abnormal and Social Psychology, 57*, 379–380. doi:10.1037/h0042296.

Tismar, K. G. (1987). Psychological aspects of temporal dominance during adolescence. *Psychological Reports, 61*, 647–654. doi:10.2466/pr0.1987.61.2.647.

Webb, J. T., & Mayers, B. S. (1974). Developmental aspects of temporal orientation in adolescents. *Journal of Clinical Psychology, 30*, 504–507. doi:10.1002/1097-4679(197410)30:4<504::AID-JCLP2270300414>3.0.CO;2-Q.

Wessman, A. E., & Gorman, B. S. (1977). *The personal experience of time*. New York: Plenum Press.

Wills, T. A., Sandy, J. M., & Yaeger, A. M. (2001). Time perspective and early-onset substance use: A model based on stress-coping theory. *Journal of Addictive Behaviors, 15*, 118–125. doi:10.1037/0893-164X.15.2.118.

Worrell, F. C., & Mello, Z. R. (2007). Reliability and validity of Zimbardo Time Perspective Inventory scores in academically talented adolescents. *Educational and Psychological Measurement, 67*, 487–504. doi:10.1177/0013164406296985.

Worrell, F.C., & Mello, Z.R. (2009). Convergent and discriminant validity of time attitude scores on the adolescent time perspective inventory. *Diskurs Kindheits- und Jugendforschung* [Research on Child and Adolescent Development], 185–196.

Worrell, F. C., Mello, Z. R., & Buhl, M. (2013). Introducing English and German versions of the Adolescent Time Attitude Scale (ATAS). *Assessment, 20*, 496–510. doi:10.1177/1073191110396202.

Zimbardo, P. G., & Boyd, J. N. (1999). Putting time in perspective: A valid, reliable individual-difference metric. *Journal of Personality and Social Psychology, 77*, 1271–1288. doi:10.1037/0022-3514.77.6.1271.

Zimbardo, P. G., & Boyd, J. N. (2008). *Time paradox: The new psychology of time that will change your life*. New York: Simon & Schuster.

Zimbardo, P. G., Keough, K. A., & Boyd, J. N. (1997). Present time perspective as a predictor of risk driving. *Personality and Individual Differences, 23*, 1007–1023. doi:10.1037/0022-3514.77.6.1271.

Learning and Future Time Perspective: The Promise of the Future – Rewarding in the Present

Jenefer Husman, Sarah K. Brem, Sara Banegas, Daniel W. Duchrow, and Shanjeedul Haque

> *Thus it is not properly said that there are three times, past, present, and future. Perhaps it might be said rightly that there are three times: a time present of things past; a time present of things present; and a time present of things future. For these three do coexist somehow in the soul, for otherwise I could not see them. The time present of things past is memory; the time present of things present is direct experience; the time present of things future is expectation.*
>
> –Augustine, Confessions, Book XI, Chapter XX

Whenever we envision someone learning, we are inherently thinking about the future (Peetsma 2000). The knowledge and skills we gain today would have little value if we did not use them at some time in the future. Whether we, as teachers and mentors are trying to improve retention in memory, instilling skills for problem solving and decision making, or encouraging a student who has stumbled to keep trying, we are, explicitly or tacitly, making them a promise that they will see a return on their efforts at some point in the future.

Funding for the current study was provided by National Science Foundation Grant, REC- 0546856, *CAREER: Connecting with the Future: Supporting Career and Identity Development in Post-Secondary Science and Engineering*

J. Husman (✉) • S.K. Brem
The T. Denny Sanford School of Social and Family Dynamics, Arizona State University, Box 3701, Tempe, AZ 85268, USA
e-mail: Jenefer.Husman@asu.edu

S. Banegas
University of Arizona, Tuscon Arizona, Austin, TX, USA

D.W. Duchrow • S. Haque
Mary Lou Teachers College, Arizona State University, Tempe, AZ 85287, USA

M. Stolarski et al. (eds.), *Time Perspective Theory; Review, Research and Application: Essays in Honor of Philip G. Zimbardo*, DOI 10.1007/978-3-319-07368-2_8,

Although learning has such a strong future focus, we spend very little time conceptualizing, operationalizing, measuring or analyzing this knotty problem, "the future." Most often, cognitive psychologists and educational researchers invoke the future in terms of student retention, by re-testing learners a week, 6 months, a year after the intervention. As Augustine realized over 1600 years ago, time is at least as much a mental phenomenon as it is a physical one; time both shapes our minds and takes it shape from our minds. This theme has permeated modern work on time perspective from Lewin's work in the 1940s to current work on prospective memory (Addis et al. 2007; Klein et al. 2011).

It is well established that being able to access and use knowledge and skills after time has passed is important, and researchers tend to turn to the easiest, least controversial way of looking at the future—the chronological passage of time (Friedman 1993). The future as it is perceived by human beings, however, is not an endless accounting of identical increments of time. We have all experienced the agony of meetings during which time slows so that each minute seems like 10; we've also been surprised to learn that an engaging conversation has been going on for 2 h, when it feels as if it could not have been more than 20 min since we first sat down. What feels distant for one person looms before another; the approaching deadline may cause excitement or anxiety, depending on how the person looks upon the looming event. At other times, we mistakenly decide that we have "plenty of time" to complete a report or learn our lines for an upcoming play; everyone has known the embarrassment and poor performance which ensue. The future may seem filled with many different situations and events, or largely empty; again, how a cluttered or sparse future affects us depends on our own tolerance for and skill in time management, and whether the events before us evoke positive emotions or cause a black mood to descend upon us. Events we envision as part of our future may be deeply interconnected or largely unrelated; we may see a clear path as to how we will arrive at an event, or have no idea how to make a desired future experience come to pass.

If we wish to have a thorough understanding of learning, actions, and the reasons people give for those actions, we need to give the future a great deal more time than it has generally received in the social sciences. As educational researchers and psychologists we need to identify ways to tease apart the many factors that affect how students perceive and react to the future, and connect their representations of the future with present-day actions, emotions, and motivations.

In search of an effective metaphor for thinking about the relationship between past, present and future, my research team and Husman has framed Time Perspective as a "time bubble." The image it is meant to elicit is of a person enclosed in a sphere. Although the person can turn and look in all directions, for the moment we will imagine her facing forward, toward the future. Behind her is the past, and to the left and right are events concurrent with her present. The size of each person's time bubble varies, as does its shape, and the bubble can be centered on the present, or positioned so that more of it lies in the past, or more in the future. Some of us have very large, round bubbles, centered on the present. We see far, equally far, into the past and future, and we can take in many things happening at once. Others might have a bubble that is long and thin; they can remember many years ago and envision many years to come, but only regarding a few events or aspects of their life. A person with a very small bubble lives primarily in the moment, making few plans and rarely consulting memory to assist them in the present. For all the possible configurations of the bubble's size, shape and positioning, there is a particular way of encountering and interacting with the world. Different resources are available, different skills are brought to bear, different events have greater or lesser import, and so on.

The time bubble gives us a figurative framework from which we can begin to determine how specific elements affect a person's perception of the future, and allows us to predict actions and outcomes based on those perceptions. Our work over the past 15 years has been to take such thought experiments and separate the factors that affect how people perceive and react to time, quantifying these as parameters and using them to predict performance, effort, persistence, perceived utility, and so on. In this chapter, we will provide an integrated overview, sketching what has, so far, served as a robust quantitative model of how people perceive the future that predicts aspects of motivation, emotion and cognition. In examining the ways in which our work and Zimbardo's overlap and intersect, as well as the gaps and missing bridges, we hope to suggest how work in Future time perspective might proceed, and discuss what we see as some of the most important next steps.

Past, Present and Future Goals

Future Time Perspective has been examined through the lens of Achievement Motivation frequently over the past 50 years (e.g., Husman and Lens 1999; Nuttin and Lens 1985; Nuttin 1964), as FTP has been shown over many studies to affect task choice, effort, and persistence, the three indexes of achievement motivation.

In our approach to FTP, goals and the structures in which goals reside are central to the way the future is conceptualized, as well as how we think about the past and present. The number of goals a person entertains within their future time space, the distance to those goals, perceived and chronological, the connections between those goals and events past and present, are some of the most important factors in predicting a person's actions and reasoning about those actions, as well as the effort and persistence they exert to progress with respect to those goals (Husman and Shell 2008). The placement and characteristics of goals play a major role in how individuals make decisions about their present tasks and the effort they put into the tasks they choose to engage (Brickman and Miller 2001).

Through our research, my colleagues and I have identified four components of the Time Bubble that influence its structure and how a person functions: connectedness, valence, distance and speed (Husman 1998, 2012). Connectedness is the cognitive piece of FTP and refers to the tendency to make connections between present activities and some future goal (Husman and Shell 2008). Using the Time Bubble analogy Connectedness is the cohesiveness of the students' pathways between present and future goals. Individuals who have a stronger FTP are more able to see the connection between their present activity and future goals. Shell and Husman (2001) found that connectedness is a predictor of student achievement in post-secondary classrooms.

de Volder and Lens (1982) defined valence as the importance individuals place on goals that were attainable in the future. Nuttin (1964) argued that less valence is attached to goals that are farther into the future. This argument has been extensively tested by Halvari (1991a, b, 1996) and time horizon researchers (Okhuysen et al. 2003). In all cases of research on the decreased valance, the more distant the goal the lower the valance, results in less effort being put toward a goal. Future Time Perspective researchers have argued FTP is the individual difference factor which moderates the relationship between the valance of a goal and its distance in physical time (Nuttin and Lens 1985). The importance of FTP is in-part due to the consistent finding that individual who have a longer FTP are more effortful regarding their long-term future goals. de Volder and Lens (1982) found that secondary students who placed higher valence towards goals in the distant future were more persistent in their daily study and obtained better academic results.

Daltrey and Langer (1984) describe distance as how far ahead an individual projects one's thoughts. Goals that exist within an individual's "time bubble" seem closer and hold greater importance than a goal outside of their "time bubble" (Husman and Shell 2008). The longer a person's FTP is, the nearer and more important long term goals will appear.

Speed is the perception of how quickly one feels the events in their imagined future advance in time space. An extended FTP has been associated with the ability to anticipate and plan for the future. Those with a shorter FTP might perceive their future events as rapidly advancing and thus may feel that they are less able to manage their future (Hilpert et al. 2012).

Perceptions of Instrumentality (or simply, PI or instrumentality), is a commonly examined future oriented, yet task specific, aspect of motivation for learning. Instrumentality is defined as a person's perception of how useful a present task is for a future goal. Instrumentality has been theoretically linked to the framework of future time perspective (Husman et al. 2004). Instrumentality has focused on the "connection between the utility of a present act for some future goal" and is measured as such (Husman et al. 2004). Research has provided evidence that students' positive perception of instrumentality is related to learning gains in the classroom (Malka and Covington 2005; Tabachnick et al. 2008). Students with a long FTP can more easily see the connection between their current class activities for the more distant future (instrumentality) and thus have an increased instrumentality for their present learning in school (Hilpert et al. 2012; Husman and Lens 1999). Researchers have argued that instrumentality may be similar to utility value as described by Eccles (1983), although this aspect of value is focused on external constraints creating the connections between learning and future goals. One example is the importance pre-medical students place on the physics courses they take, they do not think they will use the content in the future, but they know their admission to medical school is dependent upon their grades in the class. The extrinsic nature of PI has been challenged by several researchers, Miller et al. (1999) found through a study of 180 undergraduate students enrolled in an intro to psychology course that perceived instrumentality was significantly related to intrinsic and extrinsic valuing. Lens, Simons, and Vansteenkiste have thoroughly examined students' ability to differentiate between extrinsic and intrinsic future value of goals. In their work these researchers have demonstrated the importance of emphasizing intrinsic future goals, and authentic connections between current learning activities and valued future goals (Simons et al. 2003, 2004; Vansteenkiste et al. 2004a, b).

We are certain that there are aspects of the time bubble and FTP that have still not been identified, especially when we consider the structure of goals themselves. Nevertheless, before venturing on to examine where FTP research may go, this is a good place to consider where our work and Zimbardo's are positioned relative to one another.

Zimbardo and the Time Bubble: Intersections and Near Misses

As is well established by Zimbardo and his colleagues, people differ on how far they look into the future and these differences are shaped by a variety of environmental factors (sociocultural, education, religion etc.). Zimbardo has consistently found a link between time perspective to self-regulation and the ability to delay gratification (Zimbardo and Boyd 2008). Additionally, other researchers have extended Zimbardo's work, providing theoretical and empirical connections between Time Perspective and self-regulated learning frameworks such as Expectancy x Value, and Self-Determination Theory (e.g., Lens and Vansteenkiste 2008). Zimbardo and his colleagues have demonstrated that humans who have extended time perspectives are better able to resist the temptations of the immediate activities that might distract them of their long- term goals (Harber et al. 2003). From a Self-Determination Theory perspective, in the development of increasing self-reliance and taking on of greater responsibilities and a stronger identity in their culture, young people adopt extrinsic motivators as part of their own perception of themselves, moving from extrinsic motivation to introjected and then on to identified and finally integrated (Deci et al. 1994; Williams et al. 2009). The most consistent association between students extended time perspective (as measured using the ZTPI), is between introjected and identified regulation; furthermore, extrinsic pressures created by thinking about the future (as measured using the ZTPI) was correlated with less use of metacognitive strategies (de Bilde et al. 2011). Our team of researchers have consistently found positive relationships between Connectedness and Perceptions of Instrumentality, two of the key FTP variables measured in our FTP scale, and students deep cognitive strategy use (Hilpert et al. 2012), volitional strategies (Husman et al. 2000), and strategic learning (Shell and Husman 2008).

There is much about the work done by my colleagues and I that is consistent with that conducted by Zimbardo and his collaborators, particularly with respect to many of the predicted and preferred outcomes. For example, his work in delay of gratification fits well with Zaleski's (1987) finding that an extended time horizon is associated with strong achievement motivation, persistence, and greater satisfaction focusing on their present goals, knowing a positive future awaits. So, we both would agree, that having a longer view of the future is generally healthier and more likely to lead to a good ending. We both, for example, theorize and demonstrate that being able to see present activities as relevant to the future likewise supports positive outcomes.

The key difference between our two approaches, a dispute that we will have to wait for further evidence to help us to adjudicate, is that our teams are making very different wagers about how the brain and mind function to produce the outcomes we observe. Zimbardo has framed his work with each element—past, present, and future—contributing a related but distinct component to a person's overall perspective. The past is framed in terms of emotional valence, the present in terms of risk perception, and the future in terms of distance. The likely fate of a person lies in the interaction of three contributing mechanisms. Our work, in contrast, posits one, albeit rather complicated mechanism. Whether a person's time perspective is dominated by past or future, is narrow or wide, has many goals and paths within or very few, the same four parameters apply and can be measured at all points in the time landscape.

To return to the dilemma that Augustine faced as we opened, are there three different times, each making a different contribution to our cognition and affect? Alternatively, is there one time—the present—that may fix upon these different inputs? Of course, in all three cases, there is likely more of the mind engaged than a few, easily identified and isolated, components, and they may differ from one time orientation than the next. However, it is interesting that memory, both working and long-term, are central in all three cases; even the present would be one unintelligible snapshot after another without working memory to string them together, and long-term memory to infer about the things the snapshots contain.

Considering Culture and FTP

Future Time Perspective theory gives teachers a motivational framework for understanding how and why their students are motivated to participate in classroom activities. Cultural and societal expectations can significantly influence the development and structure of a student's future time perspective (Jones and Brown 2005; Seginer 2008, 2009; Seginer and Halabi 1991) and a teacher could effectively construct a range of versatile and personalized techniques that both identify and take advantage of the individual and culturally influenced FTPs of their students. Children of all ages strive to comprehend their experiences within a society. Changing norms lead to individuals changing their perceptions, potentially allowing young people to have FTP different from that of their parents or mentors. Especially when students live in societies characterized by rapid cultural, political, and economic change, their understandings of these changes can significantly influence their FTP. Societal transitions such as those which occurred during the Arab Spring may create both opportunities and challenges in the development of children's self-awareness. The students understanding of social roles and expectations for their future are therefore impacted by the societal transitions that take place (Thompson 2012).

Although few researchers have addressed the process of transition of time perspectives in relation to social and cultural change, Romero (2009) considered the question of the influence of Time Perspective, as conceptualized by Zimbardo and his colleagues, and acculturation on psychological well-being in Mexican Americans. She hypothesized that acculturation would moderate the relationship between time perspective and psychological well-being in Mexican Americans. Participants completed the Zimbardo Time Perspective Inventory, the Acculturation Rating Scale for Mexican Americans, the Ryff Psychological Well-being scale, and the Developmental Reading assessment in order to verify adequate reading ability. The results from the study suggests, contrary to her original hypothesis, is that a Positive Future time perspective was a better indicator of psychological well-being than acculturation.

Implications in the Classroom

In this section we will discuss Future time perspective and the relation of societal and cultural factors that take part in the cause of one's experiences and perceptions regarding their education and then lay out three implications of FTP theory that can lead to practical techniques that can be utilized in the classroom – the importance of students clarifying their future goals and subgoals, the utility of perceived instrumentality as a diagnostic tool for important motivational problems, and the importance of emphasizing the intrinsic goals (Tabachnick et al. 2008).

Within the context of the classroom, teachers can utilize the understandings gleaned from FTP research to positively impact learning. One of the strategies that a teacher could implement is using interventions to help develop personal goals and sub-goals for at-risk students. Daphna Oyserman and Hazel Markus (1990) have demonstrated that students who lack balanced future possible selves, future oriented self-concepts, are at higher risk of delinquency. Interventions to promote longer FTPs can be used as a strategy to overcome delinquency and retention problems. Oyserman and her colleagues have demonstrated that partnerships between mentors and students, which focus on goal setting for the future, and considering how the present links to the future supports the development of academic possible selves (Destin and Oyserman 2010; Oyserman et al. 2002). The purpose of such interventions would be to determine and develop students' future selves and goals. This is a different approach to what is done in remedial courses, which try to help foster success by teaching learning strategies and tutoring (NCES 2004). Once a teacher has recognized that a student is at risk of failing they would set up an individual conference with them. The teacher would ask the student questions such as, "What plans do you have for after high school?" and, "Where do you see yourself in five years?" The teacher could then use the responses to help the student construct a model of their future self; this could be drawn out as a chart as an aid. If the student indicates that they have a short FTP than the teacher can use the conference to help the student develop an FTP for themselves by connecting it with their current interests and priorities. The important thing is that the teacher or mentor helps to navigate the student down a path that enables them to lengthen their FTP and consider future academic possible selves.

Another way to develop students future oriented motivation is to assist students' in the development of their perceptions of instrumentality or utility value. PI is an incentive that may encourage students to persist at important activities that are not inherently pleasurable (Greene et al. 2004). A teacher can use PI as an early warning signal for student motivational problems using an informative assessment at the end of activities (Tabachnick et al. 2008). Specifically, Tabachnick et al. (2008) showed that when students write a short paragraph that answers the prompt, 'what did you learn or gain from this lesson?' or, 'how will this be useful to you in the future?' after a particular classroom activity, teachers can gauge student's PI for those activities. If a student is constantly showing through their responses that they have a low PI for the class' activities then it might be an indicator that an intervention is necessary.

Hulleman (Hulleman et al. 2008; Hulleman and Harackiewicz 2009) and his colleagues have demonstrated that asking students to write on the value of learning of activities does produce the positive motivational outcomes FTP researchers would expect from an increase in students PI. Hulleman's research is notable for the different types of activities he has demonstrated this effect. His research has included physical education, science, and mathematics students. Consistently, students who recognize the utility of their learning activities have sustained improved learning outcomes after a delay.

Teachers may also implement classroom discussion that encourages students to recognize and develop perceptions of instrumentality for succeeding in the class. The research of Vansteenkiste, Lens, and Simons reminds us of the importance of ensuring that intrinsic goals are emphasized in classroom discussions of the future utility of classroom learning activities (Vansteenkiste et al. 2004a, 2005). These researchers demonstrated that simply making connections between present and any future goal is not as effective, and may in fact be detrimental to motivation. The Intrinsic motivation has been shown to be a much more powerful contributor to success in a classroom goal-based system than extrinsic motivators (Tabachnick et al. 2008). An example of an extrinsic classroom motivator might be to complete the class to graduate and make more money. Examples of intrinsic motivation might be a student excelling in class because they want to use the skills that they learn in the class to contribute positively to their community. To help students recognize possible reasons to be intrinsically motivated about the class a teacher could set up a class debate early on in the semester. The students will have to argue why the class is or is not important to them and how the content could be used to support pro-social goals.

Zimardo's most recent work reminds us that optimal well-being can be found when we focus on where we are going (Zimbardo et al. 2012). Our own research as well as the strong work of Lens and his colleagues can assist teachers to consider the optimal approaches that may be taken to help students see their futures, guide their present, and build on their past.

References

Addis, D. R., Wong, A. T., & Schacter, D. L. (2007). Remembering the past and imagining the future: Common and distinct neural substrates during event construction and elaboration. *Neuropsychologia, 45*(7), 1363–1377. doi:10.1016/j.neuropsychologia.2006.10.016.

Brickman, S. J., & Miller, R. B. (2001). The impact of sociocultural context on future goals and self-regulation. In D. M. McInerney & S. Van Etten (Eds.), *Research on sociocultural influences on motivation and learning* (pp. 119–137). Greenwich: Information Age.

Daltrey, M. H., & Langer, P. (1984). Development and evaluation of a measure of future time perspective. *Perceptual and Motor Skills, 58*(3), 719–725.

de Bilde, J., Vansteenkiste, M., & Lens, W. (2011). Understanding the association between future time perspective and self-regulated learning through the lens of self-determination theory. *Learning and Instruction, 21*(3), 332–344. doi:10.1016/j.learninstruc.2010.03.002.

de Volder, M. L., & Lens, W. (1982). Academic achievement and future time perspective as a cognitive–motivational concept. *Journal of Personality and Social Psychology, 42*(3), 566–571.

Deci, E. L., Eghrari, H., Patrick, B. C., & Leone, D. (1994). Facilitating internalization: The self-determination theory perspective. *Journal of Personality, 62*, 119–142.

Destin, M., & Oyserman, D. (2010). Incentivizing education: Seeing schoolwork as an investment, not a chore. *Journal of Experimental Social Psychology, 46*(5), 846–849. doi:10.1016/j.jesp.2010.04.004.

Eccles, J. S. (1983). Expectancies, values, and academic behaviors. In J. T. Spence (Ed.), *Achievement and achievement motives* (pp. 75–146). San Francisco: W. H. Freeman.

Friedman, W. J. (1993). Memory for the time of past events. *Psychological Bulletin, 113*(1), 44–66.

Greene, B. A., Miller, R. B., Crowson, H. M., Duke, B. L., & Akey, K. L. (2004). Predicting high school students' cognitive engagement and achievement: Contributions of classroom perceptions and motivation. *Contemporary Educational Psychology, 29*, 462–482.

Halvari, H. (1991a). Goal distance in time and its effects on the relations between achievement motives, future-time orientation, and motor performance among girls and boys. *Perceptual and Motor Skills, 72*(2), 675–697.

Halvari, H. (1991b). Perception of goal proximity, latency and duration of action plans, and worry in relation to goal distance in time and personality characteristics. *Perceptual and Motor Skills, 72*(3, Pt 1), 707–741.

Halvari, H. (1996). Personality and educational choice of general versus vocational studies among 16- to 19-year-olds. *Psychological Reports, 78*, 1379–1388.

Harber, K. D., Zimbardo, P. G., & Boyd, J. N. (2003). Participant self-selection biases as a function of individual differences in time perspective. *Basic and Applied Social Psychology, 25*(3), 255–264.

Hilpert, C. J., Husman, J., Stump, S. G., Kim, W., Chung, W., & Duggan, A. M. (2012). Examining students' future time perspective: Pathways to knowledge building. *Japanese Psychological Association, 54*, 229–240.

Hulleman, C. S., & Harackiewicz, J. M. (2009). Promoting interest and performance in high school science classes. *Science, 326*(5958), 1410–1412. doi:10.1126/science.1177067.

Hulleman, C. S., Durik, A. M., Schweigert, S. B., & Harackiewicz, J. M. (2008). Task values, achievement goals, and interest: An integrative analysis. *Journal of Educational Psychology, 100*(2), 398–416.

Husman, J. (1998). *The effects of perceptions of the future on intrinsic motivaiton*. Dissertation, University of Texas at Austin, Austin.

Husman, J. (2012). *Using the future to stay motivated in the present: Learning in engineering*. Key note address. International conference on time perspective. Coimbra, Portugal.

Husman, J., & Lens, W. (1999). The role of the future in student motivation. *Educational Psychologist, 34*(2), 113–125.

Husman, J., & Shell, D. F. (2008). Beliefs and perceptions about the future: A measurement of future time perspective. *Learning and Individual Differences, 18*(2), 166–175.

Husman, J., McCann, E. J., & Crowson, H. M. (2000). Volitional strategies and future time perspective: embracing the complexity of dynamic interactions. *International Journal of Educational Research, 33*, 777–799.

Husman, J., Derryberry, W. P., Crowson, H. M., & Lomax, R. (2004). Instrumentality, task value, and intrinsic motivation: Making sense of their independent interdependence. *Contemporary Educational Psychology, 29*(1), 63–76.

Jones, J. M., & Brown, W. T. (2005). Any time is Trinidad time! Cultural variations in the value and function of time. In A. Strathman & J. Joireman (Eds.), *Understanding behavior in the context of time: Theory, research, and application* (pp. 305–323). Mahwah: Lawrence Erlbaum Associates Publishers.

Klein, S. B., Robertson, T. E., & Delton, A. W. (2011). The future-orientation of memory: Planning as a key component mediating the high levels of recall found with survival processing. *Memory, 19*(2), 121–139. doi: Pii 932277976.

Lens, W., & Vansteenkiste, M. (2008). Promoting self-regulated learning a motivational analysis. In *Motivation and self-regulated learning: Theory, research, and applications* (pp. 141–168). Mahwah: Lawrence Erlbaum Associates Publishers.

Malka, A., & Covington, M. V. (2005). Perceiving school performance as instrumental to future goal attainment: Effects on graded performance. *Contemporary Educational Psychology, 30*(1), 60–80.

Miller, R. B., DeBacker, T. K., & Greene, B. A. (1999). Perceived instrumentality and academics: The link to task valuing. *Journal of Instructional Psychology, 26*(4), 250–260.

National Center for Educational Statistics. (2004). *The condition of education: Student effort and educational progress.* Retrieved September 30, 2004, from http://www.nces.ed.gov/programs/coe/2004/section3/indicator16.asp and http://www.nces.ed.gov/programs/coe/2004/section3/indicator18.asp

Nuttin, J. R. (1964). The future time perspective in human motivation and learning. *Acta Psychologica, 23*, 60–82.

Nuttin, J., & Lens, W. (1985). *Future time perspective and motivation: Theory and research method.* Leuven & Hillsdale: Leuven University Press & Erlbaum.

Okhuysen, G., Galinsky, A. D., & Uptigrove, T. A. (2003). Saving the worst for last: The effect of time horizon on the efficiency of negotiating benefits and burdens. *Organizational Behavior and Human Decision Processes, 91*, 269–279.

Oyserman, D., & Markus, H. R. (1990). Possible selves and delinquency. *Journal of Personality & Social Psychology, 59*(1), 112–125.

Oyserman, D., Terry, K., & Bybee, D. (2002). A possible selves intervention to enhance school involvement. *Journal of Adolescence, 25*(3), 313–326. doi:10.1006/jado.2002.0474.

Peetsma, T. (2000). Future time perspectives as a predictor of school investment. *Scandinavian Journal of Educational Research, 44*(2), 177–192.

Romero, H. (2009). *Time perspective, acculturation, and psychological well-being in Mexican American.* Dissertation, Seattle Pacific University, Seattle Washington.

Seginer, R. (2008). Future orientation in times of threat and challenge: How resilient adolescents construct their future. *International Journal of Behavioral Development, 32*(4), 272–282. doi:10.1177/0165025408090970.

Seginer, R. (2009). *Future orientation: Developmental and ecological perspectives: New York.* New York: Springer Science+Business Media.

Seginer, R., & Halabi, H. (1991). Cross-cultural variations of adolescents' future orientation: The case of Israeli Druze versus Israeli Arab and Jewish male. *Journal of Cross-Cultural Psychology, 22*(2), 224–237.

Shell, D. F., & Husman, J. (2001). The multivariate dimensionality of personal control and future time perspective in achievement and studying. *Contemporary Educational Psychology, 26*, 481–506.

Shell, D. F., & Husman, J. (2008). Control, motivation, affect, and strategic self-regulation in the college classroom: A multidimensional phenomenon. *Journal of Educational Psychology, 100*(2), 443–459. doi:10.1037/0022-0663.100.2.443.

Simons, J., Dewitte, S., & Lens, W. (2003). "Don't do it for me. Do it for yourself!" Stressing the personal relevance enhances motivation in physical education. *Journal of Sport & Exercise Psychology, 25*(2), 145–160.

Simons, J., Vansteenkiste, M., Lens, W., & Lacante, M. (2004). Placing motivation and future time perspective theory in a temporal perspective. *Educational Psychology Review, 16*(2), 121–139. doi:10.1023/B:EDPR.0000026609.94841.2f.

Tabachnick, S. E., Miller, R. B., & Relyea, G. E. (2008). The relationships among students' future-oriented goals and subgoals, perceived task instrumentality, and task-oriented self-regulation strategies in an academic environment. *Journal of Educational Psychology, 100*(3), 629–642. doi:10.1037/0022-0663.100.3.629.

Thompson, R. (2012). Changing societies, changing childhood: Studying the impact of globalization on child development. *Child Development Perspectives, 6*(2), 187–192.

Vansteenkiste, M., Simons, J., Lens, W., Soenens, B., Matos, L., & Lacante, M. (2004a). Less is sometimes more: Goal content matters. *Journal of Educational Psychology, 96*(4), 755–764.

Vansteenkiste, M., Simons, J., Soenens, B., & Lens, W. (2004b). How to become a persevering exerciser? Providing a clear, future intrinsic goal in an autonomy-supportive way. *Journal of Sport & Exercise Psychology, 26*(2), 232–249.

Vansteenkiste, M., Simons, J., Lens, W., Soenens, B., & Matos, L. (2005). Examining the motivational impact of intrinsic versus extrinsic goal framing and autonomy-supportive versus internally controlling communication style on early adolescents' academic achievement. *Child Development, 76*(2), 483–501.

Williams, G. C., Niemiec, C. P., Patrick, H., Ryan, R. M., & Deci, E. L. (2009). The importance of supporting autonomy and perceived competence in facilitating long-term tobacco abstinence. *Annals of Behavioral Medicine, 37*, 315–324.

Zaleski, Z. (1987). Behavioral effects of self-set goals for different time ranges. *International Journal of Psychology, 22*(1), 17–38.

Zimbardo, P. & Boyd, J. (2008). *The time paradox: The new psychology of time that will change your life*. New York: Free Press.

Zimbardo, P., Sword, R., & Sword, R. (2012). *The time cure: Overcoming PTSD with the new psychology of time perspective therapy.* San Francisco: Jossey-Bass.

From Time Perspective to Psychological Distance (and Back)

Sam J. Maglio, Yaacov Trope, and Nira Liberman

To mark his retirement in 2003, Phil Zimbardo received a proper and through roasting from his colleague and friend, Gordon Bower. No gold watch, no paperweight, just a smattering of stories from a storied career. And what yarns did Bower deem worthy of spinning? He begins by flashing back "a very long way" to the year 1955 and his first meeting with classmate Zimbardo.[1] He anchors his remarks nearly 50 years in the past, and there he remains for the majority of the toast. Narrating from Stanford's Palo Alto campus, he conjures up images and events from New Haven, a continent away, where the two completed their graduate training at Yale's Psychology Department. He recounts the shenanigans of a host of characters belonging exclusively to that time and place, identifying them only by their initials ("D. D., who produced homemade beer in his bathtub that tasted like it was indeed fermented from his bath water, or that borderline personality, T.B., who'd drop by unannounced at midnight to drink up all our cheap wine and insult us"). He describes the one-in-a-million of circumstances the brought them together in the first place (Bower originally pursuing mathematics; the fact that, "kids usually got out of Phil's neighborhood in an ambulance or a paddy wagon; they got out of [his] neighborhood by back-breaking, mind-numbing work on a farm or in the coal mines"). Altogether, Bower paints a lighthearted, flattering portrait of Professor Emeritus Zimbardo. But, with a lifetime of material from which to pull, why did he share these specific memories?

[1] http://www.zimbardo.com/downloads/Phils%20Retirement%20Speech.pdf

S.J. Maglio (✉)
Department of Marketing, University of Toronto Scarborough, Toronto, ON, Canada
e-mail: sam.maglio@utoronto.ca

Y. Trope
Department of Psychology, New York University, New York, NY, USA
e-mail: yaacov.trope@nyu.edu

N. Liberman
Department of Psychology, Tel Aviv University, Tel Aviv, Israel
e-mail: niralib@post.tau.ac.il

M. Stolarski et al. (eds.), *Time Perspective Theory; Review, Research and Application: Essays in Honor of Philip G. Zimbardo*, DOI 10.1007/978-3-319-07368-2_9,

With this chapter, we identify a consistent thread running through each of Bower's recollections: They all center upon psychologically distant times, places, people, and probabilities. We will first conceptualize a formal definition of psychological distance and then review evidence supporting the association among different dimensions of distance and the interchangeability of these distances. Expanding from psychological distance to time perspective and the Zimbardo Time Perspective Inventory, we compare and contrast these frameworks. We highlight the insights to basic and applied psychology offered by both, and we propose that each has the potential to speak volumes the other. Dispatches from the interface of these perspectives reveal intriguing possibilities for future research, and the theoretical and practical implications of such investigations are discussed.

Defining Distance

The anecdotes Gordon Bower told to his audience shared many similarities. They all related to Phil Zimbardo. They portrayed character through example. They packaged flattery in verbal abuse. But, most germane for our purposes here, none of them had anything to do with where Bower himself stood as he orated (or, for that matter, where Zimbardo was standing). Rather, they all belonged to the ether outside his direct experience at that time – they all transcended his egocentric perspective. More generally, any target that is not present in the here and now, that is beyond one's immediate environment, can be conceptualized as psychologically distant.

Parsing the vast realm outside of immediate experience, construal level theory (Liberman and Trope 2008; Trope and Liberman 2010) has identified four primary avenues along which a target of representation can become psychologically distant: time, geographical space, social distance, and probability. Through this lens, let us return to the selection of stories with which we opened this chapter. The retirement party begins half a century in the past, focusing on the distant time when Bower and Zimbardo met. Fittingly, this event took place not just down the street from where the retirement party was being held, but in a spatially distant venue on the other side of the country (New Haven). This time and place was populated not by lifelong friends (save for each other), but rather by socially distant others with which they presently share very few similarities and little contact (D.D., T.B.). An air of probabilistic distance hung over all of these proceedings, as the odds that Bower and Zimbardo would cross paths at all were vanishingly low from the outset.

Associations Among Distances

We have embraced this retirement monologue because it serves as a very efficient example, illustrating not just one isolated instantiation of psychological distance, but rather invoking each of the four dimensions simultaneously. Of course, it is entirely possible to imagine a target that is distant along one – and only one – of the four avenues: People make future plans for themselves (rather than others), consider the perspective of another person sitting in the same room (rather than across town), and test probability in taking risks immediately (rather than down the road). Still, anecdotal evidence suggests that Doctor Bower may not be alone in his tendency to pair distance with distance (or the opposite – proximity with proximity). Consider how just about everybody fills in the following blank: "a long time ago in a ____ place".

Why does the distant past sync so well in our minds with a *faraway* place rather than a *next door* place? A recent investigation into this question contends that people tend to remember and anticipate their real world experiences as sharing a similar feeling of distance (Fiedler et al. 2012). In one study, research participants envisioned a situation in which two of the distance dimensions were explicitly stated and two remained unknown. For example, they considered having an argument with a close friend in a nearby location (or a distant acquaintance in a faraway location), leaving the temporal and probabilistic distance unknown. When asked to rate how far the event subjectively felt on the unknown dimensions, people gave ratings that corresponded to the known distances: The nearby argument with a good friend was expected to happen sooner and was more likely to happen, and vice versa for the distant argument. A second study documented similar positive correlations among subjective distance ratings (on all four dimensions) for actual past autobiographical events. However, people do not need an initial distance cue to impact how near or far an event feels. For example, students at the University of Colorado at Boulder were asked to write in emotional (or neutral) terms about the April, 2007, shootings at Virginia Tech (Van Boven et al. 2010). Afterward, they indicated how far they felt from when the shootings happened (time), where they happened (the Virginia Tech campus, space), and the Virginia Tech students (social). Ratings at the individual level correlated strongly across the three distances, and all aspects of the event felt close for those who wrote in emotional terms. Thus, not only does distance on one dimension imply distance on all dimensions, but subjective feelings of distance also tend to respond similarly to certain external forces.

Because the four distances tend to move together in subjective experience, it stands to reason the introduction of distance on one dimension should trigger an inference of distance on any of the other dimensions. Stephan and colleagues explored this possibility in the domain of language, using politeness as a proxy for social distance (and the reverse, with colloquial speech reflecting social closeness). Research participants read descriptions of situations that had been phrased either more politely or more colloquially, and then they estimated when that event would occur. Consistent with the hypothesis, people who read the polite description expected it to happen in the more distant future than did people who read about the same event phrased more colloquially (Stephan et al. 2010). This suggests that social distance leads to the inference of greater temporal distance; a separate study confirmed a similar effect of politeness on the inference of spatial distance. Furthermore, when research participants were charged with the task of generating a message for another person, they worded those messages more politely when that other person was believed to receive the communication in the distant future or in a distant location. This bi-directional relationship between politeness (i.e., social distance) and both time and space supports the existence of a shared meaning among these distances.

Additional research broadens the scope of these effects to include different dimensions and operationalizations of distance. For instance, inferences of social distance can be captured using a variety of measures beyond politeness. To wit, the introduction of temporal distance also makes other people feel less familiar and less similar to the self, indicative of greater social distance (Stephan et al. 2011). A more straightforward conceptualization of social distance – the binary distinction between self and other – provides a connection to the fourth and final dimension of distance, probability. When people judge what kinds of things will happen to whom, they anticipate likely, common (i.e., probabilistically close) events for themselves but less likely, rare circumstances (i.e., probabilistically distant) to befall other people (Chambers et al. 2003; Kruger and Burrus 2004). These rare events of remote probability are also expected to transpire in geographically remote locations and in remote times (Wakslak 2012). Taken together, these studies provide robust evidence that each dimension of distance has a consistent and strong impact on inferences for each of the other distances.

How basic is this association among the four dimensions of distance, and what are the downstream consequences of this interrelation? To the first question, Bar-Anan et al. (2007) reasoned that if the different distances indeed share an inherent common meaning, then they should also share a nonconscious association. They tested this hypothesis in a series of studies in which participants were presented with pictures containing depth cues to make presented words appear spatially near or far. The words themselves pertained to proximity or distality on the remaining (non-spatial) dimensions of distance (e.g., "us" or "them" as markers of social distance). Given the task to indicate as quickly as possible the location of the word (spatially close or far), participants responded fastest when the distance implied by the content of the word matched the spatial distance cue from its location (e.g., "us" presented proximally or "them" presented distally). As reaction time responses are enacted too quickly to allow for explicit deliberation, the results from this study support the idea that the four dimensions of distance share an implicit, automatic interrelationship in human cognition.

At the other end of the spectrum, we can consider how expectations based upon this relationship (i.e., that targets distant on one dimension should be distant on all dimensions) impact explicit, willful judgments and decisions. Zhao and Xie (2011) examined circumstances in which recommendations from others exerted greater impact on consumer attitudes. They found that *who* exerted more influence depended upon *when* the potential purchase was to be made: People were more strongly persuaded by a recommendation from socially close others when considering a purchase for the near future, but placed greater weight on the recommendation from a distant other person when considering a later purchase. Further, because people mentally pair improbable events with distant places and times, they indicate greater willingness to bet on underdogs (i.e., long shots) when the outcome is determined in a spatially distant (versus near) location and a greater desire to insure against unlikely mishaps in the distant (versus near) future (Wakslak 2012). Thus, there appears to exist a natural fit between the different dimensions of distance, powerful enough to shape explicit, real-world decision making.

Interchangeability of Distances

A clear association has emerged whereby time, space, social distance, and probability all tap into a unified construct of psychological distance. Thus far, we have reviewed evidence in support of this conclusion that is based on assimilation among the different distances: When the location of a target (i.e., near or far) is known on one dimension of distance, people infer a similar location of that target on each of the other dimensions, and this fit appears to be both automatic (on the implicit level) and powerful (on explicit judgment). But how would initial distancing on one dimension impact a constant, known span of distance from another dimension? For example, might we observe a shift in sensitivity to a known time delay (i.e., a given magnitude of temporal distance) depending upon whether it is framed from the outset as *spatially* near or far? More generally, what is the effect of distance on distance itself? We recently examined this exact question, predicting that an initial distance cue would cause a second, given span of distance to subjectively shrink (Maglio et al. 2013).

We based this hypothesis on previous findings that constituted, to us, within-dimension distancing, which considered how initial distancing caused further distance from the same dimension to loom less large. The vast majority of this research came from the intertemporal decision-making literature, showing that the value of a delayed reward decreases at a declining rate over longer periods of time (Frederick et al. 2002). Importantly, this phenomenon has been documented for other distances as well – namely, social distance and probability (Green and Myerson 2004; Jones and Rachlin 2006). This decreasing sensitivity with increasing distance is reflected in a variety of judgments and decisions, the most prevalent of which involves a reversal in preference between receiving a small reward sooner or a larger reward later. For example, a person may prefer $5 now over $10 the next day but would simultaneously prefer $10 in 366 days over $5 in 365 days (Thaler 1981). Such preference reversals have been explained as resulting from insensitivity to prospective duration estimates (Zauberman et al. 2009). That is, subjective judgments of how long a stretch of time will feel do not correspond to objective time but instead suggest that people are more sensitive to proximal intervals of time than to distal intervals. From our perspective, this reflects initial temporal distance reducing sensitivity to a second time delay.

In testing how psychological distance affects sensitivity to subsequent instantiations of psychological distance, all of the studies on this issue adopted a similar design: We first manipulated initial distance by framing the judgment task as either near or far (e.g., occurring in a near or far location) and thereafter assessed sensitivity to a constant, known amount of distance from another dimension (e.g., the magnitude of a given time delay). If the different distances represent a sort of common currency with an interchangeable meaning, we expected to observe a similar reduction in sensitivity when looking at the impact of an initial distance from one domain on a second distance from another. For example, a wait of 1 month should seem shorter when it pertains to a spatially more distant event, and one study tested this possibility. Research participants chose between receiving either \$50 immediately or \$65 after 3 months. They were told that their payment would be deposited into an online bank account and accessible immediately and also that the central branch of that bank was located in either a spatially near or distal location. As predicted, those with their money to be stored in a distant bank were more likely to choose the larger-later option – in keeping with the proposition that sensitivity to the delay was reduced with the introduction of initial spatial distance.

Would spatial distance have a similar impact on other distances? A separate study considered how geographical space impacts sensitivity to social distance. First, participants imagined making a list of their 100 closest friends – ranging from their best friend to a mere acquaintance – and then thought of who would fit best at positions #5 and #20. Next, they indicated the dollar amount at which they would be indifferent between giving \$75 to their fifth-closest friend and that indifference amount to their twentieth-closest friend. Utilizing the bank account manipulation, people demanded less money to attain indifference (revealed a reduced sensitivity to the social distance between #5 and #20) for the distal bank.

To further broaden our scope, another study introduced initial social distance and assessed how people evaluate probabilities. Participants imagined entering a lottery that provided a free entry but gave the reward to a member of their social network. Again, they imagined listing their 100 closest friends, and participants were randomly assigned specifically to consider #5, #45, or #95. They then indicated whether they believed that person would prefer an 80 % chance to win a \$50 reward or a 20 % chance for \$200. When deciding for a close person (#5), people proved especially sensitive to probability, preferring the safer gamble. However, when choosing for a distal person (either #45 or #95), people were less sensitive to probability and opted for the larger, less likely payoff. This suggests that people make choices for others that reflect a diminishing sensitivity to probability as a function of social distance.

While these first studies all assessed outcomes designed to reflect sensitivity to initial distance, the final study directly explored our proposed mechanism of diminishing sensitivity to other dimensions of distance. Here, we asked participants to imagine receiving free passes to a museum that was scheduled to open 27 miles from their home. We manipulated initial temporal distance by indicating that the museum was to open either in 1 week or 1 year. First, they reported how subjectively far away the museum felt to them. Next, they reported how interested they were in using the passes to visit the museum. As predicted, initial temporal distance caused the length of that 27-mile span of space to subjectively shrink, and this effect mediated the relationship between greater temporal distance and increased willingness to visit the museum.

Table 1 Overview of experiments by initial and second distance

	Initial distance			
Second distance	Spatial	Temporal	Probabilistic	Social
Spatial		Study 8 (*J*+*D*)		
Temporal	Study 3 (*D*)		Study 2 (*J*)	Studies 1A & 1B (*J*)
Probabilistic	Study 4 (*D*)			Study 7 (*D*)
Social	Study 5 (*D*)		Study 6 (*D*)	

Note: The parentheses alongside each specific study indicate the type of task performed by participants: J = judgment of subjective magnitude of second distance; D = decision designed to reflect sensitivity to second distance; J + D = both types of tasks. From Maglio et al. (2013)

Altogether, nine studies supported the hypothesis that the relevance of any span of distance is reduced when it is framed as distal. Overall, each of the four dimensions of distance were used at least once as both the initial as well as the second distance, and Table 1 provides a summary of the different distances examined in each specific study. Consistently, the experience of an initial instantiation of distance reduces sensitivity to additional instantiations of temporal, spatial, social, and probabilistic distance. These findings suggest that the dimensions of psychological distance share a common, interchangeable meaning and that the difference between far and further is much less than that between near and far.

Of course, ours was but one approach to documenting a sort of common currency among the different dimensions of distance. Looking not within a single empirical paper but rather across the corpus of literature on psychological distance provides another perspective on interchangeability: A number of separate research programs empirically manipulated different forms of psychological distance and found comparable effects across them when making similar judgments. This general link between distance and judgment has been summarized elsewhere (Trope and Liberman 2010), so we will expound upon only one example, creativity, by means of illustration. To begin, distance is theorized to broaden the scope with which people mentally construe their world. As a result, distancing not only enables links to other varieties of distance (see 'Associations Among Distances' section above) but it also makes people more inclusive in their consideration sets or the possibilities they are willing to entertain. These latter two outcomes have been predicted to enhance creative thought, and this has been found in the empirical literature across all four dimensions of distance. People who expect to perform a task in the distant (versus near) future generate more creative responses on that task (Förster et al. 2004), and people who expect that they are probabilistically unlikely (versus likely) to perform the same task show a similar boost in creative responding (Wakslak et al. 2006). When given a task ostensibly designed by a group from a spatially distant (versus close) location, people list more creative answers when they themselves perform the task (Jia et al. 2009). When primed to think about distal locations (the globe, the solar system) kids scored higher on a creativity test than when primed to think about proximal locations (their class, their desk, Liberman et al. 2012). Finally, people draw more creative figures and are more likely to solve problems requiring creative insight when performing those tasks on behalf of others rather than for themselves (Polman and Emich 2011). Thus, whether interchangeable at the level of cross-dimensional diminishing sensitivity or cross-dimensional consistent shifts in cognition, the four dimensions of psychological distance relate to one other in a fundamental way.

The Personality Perspective: Two Questions

Research from our lab and others has underscored the power of psychological distance, revealing an interconnected network of associations and a systematic impact on judgment and decision making. These findings have provided evidence for commonalities among time, space, social distance, and probability. However, they have told only the situational part of the story, manipulating distance and assessing a host of outcomes. What can be said of the situation's precursors – the personality variables that complicate the story into richer, more nuanced detail? Much has been said of and done with the Zimbardo Time Perspective Inventory (ZTPI; Zimbardo and Boyd 1999), and we will not aspire to summarize it properly here. Rather, let us consider two specific questions arising from the interface of this model and our own conceptualization of psychological distance.

First, might we extrapolate from the ZTPI in an effort to quantify individual differences in orientation on the remaining three dimensions of psychological distance (i.e., space, social distance, and probability)? Zimbardo and Boyd (1999) decomposed time in a manner quite different from the usual approach taken by psychological distance researchers, examining not strictly a binary distinction between near and far but rather a multitude of factors (five, to be exact) within this single construct: Past-Negative, Present-Hedonistic, Future, Past-Positive, and Present-Fatalistic. Might we expect a similar set of factors to underlie the natural tendencies people adopt in thinking about space, social distance, and probability? Though we only hope to raise rather than to answer this question here, an interesting point of entry may lie in the role of valence; the ZTIP distinguishes between now and then (and further between future and past) in addition to a factor marking positivity versus negativity. This hints at the possibility of dispositional differences in, for example, thinking local or global (spatially) and further in perseverating upon local tragedies versus global successes. Similar predictions could be derived for social and probabilistic distance as well.

Alternatively, the straightforward binary distinction of near versus far might prove more immediately useful in quantifying any such personality measure. The best candidate very well may be the reflection of social distance in self-construal (Singelis 1994). This construct differentiates between independence (i.e., anchoring on the perspective of the self) and interdependence (i.e., incorporating the more distant viewpoints of others). Additionally, if we take a looser interpretation of individual differences with respect to spatial distance, Maddux and Galinsky (2009) found measurable differences among people who spent more time living in a foreign country – to us, people who anchored their lives geographically far from their point of origin. It bears noting that their dependent measure assessed creativity, whereby people who had lived abroad performed better on measures of creative insight. This finding provides an important link, documenting an association between spatial distance and creativity at the dispositional level that has a parallel in situational manipulation of spatial distance boosting creativity as well.

For a variation on this theme – connecting temporal distance and self-control – we need look no further than Zimbardo's and our own research groups. An orientation toward the future, as documented by the ZTPI, predicts a host of self-control successes that range from students completing course requirements to adults coping with homelessness (Epel et al. 1999; Harber et al. 2003). In our own work (Freitas et al. 2001), we have found that people planning for the future more readily forsake short-term indulgence for their long-term interests (see also Fujita et al. 2006). If personality-level differences did indeed exist for all four dimensions of distance, a corollary of our first question should ask whether these orientations share a mutual association. That is, would future-looking individuals also tend to take the long-view on each of the other distances? After all, developmental research has established a correlation in the emergent ability to traverse each of the different distances. We have already established a similar such relationship among the four distances via experimental manipulation, and the creativity and self-control connections suggest that dispositional distance may operate in much the same way as the situational counterpart. Should this be the case, we would predict a dispositional orientation toward distance on any dimension (or, potentially, all of them at once) to evince similar consequences to the well-documented effects of a future-oriented time perspective (see this volume).

Still, a host of complications remain inherent in attempting to quantify and then unify individual difference metrics for each dimension of psychological distance. We have provided evidence for similarities among the four distance dimensions insofar as they constitute removal from an egocentric *here and now* reference point, but they also have important differences. Take the clear contrast between time and probability: The future can be seen as uncertain as it has not yet materialized, but the past (temporally distant, but in the other direction) most certainly has occurred. This dissociation may, in fact, capture the reason why the ZTPI posits two factors for the past but only one for the future, to say nothing of the two dimensions of present-orientation.

Accordingly, before considering a potential interchangeability of dispositional orientation among the four dimensions of distance, a more appropriate starting point might inquire after the classic psychological issue of how the person interacts with his or her situation. Regardless of personal tendencies or orientations, everyone at certain times reflects on the past, acts in the present, and plans for the future. Indeed, this capacity for mental time travel is a hallmark of our species. At the same time, the ZTPI acknowledges that certain individuals maintain an innate tendency or preference to anchor their minds in one of those three time perspectives (and with different appraisals thereof). What is the consequence, therefore, of matching the person to the situation? Are people who chronically live their mental lives connected to their own future better able to simulate it when the situation demands it? Conversely, are present-oriented individuals particularly successful in judgments and decisions for the here and (especially) now? And does this appropriateness or fit between disposition and situation make for a happier, healthier human?

Although the previous paragraph ended with not one but four queries, not one of them constitutes our second, overarching question framing this section. Whereas those issues relate to within-dimension fit between person and situation, our primary interest remains with the notion of commonalities shared among the different dimensions of distance. As such, we offer the following conjecture: Might individuals differ in their inclination or ability to traverse psychological distance – from near to far and back – from either the same or different dimensions? Certainly, a dispositional orientation toward the future should facilitate the simulation of future (versus sooner) outcomes given that one's chronic thoughts tend to live in that temporal venue. But, given that a person has anchored his or her thoughts in a given context of psychological distance (e.g., spatially far, socially close), how easily can that person switch to a new location within the same dimension of distance (e.g., spatially close, socially far) or across distance modality (e.g., temporally close, probabilistically far)?

This question adds a new fold to the ZTPI, asking not where individuals tend to anchor their thoughts in time, but how easily they might adopt a different temporal perspective. Of the five factors comprising the ZTPI, we see future orientation as the best potential predictor of success in mental transitions (at least within a single dimension). Not only do future-oriented individuals attune their thoughts to the higher-order goals shaping the broad scope of their lives, but they also manage to implement related behavior in the present moment that makes successful progress toward these goals (Harber et al. 2003). It stands to reason that these individuals may enjoy the best of both worlds, readily transitioning between a strong, temporally distanced awareness of their long-term interests before importing these priorities to the present moment, helping them to overcome short-term temptations in navigating their immediate environments.

If ZTPI researchers stand to learn from within-dimension (i.e., temporal) transitions, psychological distance researchers stand to learn from cross-dimension distance transitions. We have established that distance on one dimension elicits the inference of distance on all dimensions (as evidenced by the effects documented previously). However, might these effects only obtain among people who readily associate (and, necessarily, succeed in traversing between) the four established dimensions of distance? Importantly, the psychological profile of people who struggle to extrapolate from one distance to another might shed light on a question that has followed psychological distance research for decades: the issue of whether one particular distance fundamentally encapsulates the others. For instance, if space underlies how people reason about all distance because it is the only dimension experienced physically (Boroditsky 2000), might cultures for whom this space-time metaphor is not prevalent struggle to traverse between them?

Looking Backward, Looking Forward

If imitation is the sincerest form of flattery, we delight in ending this chapter in much the same way Zimbardo and Boyd concluded their seminal paper on ZTPI: with the hope that a balance in perspective – situational and dispositional – may allow for optimality in life, from its planning to its experience to its recalled highlight reel (Zimbardo and Boyd 1999). We echo their call for a balanced perspective, at the level of individual lives, in our hope of quantifying how easily people transition between distant and proximal perspectives. After all, research from both of our groups suggests that long-term interests are served best by distant-future planning, but people ultimately must make their choices in the multitude of present moments that threaten to compromise those aspirations. We hope our unique take on time as but one psychological distance frames time perspective in a broader context, allowing measures such as the ZTPI to communicate with a broader scope of possible individual differences in orientation on other distance dimensions. Just as the dynamic, real-time experience of psychological distance cannot perfectly be distilled into binary, lab-based distinctions, nor either can personality variables operate in a vacuum devoid of situational determinants. As such, if basic psychological research hopes to broaden its scope beyond the lab to inform applied, real-world issues, it must take into account both the situational and the dispositional factors that shape human behavior.

References

Bar-Anan, Y., Liberman, N., Trope, Y., & Algom, D. (2007). Automatic processing of psychological distance: Evidence from a Stroop task. *Journal of Experimental Psychology: General, 136*(4), 610–622.

Boroditsky, L. (2000). Metaphoric structuring: Understanding time through spatial metaphors. *Cognition, 75*(1), 1–28.

Chambers, J. R., Windschitl, P. D., & Suls, J. (2003). Egocentrism, event frequency, and comparative optimism: When what happens frequently is "more likely to happen to me". *Personality and Social Psychology Bulletin, 29*(11), 1343–1356.

Epel, E. S., Bandura, A., & Zimbardo, P. G. (1999). Escaping homelessness: The influences of self-efficacy and time perspective on coping with homelessness. *Journal of Applied Social Psychology, 29*(3), 575–596.

Fiedler, K., Jung, J., Wänke, M., & Alexopoulos, T. (2012). On the relations between distinct aspects of psychological distance: An ecological basis of construal-level theory. *Journal of Experimental Social Psychology, 48*(5), 1014–1021.

Förster, J., Friedman, R. S., & Liberman, N. (2004). Temporal construal effects on abstract and concrete thinking: Consequences for insight and creative cognition. *Journal of Personality and Social Psychology, 87*(2), 177–189.

Frederick, S., Loewenstein, G., & O'Donoghue, T. (2002). Time discounting and time preference: A critical review. *Journal of Economic Literature, 40*(2), 351–401.

Freitas, A. L., Salovey, P., & Liberman, N. (2001). Abstract and concrete self-evaluative goals. *Journal of Personality and Social Psychology, 80*(3), 410–424.

Fujita, K., Trope, Y., Liberman, N., & Levin-Sagi, M. (2006). Construal levels and self-control. *Journal of Personality and Social Psychology, 90*(3), 351–367.

Green, L., & Myerson, J. (2004). A discounting framework for choice with delayed and probabilistic rewards. *Psychological Bulletin, 130*(5), 769–792.

Harber, K. D., Zimbardo, P. G., & Boyd, J. N. (2003). Participant self-selection biases as a function of individual differences in time perspective. *Basic and Applied Social Psychology, 25*(3), 255–264.

Jia, L., Hirt, E. R., & Karpen, S. C. (2009). Lessons from a Faraway land: The effect of spatial distance on creative cognition. *Journal of Experimental Social Psychology, 45*(5), 1127–1131.

Jones, B., & Rachlin, H. (2006). Social discounting. *Psychological Science, 17*(4), 283–286.

Kruger, J., & Burrus, J. (2004). Egocentrism and focalism in unrealistic optimism (and pessimism). *Journal of Experimental Social Psychology, 40*(3), 332–340.

Liberman, N., & Trope, Y. (2008). The psychology of transcending the here and now. *Science, 322*, 1201–1205.

Liberman, N., Polack, O., Hameiri, B., & Blumenfeld, M. (2012). Priming of spatial distance enhances children's creative performance. *Journal of Experimental Child Psychology, 111*(4), 663–670.

Maddux, W. W., & Galinsky, A. D. (2009). Cultural borders and mental barriers: The relationship between living abroad and creativity. *Journal of Personality and Social Psychology, 96*(5), 1047–1061.

Maglio, S. J., Trope, Y., & Liberman, N. (2013). Distance from a distance: Psychological distance reduces sensitivity to any further psychological distance. *Journal of Experimental Psychology. General, 142*(3), 644–657.

Polman, E., & Emich, K. J. (2011). Decisions for others are more creative than decisions for the self. *Personality and Social Psychology Bulletin, 37*(4), 492–501.

Singelis, T. M. (1994). The measurement of independent and interdependent self-construals. *Personality and Social Psychology Bulletin, 20*(5), 580–591.

Stephan, E., Liberman, N., & Trope, Y. (2010). Politeness and psychological distance: A construal level perspective. *Journal of Personality and Social Psychology, 98*(2), 268–280.

Stephan, E., Liberman, N., & Trope, Y. (2011). The effects of time perspective and level of construal on social distance. *Journal of Experimental Social Psychology, 47*, 397–402.

Thaler, R. H. (1981). Some empirical evidence on dynamic inconsistency. *Economic Letters, 8*, 201–207.

Trope, Y., & Liberman, N. (2010). Construal level theory of psychological distance. *Psychological Review, 117*(2), 440–463.

Van Boven, L., Kane, J., McGraw, A., & Dale, J. (2010). Feeling close: Emotional intensity reduces perceived psychological distance. *Journal of Personality and Social Psychology, 98*(6), 872–885.

Wakslak, C. J. (2012). The where and when of likely and unlikely events. *Organizational Behavior and Human Decision Processes, 117*, 150–157.

Wakslak, C. J., Trope, Y., Liberman, N., & Alony, R. (2006). Seeing the forest when entry is unlikely: Probability and the mental representation of events. *Journal of Experimental Psychology: General, 135*, 641–653.

Zauberman, G., Kim, B. K., Malkoc, S. A., & Bettman, J. R. (2009). Discounting time and time discounting: Subjective time perception and intertemporal preferences. *Journal of Marketing Research, 46*(4), 543–556.

Zhao, M., & Xie, J. (2011). Effects of social and temporal distance on consumers' responses to peer recommendations. *Journal of Marketing Research, 48*(3), 486–496.

Zimbardo, P. G., & Boyd, J. N. (1999). Putting time in perspective: A valid, reliable individual-differences metric. *Journal of Personality and Social Psychology, 77*(6), 1271–1288.

Part II
Evolutionary, Cultural, and Social Context of Time Perspective

The Evolved Psychology of Time Perspective

Curtis S. Dunkel and Daniel J. Kruger

You are hungry and you have a limited supply of seed. Do you eat all of your seed to dampen the hunger pangs or do you save some with thoughts of planting next season's crops? The development of agriculture was a turning point in human cultural and phylogenetic history. These excerpts from Cochran and Harpending's (2009) book the *The 10,000 Year Explosion* are good examples of how the development of agricultural could have exerted selective pressures leading to changes in time perspective.

> At first, all these pro-agricultural behaviors must have run against the grain: It's unlikely that humans were comfortable doing things that had never made sense in the past. But over time, alleles that induced this kind of ant-like behavior must have increased in frequency, until eventually, after millennia, selfish, hardworking, self-denying people were far more common than they had been among hunter gatherers.

and

> Agriculture itself, and the particular form it took in state societies, must have selected for personalities that can only be called bourgeois, characterized by the traits that make a man successful rather than interesting. One such trait was the ability to defer gratification for long periods of time.

We believe agriculture presented new environmental pressures that selected for stronger future time orientation across many generations. This is not to say that a strongly future-oriented time perspective is ultimately superior and that preserving the seed, instead of eating it, is always the correct decision. This is to say that as the environment changed with the introduction of agriculture, the mean balance between

C.S. Dunkel (✉)
Department of Psychology, Western Illinois University, Macomb, IL, USA
e-mail: C-Dunkel@wiu.edu

D.J. Kruger
School of Public Health, University of Michigan, Ann Arbor, MI, USA
e-mail: kruger@umich.edu

M. Stolarski et al. (eds.), *Time Perspective Theory; Review, Research and Application: Essays in Honor of Philip G. Zimbardo*, DOI 10.1007/978-3-319-07368-2_10,

Future and Present time perspectives was recalibrated toward the Future time perspective. Enough variation in outcomes remained so that genetic variation between groups and individuals remained. Additionally, phenotypic variance should rely heavily on individual experiences with immediate behaviors and decisions contingent upon the interaction of concurrent environmental stimuli and the phenotypic composition.

The historical shift in human time perspective over evolutionary time is not the only reason to consider the relationship between evolutionary theory and our understanding of time orientations. More general insights into Present and Future time perspective can be gained through the application of evolutionary theory. The understanding of these individual differences in time perspective couched within the framework of evolutionary theory has guided our research in the area.

Evolutionary Psychology

Evolutionary theory is steadily gaining prominence as a foundation for a cumulative understanding of psychological science (Webster 2007a, b, c). Evolution by natural and sexual selection is the unifying theory of the life sciences and offers an unparalleled ability to integrate currently disparate research areas (Wilson 1998), creating a powerful framework for understanding the complex patterns of causality in psychological and behavioral phenomena. The incorporation of evolutionary theory into psychology has waxed and waned in the 150 years since Darwin (1859) predicted a new foundation for the field. There are many notable historical examples of psychological theories with evolutionary bases, such as Bowlby's (1969) model of attachment, though in the last three decades, the evolutionary perspective has experienced rapid maturation with considerable theoretical advances and a continually growing array of empirical studies. An evolutionary approach to psychology focuses on proximate mediation; those affects, cognitions, and behaviors that helped to solve some adaptive problem in the ancestral environment. Evolutionary Psychology is concerned with the conditions that existed in ancestral environments, the proximate mechanisms that evolved to deal with conditions in these environments, and the functions of these evolved mechanisms in our current environments.

Life History Theory

Although there are several midlevel evolutionary approaches to understanding individual psychological differences (e.g., Buss 2009; Michalski and Shackelford 2010), among these we believe Life History (LH) theory best explains individual differences in Present and Future time perspective. LH theory is based on the idea that organisms must allocate resources toward maintenance, growth, and reproduction. Originally used to explain differences in the allocation of resources given various environmental constraints (MacArthur and Wilson 1967), LH theory was then put to use to explain a wide array of co-varying characteristics between species (Promislow and Harvey 1990). Organisms' allocation of resources and the co-varying characteristics are referred to LH strategies. The differences in resource allocation can be plotted along a continuum with one pole defined by a *fast* LH strategy and the other pole defined by a *slow* LH strategy. Rapid maturation, a shortened lifespan, early and unrestrictive reproductive behavior, and relatively less parental investment in offspring define the fast pole. The slow strategy is defined by slow maturation, a lengthened lifespan, delayed initiation and more restrictive reproductive behavior, with greater parental investment in offspring.

LH Strategies as the Basis for Individual Differences

The original models of LH theory (MacArthur and Wilson 1967; Pianka 1970) predicted that species living in environments with resource instability and unpredictability of future events (due to high predation rates, for example) will tend to evolve clusters of traits associated with rapid and prolific breeding with relatively low investment in offspring. In contrast, species living in stable and predictable environments are expected to instead have a long-term strategy investing more so in somatic and parental effort with lower reproductive rates and longer intergenerational times than those in less predictable and stable environments.

Researchers originally studied variation in LH strategy exclusively between species (Figueredo et al. 2005). Figueredo and colleagues (see Figueredo et al. 2006) propose that a common hereditary LH factor underlies human reproductive, familial, and social behaviors. This factor, named the *K*-factor, represents a continuum of strategies, ranging from a focus on short-term gains at the expense of long-term costs, high mating effort, and low parenting effort to long-term strategies, selective mating, and high parental effort. Figueredo et al. (2005) argued that individual differences in LH are maintained through frequency-dependent selection on pleiotropic regulatory genes that moderate the expression of the coordinated set of LH traits. Analyses of data from monozygotic (identical) and dizygotic (fraternal) twins produced a high heritability estimate (.65) for the *K*-Factor (Figueredo et al. 2004).

Heath and Hadley (1998) argued that although the heritability of LH strategies is evident, developmental experiences and environmental circumstances such as socio-economic and cultural conditions, and physical constraints shape how humans exhibit these strategies. Rushton (1985) summarized evidence demonstrating individual differences in LH within species contingent on environmental conditions and proposed that LH theory could be useful in understanding human individual differences in psychology and behavior. Thus, LH theory is a framework for understanding variation in human behavioral strategies as evolved adaptations to socio-environmental conditions. Individuals developing in relatively less certain environments will exhibit riskier, present oriented, behavioral strategies because of the low probability of reproductive success for more cautious approaches.

The field of Behavioral Ecology studies behavioral strategies related to reproductive success and their relationship to the characteristics of the physical, economic, and social environment (Crawford and Anderson 1989). Following this approach, Belsky et al. (1991) proposed that the psychological attachment process is an evolved psychological mechanism to evaluate life conditions and guide reproductive strategy that would likely be successful in one's environment. Bowlby (1969) originated the theory of attachment noting that early and impulsive displays of sexual and aggressive behavior were most prevalent in individuals who had experienced disturbed family relations. Belsky et al. (1991) concluded that insecure attachment is a response to environmental cues that long-term monogamous relationships are not a viable strategy in the social world in which the child is growing up and that inadequate parental attention will lead to insecure attachment styles and short-term mating strategies. This theory explained empirical findings that women who grow up without father involvement, a major risk factor for insecure attachment, show earlier sexual activity, as well as a lack of interest or ability to form and/or maintain, long-term monogamous relationships (Belsky et al. 1991; Chisholm 1999).

Evolutionary theorists have described how developmental environments can shape women's behavioral strategies. The optimal age at first birth is the result of tradeoffs in fertility and mortality; the higher the adult mortality rate, the earlier the average age at first birth (Low et al. 2002). Women growing up in areas with high risks of violent death begin reproducing at an earlier age and have more children during their reproductive lifespan than do women who grow up in lower-risk areas (Wilson and Daly 1997). These strategies reflect an emphasis on current opportunities and a discounting of future possibilities.

Some researchers argue that steep discounting of the future by adolescents and young adults could be a rational response to uncertainty (e.g., Gardner 1993; Wilson and Daly 1997). Risky behavioral strategies of young males were selected for over time because they tended to aid in mating competition. The observed peak of risky behaviors in young adulthood corresponded with entrance into mating competition (Wilson and Daly 1997), with its associated consequences in mortality patterns. Cross-culturally, males die at three or more times the rate of females in late adolescence and young adulthood, predominantly from behavioral causes (Kruger and Nesse 2004, 2006). Those who develop in relatively uncertain environments will develop riskier behavioral strategies to take advantage of possibly fleeting opportunities (Chisholm 1999). Other studies suggest that humans living in chronically risky and uncertain environments are more likely to experience earlier menarche, earlier ages of reproduction, and higher reproductive rates (Chisholm 1999; Kim et al. 1997).

In unpredictable environments, the most pressing adaptive problem faced by individuals has been avoiding death. Shorter time horizons encouraging risky behaviors may have facilitated early reproduction before death occurs. In fact, community college students with shorter lifespan estimates and higher estimates of the unpredictability of the future showed a higher frequency of risk-taking (Hill et al. 1997). When mortality rates are low and predictable, a less risky, long-term strategy may have been optimal. Wilson and Daly (1997) found that neighborhood life expectancy and income inequality predicted neighborhood homicide rates. They argued that risky behaviors such as homicide are a result of steep future discounting in response to environments that did not favor cautious strategies, even if the majority of individuals exhibiting risky strategies may have detrimental outcomes. Under these conditions, men may focus more on mating effort as they may have more to gain from increasing the quantity of offspring than investing paternal effort in the quality of offspring, given their uncertain futures. These mechanisms are a legacy from times when mortality rates throughout the lifespan were considerably higher, especially in infancy; they may not promote reproductive success in modern environments.

Time Perspectives as an Element of LH Strategy

Time perspective may represent a fundamental psychological trade-off in LH strategies. Conscientiousness is known to be associated with greater longevity and long-term behavioral strategies, as well as a desire for control and dependability (Friedman et al. 1993; Schwartz et al. 1995). Psychological measures of time perspective have strong associations with the selection and pursuit of social goals (Carstensen et al. 1999). Mischel and colleagues documented the relationship between future-oriented self-control and a wide range of outcomes including social competence, educational achievement, and resilience to frustration and stress (e.g., Mischel et al. 1989). Zimbardo and Boyd (1999) consider time perspective to be a pervasive, powerful, and largely unrecognized influence on human behavior and validated an inventory assessing time perspective.

Two of Zimbardo and Boyd's (1999) psychological measures of time perspective are especially relevant to LH variation. Present orientation, or "Present-Hedonistic" in Zimbardo and Boyd's terms, reflects an orientation towards immediate outcomes and little concern for future consequences. Future orientation reflects a pattern of behavior dominated by a striving for future goals and rewards. Zimbardo and Boyd (1999) found that sensation seeking was directly related to present-hedonic orientation and inversely related to future orientation. Consideration for future consequences mirrors future orientation and is inversely related to Present-Hedonistic orientation. *Simply, we believe that a more hedonistic time perspective is a facet of a fast LH strategy and a stronger Future time perspective is a facet of a slow LH strategy.*

Correlational Data

Correlational data supports the contention that the Future time perspective is an aspect of a slow LH strategy. Dunkel and Decker (2010) found significant positive correlations between Future time perspective and two separate self-report measures of slow LH strategy. They also found that measures more tangentially associated with a LH strategy were correlated with Future time perspective. Answers to the single question, "If you had to guess, at what age do you think you will die?", and a composite of positive personality traits called the General Factor of Personality were positively correlated with Future time perspective, while interest in short-term mating orientation was negatively correlated with Future time perspective. Additionally, when factor analyzed, future time perspective, the two self-report measures of LH strategy, answers to the question concerning expected lifespan, and short-term mating orientation all loaded a single factor that was speculated to represent LH strategy.

The positive correlation between future time perspective and slow LH strategy was replicated by Dunkel and Weber (2010) and they also found significant correlations between LH strategy and past time perspectives. Slow LH strategy was positively correlated with a Past Positive time perspective and negatively correlated with a Past Negative time perspective. Contrary to predictions, a Present-Hedonistic time perspective was not associated with LH strategy, and this finding is confirmed by unpublished data analyzed when writing this chapter. Looking at individual items of the Present Hedonistic subscale, the picture appears more complex, with items concerning living and enjoying the moment being positively correlated with a slow LH strategy (e.g., I try to live my life as fully as possible, one day at a time) while items reflecting impulsivity and risk-taking (e.g., I do things impulsively) being more likely to reflect a fast LH strategy. It could also be that the relationship between LH and a Present-Hedonistic time perspective is not linear as suggested by the modest negative correlation between the Present-Hedonistic time perspective and Future time perspective.

Modeling Data

Individuals who have experienced environments in which personal safety, social support, and resource control are uncertain may be more likely to discount future outcomes in favor of present outcomes. They would score higher on the Present-Hedonistic dimension and lower on the future dimension reflecting an internalized environmental representation guiding them towards shorter-term strategies. Others who experienced more reliably supportive environments where resource control is more certain could be expected to exhibit the reverse pattern as a reflection of experiences which promote longer-term strategies.

Results from a survey of inner-city middle school students indicated that present and future orientations completely mediated the relationship of positive and negative aspects of students' neighborhood social environments with reports of interpersonal aggression and property crimes (Kruger et al. 2008). The mediation model was superior to competing models portraying time perspective as a byproduct of either phenotypic strategy or social-environmental experiences. In this analysis, present orientation played the stronger role, uniquely explaining 77 % of the variance in interpersonal aggression and 55 % of the variance in property crimes.

Future orientation only weakly accounted for interpersonal aggression, uniquely explaining about 1 % of the variance. It is possible that future orientation would evidence stronger effects in different samples. These youth live in highly disadvantaged areas and may not have had the experiences suitable for developing stronger orientations towards distal goals.

Experimental Data

Dunkel, Mathes, and colleagues have also reasoned that manipulating time perspective through changes in life expectancy would cause a corresponding change in the willingness to engage in behaviors reflective of LH strategy. Specifically, it was proposed that shorter life expectancies would cause an increase in the willingness to engage in behaviors reflective of a fast LH strategy and longer life expectancies would tilt attitudes toward a slow LH strategy. To manipulate life expectancy Dunkel, Mathes, and colleagues (Dunkel and Mathes 2011; Dunkel et al. 2010a, b, 2013) presented participants with a hypothetical situation in which participants were instructed to imagine living 5 more months, 5 more years, or at least more 50 years.

> Imagine that you have just been to the doctor for your annual checkup and find out that you are very ill and have 5 months to live. You will be pain free, have no symptoms, and be able to do all the things you do now during those 5 months. Please answer the following questions with the understanding that the doctor told you that you will have 5 months to live.

Using this methodology, differences in the willingness to engage in short-term mating, long-term mating, aggression, generativity, self-control, sexual-coercion, and criminal behavior across the life expectancies has been examined. Shortened life expectancies cause changes that reflect greater interest in short-term mating, less interest in long-term mating, greater willingness to engage in aggression, diminished generativity, decreased self-control, and increased willingness to engage in sexual-coercion and assorted other criminal acts. Taken together these findings suggest that as time horizon is reduced LH strategies shift within an individual's reaction range becoming "faster".

To test the association between life expectancy and time perspective more directly we analyzed unpublished data in which the life expectancy manipulation was used with hedonistic time perspective acting as the dependent variable. One hundred and twenty-five college students (92 female) between the ages of 18 and 35 ($M = 19.78$, $SD = 2.48$) took part in the study for class credit. A repeated measures analysis of variance (ANOVA) was calculated examine the differences in hedonistic time perspective by life expectancy. There was a violation of the assumption of sphericity and therefore Greenhouse-Geiser estimates were used. The ANOVA was significant, $F\,(1.69, 209.29) = 20.37$, $p < .001$, $\eta_p^2 = .14$. Bonferroni corrected pairwise comparisons showed that the hedonistic time perspective was greater for the 5 month and 5 year life expectancy in comparison to the 50 year life expectancy (Table 1).

Table 1 Means and Standard Deviations of Hedonistic Time Perspective by Life Expectancy

	Life expectancy		
	5 months	5 years	50 years
Present Hedonistic TP	60.14 (8.81)	59.89 (9.47)	56.38 (10.30)

Standard deviations are in parentheses
TP Time Perspective

Summary and Directions for Future Research

We propose that Future time perspective is an important psychological attribute that was selected for and simultaneously allowed for advances like agricultural or even the industrial revolution as proposed by Clark (2007), and that Future and Present Hedonistic time perspective can be understood as part of a collection of individual differences working together as different LH strategies. Within this framework, stronger Future time perspective is thought to be part of a slow LH strategy and stronger Present Hedonistic time perspective part of a fast LH strategy. The results testing these two ideas are mixed, suggesting that a more complicated picture may best represent the relationship between time perspective and LH strategy.

Measures of slow LH strategy are positively correlated with Future time perspective, but are not negatively correlated with hedonistic time perspective. However, the importance of a hedonistic time perspective in accounting for behaviors associated with LH strategy is strongly supported in the mediation model. Finally, manipulating life expectancy has the predicted impact on indicators of LH strategy suggesting that as time horizons are shortened or lengthened LH strategies respond. This interpretation is lent further credence because we found that Present Hedonistic time perspective increased with as life expectancy was shortened from 50 years to 5 years or 5 months.

As with the choice presented in the opening paragraph of whether or not to eat crop seed, choices are often mutually exclusive. In fact, the belief that every decision involves a trade-off is at the core of LH theory. Thus future research could present participants with forced choice items representing Present Hedonistic options (e.g., go to a party) in contrast to those representing future options (e.g., study for tomorrow's exam). Additionally, future research could focus on the more nuanced relationship between the Future and Present Hedonistic time perspectives and LH strategies.

Enhanced measures of the psychology related to LH trade-offs may further clarify the relationship between LH and time perspective. The 20 item Mini-K (Figueredo et al. 2005) was based on a secondary analysis of a large national dataset from the Midlife in the US (MIDUS) study. It is a composite of developmental experiences, proclivity towards risk-taking, and social support. As all of these components are related to LH, the measure has good predictive power. Yet it is also very general and combines qualitatively different predictors of LH, which also vary by timeframe. Measures that assess psychological specific LH aspects such as mating effort and parental investment may have stronger predictive power and theoretical clarity.

Other time perspectives, besides the Future and the Present-Hedonistic, proposed by Zimbardo and Boyd (1999) and Boyd and Zimbardo (1997) also warrant investigation in the context of LH theory. One would expect that the Past-Positive time perspective would be associated with positive early life events and felt security while a Past-Negative time perspective would be associated with negative early life events and insecurity, thus given the developmental trajectories (e.g., Belsky et al. 1991) of the LH strategies a slow LH strategy should be associated with a positive-past time perspective and a fast LH strategy should be associated with a negative-past time perspective. The simple bivariate correlations (Dunkel and Weber 2010) bear this out, but more extensive investigations are needed.

The relationship between the transcendental time perspective (Boyd and Zimbardo 1997) and LH strategy is especially intriguing. Does the relationship between LH strategy and Future time perspective extend to a future perspective that moves beyond physical being? The role played by LH in religion is in need of more extensive investigation and one manner in which to proceed is to look at the relationship between LH strategy and transcendental time perspective.

Naturalistic studies utilizing both archival and observational data would help bolster the evidence for relationships between environmental conditions and behavioral patterns related to time perspective. Of course, experimental methodology is the often considered the gold standard in psychological research and so the development of manipulations more directly involving time perspective, other than life expectancy, would be a favored approach.

References

Belsky, J., Steinberg, L., & Draper, P. (1991). Childhood experience, interpersonal development, and reproductive strategy: An evolutionary theory of socialization. *Child Development, 62*, 647–670.

Bowlby, J. (1969). *Attachment and loss* (Vol. 1). New York: Basic Books.

Boyd, J., & Zimbardo, P. G. (1997). Constructing time after death: The transcendental-future time perspective. *Time & Society, 6*, 35–54.

Buss, D. M. (2009). How can evolutionary psychology successfully explain personality and individual differences? *Perspectives on Psychological Science, 4*, 359–366.

Carstensen, L. L., Isaacowitz, D. M., & Charles, S. T. (1999). Taking time seriously: A theory of socio emotional selectivity. *American Psychologist, 54*, 165–181.

Chisholm, J. S. (1999). *Death, hope and sex: Steps to an evolutionary ecology of mind and morality*. Cambridge: Cambridge University Press.

Clark, G. (2007). *A farewell to alms: A brief economic history of the world*. Princeton: Princeton University Press.

Cochran, G., & Harpending, H. (2009). *The 10,000 year explosion: How civilizations accelerated human evolution*. New York: Basic Books.

Crawford, C., & Anderson, J. (1989). Sociobiology: An environmentalist discipline? *American Psychologist, 44*, 1449–1460.

Darwin, C. (1859). *On the origin of species by means of natural selection*. London: John Murray.

Dunkel, C. S., & Decker, M. (2010). Convergent validity of measures of life history strategy. *Personality and Individual Differences, 48*, 681–684.

Dunkel, C. S., & Mathes, E. (2011). The effect of individual differences and manipulated life expectancies on the willingness to engage in sexual coercion. *Evolutionary Psychology, 9*, 588–599.

Dunkel, C. S., & Weber, J. (2010). Using three levels of personality to predict time perspective. *Current Psychology, 29*, 95–103.

Dunkel, C. S., Mathes, E., & Decker, M. (2010a). Behavioral flexibility in life history strategies: Evidence for the role of life expectancy. *Journal of Cultural, Evolutionary, and Social Psychology, 4*, 51–61.

Dunkel, C. S., Mathes, E., & Papini, D. R. (2010b). The effect of life expectancy on aggression and generativity: A life history perspective. *Evolutionary Psychology, 8*, 492–505.

Dunkel, C. S., Mathes, E., & Beaver, K. M. (2013). Life history theory and the general theory of crime: Life expectancy effects on low self-control and criminal intent. *Journal of Cultural, Evolutionary, and Social Psychology, 7*, 12–23.

Figueredo, A. J., Vásquez, G., Brumbach, B. H., & Schneider, S. M. R. (2004). The heritability of life history strategy: The K-factor, covitality, and personality. *Social Biology, 51*, 121–143.

Figueredo, A. J., Vásquez, G., Brumbach, B. H., Sefcek, J. A., Kirsner, B. R., & Jacobs, W. J. (2005). The K-factor: Individual differences in life history strategy. *Personality and Individual Differences, 39*(8), 1349–1360.

Figueredo, A. J., Vásquez, G., Brumbach, B. H., Schneider, S. M. R., Sefcek, J. A., Tal, I. R., Hill, D., Wenner, C. J., & Jacobs, W. J. (2006). Consilience and life history theory: From genes to brain to reproductive strategy. *Developmental Review, 26*, 243–275.

Friedman, H. S., Tucker, J. S., Tomlinson-Keasey, C., Schwartz, J. E., Wingard, D. L., & Criqui, M. H. (1993). Does childhood personality predict longevity? *Journal of Personality and Social Psychology, 65*, 176–185.

Gardner, W. (1993). A life-span rational-choice theory of risk taking. In N. J. Bell & R. W. Bell (Eds.), *Adolescent risk taking* (pp. 66–83). Newbury Park: Sage Publications.

Heath, K., & Hadley, C. (1998). Dichotomous male reproductive strategies in a polygynous human society: Mating versus parental effort. *Current Anthropology, 39*, 369–374.

Hill, E. M., Ross, L. T., & Low, B. S. (1997). The role of future unpredictability in human risk-taking. *Human Nature, 8*, 287–325.

Kim, K., Smith, P. K., & Palermiti, A. L. (1997). Conflict in childhood and reproductive development. *Evolution and Human Behavior, 18*, 109–142.

Kruger, D. J., & Nesse, R. M. (2004). Sexual selection and the male: Female mortality ratio. *Evolutionary Psychology, 2*, 66–77.

Kruger, D. J., & Nesse, R. M. (2006). An evolutionary life-history framework for understanding sex differences in human mortality rates. *Human Nature, 17*, 74–97.

Kruger, D. J., Reischl, T. M., & Zimmerman, M. A. (2008). Time perspective as a mechanism for functional developmental adaptation. *Journal of Social, Evolutionary, and Cultural Psychology, 2*, 1–22.

Low, B., Simon, C. P., & Anderson, K. G. (2002). An evolutionary ecological perspective on demographic transitions: Modeling multiple currencies. *American Journal of Human Biology, 14*, 149–167.

MacArthur, R., & Wilson, E. O. (1967). *The theory of Island Biogeography*. Princeton: Princeton University Press.

Michalski, R. L., & Shackelford, T. K. (2010). Evolutionary personality psychology: Reconciling human nature and individual differences. *Personality and Individual Differences, 48*, 509–516.

Mischel, W., Shoda, Y., & Rodriguez, M. L. (1989). Delay of gratification in children. *Science, 244*, 933–938.

Pianka, E. R. (1970). On r- and K-selection. *American Naturalist, 104*, 592–596.

Promislow, D. E. L., & Harvey, P. H. (1990). Living fast and dying young: A comparative analysis of life-history variation among mammals. *Journal of Zoology, 220*, 417–437.

Rushton, J. P. (1985). Differential K theory: The sociobiology of individual and group differences. *Personality and Individual Differences, 6*(4), 441–452.

Schwartz, J. E., Friedman, H. S., Tucker, J. S., Tomlinson-Keasey, C., Wingard, D. L., & Criqui, M. H. (1995). Socio demographics and psychosocial factors in childhood as predictors of adult mortality. *American Journal of Public Health, 85*, 1237–1245.

Webster, G. D. (2007a). What's in a name: Is "evolutionary psychology" eclipsing "sociobiology" in the scientific literature? *Evolutionary Psychology, 5*, 683–695.

Webster, G. D. (2007b). Evolutionary theory's increasing role in personality and social psychology. *Evolutionary Psychology, 5*, 84–91.

Webster, G. D. (2007c). Evolutionary theory in cognitive neuroscience: A 20-year quantitative review of publication trends. *Evolutionary Psychology, 5*, 520–530.

Wilson, E. O. (1998). *Consilience: The unity of knowledge*. New York: Knopf.

Wilson, M., & Daly, M. (1997). Life expectancy, economic inequality, homicide, and reproductive timing in Chicago neighbourhoods. *British Medical Journal, 314*, 1271–1274.

Zimbardo, P. G., & Boyd, J. N. (1999). Putting time in perspective: A valid, reliable individual-differences metric. *Journal of Personality and Social Psychology, 77*, 1271–1288.

Time Perspective Profiles of Cultures

Anna Sircova, Fons J.R. van de Vijver, Evgeny Osin, Taciano L. Milfont, Nicolas Fieulaine, Altinay Kislali-Erginbilgic, Philip G. Zimbardo, and 54 members of the International Time Perspective Research Project

Introduction

This chapter deals with the question of cross-cultural similarities and differences in time perspective. Are there reliable similarities and differences in the way persons deal with time? Do persons from different cultures have similar or different views of the past, present, and future? This chapter is based on a large-scale study from the International Time Perspective Research Project, involving samples from 24 countries, which was designed to address these questions. In the remainder of introduction, we first describe the theoretical background and findings of related studies, followed by a short description of the main findings. We draw conclusions in the final section.

The 54 members of the International Time Perspective Research Project are listed in alphabetical order by country: Slimane Djarallah (Université of Batna, Algeria), Mohamed Seghir Chorfi (Université Ferhat Abbas – Setif, Algeria), Umbelina do Rego Leite (Universidade de Rio Verde, Brasil), Hui Lin (Peking University, China), Houchao Lv (Southwest University, China), Tomislav Bunjevac, Tena Tomaš, Jasmina Punek, Anica Vrlec, Jelena Matić, Marko Bokulić (University of Zagreb, Croatia), Martina Klicperová-Baker, Jaroslav Košťál (Institute of Psychology, Academy of Sciences of the Czech Republic, Czech Republic), Riin Seema, Arno Baltin (Tallinn University, Estonia), Themistoklis Apostolidis (Université de Provence, France), Daphne Pediaditakis (Ruprecht-Karls-University of Heidelberg, Germany), Fay Griva, Fotios Anagnostopoulos (Panteion University of Social and Political Sciences, Greece), Nurit Carmi, Marina Goroshit (Tel-Hai College, Israel), Martina Peri (Salesiana University, Rome, Italy), Yumi Shimojima (Kyorin University, Japan), Koichi Sato (Gunma University, Japan), Keita Ochi (Hosei University, Japan), Antanas Kairys (Vilnius University, Lithuania), Audrone Liniauskaite (Klaipeda University, Lithuania), Víctor Corral-Verdugo (Universidad de Sonora, Hermosillo, Mexico), Aneta Przepiorka, Agata Blachnio (The John Paul II Catholic University in Lublin, Poland), Victor E. C. Ortuño (Universidade de Coimbra, Portugal), Vítor Gamboa (Universidade do Algarve, Portugal), Olga Mitina, Nadezhda Semyenova (Moscow State University, Russia), Valentina Gerasimova (Kaluga State University of Education, Russia), Tatiana Rawski (Nepryakho) (Tver State University, Russia), Ekaterina Kuleshova (A.I. Gertsen Russian State University of Education, Russia), Natalia Polskaya (Saratov State University, Russia), Nikolaj Tulinov (Balabanovo branch of Moscow State University of Humanities, Russia), Isabella Romanko (St. Petersburg State

M. Stolarski et al. (eds.), *Time Perspective Theory; Review, Research and Application: Essays in Honor of Philip G. Zimbardo*, DOI 10.1007/978-3-319-07368-2_11,

The Concept of Time

Two dominant views of the perception of time have prevailed (McHale 1978). The first and more traditional view – and prevailing in psychology – treats time from a linear perspective. This linear perspective emphasises "life tasks" rather than something "given" and/or "unalterable" (Bauman 1999). This linear view embodies the idea of progress: human welfare, perfectibility of human institutions, and to a degree the perfectibility of the human condition. The second view is based on the life cycle and assumes that the past is unalterable and the future unknowable.

University, Russia), Yulia Semina (Moscow State Regional University, Russia), Ekaterina Nikitina (Sociology of Education Center, Russian Academy of Education, Russia), Vera Yasnaya (National Research University Higher School of Economics, Moscow State University of Psychology and Education, Russia), Irina Davydova, Elsa Utyasheva (Russian State University of Humanities, Russia), Irina Emeliyanova (Moscow State University of Psychology and Education, Russia), Regina Ershova (Kolomna State Institute of Education, Russia), Jasmina Nedeljković (Faculty of Law and Business Studies, Novi Sad, Serbia), Juan Francisco Díaz Morales (Universidad Complutense de Madrid, Spain), Maria Grazia Carelli, Britt Wiberg (Umeå University, Sweden), Ilona Boniwell (University of East London, UK), P. Alex Linley (Centre for Applied Positive Psychology, UK), and John Nathan Boyd (Google Inc., USA).

A. Sircova (✉)
Independent Researcher, Skyttegade 14, 2 th, 2200, Copenhagen, Denmark
e-mail: anna.sircova@gmail.com

F.J.R. van de Vijver
Department of Social Psychology, Tilburg University, PO Box 90153 5000 LE, Tilburg, The Netherlands

North-West University, Potchefstroom, South Africa

University of Queensland, Brisbane, Australia
e-mail: Fons.vandeVijver@uvt.nl

E. Osin
Department of Psychology, National Research University Higher School of Economics, Moscow, Russia
e-mail: eosin@hse.ru

T.L. Milfont
School of Psychology and Centre for Applied Cross-Cultural Research, Victoria University of Wellington, Wellington, New Zealand
e-mail: taciano.milfont@vuw.ac.nz

N. Fieulaine
Groupe de Recherche en Psychologie Sociale, Institut de Psychologie, Université de Lyon, 69600 Bron, France
e-mail: Nicolas.fieulaine@univ-lyon2.fr

A. Kislali-Erginbilgic
Toronto, Canada
e-mail: aerginbilgic@gmail.com

P.G. Zimbardo
Psychology Department, Stanford University, Stanford, CA 94305-2130, USA

This cyclic view of time accentuates recurrence, fatalism, and balance (e.g., in Chinese philosophy between the passive, female Yin and the dynamic, male Yang).

Going into a more detailed classification, McGrath and Tschan (2004) distinguished four processes in temporal aspects of everyday life: *time use*, *pace of life*, *time perception*, and *time orientation*. Time use refers to an individual's distribution of time over daily activities such as working, eating, leisure time, travel time, and personal care. Pace of life refers to the speed of doing everyday activities. Time perception is about how humans judge the passage of time and is often studied by asking individuals to estimate durations of specific temporal intervals and feelings about the passage of time in general. Finally, time orientation refers to how people compare the present to the future (hopes and fears).

Focusing specifically on time orientation and drawing from his anthropological work, Hall (1989) dichotomised time orientations into monochronic and polychronic. He argues that people with monochronic time orientation tend to prefer to do one thing at a time and rely on schedules and segmentation. On the other hand, people with polychronic time orientation tend to do several things at once, and they stress the completion of transactions rather than adherence to preset schedules. Hall (1989) asserts that Westerners are likely to be monochronic, whereas Latin American and Mediterranean people tend to have a more polychronic orientation. Hall's concept of time orientation has also attracted the attention of cross-cultural scholars. For example, Brislin and Kim (2003) have suggested a closely related dichotomy of clock and event time. Clock-time cultures, like the USA, adhere to schedules and punctuality, whereas event-time cultures, like Latin America, go more with the natural flow of social events. Although perhaps still prevalent, these distinctions may blur with globalisation and the advance of technology and multitasking in all developed countries.

Time perspective is another concept relevant for the perception of time and that has been gaining prominence in the last decade. Time perspective corresponds to an individual's view on his or her past and future at a given time (Frank 1939; Lewin 1942). Time perspective links past, present, and future (Hoornaert 1973), or in Zimbardo and Boyd's (1999) words: "Between the abstract, psychological constructions of prior past and anticipated future events lies the concrete, empirically centered representation of the present" (p. 1271). In addition, these researchers conceive of time perspective as the ways in which individuals partition the flow of their personal experiences into time zones or temporal categories (see also Zimbardo and Boyd 2008).

Cross-Cultural Research on Time

Our study is the first extensive cross-cultural examination focused entirely on time perspective. Previous cross-cultural studies have addressed other aspects according to McGrath and Tschan's (2004) classification of psychological time processes. Three prior large-scale survey studies have been conducted.

The first was done by Hofstede (2001), who studied work-related values in 40 countries. He did not report a temporal factor in his IBM data published in 1980, but added a long-term versus short-term orientation factor in his later work based on the Confucian Work Dynamism dimension, found in the Chinese Values Survey administered to university students in 22 countries (Chinese Culture Connection 1987). Countries with a strong short-term orientation (most Western countries) foster values involving future-oriented rewards, in particular perseverance and thrift, whereas countries with a long-term orientation (such as China and Taiwan) foster respect for tradition, preservation of "face", and fulfilling social obligations. Long-term orientation shows significant correlations with other national characteristics, notably the current economic growth.

Recently, Hofstede et al. (2010) proposed a new version of this index of long-term versus short-term orientation based on a subset of the World Values Survey items and reported a significant relation between the score calculated for 93 countries with school results and economic growth (Hofstede and Minkov 2010). A similar distinction between past and future orientations was found by Meade (1972), who asked Americans and samples from Indian subcultures to write stories. Americans tended to write more stories with future themes (involving more personal aspects of achievement) than most Indian samples who wrote more stories with past themes.

The second large cross-cultural study is the GLOBE project. This 62-country study focusing on leadership and organisational behaviour also collected data on future orientation, described as "the degree to which a collectivity encourages and rewards future-oriented behaviours such as planning and delaying gratification" (Ashkanasy et al. 2004, p. 282). Their data deal with the extent to which an organisation or society is focused on its future and reinforces future-oriented behaviours, such as planning. The scale showed good equivalence across varied nations. Societies with a stronger future orientation tend to be less hierarchical, more humane, and individualistic.

The third study conducted by Trompenaars and Hampden-Turner (1998) examined time horizon in 42 countries. Time horizon refers to the length of the planning horizon and the length of time a person uses to think about the past or future. Confucian cultures scored higher on long-term planning, whereas Western cultures scored higher on short-term planning.

The convergence of findings of the three studies is lacking. Ashkanasy et al. (2004, p. 311) computed correlations between the country scores of the three studies mentioned, and almost none of the correlations were significant. There are a number of possible reasons for this negative finding. First, correlations were computed at the country level, which implies that the number of units for computing the correlations was small (with a minimum of eight) and showed limited cultural variation (all studies involved just Western countries). Also, the different studies covered dissimilar aspects of psychological time. Finally, only the GLOBE study conducted equivalence analyses to ensure that the instrument measured the same construct in each country.

Apart from these large survey studies, three other studies could be mentioned. One focused on the pace of life in 31 countries, using behavioural observations (Levine and Norenzayan 1999). Their three measures were the average walking speed of pedestrians in a downtown location, the average time needed for a routine transaction in a post office, and the average accuracy of public clocks. The pace of life was faster in individualistic, more affluent, and colder countries. A study by Luszczynska et al. (2005) in Americans, Turkish, and Polish high-school students showed a small, positive relation between orientation towards the future, measured by a shortened version of the Consideration of Future Consequences scale (Strathman et al. 1994), and general self-efficacy (Bandura 1997). A more recent study (Milfont and Gapski 2010) integrated a number of culture-level data of time orientations from 73 countries, yielding two factors. The first factor grouped data measuring how much cultures emphasise future orientation (fast pace of life, planning and investing in the future). The second factor grouped data measuring how cultures assign different meanings to time horizons, with an emphasis on long-term orientation (enduring goals, long-standing plans). Both factor scores were compared with per capita gross national product and the Human Development Index from 2007. Only the first factor correlated strongly positively with these two indicators, indicating that only the future-oriented factor seems to be related to the countries' national wealth and level of human development.

Challenges in Cross-Cultural Research

Time orientation has been the topic of several major cross-cultural studies, which were often based on the juxtaposition of Eastern and Western time concepts. However, an integration of their findings is impossible due to the absence of an underlying general theoretical basis and a lack of methodological convergence across these studies. In our view, this is due to both substantive and methodological reasons. To start with the former, the instruments that have been used cover only parts of the domain of psychological time and do not start from a global view on the integration of these parts, thus, the essential overarching theoretical framework of psychological time is missing. Methodological shortcomings include an absence of widely employed instruments with well-established psychometric properties for the time concepts studied. In addition, almost no cross-cultural studies have conducted equivalence analyses, thus, some reported cross-cultural differences in time orientation might have been influenced by measurement anomalies, such as inadequate item content for some countries.

Why is equivalence analysis so important in this kind of cross-cultural research? When comparing groups on a measured construct, such as time perspective, an assumption is made that the instrument measures the same psychological construct in all groups. This assumption is verified by equivalence testing. Equivalence refers to the measurement invariance of the measured construct across groups. If this equivalence assumption holds, the group comparisons are valid, and differences/similarities between groups can be meaningfully interpreted. If this equivalence assumption does not hold, comparisons and interpretations are not fully meaningful (Chen 2008; Milfont and Fischer 2010; van de Vijver and Leung 1997). Establishing measurement invariance is thus a prerequisite for meaningful comparisons across groups, and four main levels of equivalence can be distinguished: functional, structural, metric, and full-score or scalar equivalence (Fontaine 2005).

The International Time Perspective Research Project tries to overcome the theoretical and methodological shortcomings of past research by using a particular theoretical frame underlying the Zimbardo Time Perspective Inventory (ZTPI; Zimbardo and Boyd 1999) and by examining the equivalence of the ZTPI across cultures. Participants completing the ZTPI are asked to indicate the extent to which each of the 56 statements are characteristic or true of them on a 5-point Likert scale ranging from 1 (*very untrue*) to 5 (*very true*). It measures five temporal orientations: Past Positive (PP), Past Negative (PN), Present Hedonistic (PH), Present Fatalistic (PF), and Future (F).

The PP dimension represents pleasurable, usually sentimental and nostalgic views of one's past while emphasising the maintenance of relationships with family and friends. In contrast, the PN dimension reflects a focus on personal experiences that were aversive, noxious, traumatic, or filled with regret. Those high on PH live in the moment, enjoy high intensity activities, sensation seeking, and act with minimal concern for the consequences of their behaviour. The PF dimension reflects helpless and hopeless attitude towards the future and one's life that seems fated and not under personal control. The Future factor represents an attitude of goal setting and working for these goals at the expense of present enjoyment and delaying gratification, while always considering the consequences of one's own actions and decisions.

Establishing Equivalence of the ZTPI Across 24 Countries

Various studies have addressed the psychometric properties of the ZTPI, and the scales reveal adequate internal consistencies (usually in the range of .63 and .84). Adequate psychometric properties were found in Algeria (Djarallah and Seghir Chorfi 2009), Brazil (Leite and Pasquali 2008; Milfont et al. 2008), the Czech Republic (Lukavská et al. 2011), Estonia (Seema and Sircova 2013), France (Apostolidis and Fieulaine 2004), Greece (Anagnostopoulos and Griva 2012), Israel (Carmi and Goroshit 2013), Japan (Shimojima et al. 2012), Latvia (Kolesovs 2009), Lithuania (Liniauskaite and Kairys 2009), Mexico (Corral-Verdugo et al. 2006), the Netherlands (van Beek et al. in preparation), the Philippines (Cebuano language; Agsoy et al. 2010), Poland (Przepiorka 2011), Portugal (Ortuño, and Gamboa 2009), Romania (Gavreliuc et al. 2012), Russia (Sircova et al. 2008), Serbia (Nedeljković 2013), South Africa (Dissel and Potgieter 2007), Spain (Diaz-Morales 2006), Sweden (Carelli et al. 2011), and Ukraine (Senyk 2012). The predictive, convergent, and discriminant validity of the instrument has also been demonstrated across a number of studies.

From these studies conducted in 15 different countries, Past Negative and Present Fatalistic orientations repeatedly appeared as negatively associated with psychological well-being and behaviours, whereas past positive and future orientations appeared to be positively associated in many cases. Present hedonistic appeared as having associations, simultaneously related to risky behaviours and to more satisfactory relations and greater psychological well-being. Recently, Boniwell and Zimbardo (2004) investigated temporal profiles based on the interrelations between the five dimensions of his model. These authors proposed that the more functional profile is a balanced time perspective with low scores on dysfunctional orientations, high scores on the functional ones, and a moderate score on the remaining present hedonistic orientation. Two studies subsequently demonstrated that balanced time perspective profiles are closely related to subjective well-being and satisfaction with life (Boniwell et al. 2010; Drake et al. 2008). Lastly, clinical investigations demonstrated that this time perspective model is effective for diagnosis and interventions (van Beek et al. 2011).

Even though studies in various countries have employed the ZTPI, only few studies adopted a comparative approach. Studies have performed comparisons of time perspective as measured by the ZTPI between countries (Russia and the UK; Boniwell et al. 2010) or ethnolinguistic samples (Kolesovs 2009), but with no or limited tests for structural equivalence. This chapter builds upon our earlier review study (Sircova et al. 2007) that presented a summary of applications of the ZTPI in Brazil, France, Italy, South Africa, Spain, Russia, and the USA. Using more refined statistical approaches, White et al. (2011) tested for structural equivalence of the ZTPI measure between three countries (Estonia, Morocco, and the USA) using principal components analysis within each country sample compared to factors extracted from a pooled matrix through Tucker coefficients of congruence. They concluded that the ZTPI showed somewhat comparable, but not completely identical factors across the three countries.

The first stage of our study aimed to examine whether the proposed five factors of time perspective (as proposed by the ZTPI) can be empirically identified across cultures and whether their meaning is fully or partially invariant across countries and gender. We performed invariance tests across a set of data ($N = 12{,}200$) from 24 countries, 17 countries from Europe (Croatia, the Czech Republic, Estonia, France, Germany, Greece, Israel, Italy, Lithuania, Poland, Portugal, Serbia, Russia, Spain, Sweden, Turkey, the UK), 3 countries from Asia (China, Japan, New Zealand) and America (Brazil, Mexico, the USA), and 1 African country (Algeria). Two independent translations were available for Brazil, China, and Greece. Details on the specific country samples, translation procedure, and the invariance analyses are presented in a special paper (Sircova et al. 2014). Here we briefly summarise the main findings and focus on some preliminary results on cultural differences that were obtained in the course of this study.

Factor Structure of the ZTPI. Correlation matrices of individual country samples were summed up (using weighting based on square root of sample size to reduce sample size bias) to form a pooled correlation matrix. The factor structure of the resulting cross-cultural matrix was similar to the original structure published by Zimbardo and Boyd (1999), with the exception of two items: 25 (loading on Past Negative, non-reverse-scored) and 52 (loading on Present Hedonistic). Both items had cross-loadings of similar magnitude on two scales in the original US sample and were assigned arbitrarily by the authors (J. N. Boyd, personal communication, May 2012). The factor loading matrix is presented elsewhere (Sircova et al. 2014).

Construct Equivalence. In order to assess the cross-cultural equivalence, originally a confirmatory factor analysis was applied. However, this approach proved too challenging because of the large number of country samples and size of the instrument (56 items), as well as its complexity due to intrinsic heterogeneity of the scales (e.g., within the Past Negative scale, two subfactors, Trauma and Regret, can be extracted). As a result, a more traditional approach using target (Procrustes) rotation was applied with subsequent calculation of factor congruence coefficients (Tucker's phi; the proportionality coefficients above .95 suggest factorial similarity, according to van de Vijver and Leung 1997).

In most cases, the proportionality coefficient values were above .90, suggesting good overall structural equivalence. Countries that showed notably low congruence coefficients were Algeria, Italy, Mexico, and both Chinese versions. The reasons may vary across countries and can include sample particulars, translation issues, limited applicability of some items, and response styles. Additionally we calculated factor congruence coefficients for each factor separately (i.e., based on five separate factor analyses rather than a single factor analysis including all items). Median values then were .99 for all five scales. This indicates that the core of the factors is well replicable across cultures. However, various factors have items with substantial secondary loadings that "walk between" factors.

Scalar Equivalence and Bias. To address the question if direct comparison of scores on the ZTPI subscales across the cultural groups is possible (scalar equivalence), the assessment of item bias, or differential item functioning (DIF), was performed using an ANOVA approach (van de Vijver and Leung 1997). The individual mean scores of the ZTPI scales were split into 3 score levels (bands) based on 33rd and 66th percentile cutoff points. Subsequently, country and score level (band) were used in two-way ANOVA as factors predicting raw scores on each respective scale.

To provide an overall DIF indicator per each item, effect sizes (partial eta-squared) for the country factor were calculated. In order to single out specific countries that resulted in DIF for each item, deviance values were calculated. They indicate absolute difference between mean item score for each score band in a specific country and the country-pooled mean for that item for each score band, divided by country-pooled standard deviation. The resulting effect size indicator was similar in nature to Cohen's *d*. Mean deviance values (for each item-country pair across the 3 score bands) above .50 were used as indication of item bias, which corresponds to a medium effect size in terms of Cohen's (1988) guidelines. We decided to consider only moderate and large effect sizes, since we expected that with our large sample size the use of conventional significance criteria would lead to an overestimation of DIF.

If a country or an item was identified as having the strongest sources of bias, they were removed, and then the analysis on the reduced item set was repeated. The iterative strategy was used to create such a subset of items and country samples, where item bias would be limited to specific item-country pairs. In order to reach this goal, countries with three or more instances of bias were removed, and items that showed medium or strong bias in two or more countries, or demonstrated effect size (partial eta-squared) values above .06 for the country factor, were removed as well. The remaining sources of bias were examined to find theoretical explanations for why specific items performed poorly in specific countries (e.g., translation artifact or cultural differences).

Three country samples were identified as outliers in terms of average item bias (in decreasing order): China 2, Japan, China 1, and Algeria. Items and country samples contributing to most bias were iteratively removed. The resulting set included 36 items and 23 country samples with one instance of strong bias (item 21 in Algeria, $d=.90$) and 12 instances of medium item bias: items 37 and 49 in China 1 ($d=.64$ in both cases), item 52 in Germany ($d=.53$), items 29 and 31 in Estonia ($d=.51$ and .61, respectively), item 51 in France ($d=.59$), item 17 in Italy ($d=.59$), items 23 and 34 in Poland ($d=.51$ and .52, respectively), item 51 ($d=.52$) in Serbia, and items 8 and 50 in Turkey ($d=.78$ and .60, respectively).

Only three country samples with more than 2 instances of bias were removed: China 2, Japan, and Greece 2. We decided to keep the two items (51 and 52) showing only marginal bias (*d* between .50 and .60) for the sake of construct representation in the item subset. Thus, data from 23 out of the 24 participating countries (except for Japan) were deemed suitable for country-level analyses, and at most a single biased item per scale remained.

Interestingly, samples from Mexico and Italy identified earlier as outliers in terms of construct equivalence did not exhibit strong item bias, suggesting that these countries differ from the cross-cultural version mostly in cross-loadings and scale intercorrelations. On the other hand, we observed China and Algeria having the highest average bias and Japan (which was removed altogether) with many item bias instances. This suggests potential differences in the structure or content of the construct of time perspective (and, as a result, limited applicability of the ZTPI) in non-Western cultures. However, our data set is mostly composed with data from European countries or cultures historically linked to them that in turn can cause the bias. More data from different cultures is needed to test this hypothesis.

The 36-Item Version of the ZTPI

The resulting subset of 36 items from ZTPI we recommend as the working instrument for cross-cultural comparison studies. The item numbers (corresponding to the full version numbering) of this subset are given in Table 1. The 36 items for any specific language can be created by extracting these items from the full version either before data collection or during the data analysis (if the 56-item version was used) and numbering from 1 to 36 in their original order.

The factor structure of this short version was similar to that of the cross-cultural 56-item version, with the exception of two items. Item 24 had a noticeably stronger

Table 1 Keys for the 36-item cross-cultural version of the ZTPI

Scale	Original ZTPI items
Past-Negative	4, 25, 27, 34, 36, 50, 54
Past-Positive	9 (reverse-scored), 10, 21, 30, 40, 45, 51
Present-Fatalistic	24, 33, 35, 37, 38, 47
Present-Hedonistic	8, 12, 17, 19, 23, 31, 42, 44, 52, 55
Future	2, 7, 11, 20, 29, 49

Table 2 Reliability coefficients for the full and short unbiased ZTPI version in different countries

		Cronbach's alpha, 56 items					Cronbach's alpha, 36 items				
Country	N	PN	PP	PF	PH	F	PN	PP	PF	PH	F
Algeria	434	.79	.68	.73	.82	.76	.67	.65	.57	.77	.73
Brazil	528	.80	.64	.68	.80	.71	.76	.63	.62	.73	.63
China 1	356	.74	.60	.62	.64	.63	.68	.56	.55	.50	.41
China 2	924	.81	.67	.78	.69	.71	.73	.64	.72	.61	.59
Croatia	357	.86	.73	.72	.77	.82	.84	.68	.62	.69	.77
Czech Rep.	1,034	.84	.70	.75	.85	.74	.80	.71	.66	.79	.64
Estonia	891	.84	.73	.70	.81	.78	.82	.74	.65	.72	.67
France	419	.74	.61	.68	.79	.76	.75	.64	.54	.70	.67
Germany	215	.81	.74	.66	.82	.76	.79	.66	.55	.72	.65
Greece 1	337	.82	.72	.70	.85	.83	.78	.70	.60	.77	.73
Greece 2	215	.84	.76	.64	.86	.76	.80	.72	.52	.80	.72
Israel	334	.84	.72	.72	.80	.76	.83	.72	.62	.70	.66
Italy	143	.82	.61	.72	.70	.68	.80	.58	.63	.55	.58
Japan	433	.76	.69	.63	.72	.74	.72	.69	.45	.60	.64
Lithuania	438	.80	.66	.72	.77	.77	.74	.66	.62	.67	.70
Mexico	293	.76	.58	.70	.73	.70	.72	.59	.59	.62	.65
New Zealand	329	.81	.75	.64	.8	.78	.77	.72	.50	.71	.61
Poland	200	.84	.62	.64	.77	.70	.83	.63	.60	.64	.60
Portugal	342	.81	.61	.71	.80	.72	.79	.63	.64	.72	.66
Russia	1,269	.84	.71	.66	.78	.70	.73	.66	.64	.69	.66
Serbia	401	.77	.68	.71	.78	.77	.83	.68	.57	.68	.57
Spain	763	.77	.65	.63	.80	.74	.73	.64	.47	.70	.63
Sweden	325	.85	.74	.66	.82	.73	.82	.73	.60	.75	.64
Turkey	475	.81	.60	.65	.76	.72	.78	.55	.56	.64	.61
UK	180	.82	.75	.69	.76	.76	.79	.77	.62	.68	.57
USA	565	.79	.70	.71	.76	.73	.74	.66	.62	.67	.58
Median value		.82	.69	.70	.78	.74	.78	.66	.60	.69	.64

Note. PN Past-Negative, *PP* Past-Positive, *PF* Present-Fatalistic, *PH* Present-Hedonistic, *F* Future

loading on Present Fatalistic. Item 33 had loadings of .38 on Past Negative and .40 on Present Fatalistic. The wording of item 33 indeed taps into both negative past experiences and fatalistic attitudes; it was decided to assign it to the Present Fatalistic scale. Table 2 presents reliability coefficients of this version for different country samples.

Table 3 Descriptive statistics for the 36-item cross-cultural version of the ZTPI scales in the balanced sample (N=7,942, age 18–35, equal weighting for gender)

	N		Mean					SD				
Country	Male	Female	PN	PP	PF	PH	F	PN	PP	PF	PH	F
Algeria	172	240	3.31	3.63	3.15	3.62	3.62	0.7	0.69	0.74	0.7	0.71
Brazil	264	237	3.04	3.47	2.68	3.26	3.53	0.78	0.69	0.7	0.65	0.6
China-1	117	204	3.04	3.4	2.86	2.88	3.51	0.59	0.54	0.54	0.42	0.42
Croatia	148	204	2.74	3.38	2.88	3.22	3.44	0.87	0.7	0.67	0.55	0.68
Czech Rep.	152	141	2.81	3.51	2.99	3.29	3.51	0.72	0.67	0.67	0.69	0.53
Estonia	624	203	2.66	3.82	2.62	3.08	3.77	0.83	0.64	0.66	0.57	0.56
France	124	288	2.76	3.33	2.9	3.33	3.45	0.77	0.65	0.63	0.61	0.61
Germany	32	132	2.47	3.4	2.56	3.21	3.67	0.72	0.53	0.52	0.47	0.53
Greece-1	109	214	2.61	3.35	2.6	3.26	3.74	0.75	0.65	0.64	0.62	0.61
Israel	88	204	2.68	3.78	2.68	3.23	3.65	0.75	0.55	0.61	0.54	0.54
Italy	47	75	2.8	3.65	2.71	3.1	3.7	0.82	0.56	0.7	0.52	0.54
Lithuania	109	263	2.83	3.56	2.89	3.18	3.64	0.75	0.63	0.64	0.58	0.59
Mexico	52	71	2.89	3.42	2.67	3.21	3.38	0.77	0.66	0.6	0.56	0.57
New Zealand	87	214	2.87	3.56	2.92	3.45	3.19	0.7	0.61	0.54	0.5	0.58
Poland	86	113	2.79	3.65	2.66	3.36	3.57	0.84	0.64	0.65	0.52	0.56
Portugal	98	190	2.64	3.61	2.7	3.31	3.86	0.79	0.63	0.64	0.58	0.56
Russia	277	457	2.67	3.71	2.53	3.28	3.69	0.75	0.69	0.67	0.6	0.63
Serbia	112	282	2.68	3.59	2.8	3.37	3.48	0.88	0.69	0.63	0.59	0.57
Spain	67	94	2.59	3.57	2.78	3.15	3.45	0.78	0.66	0.58	0.57	0.53
Sweden	37	219	2.65	3.4	2.66	3.27	3.38	0.72	0.64	0.45	0.56	0.49
Turkey	203	229	2.88	3.64	2.77	3.52	3.89	0.83	0.6	0.65	0.52	0.5
UK	26	128	2.75	3.63	2.74	3.35	3.49	0.79	0.62	0.59	0.54	0.56
USA	192	317	3.21	3.51	2.91	3.28	3.48	0.74	0.61	0.68	0.54	0.55

Note. PN Past-Negative, *PP* Past-Positive, *PF* Present-Fatalistic, *PH* Present-Hedonistic, *F* Future

As expected, the scales of the 36-item version display somewhat lower reliability than the full version of the ZTPI, with the added benefit of improved invariance. In most cases scales display reliability coefficients above .60, which is sufficient for research purposes. Thus, the 36-item version can be recommended for cross-cultural comparison studies and large-scale surveys, where shorter scales have a strong preference.

Cultural Differences in Time Perspective. In order to gain some preliminary insight into the cultural differences in time perspective, we correlated country-level scores of the ZTPI and other culture-level variables. We computed mean scores for the 36-item version of the ZTPI for a balanced sample by selecting individuals aged 18–35 and equal weighting for males and females from 23 countries (except for Japan and China 2 and Greece 2 samples). The descriptive statistics are presented in Table 3.

We used dimensions of national culture by Hofstede and Minkov (2010; power distance, individualism, masculinity, uncertainty avoidance, long-term orientation, indulgence) and the 2011 Human Development Index (Human Development Report

Table 4 Pearson correlations between the ZTPI average scores and cultural indicators

Indicator	N	PN	PP	PF	PH	FU
Power distance	22	.12	−.22	−.05	−.07	.09
Individualism vs Collectivism	22	.08	.13	.18	.19	−.27
Masculinity vs Femininity	22	.31	−.11	.05	−.07	−.13
Uncertainty avoidance	22	**−.37***	.09	−.29	.28	**.44***
Long-term orientation	23	**−.37***	−.03	−.19	**−.58****	.19
Indulgence vs Restraint	22	.15	**−.41***	−.07	.24	**−.54****
Human development index	23	**−.45***	−.09	−.14	−.10	−.28

Note. PN Past-Negative, *PP* Past-Positive, *PF* Present-Fatalistic, *PH* Present-Hedonistic, *F* Future. Significant and marginally significant correlations marked in bold
$^{*}p<.05$; $^{**}p<.01$; $^{***}p<.10$

2011). Indices of power distance, individualism, masculinity, and uncertainty avoidance were unavailable for Algeria, and the index of indulgence was unavailable for Israel. The resulting correlations are presented in Table 4.

The results suggest some convergent validity between the Hofstede dimensions and the ZTPI scales, as confirmed by the pronounced negative associations between Present Hedonistic and long-term orientation, as well as between future and indulgence. Greater long-term orientation in a country is associated with lower hedonistic focus, and greater indulgence is associated with lower Future time perspective. Interestingly, both pairs of scales from the ZTPI and Hofstede dimensions are not related significantly to each other, suggesting that the related pairs capture two different aspects of future versus present orientation (cf. Milfont and Gapski 2010).

Past negative is also negatively associated with the Human Development Index, suggesting that a greater focus on past traumatic events that individuals experience in countries is associated with lower income, educational level, and life expectancy that form the HDI. Future was positively associated with uncertainty avoidance, suggesting that in countries where people are uncomfortable with unstructured, novel, and unknown situations, they tend to have a stronger accent on planning their future and to be more committed to their goals.

Other associations emerged that may be of interest, but were marginally significant ($p<.10$) due to small sample size. Past negative was negatively associated with uncertainty avoidance and long-term orientation, suggesting that in countries where people are more inclined to focus on negative past experiences, they are also more uncomfortable with unknown situations and attach less importance to the future. The association of Past Positive with restraint suggests that in countries where people have a more positive, pleasurable, and nostalgic views of the past and are more focused on preserving traditions, need gratification is more strongly regulated by social norms.

Cultural Differences in Time Perspective Profiles. We further set out to investigate the typical TP profiles characteristic of each country. We applied cluster analysis approach at the individual level based on the scores on the five scales of the 36-item ZTPI for the above 23 countries. This approach has been successfully applied to individual country samples (e.g., Boniwell et al. 2010; Osin and Orel 2012).

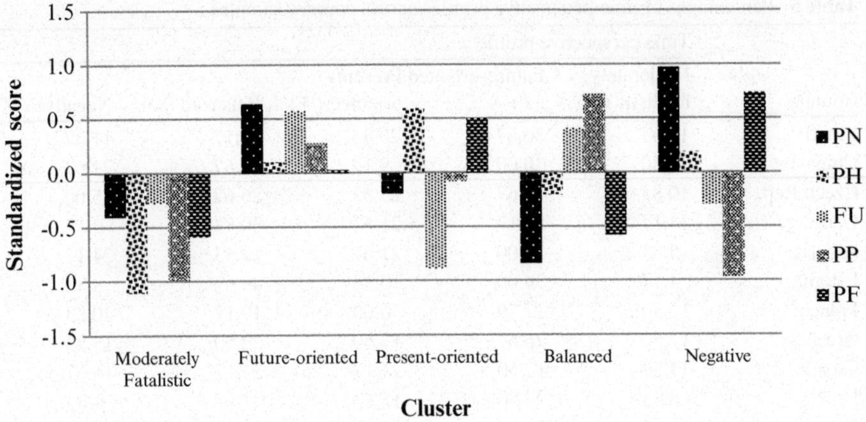

Fig. 1 Cluster profiles (in standardised ZTPI scores)

We aimed to equalise the contribution of different countries and genders to the resulting cluster structure; thus, we formed a balanced sample by selecting randomly 120 individuals aged 18–35 from each country (60 female and 60 male where available). The ZTPI scores were standardised by variable and cluster-analysed using Ward's method and squared Euclidean distance measure. A five-cluster model was chosen, consistent with previous research results. The cluster profiles are presented on Fig. 1. The clusters can be respectively labelled as moderately fatalistic ($N=322$), future-oriented ($N=738$), present-oriented ($N=587$), balanced ($N=727$), and negative ($N=386$).

The distribution of types was significantly nonuniform across genders ($\chi^2(4)=33.89$, $p<.001$), but the prevalence of persons of any gender in each cluster did not exceed 60 %, suggesting that gender differences in time perspective types are weak. Weak age differences were also observed ($F(4, 2{,}755)=15.09$, $p<.001$), with post hoc tests indicating a higher average age in the Cluster 1 ($M=23.7$) compared to the other four clusters (mean age in the 21.7–22.6 range).

According to the chi-square test, the distribution of cluster representation was not the same across countries ($\chi^2(88)=353.08$, $p<.001$). See Table 5 for cluster membership statistics, and the distribution for the overall sample is given below.

Since all country samples have equal size, percentages for the overall sample correspond to expected frequencies of each time perspective type in each sample, and differences between observed and expected frequencies can be calculated and interpreted. The results of such analysis suggest that in some countries the distribution of types is statistically different from the overall distribution. The strongest differences were found for New Zealand ($\chi^2(4)=50.28$, $p<.001$), China ($\chi^2(4)=49.40$, $p<.001$), Estonia ($\chi^2(4)=33.97$, $p<.001$), the USA ($\chi^2(4)=28.41$, $p<.001$), and Algeria ($\chi^2(4)=23.17$, $p<.001$), followed by Israel ($\chi^2(4)=18.13$, $p<.01$), Mexico ($\chi^2(4)=16.83$, $p<.01$), France ($\chi^2(4)=14.57$, $p<.01$), and Brazil ($\chi^2(4)=14.22$, $p<.01$). Weaker, yet still significant, differences were found for

Table 5 Percentages of time perspective profiles across country samples

Country	Time perspective profile				
	Moderately fatalistic (%)	Future-oriented (%)	Present-oriented (%)	Balanced (%)	Negative (%)
Brazil	16.67	36.67	20.83	14.17	11.67
China-1	27.50	30.00	9.17	11.67	21.67
Czech Rep.	10.83	21.67	25.83	26.67	15.00
Germany	14.17	24.17	21.67	30.83	9.17
Algeria	5.83	35.00	21.67	13.33	24.17
Estonia	4.17	30.00	10.83	46.67	8.33
France	12.50	17.50	30.00	19.17	20.83
Greece-1	17.50	26.67	17.50	22.50	15.83
Croatia	17.50	17.50	24.17	24.17	16.67
Israel	8.33	27.50	15.83	41.67	6.67
Italy	10.83	31.67	14.17	32.50	10.83
Lithuania	15.00	28.33	15.83	28.33	12.50
Mexico	19.17	28.33	28.33	14.17	10.00
New Zealand	5.00	13.33	45.00	17.50	19.17
Poland	7.50	26.67	17.50	35.00	13.33
Portugal	8.33	34.17	16.67	32.50	8.33
Serbia	9.17	19.17	31.67	27.50	12.50
Russia	11.67	33.33	14.17	34.17	6.67
Spain	18.33	18.33	25.83	26.67	10.83
Sweden	15.00	19.17	28.33	26.67	10.83
Turkey	2.50	31.67	17.50	30.00	18.33
UK	5.00	24.17	25.00	31.67	14.17
USA	5.83	40.00	11.67	18.33	24.17
Overall sample	*11.67*	*26.74*	*21.27*	*26.34*	*13.99*

Turkey ($\chi^2(4)=12.77$, $p<.05$), Russia ($\chi^2(4)=12.18$, $p<.05$), Sweden ($\chi^2(4)=9.78$, $p<.05$), and Serbia ($\chi^2(4)=9.57$, $p<.05$).

Scores in the countries with statistically stronger differences from expected distribution (i.e., $p<.01$ above) showed some interesting patterns. For instance, in New Zealand and France, there was an emphasis on present-oriented and negative patterns indicative of hedonistic, present-day orientation. China exhibited emphasis on moderately fatalistic and negative profiles, suggesting a rather pessimistic time perspective. In Estonia and Israel, the balanced profile was particularly pronounced. The combination of future-oriented and negative types was characteristic of the USA, Algeria, and, to a weaker extent, Turkey. The combination of present-oriented and moderately fatalistic subtypes was shown in Mexico and, to a weaker extent, in Sweden. Brazil was characterised by moderately fatalistic and future orientation. Serbia tended towards a present-oriented pattern. Russia exhibited increased prevalence of future-oriented and balanced profiles, which was marginally significant. These data suggest that some countries may be characterised by a prevalence of people with specific time perspective profiles.

However, these results should be considered only as pilot and explorative. Currently our data shows evidence only of scalar equivalence of the ZTPI. Possibly average country score reflects the cultural bias associated with the way people in different cultures react to survey questions (e.g., acquiescence bias). When the individual scores were standardised within countries in order to eliminate response bias (such as acquiescence or extreme responding), no statistically significant cultural differences emerged. However, this approach may also eliminate valid variance associated with cultural differences. We plan to further investigate these emerging cultural profiles.

Discussion

An increasing number of studies have examined time perspective and other constructs dealing with the perception of time across cultures. Trying to overcome theoretical and methodological deficiencies in past research, our International Time Perspective Research Project has systematically examined the equivalence of the ZTPI across cultures. The data we presented in this chapter allow us to address the main question we posed in the introduction. We observed important similarities across countries in time perspective. Our results suggest that five temporal orientations are invariant across many countries with diverse cultural traditions. Therefore, we now can strongly recommend the revised version of the ZTPI as the "gold standard" for further research on time perspective, as well as its utility in cross-cultural comparisons. The basic dimensions underlying time perspective, as measured by the ZTPI, do not differ across cultures. This observation is in line with general findings in cross-cultural psychology according to which basic features of psychological functioning are invariant across cultures. However, the problems we had with the equivalence of items clearly illustrated another common finding in the field. Even if the structure of psychological functioning is invariant, that does not yet mean that items always "travel well"; some items may just not be suitable to measure the basic factors (in our case mainly due to unstable secondary loadings).

Future orientation, present orientation, and a balanced orientation are the most important time perspective profiles, followed by a negative and moderately fatalistic orientation. Clearly, the more positive orientations prevail as this is the pattern found in many countries. Yet, countries also show certain differences in preferred time perspective. For example, China has relatively high scores on the latter two negative orientations whereas Israel has very low scores on these dimensions.

Future research should relate time perspective to indicators of economic development, well-being, social functioning, and sustainability in various domains. At the current time of economic crises in many countries, those with insecure economic situations tend to move away from a focus on the future of saving and investing towards a more pragmatic style: living each day as it comes. Previous research has shown that time perspective changes during economical crises, as the future becomes unpredictable and uncertain, people cannot afford to plan for the long term and thus focus more on the present (Muzdybaev 2000). The revised version of the ZTPI we propose opens the way to more integrative and cumulative research on this issue of economic and political instability as related to time perspective.

Similarly, we would expect that central to establishing a solid future orientation is a sense of trust in one's predictions of outcomes of given current behaviours. With instability in one's family, children cannot trust that parents will deliver on their promises, so it is wiser to accept lesser short-term certain gains than plan on bigger elusive future ones. Hence, individuals' time perspectives are not only antecedent of society's sustainability and growth but also consequences, and research is needed to clarify how this construct, largely considered as a personality variable, interacts with cultural contexts. It is our hope that our study will stimulate researchers to pay more attention to time perspective as a critical construct linking attitudes, values, and behaviours in cross-cultural research.

References

Agsoy, E. J. R., Cacanog, A. Q., Chiong, K. O., & Ocenar, P. A. A. (2010). *A validation study of the Zimbardo Time Perspective Inventory (ZTPI) using a Cebuano-speaking sample.* Unpublished bachelor thesis, The Faculty of the Department of Psychology, University of San Carlos, Philippines.

Anagnostopoulos, F., & Griva, F. (2012). Exploring time perspective in Greek young adults: Validation of the Zimbardo Time Perspective Inventory and relationships with mental health indicators. *Social Indicators Research, 116*(1), 41–59. doi:10.1007/s11205-011-9792-y.

Apostolidis, T., & Fieulaine, N. (2004). Validation française de l'échelle de temporalité [French validation of the time perspective inventory]. *Revue européenne de psychologie appliquée, 54*, 207–217. doi:10.1016/j.erap.2004.03.001.

Ashkanasy, N., Gupta, V., Mayfield, M., & Trevor-Roberts, E. (2004). Future orientation. In R. House, P. Hanges, M. Javidan, P. Dorfman, & W. Gupta (Eds.), *Culture, leadership, and organizations: The GLOBE study of 62 societies* (pp. 282–342). Thousand Oaks: Sage.

Bandura, A. (1997). *Self-efficacy: The exercise of control.* New York: Freeman.

Bauman, Z. (1999). *Culture as praxis* (Newth ed.). London: Sage.

Boniwell, I., & Zimbardo, P. (2004). Balancing time perspective in pursuit of optimal functioning. In P. A. Linley & S. Joseph (Eds.), *Positive psychology in practice* (pp. 165–178). Hoboken: Wiley.

Boniwell, I., Osin, E., Linley, P. A., & Ivanchenko, G. (2010). A question of balance: Examining relationships between time perspective and measures of well-being in the British and Russian student samples. *Journal of Positive Psychology, 5*, 24–40. doi:10.1080/17439760903271181.

Brislin, R. W., & Kim, E. S. (2003). Cultural diversity in people's understanding and use of time. *Applied Psychology: An International Review, 52*, 363–382. doi:10.1111/1464-0597.00140.

Carelli, M. G., Wiberg, B., & Wiberg, M. (2011). Development and construct validation of the Swedish Zimbardo Time Perspective Inventory. *European Journal of Psychological Assessment, 27*, 220–227. doi:10.1027/1015-5759/a000076.

Carmi, N., & Goroshit, M. (2013). פרספקטיבת הזמן של זימברדו: בחינת הגרסה העברית של [Zimbardo's time perspective inventory: Testing the Hebrew version]. *Megamot – Journal of Behavioral Science, 49*.

Chen, F. F. (2008). What happens if we compare chopsticks with forks? The impact of making inappropriate comparisons in cross-cultural research. *Journal of Personality and Social Psychology, 95*, 1005–1018. doi:10.1037/a0013193.

Cohen, J. (1988). *Statistical power analysis for the behavioral sciences*. Hillsdale: Erlbaum.

Chinese Culture Connection. (1987). Chinese values and the search for culture-free dimensions of culture. *Journal of Cross-Cultural Psychology, 18*, 143–164. doi:10.1177/0022002187018002002.

Corral-Verdugo, V., Fraijo-Sing, B., & Pinheiro, J. Q. (2006). Sustainable behavior and time perspective: Present, past, and future orientations and their relationship with water conservation behavior. *Interamerican Journal of Psychology, 40*, 139–147.

Diaz-Morales, J. F. (2006). Estructura factorial y fiabilitad del Inventario de Perspectiva Temporal de Zimbardo [Factorial structure and reliability of Zimbardo Time Perspective Inventory]. *Psicothema, 18*(3), 565–571.

Dissel, J., & Potgieter J. C. (2007). *Validation of a scale to measure time perspective in an African context*, Unpublished master's thesis. North-West University, South Africa.

Djarallah, S., & Seghir Chorfi, S. (2009). تكييف قائمة زمباردو لمنظور الزمن للبيئة العربية [Zimbardo Time Perspective Inventory (ZTPI) (Arabic version)]. *Arabic Journal of Psychological Science, 23*, 53–65.

Drake, L., Duncan, E., Sutherland, F., Abernethy, C., & Henry, C. (2008). Time perspective and correlates of well-being. *Time and Society, 17*(1), 47–61. doi:10.1177/0961463X07086304.

Fontaine, J. R. J. (2005). Equivalence. In K. Kempf-Leonard (Ed.), *Encyclopedia of social measurement* (Vol. 1, pp. 803–813). San Diego: Academic. doi:10.1016/B0-12-369398-5/00116-X.

Frank, L. K. (1939). Time perspectives. *Journal of Social Philosophy, 4*, 293–312.

Gavreliuc, A., Mitu, E., & Gavreliuc, D. (2012). Time perspective in relation with social axioms for a romanian young cohort. In *Proceedings of 15th European conference of developmental psychology* (pp. 131–137). Milano: Medimond.

Hall, E. T. (1989). *Beyond culture*. New York: Anchor Books Editions.

Hofstede, G. (2001). *Culture's consequences: Comparing values, behaviors, institutions, and organizations across nations* (2nd ed.). Thousand Oaks: Sage.

Hofstede, G., & Minkov, M. (2010). Long- versus short-term orientation: New perspectives. *Asia Pacific Business Review, 16*(4), 493–504. doi:10.1080/13602381003637609.

Hofstede, G., Hofstede, G. J., & Minkov, M. (2010). *Cultures and organizations: Software of the mind* (3rd ed.). New York: McGraw-Hill.

Hoornaert, J. (1973). Time perspective: Theoretical and methodological considerations. *Psychologica Belgica, 13*, 265–294.

Human Development Report. (2011). *Human development statistical annex*. New York: HDRO (Human Development Report Office) United Nations Development Programme, pp. 127–130. Retrieved July 4, 2014, http://www.undp.org/content/dam/undp/library/corporate/HDR/2011%20Global%20HDR/English/HDR_2011_EN_Tables.pdf

Kolesovs, A. (2009). Factorial validity of the Latvian and Russian versions of the Zimbardo Time Perspective Inventory in Latvia. *Baltic Journal of Psychology, 10*(1,2), 55–64.

Leite, U. R., & Pasquali, L. (2008). Estudo de validação do Inventário de Perspectiva de Tempo do Zimbardo [Zimbardo Time Perspective Inventory validation study]. *Avaliação Psicológica, 7*, 301–320.

Levine, R., & Norenzayan, A. (1999). The pace of life in 31 countries. *Journal of Cross-Cultural Psychology, 30*, 178–205. doi:10.1177/0022022199030002003.

Lewin, K. (1942). Time perspective and morale. In G. Watson (Ed.), *Civilian morale*. Houghton Mifflin: Boston.

Liniauskaite, A., & Kairys, A. (2009). The Lithuanian version of the Zimbardo time perspective inventory. *Psichologija, 40*, 66–87.

Lukavská, K., Klicperová-Baker, M., Lukavský, J., & Zimbardo, P. G. (2011). ZTPI – Zimbardův dotazník časové perspektivy [Zimbardo Time Perspective Inventory]. *Československá psychologie, 55*(4), 356–373.

Luszczynska, A., Gutiérrez-Doña, B., & Schwarzer, R. (2005). General self-efficacy in various domains of human functioning: Evidence from five countries. *International Journal of Psychology, 40*, 80–89. doi:10.1080/00207590444000041.

McGrath, J. E., & Tschan, F. (2004). *Temporal matters in social psychology: Examining the role of time in the lives of groups and individuals*. Washington, DC: American Psychological Association. doi:10.1037/10659-000.

McHale, J. (1978). Time and the future sense. *Technological Forecasting and Social Change, 12*, 1–12. doi:10.1016/0040-1625(78)90031-8.

Meade, R. D. (1972). Future time perspectives of Americans and subcultures in India. *Journal of Cross-Cultural Psychology, 3*, 93–99. doi:10.1177/002202217200300108.

Milfont, T. L., & Fischer, R. (2010). Testing measurement invariance across groups: Applications in cross-cultural research. *International Journal of Psychological Research, 3*, 112–131.

Milfont, T. L., & Gapski, E. (2010, July). *Cross-cultural differences in time orientations: Integrating culture-level data*. Paper presented at the 20th Congress of the International Association for Cross-Cultural Psychology, Melbourne, Australia.

Milfont, T. L., Andrade, P. R., Belo, R. P., & Pessoa, V. S. (2008). Testing Zimbardo time perspective inventory in a Brazilian sample. *Interamerican Journal of Psychology, 42*(1), 49–58.

Muzdybaev, K. (2000). Переживание времени в период кризисов [Experience of time in the period of crisis]. *Psikhologicheskiy Zhurnal, 21*(4), 5–21.

Nedeljković, J. (2013). Srpska verzija Zimbardovog upitnika vremenskih perspektiva (ZTPI) [Serbian version of the Zimbardo's time perspective inventory]. In A. Kostic & J. Nedeljković (Eds.), *Studije vremenskih perspektiva u Srbiji* [Studies of time perspectives in Serbia] (pp. 33–68). Serbia: PUNTA.

Ortuño, V., & Gamboa, V. (2009). Estrutura factorial do Zimbardo Time Perspective Inventory – ZTPI numa amostra de estudantes universitários portugueses [Factorial structure of Zimbardo Time Perspective Inventory – ZTPI in a sample of Portuguese university students]. *Avances en Psicología Latinoamericana, 27*, 21–32.

Osin, E. N., & Orel, E. A. (2012). Возрастная динамика временной перспективы (на материале российских женщин) [Age differences in time perspective (in Russian females)]. In: A. K. Bolotova (Ed.), *Перспективные направления психологической науки: сб. науч. ст., вып. 2* (Perspective Directions in Psychological Science: Collected Papers, Issue 2) (pp. 85–103). Moscow: Higher School of Economics.

Przepiorka, A. (2011). *The determinants of realizing entrepreneurial goals*. Unpublished doctoral thesis, The John Paul II Catholic University of Lublin, Poland.

Seema, R., & Sircova, A. (2013). Mindfulness – A time perspective? Estonian study. *Baltic Journal of Psychology, 14*(1/2), 4–21.

Senyk O. (2012). Адаптація опитувальника часової перспективи особистості Ф. Зімбардо (ZTPI) (The Ukrainian adaptation of Zimbardo Time Perspective Inventory (ZTPI)). *Соціальна психологія, 1/2*(51–52), 153–168.

Shimojima, Y., Sato, K., & Ochi, K. (2012). Factor structure of the Japanese version of the Zimbardo Time Perspective Inventory (ZTPI). *The Japanese Journal of Personality, 21*(1), 74–83.

Sircova, A., Mitina, O. V., Boyd, J., Davydova, I. S., Zimbardo, P. G., Nepryaho, T. L., Nikitina, E. A., Semyonova, N. S., Fieulaine, N., & Yasnaya, V. A. (2007). Феномен временной перспективы в разных культурах (по материалам исследований с помощью методики ZTPI) [The phenomenon of time perspective across different cultures: Review of researches using ZTPI scale]. *International Journal of Cultural-Historical Psychology, 4*, 19–31.

Sircova, A., Sokolova, E. T., & Mitina, O. V. (2008). Адаптация опросника временной перспективы личности Ф. Зимбардо [Adaptation of Zimbardo time perspective inventory]. *Psikhologigesky Journal, 29*, 101–109.

Sircova, A., van de Vijver, F. J. R., Osin, E., Milfont, T. L., Fieulaine, N., Kislali-Erginbilgic, A., & Zimbardo, P. G. (2014). A global look at time: A 24-country study of the equivalence of the Zimbardo Time Perspective Inventory. *SageOpen, 4*(1). doi: 10.1177/2158244013515686.

Strathman, A., Gleicher, F., Boninger, D. S., & Edwards, C. S. (1994). The consideration of future consequences: Weighing immediate and distant outcomes of behavior. *Journal of Personality and Social Psychology, 66*, 742–752. doi:10.1037/0022-3514.66.4.742.

Trompenaars, F., & Hampden-Turner, C. (1998). *Riding the waves of culture: Understanding diversity in global business* (2nd ed.). New York, NY: McGraw-Hill.

van Beek, W., Berghuis, J. G., & Kamphuis, J. H. (in preparation). *Validation of the Dutch ZTPI: Time perspective in a clinical and a non-clinical sample.*

van Beek, W., Berghuis, H., Kerkhof, A. J. F. M., & Beekman, A. T. F. (2011). Time perspective, personality and psychopathology: Zimbardo's time perspective inventory in psychiatry. *Time and Society, 20*(3), 364–374. doi:10.1177/0961463X10373960.

van de Vijver, F. J. R., & Leung, K. (1997). *Methods and data analysis for cross-cultural research.* Thousand Oaks: Sage.

White, L. T., Valk, R., & Dialmy, A. (2011). What is the meaning of "on time"? The sociocultural nature of standards of punctuality. *Journal of Cross-Cultural Psychology, 42*, 482–493. doi:10.1177/0022022110362746.

Zimbardo, P. G., & Boyd, J. N. (1999). Putting time in perspective: A valid, reliable individual-differences metric. *Journal of Personality and Social Psychology, 77*, 1271–1288. doi:10.1037/0022-3514.77.6.1271.

Zimbardo, P. G., & Boyd, J. N. (2008). *The time paradox: The new psychology of time that will change your life*. New York: Free Press.

Keeping Time

Robert V. Levine

In what may be the most supple of all intellectual acrobatics, Western culture has reduced time—that most obscure and abstract of all intangibles—to the most objective of all quantities—money. We live in a world where workers are paid by the hour, lawyers charge by the minute and advertising is sold by the second (over 86,667 dollars per second for the 2007 Super Bowl in the U.S.A.). With time and things on the same value scale, I can tell you how many of my working hours equal the price of the computer I am typing on.

Can I really? As a social scientist, I've spent much of the last 30 years studying how people around the world conceive, use and measure time. If I've learned anything, it is that the numbers on the clock capture only one glimpse of the human experience of time, and a most Westernly ethnocentric glimpse at that. Cultures differ profoundly in their conceptions of early and late, of waiting and rushing, of the past, the present, and the future. With no formal dictionary to spell out a culture's rules, the unsuspecting visitor often stumbles into temporal confusion.

I learned this first-hand early in my career when I was a visiting Professor of Psychology at the Federal University in Niteroi, Brazil, a mid-sized city across the bay from Rio de Janeiro. I arrived anxious to observe first-hand just what characteristics of this alien environment would require my greatest readjustment. From my past, more limited, travel experiences, I anticipated difficulties with such issues as the language, my privacy, and standards of cleanliness. But these turned out to be a piece of cake compared to the distress that Brazilians' ideas of time and punctuality were to cause me.

I was aware before arriving, of course, of the stereotype of the *amanhã* attitude of Brazilians (the Portuguese version of *a mañana*), whereby it is said that whenever it is conceivably possible the business of today is put off until tomorrow. I knew I'd need to slow down and to reduce my expectations of accomplishment. But I was

R.V. Levine (✉)
Department of Psychology, California State University,
Fresno, CA 93740-0011, USA
e-mail: robertle@csufresno.edu

M. Stolarski et al. (eds.), *Time Perspective Theory; Review, Research and Application: Essays in Honor of Philip G. Zimbardo*, DOI 10.1007/978-3-319-07368-2_12,

a kid from Brooklyn, New York, where one is taught at an early age to move fast or get out of the way, who years ago had learned to survive life in the foreign culture of Fresno, California, a city where even laid-back Los Angelenos must learn to decelerate. Adjusting to the pace of life in Brazil, I figured, would call for no more than a bit of fine tuning. What I got instead was a dose of culture shock that changed my life.

My lessons began soon after arriving. My first class was scheduled from 10 a.m. until noon. I arrived on schedule. I was greeted outside the door by a group of friendly students in animated conversation, sipping *cafezeinho*'s (the traditional Brazilian buzz-drink consisting of one-half thick coffee and one-half sugar). The students assured me they'd be in momentarily. They finally settled into their seats 10 min after the hour. Other students straggled in later. Several arrived after 10:30. A few showed up closer to eleven and two others after that. The latecomers wore the relaxed smiles I later came to enjoy. Each greeted me, and although a few apologized briefly, none seemed terribly concerned about being late. They seemed to assume that I understood. I made a smug mental note that the *amanhã* stereotype was everything I'd anticipated.

My confusion began, however, when the class came to a close. Back home in California, I never need to look at a clock to know when the class hour is ending. The shuffling of books is accompanied by strained expressions screaming: "I'm hungry/I'm thirsty/I've got to go to the bathroom/I'm going to suffocate if you keep us one more second."

But when noon arrived for my first Brazilian class, only a few students left right away. The ones who stayed were full of questions for me, about life in California, universities in the United States, pro basketball players, Las Vegas—about seemingly everything other than the course material I'd been boring them with. A few drifted out slowly during the next 15 min. Some continued asking questions long after that. Some who'd left earlier came back. After a good half hour of this, I excused myself. Their curiosity had worn me out.

These experiences were repeated in many variations over the course of the year. Brazilians did, most definitely, often show up late for appointments. But they were just as likely to show up when I didn't expect them, to arrive early or stay late, or to show up on time but with a completely different agenda. I even ran studies that supported these anecdotal observations. Initially, I was bewildered and frustrated by this seemingly undisciplined attitude. Eventually, it taught me a profound lesson: There are many ways to tell time. Brazilians' rules of punctuality, I came to realize, went well beyond a simplistic *amanhã* casualness. Their relationship to time was, in fact, completely different than what I assumed was normal.

• • •

Philip Zimbardo, who we honor in these chapters, has done more than anyone to both help us understand these differences and to use to this knowledge to enhance the quality of our lives. Zimbardo, along with talented colleagues like Alex Gonzalez and John Boyd, have demonstrated that how we think about the past, present and future, or very conception of time, effects virtually every aspect of our life—our relationships, careers, successes and failures, the decisions we make, the emotions we feel and, in the end, the very texture of our life experience. Zimbardo and his colleagues have also showed how interrelated our views of time are with the world around us. The way we think about time is mirrored in our culture, geography, climate, religion, social class, educational level and the political and economic stability of our surroundings; it is effected by our social models—family, friends, society—as well as our gender, age and seemingly every other aspect of our lives (e.g. Gonzalez and Zimbardo 1985; Zimbardo and Boyd 2008). Their work has been the inspiration for virtually every aspect of my own work on the subject of time.

My work has focused on cultural differences in time, what we can learn from these differences and—taking a page straight out of Zimbardo—how this understanding can be applied to our lives.[1]

During my year in Brazil, I was repeatedly bewildered, frustrated and, eventually, fascinated by the customs and ideas of social time sent my way. The reason that Brazilians' rules of punctuality so confused me, I was to learn, is they were operating with a completely different relationship to time than I was used to. I was living on clock time. My Brazilian hosts were on event time.

Under clock time, the hour on the timepiece governs the beginning and ending of activities. When event time predominates, scheduling is determined by activities. Events begin and end when, by mutual consensus, participants "feel" the time is right. The distinction between clock and event time is profound. Sociologist Robert Lauer, in his book *Temporal Man*, concluded that the most fundamental difference in timekeeping throughout history has been between people operating by the clock versus those who measure time by social events. What's more surprising to travelers like myself is how diverse the world remains today.

Many countries exhort event time as a philosophy of life. In Mexico, for example, there is a popular adage to "Give time to time" (*Darle tiempo al tiempo*). Across the globe in Africa, it is said that "Even the time takes its time." In Trinidad, it is a cultural bedrock that "Any time is Trinidad time." In his book of that name, anthropologist Kevin Birth found that rural residents and farmers there are still—despite having access to cable TV and being familiar with industrialized Western culture—baffled by phrases like "time is money," "budget your time," or "time management (Birth 1999)."

Even the most radical clock-timers sometimes operate on event time. In typical clock time fashion, for example, people from the United States tend to arrive much more punctually to parties than Brazilians. (In one of our studies, Brazilians said they would arrive, on average, a little over one-half hour late for a nephew's birthday party; the average for U.S. respondents was 3 min late). But once at the party, not even the most compulsive U.S. guests will schedule conversations by the clock. No one says, "I'll pencil you for a chat from 7:18 to 7:31." When do conversations

[1] Parts of this chapter are taken from: Levine (1997).

begin and end? By unstated mutual consensus, when it "seems the right time" or "just happens." This is event time.

There is a third type of timekeeping, nature time, when scheduling by clocks becomes virtually impossible. One of my former graduate students, Salvatore Niyonzima, described a good example of this in his home country of Burundi. Life in Burundi, as in most of Central Africa, is guided by the seasons. More than 80 % of the population of Burundi are farmers. As a result, "people still rely on the phases of nature," Niyonzima explains. "When the dry season begins it is time for harvesting. And when the rainy season comes back—then, of course, it's time to return to the fields and plant and grow things, because this is the cycle."

"Appointments are not necessarily in terms of a precise hour of the day. For people who grew up in rural areas, and who haven't had very much education, they might make an early appointment by saying, 'Okay, I'll see you tomorrow morning when the cows are going out for grazing.'" If they want to meet in the middle of the day, "they set their appointment for the time 'when the cows are going to drink in the stream,' which is where they are led at mid-day." In order to prevent the youngest cows from drinking too much, Niyonzima explains, farmers typically spend 2 or 3 h with them back in a sheltered place, while their elders are still drinking from the stream. "Then in the afternoon, let's say somewhere around 3 o'clock, it's time again to get the young cows outside for the evening graze. So if we want to make a late appointment we might say 'I'll see you when the young cows go out.'"

Being any more precise—to say, for example, "I'll meet you in the latter part of the time when the cows are out drinking"—would be, Niyonzima says, "just too much. If you arrange to come to my place when the cows are going to drink water, then it means it's around the middle of the day. If it's an hour earlier or an hour later, it doesn't matter. He knows that he made an appointment and that he'll be there." Precision is difficult and mostly irrelevant because it is hard to know exactly what time people will be leading the cows out in the first place. "I might decide to lead them to the river one hour later because I either got them out of the home later or it didn't look like they really had that much to eat because the place where they were grazing didn't have very much pasture."

People in Burundi use similarly tangible images to mark the night time. "We refer to a very dark night as a 'Who are you?' night," Niyonzima explains. "This means that it was so dark that you couldn't recognize anybody without hearing their voice. You know that somebody is there but can't see them because it is so dark, so you say 'Who are you?' as a greeting. They speak and I hear their voice and now I recognize who they are. 'Who are you?'-time is one way to describe when it gets dark. We might refer back to an occasion as having occurred on a 'Who are you?' night."

Specifying precise nighttime appointments, Niyonzima says, "gets difficult. 'Who are you?' simply refers to the physical condition of darkness. I certainly wouldn't give a time—like 8 p.m. or 9 p.m. When people want to name a particular time of the night, they might use references to aspects of sleep. They may, for example, say something occurred at a time 'When nobody was awake' or, if they wanted to be a little more specific, at the time 'When people were beginning the first period of their sleep.' Later in the night might be called 'Almost the morning light' or the time 'When the rooster sings;' or, to get really specific, 'When the rooster sings for the first time' or the second time, and so on. And then we're ready for the cows again."

• • •

Social psychologists like to measure things and I have tried to do this with peoples' sense of time. For the past three decades my students and I have been conducting cross-cultural studies on the speed component of everyday life. In our most recent studies, we conducted several field experiments in the largest or other major city in each of 31 countries around the world. In one experiment, for example, we timed the average walking speed of randomly selected pedestrians over a distance of 60 ft. Another experiment sampled speed in the workplace; specifically, how long it took postal clerks to fulfill a standard request for stamps. Each of the measurements were taken during main business hours in main downtown areas.

We found large cross-national differences. Most of these mirrored popular stereotypes. The fastest big cities, for example, tended to come from Western Europe and industrialized Asia while those in economically struggling nations (such as Mexico, Brazil, and Indonesia) tend to be slowest. The differences were often substantial. For example, on the walking speed measure we found that pedestrians in Rio de Janeiro walk only two-thirds as fast as do pedestrians in Zurich, Switzerland.

Next we asked whether there are characteristics of places and cultures that might be related to their tempo. Are there elements in the "personality" of a place that determine, or at least to some degree predict, how fast or slow people move? From our experiments and the research of others, there appear to be five principal factors that determine the tempo of cultures around the world: People are prone to move faster in places with vital economies, a high degree of industrialization, larger populations, cooler climates and a cultural orientation toward individualism.

Our conclusions were clear: Countries and cultures differ markedly in their overall speed of life and these differences are to at least some degree predictable by demographic, economic and environmental characteristics of these places. These differences, we also found, were reflected in many other characteristics of these places, including their psychological, physical and social well-being. (For more details of these results, see, e.g.: Levine 1997).

Of course, like most science, the findings from our studies are limited. As Zimbardo would be the first to point out, it is important to note what we have not studied. We measured the speed of workday life. But what about the duration of this tempo? To what extent do people pause between activities? How long are their off-hours? Do they take vacations? What is the balance between hard work and leisure?

It is informative, for example, to compare the work-hour patterns of industrialized nations. In these places, it may be assumed, at least some degree of personal decision-making underlies the number of hours people work and, consequently, these patterns may reflect on the cultural values of these places.

Perhaps the best example is the United States. One of the most surprising results in our speed studies found that the United States, represented by its classic speedster New York City, scored an unexpectedly slow sixteenth in overall pace—right in the middle of the list. We were so surprised by the relative slowness of New York's scores that, as a reliability check, we sent out a second experimenter to collect a new set of observations; these turned out to be virtually identical to the first. We were initially frustrated by the New York data because they muddied our pre-experimental hypotheses. Could the stereotype *of La Dolce Vita* that has characterized European life (at least in the eyes of Americans) now be more aptly applied to New Yorkers? This conclusion becomes unlikely when we look at work-hour data. There is considerable evidence that in this realm the United States outpaces most of the world.

The average workweek in the United States is the longest of all industrialized countries. A 1999 report by the International Labor Organization found that the average annual paid working hours in the United States was 1,966, compared, for example, to 1,656 h in France, 1,560 h in Germany, and 1,399 h in Norway (*ILO News* 1999). Workers in the United States, in other words, put in an annual average of 310 more hours than their counterparts in France, 406 more than workers in Germany, and 567 more than those in Norway. Taking a 40-h week as a base, these figures indicate that the average U.S. worker labors almost 8 weeks more than workers in France, 10 more weeks than those in Germany, and more than 14 more weeks—over 3 months—than those in Norway.

It is notable that the difference in working hours between western Europe and the United States is widening. Until the 1940s the average hours in both Europe and the United States had been declining in tandem for nearly a century (Hunnicutt 1988). But the average U.S. workweek has remained unchanged for more than half a century. In fact, many experts believe that leisure time has actually been decreasing. Historian Juliet Schor, for example, in her widely publicized book, *The Overworked American*: *The Unexpected Decline of Leisure*, argued persuasively that the average American has less time than 20 years ago. Schor presents evidence that this loss of leisure is not an accident and one reason is the lack of attention unions in the United States have focused on the question of work time (Schor 1991).

In Europe, on the other hand, the downward trend in work hours has persisted, albeit with increasing challenges. Unlike the United States, organized labor in Europe has kept the issue of shorter working hours at the top of its agenda throughout the postwar period. When economic crises hit, workers have fought the pressure for longer hours. In Germany, a series of bitter strikes in the 1980s earned a contract for a 35-h workweek for members of the large German union IG Metall. This standard subsequently spread to much of the German labor force (Schor 1991). The French successfully fought for even more lenient contracts. In 1996, after French truck drivers snarled the country with a series of bitter strikes, the government conceded to lower their retirement age to 55. (For people like dancers and musicians in opera companies, the retirement age in France is now as low as 45 years). With that issue settled, unions focused their attention on the length of the workweek. In January 2000, a 35-h workweek was adopted (Smith 2003).

In the United States, strikes are virtually always about more money, rarely about more time. Contrary to labor trends in France, the percentage of Americans over

65 who still work has been rising in the last two decades. In 2000, it was higher than at any time since 1979, according to government statistics (Walsh 2001). And so, after nearly 100 years of simultaneous decline, U.S. work hours, days, and years have at best remained flat over the last half century, while in Europe they have persisted in declining.

If we look at vacation time, the gap between western Europe and the United States is even wider. In Switzerland, for example, agreements mandate between 4 and 5 weeks of paid vacation for workers. Every country in Europe has collective bargaining agreements which guarantee minimum paid vacations ranging from four to five and one-half weeks. In most cases, these mandated vacation periods are for as much as 6 weeks. In Sweden, it ranges up to 8 weeks. According to recent statistics from the World Tourism Organization, Italy currently leads the world in average vacation time at 42 days a year (Infoplease 2004), it is official national policy to allow women 22 weeks of paid maternity leave and an additional year of unpaid leave (Levine 1997). The social welfare states of Scandinavia, where enhancing the psychological quality of life has long been a focus for both officials and the populace, go even further. In Sweden, new parents have in the past been entitled to a combined 12 months leave of absence at virtually full pay, and another 3 months at reduced pay. Swedish parents are also entitled to 60 days per year (120 days in some cases) at 80 % of their normal pay to care for a sick child (Hadenius and Lindgren 1992). Policies like these have become increasingly difficult to maintain with the new economic demands of the European Union. However, they persist. In the United States, vacation time for most workers remains limited to the traditional 2 weeks—that is, if the employee has been fortunate enough to avoid being shifted to seasonal contracts, in which case they may get no paid vacation at all (Levine 1997).

• • •

How does Zimbardo's work on time perspective relate to my observations on the larger social level? The discipline of social psychology casts a wide net. Unlike our colleagues in the fields of personality psychology and sociology—the first of whom tend to focus on the private, internal functioning of people; the latter on their social groups—social psychologists are concerned with the give and take between individuals *and* the groups that guide their behavior. We study—with no small arrogance—what our founding father Kurt Lewin called the "life space," the sum total of the behavior of individuals as they exist in their environments.

I believe our two approaches fit elegantly into this life space. Zimbardo emphasizes individual differences. My work focuses on places. But the underlying assumption of my work is that places, like people, have their own personalities and it is here that I have profited deeply from Zimbardo's insights into the personalities of people. I can only hope that a smattering of my approach has been of some value to his work.

Time is the slipperiest of beasts. As St. Augustine observed: "What, then, is time? If no one asks me, I know. If I wish to explain it to someone who asks, I know it not."

A 2006 study by the publishers of the Oxford Dictionary found that the word "time" is the most commonly used noun in the English language (Levine 2008). But what that word means to different people is something else again. "Each culture believes that every other kind of space and time is an approximation to or a perversion of the real space and time in which *it* lives," Lewis Mumford wisely noted (Keyes 1991). The way people conceive, use and measure time is intertwined with their fundamental cultural values and, by definition, all cultural values are arbitrary.

Our rules of social time are, as the anthropologist Edward Hall observed, a silent language, but one which often speaks louder than words (Hall 1959). No one type of time reckoning is better than another. Each has its place. But it is worth recognizing that no particular rules of social time are cut in stone. As Philip Zimbardo has shown us, the way people conceive, use and measure time is intertwined with their fundamental cultural values and, by definition, all cultural values are arbitrary. How we approach time defines nothing less than the texture of our days and the grammar of our social relationships. Learning how others' count their time teaches new options for counting our own.

References

Birth, K. (1999). *Any time is Trinidad time: Social meanings and temporal consciousness.* Gainesville: University Press of Florida.

Gonzalez, A., & Zimbardo, P. G. (1985, May). Time in perspective: A Psychology Today survey report. *Psychology Today*, 21–26.

Hadenius, S., & Lindgren, A. (1992). *On Sweden.* Helsingborg: The Swedish Institute.

Hall, E. (1959). *The silent language.* New York: Doubleday.

Hunnicutt, B. J. (1988). *Work without end.* Philadelphia: Temple University Press.

ILO News. (1999, September 6). *Americans work longest hours among industrialized countries.* http://www.hartford-hwp.com/archives/26/077.html

Infoplease. (2004, September 21). *Average number of vacation days around the world per year.* http://www.infoplease.com/ipa/A0922052.html

Keyes, R. (1991). *Timelock* (p. 192). New York: Ballantine.

Levine, R. (1997). *A geography of time.* New York: Basic Books.

Levine, R. (2008). Keeping time. *SuperConsciousness, 2*, 18–21.

Schor, J. B. (1991). *The overworked American: The unexpected decline of leisure.* New York: Basic Books.

Smith, C. S. (2003, January 10). Shortened workweek shortens French tempers. *New York Times.* Retrieved from http://www.nytimes.com/2003/01/10/world/shortened-workweek-shortens-french-tempers.html

Walsh, M. W. (2001, February 26). Reversing decades-long trend, Americans retiring later in life. *New York Times.* Retrieved from http://www.nytimes.com/2001/02/26/business/reversing-decades-long-trend-americans-retiring-later-in-life.html

Zimbardo, P. G. & Boyd, J. N. (2008). *The time paradox. The new psychology of time that will change your life.* New York: Free Press.

The Sankofa Effect: Divergent Effects of Thinking About the Past for Blacks and Whites

James M. Jones and Jordan B. Leitner

Introduction

Time Perspective is… "the often nonconscious process whereby the continual flows of personal and social experiences are assigned to temporal categories, or time frames, that help to give order, coherence, and meaning to those events" (Zimbardo and Boyd 1999, p. 1271). This view comes from an individualist perspective, a personal narrative of the self. While this is no doubt an important guide to the meaning a person attaches to her life, one may also derive meaning from a collective narrative (Markus and Kitayama 1991).

Culture and the meanings that attach to it also give order, coherence and meaning to events. As the African aphorism goes, "I am because we are, and because we are therefore I am." (Mbiti 1970, p. 351). Or, as Shweder and Sullivan (1993) argue, "culture and psyche make each other up." An important question for this paper is how does a collective time perspective affect individual behavior. More specifically, how does belonging to a cultural group affect time perspective and how it shapes responses to marginalization, prejudice and discrimination?

In our view of time perspective, the individual and the collective merge in an individual's psyche. This is particularly true when the collective is a marginalized group or culture living in the context of a dominant and discriminatory majority. Time perspective reflects not only one's autobiographical time experience or sense, but how one's beliefs about the collective historical as well as contemporary narrative intersect and influence the person's time travel forward and backward.

J.M. Jones (✉)
Department of Psychology, University of Delaware, Newark, DE, USA
e-mail: JJones@psych.udel.edu

J.B. Leitner
Department of Psychology, University of California, Berkeley, CA, USA
e-mail: jleitner@psych.udel.edu

M. Stolarski et al. (eds.), *Time Perspective Theory; Review, Research and Application: Essays in Honor of Philip G. Zimbardo*, DOI 10.1007/978-3-319-07368-2_13,

Collective Time Perspective

Culture and Time

Cultures have been characterized by their orientation to time. Western cultures have been described as *temponomic*—time is a valuable asset and must be managed judiciously like any other asset (McGrath 1988). By contrast, Jones, based on his research in Trinidad, refers to a *tempoagnostic* view of time—time has no inherent value and cannot be saved, wasted or invested. This idea is reflected in the Trinidadian notion that "Any time is Trinidad time." (Jones and Brown 2005). Anticipating Shweder and Sullivan, Hall (1983) argues that "Because time is a core system of all cultures, and because culture plays such a prominent role in the understanding of time as a cultural system, it is virtually impossible to separate time from culture…" (p. 4). Hall distinguishes cultures on the basis of their orientation toward time: *monochronic time* (M-time)—characterized by doing one thing at a time, following schedules, and considering time to be tangible, and *polychronic time* (P-time) characterized by "doing many things at once." The concept of *Confucian Dynamism*—variable orientation to the past or the future—was proposed as a fifth dimension of the influential Hofstede dimensions of culture (Hofstede and Bond 1988).

Time perspective is thus a characteristic of cultures and their members. Furthermore, cultural variations strongly suggest that time perspective is not static, and constraining it by an individual difference measurement—which can be useful theoretically, empirically and practically—may nevertheless limit our understanding of the multiple ways in which time perspectives influence human behavior.

Collective Variations in Time Perspective

We propose an approach to time perspective that focuses on ways that culture defines the relationship of the past, present and future. Specifically, we argue that Blacks and Whites use different psychological means to integrate the personal and collective pasts into the present and future. The past-present and past-future relationships may differ between Blacks and Whites because of the divergent cultural narratives that provide meaning and coherence to these events. Further, these divergent narratives influence the interpretation of the present and expectations for the future.

Cultural Reflections on Time

How do narratives about personal and collective experiences get assigned to temporal categories? One's perception and experience of time is subjective. The nature of the subjective experience of time derives in part from the motivations one brings to its construal. One's need for order, coherence and meaning dictates how events are placed in time and subsequently interpreted. Motivations, memories and coherence are influenced by one's own experiences as well as those of the group to which one belongs. The more clearly defined the group narrative, the more likely the past is to influence present and future cognitions and affect. If a person is identified with the collective, then that is part of their personal awareness, consciousness and self-definition (see measures of Collective Self-Esteem, Luhtanen and Crocker 1992; Nationalist Ideology, Sellers et al. 1997; African Self-Consciousness, Baldwin and Bell 1985; or Afrocentrism, Vandiver et al. 2002). The coherence of the self must include the ways in which the referent others in the group cohere or fit; the collective narrative has meaning, and is useful to achieving personal order and coherence of self.

Importantly, the temporal categorization of the collective narrative influences whether a person integrates or dissociates the past with the present. For example, young Whites often argue that the atrocities of slavery and racism are behind us, and most importantly are not something they had any involvement with. That is in the past. When Blacks and other supporters insist that racism is *not* a thing of the past, but is currently an active determinant of racial injustice, racial resentment among Whites may arise (Wilson and Davis 2011). Two items used to assess racial resentment are: "African Americans do not need any special consideration because racism is a thing of the past;" and "For African Americans to succeed they need to stop using racism and slavery as excuses." Clearly, there is a temporal comparative process here that it is triggered when race becomes salient and challenges one's White racial or cultural identity.

By contrast, Blacks often argue that the racist attitudes of the past persist in today's world. Research in our lab illustrates these divergent racial effects. We showed pictures of historical oppression of Blacks (lynchings, White only signs, fire hoses and dogs during the civil rights era) to White and Black students. Compared to those who saw control pictures depicting various nature scenes, Whites who saw these oppression pictures were *less* likely to perceive an ambiguously discriminatory scenario of racial injustice as wrong and unfair. Blacks who saw the oppression pictures, by contrast were *more* likely to perceive it as unfair (Turner and Jones 2004).

Just as the meaning of the present is shaped by one's construal of the past, the meaning of the past is shaped by the content of experiences, the cultural narratives they are embedded in, and the contemporary psychological motivations they engender. As a consequence, we argue that the past for members of marginalized and oppressed groups will have a different meaning and play a different role in the construction of present cognitions, motives, meanings and behaviors.

Collective Time Perspective Scale: An Idea

At the individual level, the ZTPI approach (Zimbardo and Boyd 1999) has captured the full attention of time perspective researchers. In the ZTPI approach, the past is *positive*—containing happy and desirable images and recollections of an earlier time ("I get nostalgic about my childhood"), or *negative*—filled with recurring unhappy memories and reflections ("I've taken my share of abuse and rejection in the past"). Similarly the present perspective is the residue of fate-hedonically *negative*—"My life path is controlled by forces I cannot influence," or of self-indulgence—hedonically *positive*—"I often follow my heart more than my head." Future perspective, however, is one-dimensional and is dominated by striving, achievement and restraint, and the conscientious planning for and attention to goals and possibilities for one's life. These perspectives are generally limited to a person's individual biography-their personal narrative.

On the other hand, taking the collective into account may alter the representations of the past and the future. Consider for example the Past Positive and Past Negative items from the ZTPI. What if they were framed in a collective framework? For example, "My group has taken its share of abuse and rejection in the past." In its individual form, its connotation is negative. From a collective Black narrative of slavery, discrimination, and oppression over several centuries, it could be *either* negative—guiding black individuals to low self-esteem, shame, uncertainty, or positive—producing self- esteem, pride and self-confidence, and moral certitude by focusing attention on the resilience, coping, and accomplishment of black people over time. Thus, past-present and past-future relationships critically depend on both the *locus* of these memories—individual or collective, and their *valence*—whether they are construed positively or negative in the individual's psyche.

We propose—and are in the process of developing—a measure of collective time perspective that captures the degree to which a person views the past through an individual and/or collective lens. Such a measure should integrate time perspective and collective identity, as collective identity is linked to the content and meaning of a person's collective narrative. One example of a similar integration of individual and collective perspectives is the Collective Self-Esteem Scale (CSE; Luhtanen and Crocker 1992). The CSE expands traditional measures of self-esteem such as Rosenberg (1965), by including a social identity perspective in which self-esteem is a importantly influenced by one's connections with one's social groups (Turner et al. 1979). The individual collective integration is assessed by the extent to which individuals (a) feel they are a member of their social group, (b) personally view their groups positively, (c) integrate group membership into personal identity, and (d) believe that others view their groups positively.

We hypothesize that the importance of a collective narrative on time perspective increases when a person feels strong group membership, views the group positively, and integrates group membership into personal identity. To measure collective time perspective directly we suggest asking respondents how they think about their *collective* past, present, and future. Consistent with the past dimensions on the ZPTI (Zimbardo and Boyd 1999), it is important to capture the collective Past-Positive (e.g., "I like rituals and traditions of my group that are regularly repeated") and collective Past-Negative (e.g., "It is hard for me to forget unpleasant images of my group's past"). It would be important also to measure the degree to which a collective past is integrated into an individual present (e.g., "In order to understand who I am today, I must understand my group's past") and future (e.g., "In order to plan for the future, I must consider my group's past"). Critically, such a measure might reveal ways in which thinking about the past through a collectivistic frame affects the perceptions of the present and future.

Individuals belong to many groups (e.g., racial, ethnic, religious, professional, etc.). As typically employed by the CSE, groups remain unspecified with the assumption that references to "my group" will make salient one's most personally significant groups. When measuring collective time perspective, we believe that the group about which there is a rich historical narrative should be specified. For example, a Black professor may not have a rich historical narrative about being a professor, but likely would about being black. Thus the impact of collective identity on time perspective would depend both on the salience, significance of and identification with the group, and the nature of the group's historical narrative. Ultimately, past-present and past-future relationships are defined by the interaction between a collective narrative and person's collective time perspective. This interaction is at the center of Sankofa.

Sankofa Effect

Sankofa is an Akan language word from Ghana that suggests one should look to the past to prepare for the future; literally, "go back and get it." Sankofa is represented by Adrinka symbols of a backward facing bird plucking an egg from its back, or a heart-shaped connection of past and present (see Fig. 1) (*The Spirituals Project*, University of Denver 2012).

In 1993, the significance of Sankofa was dramatized in a film by Ethiopian filmmaker Haile Gerima. His story of *Sankofa* follows Mona, a contemporary African American model, on a film shoot in Ghana at Elmina Castle. Mona does not know Elmina Castle was a central depot for the Atlantic slave trade in the seventeenth century. There she encounters a mysterious old man, *Sankofa*, and is transported to

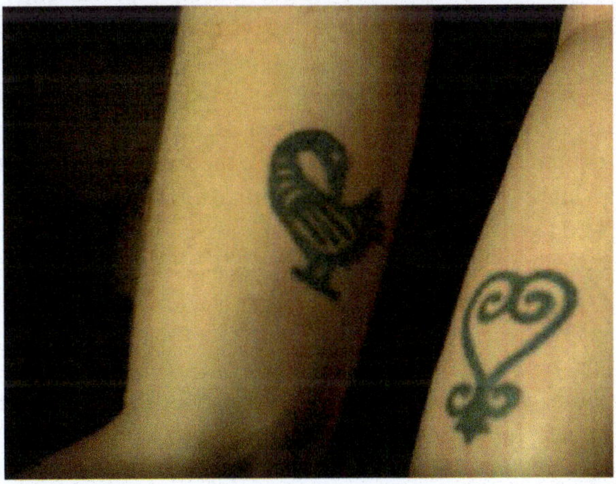

Fig. 1 Sankofa bird, and heart-shape Adrinka symbols of the importance of the past in the present and future

the past where, as a house servant named Shola on a plantation in the Southern United States, she is abused by her slave masters. Nunu, an African-born field hand, and Shango, Shola's West Indian lover, resist and rebel against the slave system. Inspired by Nunu and Shango's determination to defy the slave system, Shola joins them in fighting back against her masters. After her trials, Shola returns to the present as Mona, determined to live a life of understanding and meaning motivated by her newfound awareness of her African roots.

The Sankofa story affirms an African cultural proverb that ascribes value and importance to the past in contemporary life "It is not wrong to go back for that which you have forgotten." (*The Spirituals Project* 2012). The Akan believe that the past illuminates the present and that the search for knowledge is a life-long process. In this view of the past, it is not merely hedonic (pleasurable or painful), but crucial to understanding the present and designing a course for one's future. It is necessary to find one's "true self" (the *daimon*, see Waterman 1993) and thus involves self-awareness, seeking a meaningful life, developing positive relationships with others, and finding purpose, direction and mastery in life (Ryff and Keyes 1995).

For Blacks, when race becomes salient and is attached to injustice and racial hierarchy, its interpretation hinges to some extent on retrieving the past, "going back and getting it." It is the prominence of one's past individual and collective psychological life *in the present* and its influence on the thoughts and feelings directed at the future that we label the *Sankofa Effect*.

Drawing on lessons of the past is not a simple process, however. The past does not exist as an objective fact, but as a collection of thoughts, memories and stories that are subject to one's current affective state and motivational goals. Striving to maintain psychological health and well-being are prominent among these motivational goals. Mona encountered Sankofan time-travel and learned of the importance of her African roots. But what does this mean for her contemporary psychological processes, her sense of self, her individual or collective identities?

We propose that the past activated by thoughts of race has greater Sankofan significance for Blacks than for Whites, in particular, and more generally for members of any group whose collective narrative prominently includes oppression at the hands of a dominant out-group. Members of a racially dominant group, may dissociate themselves from the past, or rationalize the dominance as justifiable based on a racial or cultural narrative. For example, research on the *Marley hypothesis*—that group differences in perception of racism reflect dominant-group denial of and ignorance about the extent of past racism—shows that relative to Black participants, White participants perceived less historical racism and these differences were mediated by differences in historical knowledge (Nelson et al. 2013). Further, relevant to our approach, racial differences were stronger among participants who scored higher on a measure of racial identity.

We note though that in some cases the past is valued for its own sake! For example, research has shown that Chinese Canadians place greater value on events from the past, relative to events projected in the future, whereas European Canadians valued future over past events (Guo et al. 2012). Similarly, in Swahili language there is no word for future, only past (Zamani) and present (Sasa). The important point here is whether the events are primarily hedonic (positive or negative, enjoyable and so forth), or psychologically meaningful (Eudaimonic) they are the basis for constructing a contemporary self and possible future self. We argue that a Sankofan process evolves from a Eudaimonic perspective.

Beyond the differential significance of the past, we propose three characteristics that determine the influence of a past-focus on the present: (1) the *socio-emotional content* may be positive or negative, a source of pride or shame or self-doubt; (2) the past-present *comparative frame* may involve assimilation, by which the past is assimilated to and judged to be similar to or continuous with the present, or contrasted by which the past is compared to the present and differences in thoughts and feelings distinguish the present from the past. If the past is very positive, the present may be perceived as less positive by contrast. If the past is exceedingly negative, the present may, again by contrast, be perceived more positively (cf., Strack et al. 1985); and (3) the *hedonic vs. eudaimonic basis of well-being* where the emphasis rests on the degree to which one feels happy or satisfied or the desire to understand the "true self" or one's group brings coherence and meaning to one's life. Figure 2 traces the 8 potential consequences of these three main factors that influence the impact

		Temporal Psychological Processes	
Bases of Psychological well being	Valence of Temporal Experience	Temporal Continuity (past assimilated to present)	Temporal Discontinuity (past detached from or contrasted to present)
Hedonic (affective)	Positive	emotionally positive past leads to positive present affect and positive expectations for the future	emotionally positive past has no or opposite impact on affective state in the present
	Negative	emotionally negative past leads to negative present affect and negative expectations for the future	emotionally negative past has no or opposite impact on affective state in the present
		Sankofan Process (past assimilated to present)	Self-Justification Process (past detached from or contrasted to present)
Eudaimonic (self/collective knowledge)	Positive	critical assessment of past provides knowledge and guidance for reproducing success in the present and positive expectations for the future	No critical assessment of past, and no knowledge is derived from past successes
	Negative	critical assessment of past provides knowledge and guidance for avoiding or benefitting from past failures in the present and formulating expectations for the future	No critical assessment of past, and no knowledge is derived from past failures

Fig. 2 Structure, processes and outcomes of Sankofa effect

of the past on the present. The Sankofan effect, we propose, is more likely to be Eudaimonic than hedonic, to employ an assimilation strategy whether the past is positive or negative.

We thus argue that Sankofan approaches generally lead to positive psychological well-being in the present. However, when racism is made salient, Sankofan processes diverge for Blacks and Whites—Blacks, compared to Whites are more likely to *assimilate* negative past experiences of racial injustice to the present and perceive it as more prevalent. Whites, on the other hand, are more likely to *contrast* past racial injustice with the present and perceive the present as less unjust (cf. D'Souza's *The end of racism* 1995). This is the pattern of results described earlier that Turner and Jones (2004) obtained. This is a self-protective pattern that prepares one for a world of prejudice and discrimination.

Thus, when race based assault or oppression occurs, Blacks assimilate them to the historical context of oppression that provides meaning and coherence to the events. Countless examples of race-based violence or unfairness directed at Blacks reinforce this assimilation tendency. The assimilation strategy is evidence for a Sankofa effect. The critical question is how does it affect cognitions and affect in the present and projected future?

As the saying goes, what doesn't kill me makes me stronger. This aphorism could easily suggest a contrast tendency. It was very bad in the past, but I(we) survived so now I am better off because of the adversity. Research has shown that some individuals respond to major life altering and traumatic events by engaging in mental processing that produce a range of positive outcomes, including positive changes in self-esteem, coping skills, spirituality, and social support (Park et al. 1996). This stress-related growth effect has also been demonstrated as a coping response to daily stressors (LoSavio et al. 2011). So a Sankofa effect would stress the positive consequences of reflecting on and learning from negative events in the past—a eudaimonic outcome.

However research has generally shown that a past orientation or bias is associated with negative psychological outcomes and processes that precipitate and sustain them (Holman and Silver 1998; Zimbardo and Boyd 1999; Jones et al. 2012). These outcomes have more to do with happiness and satisfaction and are classified as hedonic. So the question arises, under what conditions do past thoughts have positive or negative effects on the present and future? And, to what extent do these conditions and processes vary between Blacks and Whites? And finally, how does the personal past compare to the collective past as influences on individual thoughts about the present or future?

Racial Differences in Sankofan Processes

What happens when race becomes salient for Blacks and Whites? For Whites, explaining life events in terms of race may reflect concern with affirmative action and current manifestations of "reverse-racism". Accordingly, Whites who interpret life events through a racial lens are more likely to see the current racial landscape as threatening to psychological control. They contrast the present with the past and conclude that racism is no longer operative, and efforts to combat it give Blacks an unjust advantage. Having made this comparative temporal judgment, Whites then portray the past as irrelevant.

Blacks, however, viewing life events through a racial lens likely arouses a historical narrative of oppression and denigration which is assimilated to and contextualize contemporary race relations. Thus, for Blacks, thinking about race evokes cognitions about the past. Recalling a painful historical narrative should have different effects on different aspects of well-being. Integrating a negative past into the present should diminish hedonic well-being, as past wounds become reopened. In contrast, eudaimonic well-being and self-knowledge should increase, since learning from the past gives one a richer understanding of their roots and the challenges they face.

We tested these ideas in a sample of 712 Black (n = 35) and White (n = 577) introductory psychology students. We assessed the degree to which race was salient, their past orientation, and a measure of eudaimonic well-being. Participants completed the Universal Context of Racism scale (Jones 2003), eight-items that assess the extent to which an individual uses race as an explanatory construct in understanding life events (e.g., "Situations I am in are often determined by my race", $\alpha = .92$); the past orientation dimension of the Temporal Orientation Scale (Jones et al. 2012), five-items that assess tendency to focus on the past (e.g., "I think about the past a lot", $\alpha = .78$), and the environmental mastery dimension of the Psychological Well-Being scale (Ryff 1989), 3-items that assess the degree to which one feels in control of one's external environment (e.g., "In general, I feel I am in charge of the situation in which I live", $\alpha = .58$).

Race Salience, Sankofa Processes, and Environmental Mastery

In a hierarchical linear regression analysis we regressed environmental mastery on UCR, race (0 = Black, 1 = White) and their interaction. For both Blacks and Whites, greater concern with race decreased environmental mastery, $b = -.24$, $SE = .12$, $\beta = -.06$, $t = -2.05$, $p = .04$ (See Fig. 3).

Should Blacks, relative to Whites, be more likely to exhibit Sankofa processes in response to race salience, we would expect UCR to predict past orientation for Blacks, but not Whites. To examine this possibility, we regressed past orientation on the model described above and found that the interaction was significant, $b = -.37$, $SE = .16$, $\beta = .09$, $t = -2.27$, $p = .023$ (See Fig. 3). Among Black participants, greater race salience significantly predicted greater past orientation, $b = .46$, $SE = .16$, $t = 2.88$, $p = .004$. Among White participants, however, race salience was only marginally significantly related to past orientation, $b = .09$, $SE = .04$, $t = 1.90$, $p = .058$.

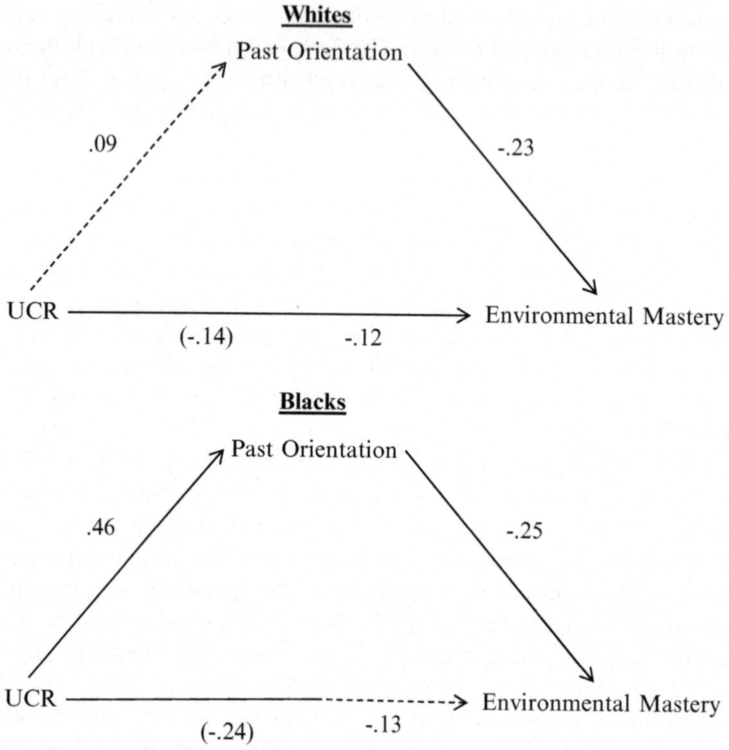

Fig. 3 Moderated mediation model showing simple paths between UCR, past orientation, and environmental mastery for White and Black participants

The Mediating Role of Past Orientation

These results suggest that, when race becomes salient, Blacks assimilate past injustices into perspectives on the present. While this Sankofan process should increase eudaimonic well-being, it might also reduce current feelings of environmental control. To determine whether data supported this hypothesis, we tested for moderated mediation (Muller et al. 2005). In a hierarchical linear regression analysis we regressed environmental mastery on race (0=Black, 1=White), and the UCR x race interaction term in Step 1. In Step 2, we entered past orientation. As hypothesized, past orientation correlated with decreased environmental mastery, $b=-.25$, $SE=.03$, $\beta=-.06$, $t=-8.77$, $p<.001$. However, when past orientation was entered in the model, the relationship between UCR and environmental mastery remained significant for Whites, $b=-.12$, $SE=.03$, $t=-3.76$, $p<.001$, but became non-significant for Blacks, $b=-.13$, $SE=.11$, $t=-1.11$, $p=.27$ (See Fig. 3). Confirming the presence of moderated mediation, a Sobel (1982) test indicated that the indirect path between the race x UCR interaction and environmental mastery was significant, $z=2.21$, $p=.03$. These results are consistent with our hypothesis that past orientation is a mechanism through which UCR affects environmental mastery for Blacks, but not Whites.

Making racial injustice salient among Blacks diminished current perceptions of environmental mastery. Blacks may have assimilated past injustices into the present, thereby perceiving the present environment as less controllable. However, this effect was mediated by past orientation. While such assimilation may reduce feelings of environmental mastery, it also may increase facets of eudaimonic well-being. For instance, assimilating the struggle and perseverance of slave ancestors into the present may increase pride. Thus, assimilation strategies can produce both positive and negative effects. Parsing the meaning of the past may be necessary to make precise predictions about Sankofan processes and their outcomes.

In sum, these findings suggest that Blacks are more likely than Whites to think about the past when race becomes salient. Other research in our lab found that when Whites are exposed to historical compared to contemporary images of black oppression, they are *more likely* to legitimate inequality and injustice, providing some evidence that recent injustices may be more difficult for people to legitimize than past injustices (Engelman 2010).

An interesting approach to time perspective considered *place* as an extension of self and group (Lewicka, 2014, personal communication). Participants from Poland reported the extent to which they had taken interest in the past of their city of residence, or denied the need to take the past into account. Past versus present city focus was related to a variety of measures of openness towards other ethnic groups. She found that people who explicitly deny the need to preserve or discover the city/town past are the most closed to other ethnic groups and are the most prejudiced. Whereas Engleman's research showed more negative effects of a salient past orientation, Lewicka's findings, congruent with the Sankofa hypothesis, linked a past-focus to greater tolerance of out-groups. Clearly there are many interactions of person and place, past and present that influence one's time perspective and its consequences.

Values represent unstandardized coefficients. Values in parentheses represent the coefficient before the mediator was entered in the model. Solid lines represent significant relationships, whereas dotted lines represent non-significant relationships.

A Boundary Condition to the Sankofa Effect: Mortality Salience

Although Sankofa involves integrating the past into the present and projecting onto the future, certain conditions may preclude the activation of Sankofan processes. One such condition may be when mortality is salient. Mortality salience is theorized to increase existential anxiety about one's finite existence (Pyszczynski et al. 2004). Thinking about death may disrupt the integration of past temporal frames into the present, increase hedonic well-being, while decreasing eudaimonic well-being motivations (see Holman and Silver 1998). The collective narrative of oppression,

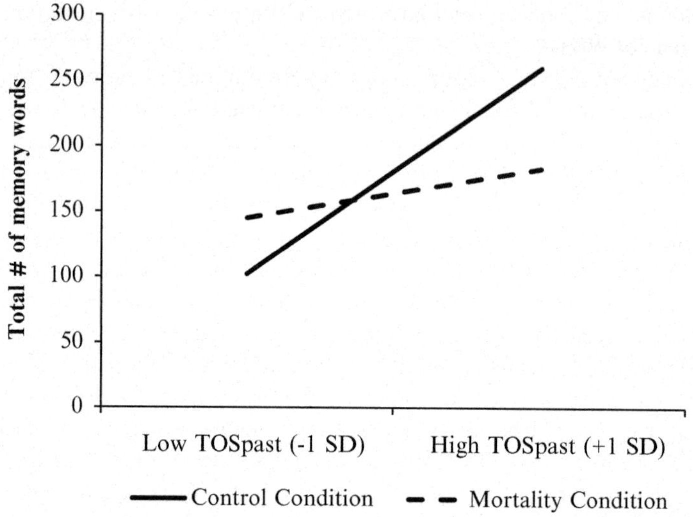

Fig. 4 Effects of past temporal orientation and mortality salience on memories of past events

may have a symbolic relationship to death, but more generally, stand as a narrative of loss, inferiority, threat and lowered individual and collective self-esteem. We suggest that mortality salience shifts temporal focus away from the past and towards the present.

To test this hypothesis, we manipulated mortality salience and measured past temporal orientation and the accessibility of past memories. White introductory psychology students (n = 186) completed a measure of past temporal orientation (Jones et al. 2012) and described their five most salient memories. We predicted that past orientation would be related to greater accessibility and density of past memories, but that this relationship would be significantly attenuated when one's mortality was salient. The dependent variable was memory elaboration which we operationalized as the total number of words participants used to describe their memories.

We regressed the total number of memory description words on mortality salience condition, centered Past orientation, and the interaction in a regression model. The interaction was significant, $b = -33.92$, $SE = 10.70$, $p = .002$ (see Fig. 4). Simple slope analyses revealed that greater Past orientation predicted greater memory elaboration in the control condition, ($b = 70.91$, $SE = 21.97$, $p < .001$), but Past orientation was unrelated to memory elaboration in the mortality salience condition. The existential anxiety related to mortality salience limits "time-travel" to the past. However, this is at an individual psychological level. Does collective mortality salience have the same effect? Instead of thinking about your own death, think about the death of your ancestors. While these results indicate that mortality salience draws the temporal focus of chronically past oriented people to the present, we do not know whether this same results would occur for collective mortality salience.

Mortality Salience as a Coping Strategy

Mortality salience interferes with the Sankofan process of looking to the past, and brings temporal focus to the present. Although present focus increases hedonic drives (Zimbardo and Boyd 1999), it may also diminish eudaimonic well-being. Thus, the Sankofa effect and eudaimonic well-being are less likely in cultural contexts where death plays a prominent role. This logic presents an interesting case for groups that have both a historical narrative of oppression (a condition that facilitates Sankofa) and cultural practices that make death salient (a condition that inhibits Sankofa). African American culture, for example, is defined by a historical narrative of oppression and denigration (Jones 1997). Additionally, Blacks often view the world in racial terms and anticipate that outcomes in their lives will be defined by their race (Jones 2003). Yet, mortality salience plays a central role in popular Black music. At the time of writing this chapter, the most popular rap song on the Billboard music charts (Billboard 2012) is "Mercy" by Kanye West, which includes the lyrics "Let the suicide doors up/I do suicides on the tour bus/I do suicides on the private jet/You know what that mean, I'm fly to death". Explicit reference to death is also prominent in the lyrics of the second most popular rap song on the Billboard charts, "No Lie", by 2 CHAINZ: "A skeleton in my closet/it's probably one of these dead ass rappers/it's probably one of these pussy ass niggas/ don't try me I'll pull that trigga".

We suggest that the ubiquity of death salience in contemporary Black culture illustrates a boundary condition of the Sankofa Effect. When the possibility of death is explicit, Blacks may be less likely to engage in Sankofan processes. Though present temporal focus contributes to hedonic well-being, as illustrated by many hip-hop lyrics that celebrate indulgence, excessive death salience also severs the link between the past and present. Thus, we expect the Sankofa Effect and eudaimonic well-being to be the greatest among Blacks who are in situations in which mortality threat is *not* salient.

References

Baldwin, J. A., & Bell, Y. R. (1985). The African self-consciousness scale: An Africentric personality questionnaire. *The Western Journal of Black Studies, 9*, 61–68.

Billboard Music. (2012, August 23). *Rap songs*. Retrieved from http://www.billboard.com/charts/rap-songs#/charts/rap-songs

D'Souza, D. (1995). *The end of racism: Principles for a multiracial society*. New York: Free Press.

Engelman, S. (2010) *Justice vs. justification: Divergent responses among Whites to anti-Black injustice*. Doctoral dissertation, University of Delaware.

Guo, T., Li-Jun, J., Spina, R., & Zhang, Z. (2012). Culture, temporal focus, and values of the past and the future. *Personality and Social Psychology Bulletin, 38*(8), 1030–1040.

Hall, E. T. (1983). *The dance of life: The other dimension of time*. Garden City: Anchor Press/Doubleday.

Hofstede, G., & Bond, M. H. (1988). The confucius connection: From cultural roots to economic growth. *Organizational Dynamics, 16*(4), 4–21.

Holman, E. A., & Silver, R. C. (1998). Getting "stuck" in the past: Temporal orientation and coping with trauma. *Journal of Personality and Social Psychology, 74*, 1146–1163.

Jones, J. M. (1997). *Prejudice and racism* (2nd ed.). New York: McGraw Hill.

Jones, J. M. (2003). TRIOS: A psychological theory of African legacy in American culture. *Journal of Social Issues, 59*, 217–241.

Jones, J. M., & Brown, W. (2005). Any time is Trinidad time: Cultural variations in the value and function of time. In A. Strathman & J. Joireman (Eds.), *Understanding behavior in the context of time* (pp. 305–323). Hillsdale: Lawrence Erlbaum Publishers.

Jones, J. M., Banicky, L., & Lasane, T. P. (2012) *A temporal orientation scale: Focusing attention on the past, present and future*. Unpublished manuscript, University of Delaware.

LoSavio, S. T., Cohen, L. H., Laurenceau, J. P., Dasch, K. N., Parrish, B. P., & Park, C. L. (2011). Reports of stress-related growth from daily negative events. *Journal of Social and Clinical Psychology, 30*(7), 760–785.

Luhtanen, R., & Crocker, J. (1992). A collective self-esteem scale: Self-evaluation of one's social identity. *Personality and Social Psychology Bulletin, 18*, 302–318.

Markus, H. R., & Kitayama, S. (1991). Culture and the self: Implications for cognition, emotion, and motivation. *Psychological Review, 98*(2), 224–253.

Mbiti, J. S. (1970). *Concepts of God in Africa*. New York: Praeger.

McGrath, J. E. (Ed.). (1988). *The social psychology of time*. Newbury Park: Sage.

Muller, D., Yzerbyt, V. Y., & Judd, C. M. (2005). Adjusting for a mediator in models with two crossed treatment variables. *Organizational Research Methods, 11*(2), 224–240.

Nelson, J. C., Adams, G., & Salter, P. S. (2013). The Marley hypothesis: Denial of racism reflects ignorance of history. *Psychological Science, 24*(2), 213–218.

Park, C. L., Cohen, L. H., & Murch, R. L. (1996). Assessment and prediction of stress-related growth. *Journal of Personality, 64*, 71–105.

Pyszczynski, T., Greenberg, J., Solomon, S., Arndt, J., & Schimel, J. (2004). Why do people need self-esteem? A theoretical and empirical review. *Psychological Bulletin, 130*, 435–468.

Rosenberg, M. (1965). *Society and the adolescent self-image*. New York/Princeton: Princeton University Press.

Ryff, C. D. (1989). Happiness is everything, or is it? Explorations on the meaning of psychological well-being. *Journal of Personality and Social Psychology, 57*, 1069–1081.

Ryff, C. D., & Keyes, C. L. (1995). The structure of psychological well-being revisited. *Journal of Personality and Social Psychology, 69*(4), 719–727.

Sellers, R. M., Rowley, S. A. J., Chavous, T. M., Shelton, J. N., & Smith, M. A. (1997). Multidimensional inventory of black identity: A preliminary investigation of reliability and construct validity. *Journal of Personality and Social Psychology, 73*(4), 805–815.

Shweder, R. A., & Sullivan, M. (1993). Cultural psychology: Who needs it? *Annual Review of Psychology, 44*, 497–523.

Strack, F., Schwarz, N., & Gschneidinger, E. (1985). Happiness and reminiscing: The role of time perspective, affect, and mode of thinking. *Journal of Personality and Social Psychology, 49*(6), 1460–1469.

The Spirituals Project, University of Denver, http://ctl.du.edu/spirituals/Literature/sankofa.cfm. Downloaded 12 Aug 2012.

Turner, C., & Jones, J. M. (2004). *TRIOS and the influence of intergroup encounters on psychological well-being and state anxiety*. Poster, Eastern Psychological Association Meeting, Washington, DC.

Turner, J. C., Brown, R. J., & Tajfel, H. (1979). Social comparison and group interest in in-group-favouritism. *European Journal of Social Psychology, 9*(2), 187–204.

Vandiver, B. J., Cross, W. E., Worrell, F. C., & Fhagen-Smith, P. E. (2002). Validating the cross racial identity scale. *Journal of Counseling Psychology, 49*(1), 71–85.

Waterman, A. S. (1993). Two conceptions of happiness: Contrasts of personal expressiveness (eudaimonia) and hedonic enjoyment. *Journal of Personality and Social Psychology, 64*(4), 678–691.

Wilson, D. C., & Davis, D. W. (2011). Reexamining racial resentment: Conceptualization and content. *The Annals of the American Academy of Political and Social Science, 64*(4), 678–691.

Zimbardo, P. G., & Boyd, J. N. (1999). Putting time in perspective: A valid, reliable individual-differences metric. *Journal of Personality and Social Psychology, 77*, 1271–1288.

Precariousness as a Time Horizon: How Poverty and Social Insecurity Shape Individuals' Time Perspectives

Nicolas Fieulaine and Thémis Apostolidis

From the very earliest studies in this field, time perspective (TP) has been regularly and centrally posited as being deeply rooted in – and shaped by – living conditions. The first known article concerning TP, as it is currently defined, already highlighted that "whole social classes may be described by the time perspectives that dominate their lives as revealed in the range of their planning, their prudential calculations, their foresight, and so on…" (Frank 1939, p. 297). However, the first person to stress this social dimension of TP was none other than Kurt Lewin, the pioneer of the concept. In order to introduce his theory on time perspective, Lewin based his work on the studies being produced at that time on unemployment, which showed how joblessness impacted on a person's morale, revealing a strong inclination for desperation, desolation and reduced aspiration for the future: "the character of the psychological future vacillates between hope and despair. But, regardless of whether the individual's picture of the future is correct or incorrect at a given time, this picture deeply affects the mood and the action of the individual at that time (…) The conduct of the unemployed, then, is an example of how time perspective may lower morale" (Lewin 1942, pp. 103–104).

A Lewinian View on the Social Roots of Time Perspective

Although Lewin considered TP as a key determining factor for a high morale when faced with difficulties, he stated: "If morale means the ability to "take it", to face disagreeable or dangerous situations, one must ask first, "What constitute

N. Fieulaine (✉)
Groupe de Recherche en Psychologie Sociale, Institut de Psychologie,
Université de Lyon, 69600 Bron, France
e-mail: Nicolas.fieulaine@univ-lyon2.fr

T. Apostolidis
Aix-Marseille Université, LPS EA 849, 13621, Aix-en-Provence, France
e-mail: Themistoklis.Apostolidis@univ-amu.fr

M. Stolarski et al. (eds.), *Time Perspective Theory; Review, Research and Application: Essays in Honor of Philip G. Zimbardo*, DOI 10.1007/978-3-319-07368-2_14,

disagreeable or dangerous situations for an individual?"" (Lewin 1942, p. 106). As an illustrative example, Lewin drew on the works of his student, M.L. Farber, a study of suffering in prison (Farber 1944). This study revealed that the levels of suffering declared by inmates appeared to be related less to the objective nature of their situations (which varied according to the privileges they had obtained) and more to certain factors connected with the future or past, such as the rumination of an unjust sentence, or the hope of "getting a break" in regard to release. Lewin concluded that "not present hardships in the usual sense of the term, then, but rather certain aspects of the psychological future and the psychological past (…) are most important in determining the amount of one's suffering. (…) In solitary confinement, too, it has been frequently reported, one of the most painful experiences is the uncertainty as to how much time has elapsed. Once again, it is not a present hardship but certain characteristics of the time perspective which lend the situation its anguish" (Lewin 1942, p. 107).

TP therefore depends on the situations in which an individual or a group may find themselves, and in parallel, the psychological significance of these situations as well as their consequences are established as a result of the time perspective which individuals and groups adopt. TP is therefore, as a dimension of the psychological field, part of the circular relationships of interdependence that people maintain with the environment (Lewin 1943, pp. 306–309). This circular interdependence not only concerns the physical environment but also the social environment; *e.g.* the group's social climate, standards and values (Lewin 1942, p. 120). This is what Lewin called as a *dynamic* theory of personality (Lewin 1926/1935), which while not denying that relatively stable psychological traits can describe a person, or that habits become stable psychological constructs, assumes that the aim of psychology is not to characterize idiosyncratically individuals, but to understand the dynamic connections which govern the relationships between individuals and the situations in which they exist. On this basis, as Lewin stated on the subject of morale, "the problem of individual [time perspective] is to a large extent a social-psychological problem" (p. 115).

This dynamic and situated approach to personality is also that which characterizes the model proposed by Zimbardo and Boyd in 1999. The origins of Phil Zimbardo's interests for psychological time (the Bronx, prison, hypnosis, cf. "Foreword" by Maslach, this volume) attests to the fact that his model is anchored in a social-psychological approach, with a strong concern for situations and contexts. This is a reminder that the ZTPI, often presented as a tool intended to measure the individual differences in orientation and attitudes towards the past, present and future, was proposed by a social psychologist well known for his awareness of the power of situations over individuals. ZTPI was introduced as an extension to the Lewinian theory of TP based on the famous equation of interdependence B = f(P, E). By this formula Lewin has encouraged researchers to articulate the ways that persons (the P term in the formula) and environment (the E term) interact to determine behaviour (the B term). Whereas the *P* term is the focus of *personality* psychology, the *E* term (and the effects of *E* on *B*) is the target of *social* psychology. Lewin claimed for taking into account *both* persons *and* situations, and moreover the *interplay* and *interdependence* of persons and situations (the f function, see Snyder 2013 for an actual debate on this issue).

It is significant that one of the first publications to mention the ZTPI concerns the influence of TP on ways of coping with homelessness (Epel et al. 1999). In this article, the authors relied on the hypothesis that "Homeless people tend to fall at the lower end of the socioeconomic spectrum which, as noted, is usually associated with a present orientation. However, immersion in the daily battle for survival, facing deprivation of basic needs such as shelter, could also induce a situationally based present orientation, regardless of one's dispositional temporal orientation. Thus, present orientation can be both a cause and a consequence of homelessness" (p. 577). The surprising results, showing that highly present-oriented homeless are more likely to find housing, lead authors to highlight the limits of the existing research on TP. Hence, although research has demonstrated the benefits of being future oriented, this has been according to middle-class standards, within a stable predictable environment (p. 590). In time of crisis and in insecure contexts, a present orientation is necessary and perhaps more adaptive. Therefore, as Epel et al. wrote, "the optimal time perspective depends upon the demands of the situation and its tasks and reward structure" (Ibid.).

This statement appears to be thoroughly consistent with Lewin's ideas concerning the effect of frustration on TP. According to Lewin, a frustrating situation (one which prevents the achievement of goals or completion of actions) results in a narrowing of TPs and a greater focus on the present (Lewin 1946, 1951). The socio-economic conditions of disadvantaged groups will therefore engender numerous moments of frustration, and in consequence, a limited TP; which becomes less oriented towards the past and the future. Lewin discusses the processes of 'regression' in connection to frustration, which are characterized by a decreased variance in behaviours, the disorganization and dedifferentiation of the psychological domains as well as the contraction of the life space (Lewin 1959, pp. 92–135). It is this last point which most directly concerns TP, since the extension of life space is defined in part by the dimension of "time perspective in the direction of the psychological past and the psychological future" (Lewin 1946, p. 797). In his work, Lewin discusses the topic of unemployment on several occasions (*e.g.* 1936, pp. 15–16, 1942, pp. 103–104) and stresses in this regard that for the unemployed, and even for his children, time perspective becomes narrow and his behaviour is depending only on the immediate situation.

Nuttin, who also carried out ground-breaking work in the field, notes the variations which can affect TP depending on social and cultural backgrounds (Nuttin 1977, pp. 346–347, 354–356). As he noted "for the members of certain sociocultural groups, the most realistic time perspective; and the optimum adaptation to the type of life thrust upon them, consists of not making plans for the future. Diverse external conditions – in particular, economic and political conditions - significantly affect the predictability of their future" (p. 324). According to Nuttin, these observations open "a perspective on the social and cultural dimension of the variable [TP] that we have studied here in the context of individual psychology" (ibid., p. 356).

TP and Socio-economic Positions

Based on the original propositions of Franck (1939) concerning the interdependent relation between individuals and their environment, studies have mainly been focused on the differences observed in the TPs of individuals and groups according to social class and socio-economic status. The first evidence of the differences in TP according to social class appeared in a study by LeShan (1952), based on the hypothesis that the most disadvantaged social classes were characterized by a contraction of TP; less oriented towards the future and the past and more oriented towards the present. Wallace (1986) also found that homeless men were more present-oriented, mainly because of the urgency of daily survival and the cyclical schedules of night shelters, soup kitchens, and welfare checks.

These studies, as well as those of Cottle and Pleck (1969), Lomranz et al. (1983), Koenig et al. (1981), Lamm et al. (1976), Schmidt et al. (1978), O'Rand and Ellis (1974), Nurmi (1987) or Bouffard et al. (1989), in spite of their methodological differences, all agree on a reduction in orientation towards the future amongst the most disadvantaged social groups and classes. More recent studies have also highlighted this link between FTP and socio-economic status (Freire et al. 1980; Fuchs 1982; Leigh 1986; Nurmi 1987; Lawrence 1991; Green et al. 1996; Bosma et al. 1999; Peetsma 2000; Wardle and Steptoe 2003; Jaroni et al. 2004). Overall, findings from these studies support the broad statement that the most privileged socio-economic situations engender TPs characterized by aspects that have positive connotations: orientation and depth towards the future, more numerous and more realistic aspirations and goals (Thiébaut 1997, p. 126).

These variations according to social class and socio-economic status, although repeatedly evidenced, gave rise a certain number of studies which brought these results into question (e.g. Judson and Tuttle 1966; Kendall and Sibley 1970; Perlman 1976). This might be due to the various definitions of socio-economic positions (occupational status, diploma, relative deprivation, social deprivation, anomia). Agarwal et al. (1983), observing these contradictory results, used another indicator for socio-economic status, based on a multi-dimensional approach of deprivation (Prolonged Deprivation Scale; Misra and Tripathi 1977), and focusing on both material and experiential deprivation (social support, family relationships, learning experiences, travel and leisure etc.). This deprivation indicator, taken as a whole, appeared to be linked to both the orientation and the extension of perspectives towards the future and the past. The less disadvantaged groups appear more oriented towards a more distant future, and the same for the past. On the other hand, when considering separately the dimensions of deprivation, it appears that the disparity in FTP between groups is lower in relation to the material dimension than to the experiential dimension (Agarwal et al. 1983, p. 372). Ahadyar (1976), Schmidt et al. (1978), D'Alessio et al. (2003) as well as Fieulaine et al. (2006) have, moreover, demonstrated the effect of education levels on TP, a lower level being linked to a lower orientation towards the future; to a more pessimistic view of the future and a more fatalistic view of the present. In an experimental study, Twenge et al. (2003) revealed the specific impact of social exclusion on TP. Thus, those subjects who were socially excluded (those who were not chosen during an exercise in which individuals were asked to choose a partner) appeared to be more centered on the present and less on the future. Other studies have demonstrated the specific impact of unemployment and job loss on TP drawing on cross-sectional (Bouffard et al. 1983; Viinamaki et al. 1994), as well as longitudinal study designs using constructs closely related to TP (Time structure; Wanberg and Griffiths 1997; Waters and Muller 2003). Finally, some studies on impaired living conditions or situations or minority groups, demonstrate the significant effect of these situations on TP, (Illness, Levy 1978; Toombs 1990; institutionalization, Landau 1976; Trommsdorff and Lamm 1980; Imprisonment, Sapsford 1978; Black and Gregson 1973; Homelessness, Epel et al. 1999; Barndt and Johnson 1955; Stein et al. 1968; Alcoholism and drug addiction, Hulbert and Lens 1988; Henick and Domino 1975).

Unfortunately, very few of these studies addressed the past dimension. However, LeShan (1952) revealed from the beginning the variations on this dimension according to social class; demonstrating that subjects from the middle classes situated themselves in a broader TP, in terms of both past and future. This result reflects those of Cottle and Pleck (1969), revealing a greater sense of historicity amongst the middle classes; which implies both a broader TP and a strong sense of time continuity (cf. also Cottle 1968). Lévy (1978) also observes differences in time continuity according to social class, the 'lower' classes presenting a greater disconnection between the past, the present and the future. Van Der Keilen (1982) highlighted that attitudes towards the past, present and future are more positive amongst privileged groups ('normal' adolescents) than amongst disadvantaged groups (adolescents who were part of a social inclusion program). She also revealed a greater continuity in attitudes towards the three temporal zones amongst privileged adolescents than amongst the others, for whom the quality of the present appears to be less related to that of the past or the future. This past dimension, under-considered in many studies, will nevertheless appear crucial in various studies, in particular in the link between socio-economic position and mental health (Fieulaine et al. 2006).

How and Why SEP Impacts on Time Perspective?

Although the variations in TP according to social position have been well established, the theoretical interpretations of these variations are multiple. Personality models, depicting TP as a stable personality trait, can theoretically lead to neo-Darwinian interpretations, stating that social positions are the result of cognitive deficiencies or bias, considered as a basis for a social selection. An opposed hypothesis of causality (cf. Dohrenwend et al. 1992) highlights the role played by socialization and social experiences on TP. In these approaches, TP is considered as the result of the temporal characteristics of social situations that significantly participate in shaping individual perspectives. Trommsdorff (1983) thus underlined the importance of the socialization processes in the development of TP, by presenting results that demonstrate that this development, far from being uniquely determined by cognitive maturation, mainly depends on social learning.

Hence, TP differences between the social classes seem to be established and reinforced during the process of socialization. Although middle-class school children appear to be more optimistic and oriented towards the future than their higher-class peers, this relationship is gradually reversed during their school career (Füchsle and Trommsdorff 1980, cited by Trommsdorff 1983). The authors conclude "it seems that the school does not compensate for possible socialization defects but rather contributes to increasing differences in socialization and resulting effects on future orientation" (Trommsdorff 1983, p. 392). This effects of class-differentiated socialization on TP has been highlighted on several occasions. The study by LeShan (1952), which in our opinion is greatly under-estimated and often reduced to its most simplistic results, is a fascinating demonstration of how this temporal class-differentiated socialization exists from a very young age. By studying child-rearing practices as revealed in a variety of monographic descriptions of various social classes everyday life, she observed systematic variations in parental control in their temporal tense. In the lower classes, parental control methods were focused on the present, with no reference to the past or to the future ("put down that bottle") and were based on immediate punishment or reward. Amongst the middle classes, on the other hand, these methods were based on the possible consequences in a more or less distant future ("Santa Claus won't come if you're bad"), and amongst the upper classes, these were above all based on the past traditions of the family ("what would your grandmother say?"). Concerning the lower classes, LeShan (ibid.) concludes that "children of the lower-lower class soon learn that major changes in their lives often occur suddenly and unpredictably", and that "there seems to be a circular phenomenon at work. The parents' training is inconsistent because of their inability to work for long-range goals, and this prevents them from breaking out of the economic trap they are in. Economic pressures further decrease stability. Children who go through this training will also emerge unable to work for long-range goals and so on." (LeShan 1952, pp. 590–591). This conclusion concerning the relatively direct influence of family background on TP is supported by various studies that highlight the role of social 'background' on orientation and attitudes towards the future, whether this is socio-economic status, size of family unit, parental occupation (Cassidy 2000) or the professional experiences of parents (Gardner 2004). This role of socialization (for a review, cf. Trommsdorff 1983) therefore depends not only on family situation and practices and integration into the school system but also on adult age, according to professional inclusion (Trommsdorff et al. 1979; Fingerman and Perlmutter 1995).

Additional analysis on the relations between TP and socio-economic status is centered on TP as arising from adaptive strategies in face of social situations. In this sense, a reduction of Future TP in a socially disadvantaged context constitutes "an optimum adaptation to imposed living conditions" (Nuttin 1977, p. 324). The living conditions of individuals from disadvantaged backgrounds fundamentally affect their ability to foresee the future; they therefore adopt a realistic attitude excluding all plans for the future (Cottle and Klineberg 1974; Koenig et al. 1981). TP plays in this case an adaptive role in situations that are chronically difficult (poverty, exclusion) as well as those of a temporary nature (imprisonment, illness and traumatic events). In this sense, TP is more readily considered as an active resource for dealing with difficult situations than as a mechanical result of living conditions. The role of TP as a method of coping when confronted with traumatic events (Holman and Silver 1998; Beiser and Hyman 1997; chapter "Time Perspective and Social Relations: A Stress and Coping Perspective" by Holman, this volume), as well as in the strategies used for the preservation of self-image (Melges 1982; Lang and Carstensen 2002), suggests the existence of 'temporal strategies', in adverse situations, to adapt TP according to external conditions (faced with homelessness: Epel et al. 1999; traumatic events: Holman and Silver 1998; unemployment: Viinamaki et al. 1994; in a social context: Cassidy 2000; with illness: Davies 1997; with imprisonment: Sapsford 1978).

Some studies have also showed the roots of TP in cultures and the social roles they define, in line with the early propositions of Frank (1939). In this respect, O'Rand and Ellis (1974) stressed that the established differences on FTP according to social classes "have been shown to be systematically related to the effectiveness with which youth can meet institutionalized role demands." (p. 60), in particular when deeply rooted in a culture of foresight and planning for the future, as it is the case for school and education. This division of role demands between upper and lower classes reflects the observations made by Bourdieu (1997) and makes it possible to further our understanding of the differences that arise and are maintained between social classes, given that TP caused by socialization can become an implicit criteria for social, educational or professionnal selection. Bourdieu (1966) thus describes the underlying mechanism in his theory of social reproduction using what he refers to as the '*relationship to time*', which he examines in the light of Lewin's article on TP (Bourdieu 1966). The findings reported by Koenig et al. (1981) are, in this respect, revealing. Using an indicator for anomia (dissatisfaction, feelings of exclusion and uselessness; Scale of anomia, Srole 1956), these authors demonstrated that TP is (in addition to being directly linked to social class) not only related to anomia, but also and most importantly, that this anomia is highest in those subjects that are most orientated towards the future. They provide specific evidence of this by showing that anomia is at its highest amongst subjects from disadvantaged social classes - and who are simultaneously the most future-oriented (Koenig et al. 1981, pp. 126–127). They have thus drawn the conclusion that "future dominance avoidance can function as a defense mechanism for members of the lower social classes. Those who are predominantly oriented towards the future and from lower classes are more likely to experience higher states of anomia" (Koenig et al. 1981, p. 127). This study not only demonstrated the possible effect of the disadjustment between an individual's TP, and that which would be considered 'normal' in a particular social context, but it also suggested how TP can be part of a strategy to adapt to the conditions in which people live.

Within this framework we can see that the approaches centered on adaptation and socialization are complementary. On one hand, the effect of social position on TP is explained on one hand by differential socialization, through the transmission of time orientations by family interaction, the effects of which are reinforced by the implicit selection in the school environment. On the other hand, frustrating, stressful or destabilizing situations regularly faced by those from disadvantaged groups lead to unpredictability and loss of control over one's environment and then reduce the propensity to develop thoughts about, or set goals for, the future (Pham et al. 2001).

Time Perspective in an Era of Precariousness

In a recent paper, Carvounas and Ireland (2008) highlighted the effects of lived precariousness (social and economic) on societies' time perspectives. They stressed the extent to which the social and economic insecurity, resulting from the generalization of McJobs, fixed-term contracts and interim labor, by "eroding a sense of security, have led to a contraction of temporal horizons" (Carvounas and Ireland 2008, p. 173).

Precariousness is in our view one of the most important social issues we are dealing with nowadays, an issue for which time perspective concept is of a crucial interest. Hence, beyond its conceptual significance when analyzing recent social evolutions in developed countries, socio-economic *precariousness* represents a very concrete and actual phenomena especially critical when related to public health (Benach and Muntaner 2007). Situations characterized by income and resource instability, job insecurity, weakened provision of social welfare and therefore difficulties in envisioning and planning the future are primarily defined as *precarious*, socio-economically speaking (Bourdieu 1998; Paugam 1995). In Europe, growing flexibility in the labor market, together with the decreasing efficiency of welfare policies, lead to instable social trajectories, insecure situations, and unpredictable futures. All over the world, economic crises repeatedly destabilize societies and disrupt temporal horizons and coherence, at both collective and individual levels. At almost all levels of our social lives, lies the shadow of instability and insecurity (Sennett 2004).

This "new landscape of precariousness" (Forrest 1999; Nettleton and Burrows 2001) is a major issue in many countries for welfare and healthcare policies (cf. Carter 1998) because numerous studies have evidenced its specific and strong links with adverse health outcomes (Benavides and Benach 1999; Platt et al. 1999). French epidemiological surveys among others have demonstrated that physical, subjective and mental health is seriously impaired by precarious situations (Lebas and Chauvin 1998; Joubert et al. 2001), and it has been repeatedly suggested that social-psychological factors may play a central role in social disparities in health (Adler et al. 1999; Gallo 2009), and in the connection between low SES and poor health (Henry 2001; Kokko and Pulkkinen 1998; Hepworth 1980). Among these variables, time perspective and psychological time were proposed as crucial (Singh-Manoux and Marmot 2005; Fieulaine et al. 2006; Adams and White 2009), potentially playing a generative role in health outcomes linked to unemployment (Jahoda 1982; Feather and Bond 1983; George 1991) or job insecurity (cf. Quinlan et al. 2001).

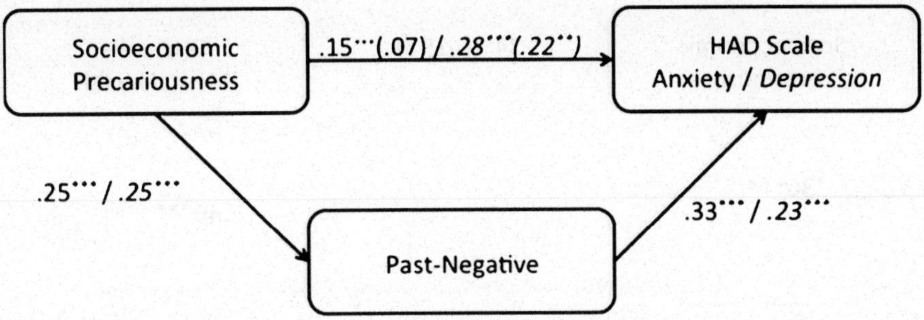

Fig. 1 Mediating effect of Past Negative TP on depression and anxiety (From Fieulaine et al. 2006). N=275; R2=.15/.14 (ΔR^2=.10/0.5); z (sobel test)=3.54***/2.98**. Note: *≤.05; **≤.01; ***≤.001; standards coefficient; ΔR^2=change in explanation rate when mediator is added; z=test for the indirect effect (See Sobel 1982)

Until recently, few studies have empirically investigated this hypothetical role of time perspective in the link between socio-economic status and health - and these studies provided evidence that TP plays a mediating role in the relation of socio-economic status to various health behaviours or outcomes (Adams 2009), such as smoking, physical activity, diabetes screening or obesity (Adams and White 2009; Crockett et al. 2009; Guthrie et al. 2009; Schunck and Rogge 2010). In a previous study, we tested the hypothesis of a mediating role of TP in the link between socio-economic *precariousness* and psychological health (Fieulaine et al. 2006). Using a sample of users of free health check centers (N=275), we showed a relation of precariousness to Future time perspective, suggesting a negative impact of socioeconomic precariousness on future orientation, and we also found a mediating role of Past-Negative time perspective in the impact of socio-economic precariousness on depression and anxiety symptoms as measured by the HAD scale (Zigmond and Snaith 1983; see Fig. 1).

Recently, these results were replicated using a more reliable measure of time perspective (56-items ZTPI instead of a selected set of items) and another assessment of psychological distress. In this study, we recruited a community sample in healthcare and welfare settings in an urban area located in central France. 182 people (mean age=39.64; *SD*=17.08, ranging from 17 to 77 years old), 83 men and 99 women, completed a self-administered questionnaire measuring time perspective using the Zimbardo Time Perspective Inventory (ZTPI; Zimbardo and Boyd, 1999) in its French validated version (Apostolidis and Fieulaine 2004); Psychological health, on the basis of subscales of the Duke Health Profile (DHP; Pakerson et al. 1991; Guillemin et al. 1997), and Socio-economic Precariousness (SEPc) using a multiple deprivation index validated in France, the EPICES (Evaluation of Precariousness and Inequalities in Health Examination Centers [EPICES]) score (Bihan et al. 2005; LaRosa et al. 2008; Nahon et al. 2009). Results confirmed that socioeconomic precariousness is closely related to past time perspective (negatively to Past Positive and positively to Past Negative), and that TP operates as a mediating

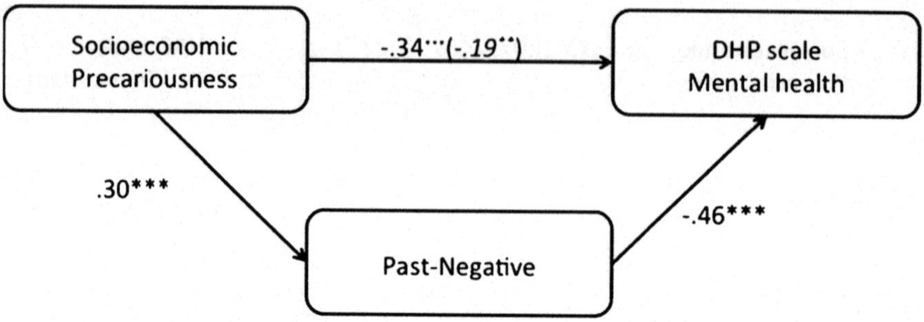

Fig. 2 Mediating effect of Past Negative TP on mental health. N=182; *≤.05; **≤.01; ***≤.001; R2=.28 (ΔR^2=.18); z (sobel test)=3.21***. Note: standards coefficient; ΔR^2=change in explanation rate when mediator is added; z=test for the indirect effect (See Sobel 1982)

factor in the sociogenesis of psychological distress. As depicted in Fig. 2, the relationship of SEPc to psychological health occurs through association with negative views—and rumination—of past experiences. Hence SEPc has an impact on psychological health partly because it acts on, or as a result of its action on, negative past time perspective. Focusing on a negative past appears to be a potential vector of '*biographical vulnerability*' and as essential to understand the lived experience of precarious living conditions.

From these findings, it could be hypothesized that one of the possible effects of the social place of precariousness is to get stuck in rumination mode as a self-reflection form (e.g. feeling of regret or guilt for not being what I should have been in terms of social career). In this line, time experience could be considered as a primary psychosocial dimension for analyzing the interiorization of the social order by individuals, as early stated by Bourdieu (1966).

Precariousness, TP and the Sustainable Societies

In conclusion, we claim for more consideration to TP as a socially grounded psychological construct. Although time perspective is a result of personal lived experiences of time, it is deeply related to individual's social position. In precarious socioeconomic conditions, people are more prone to focus on their past in a negative attitude, and to ruminate their bad experiences. And this time orientation facilitates the occurence of anxious and depressive symptoms. In lower social classes, people are less future-oriented, due to their unpredictable living conditions, and this can explain partly health and other disparities. As studies evidenced that TP is related to various socioeconomic indicators, more research is needed to deeper our understanding of how social status and living conditions impact psychological time. Granted to the ZTPI model that considers orientation and attitudes towards the three time frames, we were able to assess how TP can be a vector for the psychological suffering linked to precarious living conditions. More broadly, findings suggest that when facing danger or uncertainty, people leave out the psychological future and sometimes invest the past in a negative view. Relying on lewinian field theory, this rumination of a negative past could be understood as a way to redirect intentions from the future to the past. If the psychological field is narrowed by uncertainty, psychological forces may find a way to sustain intentions, but directed towards the past, in rumination and regret. This shrinking of the temporal dimension of the psychological field when facing danger and uncertainty is an avenue for future research, in relation with other dimensions along which psychological distance may operate (social, spatial and probability; cf. chapter "From Time Perspective to Psychological Distance (and Back)" by Maglio et al., this volume). Moreover, these considerations point to a crucial issue for research, but also for policy makers, stakeholders and citizens. In a time of financial, ecological and often political crises, uncertainty and danger are the living conditions of a growing number of countries and people. Under these conditions, how can we sustain a Future time perspective? How can we articulate the uncertainty needed to envision the possibility of a change and a future orientation to plan and achieve our goals? How can we share more fairly the present and the future, to avoid temporal inequalities and the many disparities it create?

More basically, these findings on the social roots of TP are also helpful to specify its theoretical status. In a perspective at the crossroads of personality and social psychology, time perspective can be related to the concept of habitus defined by Bourdieu as "*systems of durable and transposable dispositions, structured structures which are predisposed to function as structuring structures*" (Bourdieu 1980, p. 89). Hence, time perspective is for a part a stable dispositional construct resulting from the early and continued socialization process, and is also a dynamical factor active in the relations persons maintain with their environment at the symbolic, cognitive or behavioral levels. As such, time perspective operates as an intervening factor between the system of objective positions and subjective dispositions. Future research will have to clarify the definition of time perspective, or to explore the various facets of time perspective, to make the distinction between the personal and the situational time perspectives and their interaction in determining meanings and behaviours. In this interactionist view TP can play a moderating and/or a mediating role, depending on the situation and the behaviour under study. As a general approach, we referred to a *double contextualization* process (Fieulaine 2007) by which people are situated in concrete, historical and symbolic contexts that determine their time perspective, and by which events and situations take place in a particular time perspective that determine their meanings and behavioural consequences.

In an era of environmental, social and economic crises caused by the evolutions of the modern capitalism, it is crucial to act to avert these threats in the long term rather than only implementing stopgap solutions in the immediate present. Moreover, maintaining future orientation despite the unpredictability of the present, is a condition to become conscious and to struggle injustice or inequalities. These concerns for the long term are, as shown by the construal level theory, often related to concerns for other people and remote places. Balanced by past memories a consideration for the present and an acceptance of social change, Zimbardo's time perspective theory is not only a model and a measure of psychological time, but also a pathway from alienation to emancipation, and this constitutes the legacy of Professor Zimbardo.

References

Adams, J. (2009). The role of time preference and perspective in socio-economic inequalities in health related behaviours. In S. Babones (Ed.), *Social inequalities and public health* (pp. 9–24). Bristol: Policy Press.

Adams, J., & White, M. (2009). Time perspective in socio-economic inequalities in smoking and body mass index. *Health Psychology, 28*, 83–90.

Adler, N., Marmot, M., McEwen, B., & Stewart, J. (1999). *Socioeconomic status and health in industrial nations: Social, psychological and biological pathways*. New York: The New York Academy of Science.

Agarwal, A., Tripathi, K. K., & Srivastava, M. (1983). Social roots and psychological implications of time perspective. *International Journal of Psychology, 18*, 367–380.

Ahadyar, N. M. (1976). Orientation toward time among educated vs uneducated Afghans. *Dissertation Abstracts International, 36*, 7940–7941.

Apostolidis, T., & Fieulaine, N. (2004). French validation of the temporality scale: The Zimbardo time perspective inventory. *European Review of Applied Psychology, 54*, 207–217.

Barndt, R. J., & Johnson, D. N. (1955). Time orientation in delinquents. *Journal of Abnormal and Social Psychology, 51*, 343–345.

Beiser, M., & Hyman, I. (1997). Refugees' time perspective and mental health. *American Journal of Psychiatry, 154*, 996–1002.

Benach, J., & Muntaner, C. (2007). Precarious employment and health: Developing a research agenda. *Journal of Epidemiology and Community Health, 61*, 276–277.

Benavides, F. G., & Benach, J. (1999). *Precarious employment and health-related outcomes in the European Union*. Dublin: European Foundation for the Improvement of Living and Working Conditions.

Bihan, H., Laurent, S., Sass, C., Nguyen, G., Huot, C., Moulin, J. J., et al. (2005). Association among individual deprivation, glycemic control, and diabetes complications. The EPICES score. *Diabetes Care, 11*, 2680–2685.

Black, W. A., & Gregson, R. A. (1973). Time perspective, purpose in life, extraversion and neuroticism in New-Zeeland prisoners. *British Journal of Social and Clinical Psychology, 12*, 50–60.

Bosma, H., Van De Mheen, H., & Mackenbach, J. (1999). Social class in childhood and general health in adulthood: Questionnaire study of contribution of psychological attributes. *British Medical Journal, 318*, 18–22.

Bouffard, L., Lens, W., & Nuttin, J. R. (1983). Extension de la perspective temporelle future en lien avec la frustration. *International Journal of Psychology, 18*, 429–442.

Bouffard, L., Lapierre, S., & Bastin, E. (1989). Extension temporelle des projets personnels au cours de la vieillesse. *International Journal of Psychology, 3*, 265–291.

Bourdieu, P. (1966). L'école conservatrice: les inégalités devant l'école et devant la culture. *Revue Française de Sociologie, 7*, 325–347.

Bourdieu, P. (1980). *Le sens pratique*. Paris: Editions de Minuit.

Bourdieu, P. (1997). L'être social, le temps et l'existence. In P. Bourdieu (Ed.), *Méditations Pascaliennes* (pp. 247–288). Liber: Paris.

Bourdieu, P. (1998). *Counterfire: Against the Tyranny of the market*. London: Verso.

Carter, J. (Ed.). (1998). *Postmodernity and the fragmentation of welfare*. London: Routledge.

Carvounas, D., & Ireland, C. (2008). Precariousness, the secured present and the sustainability of the future. *Time and Society, 17*, 155–178.
Cassidy, T. (2000). Social background, achievement motivation, optimism and health: A longitudinal study. *Counseling Psychology Quarterly, 13*, 399–412.
Cottle, T. J. (1968). The location of experience: A manifest time orientation. *Acta Psychologica, 28*, 129–149.
Cottle, T. J., & Klineberg, S. L. (1974). *The present of things future: Exploration of time in human experience*. New York: Free Press.
Cottle, T. J., & Pleck, J. H. (1969). Linear estimation of temporal extension: The effect of age, sex, and social class. *Journal of Projective Techniques and Personality Assessment, 31*, 58–71.
Crockett, R. A., Weinman, J., Hankins, M., & Marteau, T. (2009). Time orientation and health-related behaviour: Measurement in general population samples. *Psychology and Health, 24*, 333–350.
D'Alessio, M., Guarino, A., DePascalis, V., & Zimbardo, P. G. (2003). Testing Zimbardo's Stanford Time Perspective Inventory (STPI) short form: An Italian study. *Time and Society, 12*, 333–347.
Davies, M. L. (1997). Shattered assumptions: Time and the experience of long-term HIV positivity. *Social Science and Medicine, 5*, 561–571.
Dohrenwend, B. P., Levav, I., Shrout, P., Schwartz, S., Naveh, G., Link, B., Skodol, A., & Stueve, A. (1992). Socioeconomic status and psychiatric disorders: The causation-selection issue. *Science, 255*, 946–952.
Epel, S. E., Bandura, A., & Zimbardo, P. G. (1999). Escaping homelessness: The influences of self-efficacy and time perspective on coping with homelessness. *Journal of Applied Social Psychology, 29*, 575–596.
Farber, M. L. (1944). Suffering and time perspective of the prisoner. *University of Iowa Studies: Child Welfare, 20*, 153–227.
Feather, N. T., & Bond, M. J. (1983). Time structure and purposeful activity among employed and unemployed university graduates. *Journal of Occupational Psychology, 56*, 241–254.
Fieulaine, N. (2007). *Time perspective, socioeconomic precariousness and health: A social-psychological approach*. Unpublished doctoral thesis, University of Provence.
Fieulaine, N., Apostolidis, T., & Olivetto, F. (2006). Précarité et troubles psychologiques: l'effet médiateur de la perspective temporelle' [Precariousness ans psychological distress: The mediating effect of time perspective]. *Les Cahiers Internationaux de Psychologie Sociale, 72*, 51–64.
Fingerman, K. L., & Perlmutter, M. (1995). Future time perspective and life events across adulthood. *The Journal of General Psychology, 122*, 95–111.
Forrest, R. (1999). The new landscape of precariousness. In P. Kennett & A. Marsh (Eds.), *Homelessness: Exploring new terrain* (pp. 17–37). Bristol: Policy Press.
Frank, L. K. (1939). Time perspectives. *Journal of Social Philosophy, 4*, 293–312.
Freire, E., Gorman, B., & Wessman, E. (1980). Temporal span, delay of gratification, and children's socioeconomic status. *Journal of Genetic Psychology, 137*, 247–55.
Fuchs, V. R. (1982). Time preference and health: An exploratory study. In V. R. Fuchs (Ed.), *Economic aspects of health* (pp. 93–120). Chicago: The University of Chicago Press.
Gallo, L. C. (2009). Socioeconomic status and health. *Current Directions in Psychological Science, 18*(5), 269–274.
Gardner, N. P. (2004). *Linking parental work experience to adolescent's future orientation*. Unpublished PhD dissertation, University of Michigan.
George, J. M. (1991). Time structure and purpose as mediator of work-life linkages. *Journal of Applied Social Psychology, 21*, 296–314.
Green, L., Meyerson, J., Lichtman, D., Rosen, S., & Fry, A. (1996). Temporal discounting in choice between delayed rewards: The role of age and income. *Psychology and Aging, 11*, 79–84.
Guillemin, F., Paul-Dauphin, A., Virion, J. M., Bouchet, C., & Briançon, S. (1997). The duke health profile: A generic instrument to measure the quality of life tied to health. *Santé Publique, 9*, 35–44.

Guthrie, L. C., Butler, S. C., & Ward, M. M. (2009). Time perspective and socioeconomic status: A link to socioeconomic disparities in health? *Social Science and Medicine, 68*(12), 2145–2151.

Henick, W., & Domino, G. (1975). Alterations in future time perspective in heroin addicts. *Journal of Abnormal and Social Psychology, 78*, 557–564.

Henry, P. (2001). An examination of the pathways through which social class impacts health outcomes. *Academy of Marketing Science Review, 3*, 1–24.

Hepworth, S. J. (1980). Moderating factors of the psychological impact of unemployment. *Journal of Occupational Psychology, 53*, 139–145.

Holman, E. A., & Silver, C. S. (1998). Getting "stuck" in the past: Temporal orientation and coping with trauma. *Journal of Personality and Social Psychology, 74*, 1146–1163.

Hulbert, R. J., & Lens, W. (1988). Time perspective, time attitude, and time orientation in alcoholism: A review. *International Journal of Addictions, 23*, 279–298.

Jahoda, M. (1982). *Employment and unemployment*. Cambridge: University Press.

Jaroni, J., Wright, S., Lerman, C., & Epstein, L. (2004). Relationship between education and delay discounting in smokers. *Addictive Behaviors, 29*, 1171–5.

Joubert, M., Chauvin, P., Facy, F., & Ringa, V. (2001). *Précarisation, risque et santé* [Precariousness, risks and health]. Paris: INSERM.

Judson, A. J., & Tuttle, C. E. (1966). Time perspective and social class. *Perceptual and Motor Skills, 23*, 1074.

Kendall, M. B., & Sibley, R. F. (1970). Social class differences in time orientation: Artifact? *Journal of Social Psychology, 82*, 187–191.

Koenig, F., Swanson, W., & Harter, C. (1981). Future time orientation, social class and anomia. *Social Behavior and Personality, 9*, 123–127.

Kokko, K., & Pulkkinen, L. (1998). Unemployment and psychological distress: Mediator effects. *Journal of Adult Development, 5*, 205–217.

Lamm, H., Schmidt, R. W., & Trommsdorff, G. (1976). Sex and social class as determinants of future orientation in adolescents. *Journal of Personality and Social Psychology, 34*, 317–326.

Landau, S. F. (1976). Delinquency institutionalization and time orientation. *Journal of Consulting and Clinical Psychology, 44*, 745–759.

Lang, F. R., & Carstensen, L. L. (2002). Time counts: Future time perspective, goals, and social relationships. *Psychology and Aging, 17*, 125–139.

LaRosa, E., Le Clésiau, H., & Valensi, P. (2008). Metabolic syndrome and psychosocial deprivation. Data collected from a Paris suburb. *Diabetes and Metabolism, 34*(2), 155–161.

Lawrence, E. (1991). Poverty and the rate of time preference: Evidence from panel data. *Journal of Political Economy, 99*, 54–77.

Lebas, J., & Chauvin, P. (1998) *Précarité et santé* [Precariousness and health]. Paris: Flammarion.

Leigh, J. (1986). Accounting for tastes: Correlates of risk and time preferences. *Journal of Post Keynesian Economics, 9*, 17–31.

LeShan, L. L. (1952). Time orientation and social class. *Journal of Abnormal and Social Psychology, 47*, 589–592.

Levy, S. M. (1978). Some determinants of temporal experience in the retired and its correlates. *Genetic Psychology Monographs, 98*, 181–202.

Lewin, K. (1926/1935). On the structure of mind. In K. Lewin (Ed.), *A dynamic theory of personality* (pp. 43–65). London: McGraw-Hill.

Lewin, K. (1936). *Principles of topological psychology*. New York: McGraw-Hill.

Lewin, K. (1942). Time perspective and morale. In G. W. Lewin (Ed.), *Resolving social conflicts* (pp. 103–124). Boston: Houghton Mifflin.

Lewin, K. (1943). Defining the field at a given time. *Psychological Review, 50*, 292–310.

Lewin, K. (1946). Behavior and development as a function of the total situation. In L. Carmichael (Ed.), *Manual of child psychology* (pp. 791–844). New York: Wiley.

Lewin, K. (1951). *Field theory in social sciences*. New York: Harper.

Lewin, K. (1959). *Psychologie Dynamique: Les relations humaines*. Paris: PUF.

Lomranz, J., Shmotkin, D., & Katznelson, D. B. (1983). Coherence as a measure of future time perspective in children and its relationship to delay of gratification and social class. *International Journal of Psychology, 18*, 407–413.

Melges, F. T. (1982). *Time and the inner future*. New York: Wiley.

Misra, G., & Tripathi, L. B. (1977). *Manual for prolonged deprivation scale*. Agra: National Psychological Corporation.

Nahon, S., Lahmek, P., Macaigne, G., Faurel, J. P., Sass, C., Howaizi, M., & Poupardin, C. (2009). Socioeconomic deprivation does not influence the severity of Crohn's disease: Results of a prospective multicenter study. *Inflammatory Bowel Diseases, 15*(4), 594–598.

Nettleton, S., & Burrows, R. (2001). Families coping with the experience of mort-gage repossession in the 'new landscape of precariousness'. *Community, Work and Family, 4*, 253–272.

Nurmi, J. E. (1987). Age, sex, social class, and quality of family interaction as determinants of adolescents' future orientation: A developmental task interpretation. *Adolescence, 12*, 977–991.

Nuttin, J. (1977). La perspective temporelle dans le comportement humain. In P. Fraisse et al. (Eds.), *Du temps biologique au temps psychologique* (pp. 307–363). Paris: PUF.

O'Rand, A., & Ellis, R. A. (1974). Social class and social time perspective. *Social Forces, 53*, 53–62.

Pakerson, J. R., Broadhead, W. E., & Tse, C. K. (1991). Development of the 17-item Duke health profile. *Family Practice, 8*, 396–401.

Paugam, S. (1995). The spiral of precariousness: A multidimensional approach to the process of social disqualification in France. In G. Room (Ed.), *Beyond the threshold: The measurement and analysis of social exclusion* (pp. 49–79). Bristol: Policy Press.

Peetsma, T. T. (2000). Future time perspective as a predictor of school investment. *Scandinavian Journal of Educational Research, 44*(2), 177–192.

Perlman, L. M. (1976). Temporal extension and orientation: A methodological Study. *Perceptual and Motor Skills, 43*, 775–785.

Pham, L. B., Taylor, S. E., & Seeman, T. E. (2001). Effects of environmental predictability and personal mastery on self-regulatory and physiological processes. *Personality and Social Psychology Bulletin, 27*(5), 611–620.

Platt, S., Pavis, S., & Akram, G. (1999). *Changing labour market conditions and health: A systematic literature review (1993–1998)*. Dublin: European Foundation for the Improvement of Living and Working Conditions.

Quinlan, M., Mahew, C., & Bohle, P. (2001). The global expansion of precarious employment, work disorganization, and consequences for occupational health: A review of recent literature. *International Journal of Health Services, 31*, 335–414.

Sapsford, R. J. (1978). Life-sentence: Prisoners psychological changes during sentence. *British Journal of Criminology, 18*, 128–145.

Schmidt, R. W., Lamm, H., & Trommsdorff, G. (1978). Social class and sex as determinant of future orientation in adults. *European Journal of Social Psychology, 8*, 71–90.

Schunck, R., & Rogge, B. G. (2010). Unemployment and its association with health-relevant actions: investigating the role of time perspective with German census data. *International Journal of Public Health, 55*(4), 271–278.

Sennett, R. (2004). *The culture of the new capitalism*. New Haven: Yale University Press.

Singh-Manoux, A., & Marmot, M. (2005). Role of socialization in explaining social inequalities in health. *Social Science and Medicine, 60*, 2129–2134.

Snyder, M. (2013). B=f (P, S): Perspectives on persons and situations, from Lewin to Bond and beyond. *Asian Journal of Social Psychology, 16*(1), 16–18.

Sobel, M. E. (1982). Asymptotic confidence intervals for indirect effects in structural equation models. *Sociological Methodology, 13*(1982), 290–312.

Srole, L. (1956). Social integration and certain corollaries. *American Sociological Review, 21*, 709–716.

Stein, K. B., Sarbin, T. R., & Kulik, J. A. (1968). Future time perspective: Its relation to the socialization process and the delinquent role. *Journal of Consulting and Clinical Psychology, 32*, 257–264.

Thiébaut, E. (1997). *La perspective temporelle – l'objet de mesure : vers une élucidation conceptuelle.* Thèse de doctorat de 3ème cycle, Université Nancy 2.

Toombs, S. K. (1990). The temporality of illness: Four levels of experience. *Theoretical Medicine, 11*, 227–241.

Trommsdorff, G. (1983). Future orientation and socialization. *International Journal of Psychology, 18*, 381–406.

Trommsdorff, G., & Lamm, H. (1980). Future orientation of institutionalized and noninstitutionalized delinquents and nondelinquents. *European Journal of Social Psychology, 10*, 247–278.

Trommsdorff, G., Lamm, H., & Schmidt, R. W. (1979). A longitudinal study of adolescents future orientation (time perspective). *Journal of Youth and Adolescence, 8*, 131–147.

Twenge, J. M., Catanese, K. R., & Baumeister, R. F. (2003). Social exclusion and the deconstructed state: Time perception, meaninglessness, lethargy, lack of emotion and self-awareness. *Journal of Personality and Social Psychology, 85*, 409–423.

Van Der Keilen, M. (1982). L'étendue de la perspective temporelle future et l'attitude à l'égard du présent, du passé et de l'avenir chez les adolescents normaux et handicapés sociaux : Influence du succès et de l'échec expérimental. *Psychologica Belgica, 22*, 161–183.

Viinamaki, H., Koskela, K., Niskanen, L., & Tahka, V. (1994). Mental adaptation to unemployment. *European Journal of Psychiatry, 8*, 243–252.

Wallace, C. J. (1986). Functional assessment in rehabilitation. *Schizophrenia Bulletin, 12*, 604–624.

Wanberg, C. R., & Griffiths, R. F. (1997). Time structure and unemployment: A longitudinal investigation. *Journal of Occupational and Organizational Psychology, 70*, 75–90.

Wardle, J., & Steptoe, A. (2003). Socioeconomic differences in attitudes and beliefs about healthy lifestyles. *Journal of Epidemiology and Community Health, 57*, 440–443.

Waters, L., & Muller, J. (2003). Money or time ? Comparing the effects of time structure and financial deprivation on the psychological distress of unemployed adults. *Australian Journal of Psychology, 55*, 166–175.

Zigmond, A. S., & Snaith, R. P. (1983). The hospital anxiety and depression scale. *Acta Psychiatrica Scandinavica, 67*, 361–370.

Zimbardo, P. G., & Boyd, J. N. (1999). Putting time in perspective: A valid, reliable individual-differences metric. *Journal of Personality and Social Psychology, 77*, 1271–1288.

Part III
Cognitive, Emotional, and Motivational Processes in Time Perspective

Neural Correlates of Time Perspective

Maria Grazia Carelli and Carl-Johan Olsson

Introduction

Both behavioral and neuropsychological studies on temporal processing suggest a discontinuity in our sense of time (Fraisse 1963). For example, Lewis and Miall 2003 (see also Lewis and Miall 2006, for an overview) suggested that timing in the shorter range is 'automatic', reflecting the engagement of processes associated with the production of skilled movements. In this view, motor timing refers to the timing aspects of the output of behavior, such as the temporal organization of motor, speech or cognitive acts. (e.g., finger tapping, rhythm production). The time range used with these methods range from milliseconds to seconds and minutes. Longer range timing is hypothesized to be 'cognitive', dependent on (fronto-parietal) neural systems associated with attention and working memory. The time range in these tasks range from seconds and minutes and even hours, and include tasks of time estimation and time (re)production. Extending this discontinuity of temporal information processing to the domains of personality and social psychology, as illustrated by the present volume, several lines of research investigate how behavior is shaped by time, including topics such as time management, time perspective, and time orientation (Francis-Smythe and Robertson 1999; Carstensen et al. 1999; Zimbardo and Boyd 1999).

During the last decades, patient studies and brain-imaging studies, using a variety of tasks and methods, have identified neural correlates of different levels of temporal processing. The primary focus of these studies has been on the neural

M.G. Carelli (✉)
Department of Psychology, Umeå University, SE-901 87 Umeå, Sweden
e-mail: grazia.carelli@psy.umu.se

C.-J. Olsson
Umeå Center for Functional Brain Imaging and Centre for Population Studies, Ageing and Living Conditions Programme, Umeå University, Umeå, Sweden
e-mail: cj.olsson@ddb.umu.se

M. Stolarski et al. (eds.), *Time Perspective Theory; Review, Research and Application: Essays in Honor of Philip G. Zimbardo*, DOI 10.1007/978-3-319-07368-2_15,

mechanisms of motor and interval timing, mainly driven by the hypothesis that time perception involves the presence of a central device, a "mental clock," often combined with the assumption that there is a specialized brain system for representing this dedicated mechanism. Nevertheless, the neural correlates of timing processes remain highly elusive, partly because there are no dedicated sensors for time. As noted by Grondin (2010) in his recent review of brain-imaging studies on motor timing and time perception, only limited conclusions can be drawn about the brain structures involved in the processing of temporal information, partly due to the variations of timing tasks and duration ranges in past work.

Although we have some knowledge about lower-level timing functions and their neural correlates, time perspective, conceptualized as "individual's orientation of psychological past and future existing at a given time" (Lewin 1951, p. 71), has gained minimal attention in neuropsychological studies. The primary aim of this chapter is to summarize our present knowledge about neural correlates of time perspective and related constructs (see Grondin 2008, 2010; Meck 2005; Rubia 2006; Penney and Vaitilingam 2008, for more comprehensive overviews of neuroimaging studies on motor timing and time perception). The following sections of the chapter will first present a brief introduction to neuroimaging methodology in the context of time perspective, with a primary focus on the functional magnetic resonance imaging (fMRI) technique. The next section summarizes brain-imaging studies involving similar, but not identical constructs as the concept of time perspective, followed by a summary of our own ongoing work on neural correlates of time perspective in the context of Zimbardo and colleagues framework. The final section presents more general conclusion and suggestions about future research on neural correlates of temporal processing.

What Functional Brain Imaging Can Tell Us About the Neuropsychology of Time Perspective?

With the use of various neuroimaging techniques it is possible to design studies with the intention to reveal the structural and functional brain architecture underlying specific abilities. Thus, it is possible to increase the knowledge regarding different sets of structures and processes within the central nervous system that are used to perform certain tasks or associated with certain phenomena such as time and temporal processing. Those particular regions recruited while one performs a certain task are seen as a reflection of a specific role for that region in a specific brain process. However, in order for these techniques to be useful, a continual interplay between behavioral and neuroimaging studies are necessary, thus it is important to integrate behavioral data in order to make sense out of brain imaging data. Hence, without behavioral measures and theory, the design and the following interpretation of the brain-imaging data will be difficult (see Kosslyn 1999). Related to the specific focus of this chapter, and to fully appreciate the meaning of the *past*, the *present* and the future in the context of neural correlates, it is necessary to combine brain-imaging data with functional levels of explanation. Thus, if we aim to investigate the neural mechanisms of time perspective, we must design a paradigm that induces systematic changes in the individual's temporal focus while simultaneously measuring the functional brain response.

The interpretation of neuroimaging data is often more complex than the interpretation of behavioral data. The reason for this is because one needs to be concerned not only about the nature of the task itself, but also about the relation between performance and the underlying physiology. However, executed correctly it provides valuable information about the underlying mechanisms for a behavior and also about how different processes and structures are working together. Moreover, a benefit with neuroimaging techniques is that the data provided are not easily explained as an artifact of experimental demand characteristics since it is difficult to voluntarily manipulate which brain regions one uses, therefore it offers a potential bridge between psychology and biology (Senior et al. 2006).

One of the most frequently used brain-imaging methods is the *functional magnetic resonance imaging (fMRI)* technique. This method is a non-invasive neuroimaging technique relying on regional cerebral blood flow (rCBF). The use of fMRI offers not only the understanding of brain organization, it is also frequently used in medical practice complementing clinical diagnoses (e.g., pre-surgical mapping) as well as characterizing neurological and psychiatric disorders. In fMRI, brain activation is based on an endogenous contrast called blood oxygenation level depend (BOLD) signal. It has been shown that the BOLD signal has a linear relationship with brain activity. Hence, an increase in BOLD signal is associated with an increase in brain activation. It was early shown that BOLD signal change follows the level of brain activation in the visual system, auditory system and the motor system and can be used as a reliable approximation for brain activity (See Logothetis et al. 2001; Logothetis 2008). The reason why the BOLD contrast offers this feature is because of the different magnetic characteristics between oxygenated blood (blood rich of oxygen) and de-oxygenated blood (blood with poor concentration of oxygen). When a subject is put in the scanner, the different characteristics create a magnetic field distortion. During activation, cerebral blood flow increases locally so that there is an overabundance of oxygenated blood delivered to the active regions. This causes a change of the magnitude of the magnetic field distortions, which leads to a change in the signal that is interpreted as a change in brain activation. fMRI has good spatial resolution and is useful for network analysis. However, the temporal resolution is poor giving difficulties to interpret the relative timing of events. Brain imaging data from fMRI should be viewed as time series data in which different tasks are induced at different time points creating a model from which one can compare activity between different conditions. Thus, its nature is comparative, meaning that you don't measure brain activation in absolute measures, you always compare with a baseline, e.g., a different task, or rest. One should bear in mind that the MRI environment is quite special, which limits the things you can do within the scanner. However, in most studies, while in the scanner, participants are viewing a mirror attached to the head coil and thereby can view a computer screen onto which it is possible to present stimuli.

Moreover, there are special response pads used which gives valuable information regarding performance on different tests.

It is necessary to mention some *shortcomings of fMRI*. Since it is an indirect method of measuring brain activity, certainly this must be taken into consideration when interpreting the results leading to limitations foremost regarding the temporal resolution. It is also sensible to subject motions, this is controlled for in as many ways as possible including cushions to stabilize the head as well as using movement parameters as covariates in the analysis. However, motions do create artifacts. Nevertheless, with a good fMRI design differences of brain activity between two tasks can be examined with the hope of isolating brain regions associated with that task in particular. Thus, to identify regions that are important for time perspective, one must create a task in which participants are put into different time perspectives and differences in brain activity between time perspectives can be assessed. Hence, by using brain imaging methods (here the focus has been on fMRI, but other methods are available too) a new dimension would be added towards understanding a remarkable feature of the human mind, the concept of time.

Neural Correlates of TP in Neuroimaging Studies

In the neuroscience community the concept of time perspective is recognized as an emerging area of interest. In fact, several neuroimaging studies have examined the concept of time especially referring to the construct of *mental time travel*, (MTT; Suddendorf and Corballis 1997; Abraham et al. 2008; Buckner 2010; Addis et al. 2007; Nyberg et al. 2010; Okuda et al. 2003). In these studies, brain activity has been measured while participants are asked to mentally envision themselves in different temporal contexts. For example, imagine your high-school graduation (past time) or imagine your 70th birthday party (future time). The results of these studies have shown a widespread neural network recruited during MTT, with both common regions across the time perspective as well as diverse regions. Specifically, these studies have revealed that a few core regions are recruited when the brain handles MTT, including the *pre-frontal cortex*, the *parietal cortex* (e.g., *posterior cingulate cortex*), and the *medial temporal lobe* (e.g., *hippocampus*). Interestingly, regions within the core network have been shown to play an important role in the retrieval of personal memories suggesting that when individuals are asked to think about future events, past events are used to complete the task. Thus, as noted earlier, it appears *that past and the future may share neural substrates* (see e.g., Szpunar et al. 2007).

The regions *within* the core brain network of time have both similar and different functions. The *medial pre-frontal cortex* has been interpreted as a region reflecting *the self*. As a support for this hypothesis, several patient studies suggest that individuals with damage to the *prefrontal cortex* have problems to think about their continued existence (Wheeler et al. 1997). More recently, findings suggest that this region is engaged during self-referential processing (Hassabis et al. 2007) as well as during constructive processes (Addis et al. 2007). This can be linked towards future thinking when one has to construct an event that will appear in the future. However, the precise function of this region in relation to time is not well understood. The *medial temporal lobe* has been suggested to reflect the critical role in retrieving episodic memories of the past (Cabeza and St Jacques 2007). Moreover, the *hippocampus* has received a lot of interest regarding its importance during the consolidation of new memories (e.g., Wang and Morris 2010), and to facilitate predictions of the future (Buckner 2010). Related to MTT, the function of the *parietal lobe* has also been proposed to be linked to episodic memory. Activation in the *parietal lobe* has also been associated with both future (dorsal parts) and past (ventral parts), (Abraham et al. 2008). Other important functions of the parietal lobe in relation to time are the involvement in visuospatial perspective taking (Abraham et al. 2008) and understanding goal-directed intentions (Fogassi et al. 2005).

Relatively few studies have investigated the neural correlates of *temporal foresight*, probably due to measurement difficulties, laboratory settings and task impurity problems related to relatively long temporal intervals. According to Rubia (2006), the *right lateral prefrontal cortex* and *fronto-striatal* brain areas are particularly involved in temporal foresight, similar to their involvement in the estimation of longer time intervals. The *right prefrontal cortex* appear to be particularly important in the discrimination of long intervals, consistent with the results of studies showing that damage to the prefrontal cortex impairs the discrimination of longer durations more than that of short durations (Droit-Volet 2013). Moreover, more specific brain regions related to temporal foresight, but not in time estimation, have been found related to the *ventromedial prefrontal* brain areas.

In general, little attention has been put towards the *present time perspective*. Recently though, Nyberg et al. (2010) reported that, relative to the present temporal orientation, brain activity during past, future and remembering, respectively, showed elevated signal changes within the *parietal cortex*. Similar patterns of activation were also observed for *thalamus* and the *frontal cortex*, whereas *hippocampus* showed no systematic changes in activation. Even though each region of the core network has distinct functions, they are proposed to reflect combined processes of long term memory function.

In an attempt to distinguish between these different regions in relation to one's own experience, Abraham and colleagues (2008) conducted a study in which they managed to separate between *thinking about events (future or past) in relation to personal or non-personal contexts*. The results showed that there was no specific region for non-personal events, however the core brain network for time was stronger associated with personal events compared to non-personal events. This pattern of neural activations emphasizes the relation between mental time travel and autobiographical memory, suggesting that experience most likely shapes brain response in relation to time. When analyzing past vs. future events in relation to personal or non-personal context (Abraham et al. 2008) an increase *in the right inferior frontal gyrus* was observed for *non-personal past events*, perhaps indicating the need for semantic retrieval. In contrast, *personal past events* were more strongly associated with *ventral posterior cingulate cortex* and *hippocampus. Future thinking* also diverged when analyzing differences between personal and non-personal context. Here it was shown that future was in general more associated with *frontal regions* and even more so for the *middle prefrontal cortex* in relation to personal experience, which others also have supported (Addis et al. 2007; Okuda et al. 2003). All together, these studies suggest that on creating adequate brain imaging paradigms to study time, might be relevant to incorporate additional information regarding personal experiences. We also believe that in order to fully appreciate the neural correlates of time, it is important also to consider the participants own time perspective profile, something that no study yet has addressed. That is, if a person is future oriented, according to the ZTPI scale, are the same brain regions engaged while thinking about the future as for a person that is more oriented towards the past?

Neural Correlates of Time Perspective: An fMRI Study

Although the relationship between some aspects of timing functions and their underlying neural substrates are well documented, *there are no studies concerning the neural underpinnings of temporal orientation as a personality-like construct.* In this attempt to include personality into the study of time perspective, we examined differences in neural (fMRI) activation between individuals with different temporal orientations as indexed by the Zimbardo Time Perspective Inventory (ZTPI; Zimbardo and Boyd 1999). Further focus of this study was to test the *suitability* of the ZTPI questionnaire as a method to incorporate time-profile information with fMRI data.

In this study, participants first completed the short version of the S-ZTPI (Carelli et al. 2011; see also chapter "Broadening the TP Profile" in this volume) while scanned. Five statements from each of its six profiles (Past Positive, PP; Past Negative, PN; Present Hedonistic, PH; Present Fatalistic, PF; Future Positive; Future Negative, FN) were selected. Based on a separate validation study (Carelli et al. 2011), these target statements showed the strongest association with each time frame. A total of 21 participants were tested (mean age = 25.7 years), with no earlier experience of fMRI or ZTPI. All participants were tested at *Umeå Center for Functional Brain Imaging, Umeå University*.

Specifically, while scanned, participants responded to 5×6 blocks of S-ZTPI items by providing a response at three levels of agreement. After the scanning phase, participants completed the full version of the S-ZTPI, and a set of cognitive measures. The primary hypothesis of this exploratory study was that responding to items referring to different temporal perspectives activates distinct neural regions.

Preliminary findings of the fMRI data show an overall general activity within the *core brain network for time*, with *medial and superior pre-frontal* regions, including *BA 32, parietal regions,* including *BA 39 (angular gyrus)* and *middle and superior temporal* regions with *BA 21/22* and *BA 48* jointly recruited for all different time perspectives (see Fig. 1).

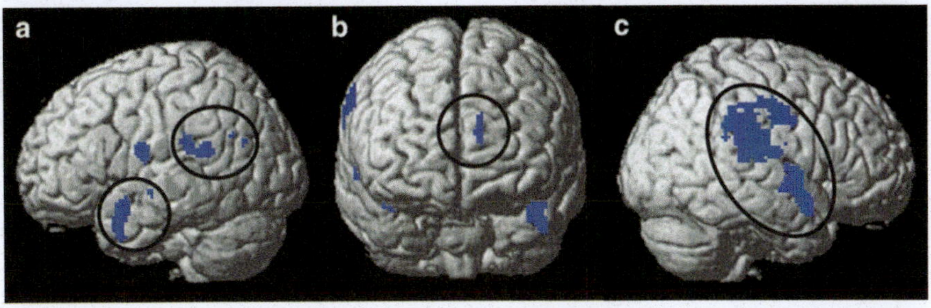

Fig. 1 Jointly recruited brain regions associated with ZTP regardless of specific time perspective. (**a**) *left side view* showing middle and superior temporal lobe (BA 21/22) as well as parietal activity in the angular gyrus (BA 39). (**b**) *anterior view* showing superior middle pre-frontal cortex activity (BA 32). (**c**) *right side view* showing middle and superior temporal lobe activity (BA 21/22)

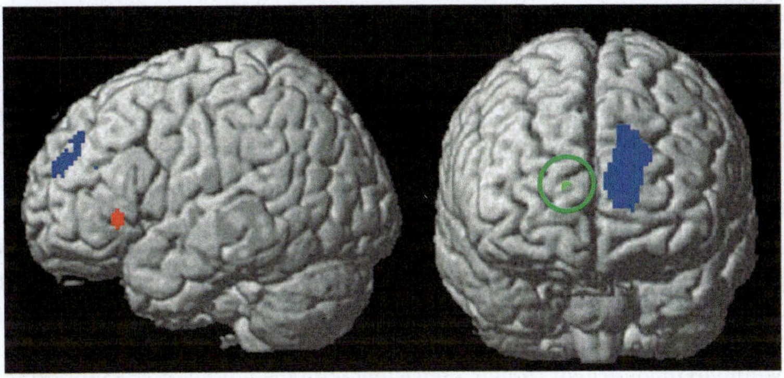

Fig. 2 Isolated brain regions recruited for past, medial frontal cortex (BA10), present, superior medial frontal cortex (BA32) and future, inferior frontal gyrus (B47) time perspectives respectively

Moreover, and perhaps more interestingly, these data suggested selective effects with distinct neural correlates for the each of the time frames, as defined by the S-ZTPI. For example, for the past and present time perspectives, the frontal activity was more associated towards *medial parts* (*BA 10* for past time perspective and *BA 32* for present time perspective) in comparison with the Future time perspective, which was more active in *ventral parts* (*ventrolateral prefrontal cortex, BA 47*) of the *pre-frontal cortex* (see Fig. 2). Furthermore, and consistent with earlier brain-imaging studies, the past time scales (Past Negative Scale, PN, and Past Positive Scale, PP) of the S-ZTPI show an activation of the *medial frontal cortex* (*BA10, frontopolar prefrontal cortex* or *rostral* PFC).

Understanding the functions of *rostral prefrontal cortex* (approximating Brodmann's area 10) presents one of the greatest scientific challenges to cognitive neuroscience. Lesions to this region in humans typically leave performance on tests of intellectual, language, memory, visual perception, motor skills, and many problem-solving abilities virtually intact. However, lesions seem to cause impairments in two specific situations (Burgess et al. 2007). The first type is open-ended situations, which require self-organized behavior, and the second class of situation is where sustained, self-maintained attending behavior is required, such as when maintaining response consistency (Bird et al. 2004).

Others studies have reported similar results in that this region has been interpreted to reflect the self and is engaged in self-referential processing (Hassabis et al. 2007). Christoff and colleagues implicated activation of the rostral PFC also during 'spontaneous thought processes' and 'evaluating self-generated information' (Christoff et al. 2004). More recently, *BA10* has also been associated with prospective memory, and especially in the maintenance and realization of delayed intentions that are triggered by event cues (i.e., event-based prospective memory) as well as processes associated with the use of time cues (time-based prospective memory). However, the exact nature of these processes has been controversial (see Okuda et al. 2007).

Furthermore, our results are consistent with previous studies suggesting that the medial temporal lobe has a critical role in *retrieving episodic memories of the past* (Cabeza and St. Jacques 2007). This line of reasoning is in agreement with the past statements of the S-ZTPI which refer to remembering past events ("*Happy memories of good times spring readily to mind*"; "*I get nostalgic about my childhood*").

Another central finding of our study was that the present scales (Present-Fatalistic, PF and Present-Hedonistic, PH) recruited specific regions of the anterior cingulate cortex, BA 32, the *superior medial frontal cortex*. Past studies related to functions of BA 32 show that the *anterior cingulate cortex* is more active when responding to *incongruent stimuli*, consistent with the notion of its monitoring function (Mac Donald et al 2000; Ridderinkhof et al. 2004). The ability to monitor and compare actual performance with internal goals and standards is critical for optimizing behavior. Flexible goal-directed behavior requires an adaptive cognitive control system for selecting contextually relevant information and for organizing and optimizing information processing (see Ridderinkhof et al. 2004). The superior medial frontal cortex has also been shown having an important *inhibitory control* of prepotent actions. The importance of such control can be seen in the inhibition of aggressive behavior, considering how meaningful for the society might be an inefficiency of inhibitory control (Chen et al. 2009). Behavioral studies suggested that individuals with high score in the present scale of ZTPI (especially the hedonistic one) show lack of inhibitory control and risky behavior (Boyd and Zimbardo 2005; Alvos et al. 1993). However, to translate such observation into neural correlates is difficult, because with the current paradigm we cannot disentangle whether the neural activity in those regions implies lack of inhibitory control or the opposite be in control of the situation. At the moment with the present data we are unable to rule out one or the other possible interpretations, but certainly that will be an interesting avenue for future studies.

Finally, our findings suggested that the Future time scale (Future-Positive and Future-Negative) activated the *inferior frontal gyrus* (BA 47/VLPFC). Interestingly, this results support other studies *using different time paradigm*. According to Addis et al. (2007) future events recruits regions involved in prospective thinking and generation processes, such as the *right frontopolar cortex* and *left ventrolateral PFC*. Further, the activation of the VLPFC has also been found in studies investigating temporal foresight (Rubia 2006), MTT (Nyberg et al. 2010), and temporal coherence (e.g. in language and music, Vuust et al. 2006). BA 47 is usually associated with language-related functions (e.g., semantic and phonological processing, De Carli et al. 2007; McDermott et al. 2003), and seems to be involved in deductive reasoning (Goel et al. 1998) and emotional related activities (e.g., adverse emotional inhibition, Berthoz et al. 2002).

It should also be noted that, although many converging lines of evidence suggest a great deal of overlap between the retrieval of past events and the imagining of future, our results are consistent with more recent findings suggesting both unity and diversity of neural mechanisms for the Past and Future time perspectives (Addis et al. 2007; Squire et al. 2010).

Conclusions

Evidence from different types of neuroimaging methods suggest that temporal processing reflects a complex neural network (see Wiener et al. 2010 for a review). By contrast, research on neural correlates of time as a personality-like construct (as illustrated by the notion of time perspective; Zimbardo and Boyd 1999) is virtually nonexistent.

In this chapter, we summarized our first attempts in this promising area of research. These findings suggest that time perspective, as indexed by the subscales of the S-ZTPI (Carelli et al. 2011) reflects both the unity and diversity of neural activations. Concerning the former, a central finding of our study was that the S-ZTPI items activated a common time-related network in that the temporal cortex and parts of the parietal and frontal areas were jointly recruited. A more specific finding was that differences in time orientation were associated with selective neural correlates, with distinct areas of neural activations for the three time frames of past, present and future. Our data also indicate that differences in agreement, at the level of individual S-ZTPI statements, recruited distinct cortical regions, suggesting that the scales were sensitive enough to be used in this context. Our attempts to use fMRI methodology was then successful in providing additional information about the underlying neural correlates of time perspective by taking into account differences in the individual time profile. For example, the ventromedial prefrontal cortex has been implicated in Future-Positive thinking. Here our preliminary data suggest that this region was indeed engaged during the processing Future-Positive oriented S-ZTPI statements.

In more general terms, the observed consistency in the patterns of neural activation provides additional validity for the time-perspective framework outlined by Zimbardo and colleagues. This is interesting, not only in terms of brain structure and function, but it also increases the validity of the time perspective construct.

Our next step in this ongoing project is to examine how individual profiles in TP and within-frame differences (positive vs. negative; fatalistic vs. hedonistic) recruits specific brain regions. Another interesting avenue for future work in this context would be to investigate the extent to individuals with balanced time perspective (BTP; Boniwell and Zimbardo 2004; Wiberg et al. 2012; chapter "Assessing Temporal Harmony: The Issue of a Balanced Time Perspective" by Stolarski et al., this volume) show systematic differences in neural activation when contrasted with individual with a less balanced perspective.

References

Abraham, A., Schubotz, R. I., & von Cramon, D. Y. (2008). Thinking about the future versus the past in personal and non-personal contexts. *Brain Research, 1233*, 106–119.

Addis, D. R., Wong, A. T., & Schacter, D. L. (2007). Remembering the past and imaging the future: Common and distinct neural substrates during event construction and elaboration. *Neuropsychologia, 45*, 1363–1377.

Alvos, L., Gregson, R. A., & Ross, M. W. (1993). Future time perspective in current and previous injecting drug users. *Drug and Alcohol Dependence, 31*, 193–197.

Berthoz, S., Armony, J. L., Blair, R. J., & Dolan, R. J. (2002). An fMRI study of intentional and unintentional (embarrassing) violations of social norms. *Brain, 125*, 1696–1708.

Bird, C. M., Castelli, F., Malik, O., Frith, U., & Husain, M. (2004). The impact of extensive medial frontal lobe damage on "theory of mind" and cognition. *Brain, 127*, 914–928.

Boniwell, I., & Zimbardo, P. G. (2004). Balancing time perspective in pursuit of optimal functioning. In P. A. Linley & S. Joseph (Eds.), *Positive psychology in practice* (pp. 165–178). Hoboken: Wiley.

Boyd, J. N., & Zimbardo, P. G. (2005). Time perspective, health, and risk taking. In A. Strathman & J. Joireman (Eds.), *Understanding behavior in the context of time* (pp. 85–107). Mahwah: Erlbaum Publishers.

Buckner, R. L. (2010). The role of the hippocampus in prediction and imagination. *Annual Review of Psychology, 61*, 27–48.

Burgess, W. P., Dumontheil, I., & Gilbert, S. J. (2007). The gateway hypothesis of rostral prefrontal cortex (area 10) function. *Trends in Cognitive Sciences, 11*, 290–298.

Cabeza, R., & St Jacques, P. (2007). Functional neuroimaging of autobiographical memory. *Trends in Cognitive Sciences, 11*, 219–227.

Carelli, M. G., Wiberg, B., & Wiberg, M. (2011). Development and construct validation of the Swedish Zimbardo Time Perspective Inventory. *European Journal of Psychological Assessment, 27*(4), 220–227.

Carstensen, L. L., Isaacowitz, D. M., & Charles, S. T. (1999). Taking time seriously: A theory of socioemotional selectivity. *American Psychologist, 54*, 165–181.

Chen, C. Y., Muggleton, N. G., Tzeng, O. J., Hung, D. L., & Juan, C. H. (2009). Control of prepotent responses by superior medial frontal cortex. *NeuroImage, 15*(44), 537–545.

Christoff, K., Ream, J. M., & Gabrieli, J. D. (2004). Neural basis of spontaneous thought processes. *Cortex, 40*, 1–9.

De Carli, D., Garreffa, G., Colonnese, C., Giulietti, G., Labruna, L., Briselli, E., Ken, S., Macrì, M. A., & Maraviglia, B. (2007). Identification of activated regions during a language task. *Magnetic Resonance Imaging, 25*, 933–938.

Droit-Volet, S. (2013). Time perception in children: A neurodevelopmental approach. *Neuropsychologia, 51*, 220–234.
Fogassi, L., Ferrari, P. F., Gesierich, B., Rozzi, S., Chersi, F., & Rizzolatti, G. (2005). Parietal lobe: From action organization to intention understanding. *Science, 308*(5722), 662–667.
Fraisse, P. (1963). *The psychology of time*. New York: Harper & Row.
Francis-Smythe, J. A., & Robertson, I. T. (1999). On the relationship between time management and time estimation. *British Journal of Psychology, 90*, 333–347.
Goel, V., Gold, B., Kapur, S., & Houle, S. (1998). Neuroanatomical correlates of human reasoning. *Journal of Cognitive Neuroscience, 10*(3), 293–302.
Grondin, S. (2008). *Psychology of time* (p. 276). Bingley: Emerald.
Grondin, S. (2010). Timing and time perception: A review of recent behavioral and neuroscience findings and theoretical directions. *Attention, Perception, & Psychophysics, 72*(3), 561–582. doi:10.3758/APP.72.3.561.
Hassabis, D., Kumaran, D., Vann, S. D., & Maguire, E. A. (2007). Patients with hippocampal amnesia cannot imagine new experiences. *Proceedings of the National Academy of Sciences of the United States of America, 104*(5), 1726–1731.
Kosslyn, S. M. (1999). If neuroimaging is the answer, what is the question? *Philosophical Transactions of the Royal Society, 354*, 1283–1294.
Lewin, K. (1951). *Field theory in the social sciences: Selected theoretical papers*. New York: Harper.
Lewis, P. A., & Miall, R. C. (2003). Brain activation patterns during the measurement of sub- and supra-second intervals. *Neuropsychologia, 41*, 1583–1592.
Lewis, P. A., & Miall, R. C. (2006). Remembering the time: A continuous clock. *Trends in Cognitive Sciences, 10*, 401–406.
Logothetis, N. K. (2008). What we can do and what we cannot do with fMRI. *Nature, 453*(7197), 869–878.
Logothetis, N. K., Pauls, J., Augath, M., Trinath, T., & Oeltermann, A. (2001). Neurophysiological investigation of the basis of the fMRI signal. *Nature, 412*(6843), 150–157.
Mac Donald, A. W., Cohen, J. D., Stenger, V. A., Cameron, S., & Carter, C. S. (2000). Dissociating the role of the dorsolateral prefrontal and anterior cingulate cortex in cognitive control 2000. *Science, 288*(5472), 1835–1838.
McDermott, K. B., Petersen, S. E., Watson, J. M., & Ojemann, J. G. (2003). A procedure for identifying regions preferentially activated by attention to semantic and phonological relations using functional magnetic resonance imaging. *Neuropsychologia, 41*(3), 293–303.
Meck, W. H. (Ed.). (2005). Neuropsychology of timing and time perception [Special issue]. *Brain & Cognition, 58*(1). doi:10.1016/j.bandc.2004.09.004
Nyberg, L., Kimc, A., Habibd, R., Levinec, B., & Endel Tulving, E. (2010). Consciousness of subjective time in the brain. *Proceedings of the National Academy of Sciences of the United States of America, 107*(5), 22356–22359.
Okuda, J., Fujii, T., Ohtake, H., Tsukiura, T., Tanji, K., Suzuki, K., Kawashima, R., Fukuda, H., Itoh, M., & Yamadori, A. (2003). Thinking of the future and the past: The roles of the frontal pole and the medial temporal lobes. *NeuroImage, 19*(4), 1369–1380.
Okuda, J., Fujii, T., Ohtake, H., Tsukiura, T., Yamadori, A., Frith, C. D., Paul, W., & Burgess, P. W. (2007). Differential involvement of regions of rostral prefrontal cortex (Brodmann area 10) in time- and event-based prospective memory. *International Journal of Psychophysiology, 64*, 233–246.
Penney, T. B., & Vaitilingam, L. (2008). Imaging time. In S. Grondin (Ed.), *Psychology of time* (pp. 261–294). Bingley: Emerald Group.
Ridderinkhof, K. R., Ullsperger, M., Crone, E. A., & Nieuwenhuis, S. (2004). The role of the medial frontal cortex in cognitive control. *Science, 306*, 443–447.
Rubia, K. (2006). The neural correlates of timing functions. In J. Glicksohn & M. Myslobodsky (Eds.), *Timing the future: The case for time-based prospective memory* (pp. 213–238). London: World Scientific Publishing.

Senior, C., Russel, T., & Gazzaniga, M. S. (Eds.). (2006). *Methods in mind*. Cambridge, MA: MIT Press.

Squire, L. R., van der Horst, A. S., McDuff, S. G. R., Frascino, J. C., Hopkins, R. O., & Mauldin, K. N. (2010). Role of the hippocampus in remembering the past and imagining the future. *Proceedings of the National Academy of Sciences of the United States of America, 107*(44), 19044–19048.

Suddendorf, T., & Corballis, M. C. (1997). Mental time travel and the evolution of the human mind. *Genetic, Social, and General Psychology Monographs, 123*, 133–167.

Szpunar, K. K., Watson, J. M., & McDermott, K. B. (2007). Neural substrates of envisioning the future. *Proceedings of the National Academy of Sciences of the United States of America, 104*, 642–647.

Vuust, P., Roepstorff, A., Wallentin, M., Mouridsen, K., & Østergaard, L. (2006). It don't mean a thing… Keeping the rhythm during polyrhythmic tension, activates language areas (BA47). *NeuroImage, 31*(2), 832–841.

Wang, S.-H., & Morris, G. M. (2010). Hippocampal-neocortical interactions in memory formation, consolidation, and reconsolidation. *Annual Review of Psychology, 61*, 49–79.

Wheeler, M. A., Stuss, D. T., & Tulving, E. (1997). Toward a theory of episodic memory: The frontal lobes and autonoetic consciousness. *Psychological Bulletin, 121*, 331–354.

Wiberg, M., Sircova, A., Wiberg, B., & Carelli, M. G. (2012). Operationalizing balanced time perspective in a Swedish sample. *International Journal of Educational and Psychological Measurement, 12*, 95–107.

Wiener, M., Turkeltaub, P., & Coslette, H. B. (2010). The image of time: A voxel-wise meta-analysis. *NeuroImage, 49*, 1728–1740.

Zimbardo, P. G., & Boyd, J. N. (1999). Putting time in perspective: A valid, reliable individual-differences metric. *Journal of Personality and Social Psychology, 77*(6), 1271–1288.

Cognitive Processes in Time Perspective

Marcin Zajenkowski, Maria Grazia Carelli, and Maria Ledzińska

Introduction

Many research has been conducted to establish how personality and emotional factors affect our thinking. It was shown that psychological states, such as mood dimensions, may influence our cognition. For instance, the high level of energetic arousal (feelings of being activated and fully awaked versus fatigued) is beneficial for many tasks requiring attentional resources (e.g. Matthews et al. 2010; Zajenkowski 2013). On the other hand, personality traits often interact with the situational factors and by that affect cognitive performance. Researchers have revealed that extraverts act differently with respect to the demands of the situation, while neurotics are more sensitive to threatening stimuli (e.g. Matthews et al. 2009).

One of the factors that influences intellectual processes is subjective time perception. This chapter is mainly focused on time perspective (TP) understood in the way proposed in Zimbardo and Boyd's (1999, 2008) theory. Within time perspective paradigm, few studies concerned cognitive performance were conducted. For instance, interesting investigations were reported by Zimbardo and Maslach (1992). In two experiments, the authors found effects of biased time perspective on problem solving. College students who differed in dispositional time perspective, high future-oriented vs. high present-oriented, attempted to, solve complex mazes as quickly as possible. In the second study, comparable subjects tried to solve this cognitive task after half of a future-oriented group had been given a post-hypnotic suggestion to alter their time perspective to be in the 'expanded present'. In both

M. Zajenkowski (✉) • M. Ledzińska
Faculty of Psychology, University of Warsaw, Warsaw, Poland
e-mail: zajenkowski@psych.uw.edu.pl; marial@psych.uw.edu.pl

M.G. Carelli
Department of Psychology, Umeå University, SE-901 87 Umeå, Sweden
e-mail: grazia.carelli@psy.umu.se

M. Stolarski et al. (eds.), *Time Perspective Theory; Review, Research and Application: Essays in Honor of Philip G. Zimbardo*, DOI 10.1007/978-3-319-07368-2_16,

studies, statistically significant effects emerged: problem solving was adversely affected by present time perspective, whether natural or manipulated.

Although the TP effects on cognition were obtained in some previous investigations, this issue still requires further studies. Here we present our own data concerning time perspective and intellectual functioning. First, we show how the subjective perception of time is related to the most general ability – intelligence. Extending these findings, the second section of the chapters focuses on a central assumption of the framework by Zimbardo and colleagues, namely, that individual differences in time perspective may have clear implications for goal-directed behavior in general, and risk taking in particular. Finally, we describe the associations between metacognitive abilities and various time perspective.

Time Perspective and Intelligence

Studies devoted to subjective time shows that Zimbardo and Boyd's (1999) dimensions of time perspective are associated with various psychological variables. For instance, Past Positive and Future tend to positively correlate with subjective well-being (Zhang and Howell 2011; Zhang et al. 2013b), emotional intelligence (Stolarski et al. 2011), delayed award (Stolarski et al. 2011; Zimbardo and Boyd 2008), while Past Negative and Present Fatalism are rather negatively related to these factors. Broadly speaking, one can conclude from these findings that an individual's time perspective may be classified as more or less adaptive.

One of the most important factors determining human adaptive behavior is intelligence. It was shown that this variable is associated with many life outcomes, such as earning, educational achievements, even longevity and health (Gottfredson 1997). It is also correlated with personality traits: positively with extraversion, openness to experience, and negatively with neuroticism (cf. Ackerman and Heggestad 1997). Austin et al. (2002) noticed that personality correlates of intelligence could be divided into two groups. The first group is positively linked with abilities and consists of traits which could be described as adaptive, whilst the traits classifiable as maladaptive are usually negatively correlated with intelligence. Taking this classification into account together with the claim that higher intelligence helps people to deal with the demands of the environment (Gottfredson 1997), it is possible that more intelligent individuals developed more adaptive profile of their TP.

Zajenkowski and Stolarski (in preparation) decided to examine the above assumption. We tested a total of 249 subjects (140 female and 109 male), undergraduate students from the University of Warsaw. Participants were given two tests. First, they were asked to fill a short measure of the Zimbardo Time Perspective Inventory (Zhang et al. 2013a). It consists of 15 items and has five scales measuring the following time perspectives: Past Negative, Past Positive, Present Fatalistic, Present Hedonistic and Future. After that, subjects solved Raven's Advanced Progressive Matrices (APM), the paper-and-pencil test of fluid intelligence (Raven et al. 1983).

Table 1 Correlations between APM and five time perspectives

	Past negative	Past positive	Present fatalistic	Present hedonistic	Future
APM	**0.056**	**−0.059**	**−0.270****	**−0.102**	**0.127***
Past Negative		−0.090	0.191**	−0.035	−0.200**
Past Positive			0.222**	0.193**	0.133*
Present Fatalistic				0.068	−0.163**
Present Hedonistic					−0.082

Note: *APM* advanced progressive matrices
*$p<0.05$; **$p<0.01$

Table 2 Regression analysis with five time perspectives

	β	*t*	*p*	Regression parameters
Past Negative	0.125	1.973	=0.050	R=0.32; adjusted $R^2=0.09$
Past Positive	0.014	0.214	=0.831	$F(5, 243)=5.38$; $p<0.001$
Present Fatalistic	−0.274	−4.229	<0.001	
Present Hedonistic	−0.073	−1.169	=0.244	
Future	0.098	1.535	=0.126	

Table 1 presents simple correlation coefficients between all variables used in the study. APM score tended to be quite highly and negatively associated with Present Fatalistic scale, while with Future TP it was positively correlated, however the latter relationship was marginal. Moreover, time perspectives were intercorrelated such as it was in the previous investigations (Zimbardo and Boyd 1999, 2008).

Further, we tried to examine how strongly are time perspectives related to intelligence when taken jointly in one regression model. Table 2 presents the results of this analysis. The model was significant and accounted for about 10 % of the variance.

The strongest predictor of intelligence was Present Fatalistic TP. When time perspectives were taken jointly, the Future scale was no longer related to intelligence. The latter result was rather surprising, however, one should keep in mind, that Past Negative orientation was positively correlated with Present Fatalistic perspective (see Table 1) – the strongest predictor of intelligence. It seems then, that Present Fatalistic is most strongly tied up with general ability.

The analyses revealed that Present Fatalistic dimension is in a strong relationship with intelligence. This association is also negative, and it could be explained in two ways. First, it is necessary to recall the definition of the discussed disposition. According to Zimbardo and Boyd (1999) it "reveals a belief that the future is predestined and uninfluenced by individual action, whereas the present must be borne with resignation because humans are at the whimsical mercy of 'fate'" (Zimbardo and Boyd 1999, p. 1278). If time perspectives are general dispositions (Zimbardo and Boyd 2008), then we may expect that they refer to wide spectrum of behaviors, including cognitive processes. The belief that we can't influence our abilities, associated with Present Fatalistic dimension, is conceptually close to the construct of implicit theory of intelligence (Dweck 1999; Hong et al. 1995). Dweck (1999) distinguished between the belief that human attributes are fixed or malleable. Individual's implicit theory about human attributes structure the way he or she understands and reacts to human actions and outcomes. Empirical studies have shown that implicit theories about intelligence are associated with adaptive or maladaptive cognitive performance, affect, and behavior in difficult achievement situations (Dweck 1999). The belief that intelligence is a fixed trait is associated with helpless reactions to achievement setbacks, whereas the belief that intelligence is malleable is connected with mastering behavior in the face of difficulties. Dweck (1999) argues that the previous option entails the tendency to seek the reasons for achievement setbacks in one's own ability, while people taking the latter perspective tend to see those reasons in a lack of effort or adequate strategy. We may wonder, whether subjects with high Present Fatalistic time perspective believe also that their intellectual abilities are fixed, and because of that they give up when encounter difficulties. In the present study, an advanced version of intelligence test was used, so it is possible that these individuals didn't put much effort to challenge with hard task, thinking that they are not able to manage. The above considerations are rather speculative in nature and require empirical verification.

Second explanation of the obtained results refers to the negative emotionality. Present fatalistic perspective is associated with low extraversion and high neuroticism (Zhang and Howell 2011). The previous is defined in terms of positive emotionality, while the latter is regarded as a tendency to experience negative affective states (Eysenck 1967; Zajenkowski et al. 2012). Moreover, people with high Present Fatalistic dimension tend to experience high negative affect and low positive affect (Zhang and Howell 2011). This combination of psychological states have usually negative influence on cognitive performance (Mitchell and Phillips 2007). It is worth mentioning that in the metaanalysis of the personality-intelligence relations, extraversion was in a positive, while neuroticism was in a negative relationship with abilities (Ackerman and Heggestad 1997). It was assumed that high intelligence helps people to efficiently regulate their emotions (Ackerman and Heggestad 1997).

As regards positive link between future perspective and intelligence, the control function seem to be the most probable explanatory mechanism. Subjects with high Future scale are described as better in self-control (Zimbardo and Boyd 1999). On the other hand, intelligence is strongly related to executive functions, such as control attention or prepotent response inhibition (Conway et al. 2003). It is possible then, that some aspect of general control may underlie the intelligence-future orientation relation. However, as our data suggest, it is not clear whether Future time perspective is correlated with intelligence because it shares some aspects with Present fatalistic disposition. Therefore, further studies should examine the unique contribution of the Future scale to intelligence.

Time Perspective, Goal-Directed Behaviour and Executive Control Functions

A central prediction of the framework by Zimbardo and colleagues is that biases in time perspective are assumed to have selective effects on goal-directed behavior. As the relevant past research suggests, including the studies summarized above, individual differences in time perspective may have clear implications for goal-directed behavior in general, and risk taking in particular. However, virtually, no studies have provided direct support for the hypothesis that individual differences in time perspective are systematically related to risk taking. Zimbardo et al. (1997) reported indirect support by testing the hypothesis that time perspective is a significant predictor of risky driving (see also Keough, Zimbardo and Boyd 1999; and related references on cancer screening, drug abuse etc. here). Specifically, they predicted that more present-oriented individuals would self-report more risky driving and those who were more future-oriented was expected to report less risk taking. This hypothesis was based on the notion that "Individuals that score higher on the present subscale of the ZTPI should report more risky driving, because their behavior is less under the control of past experience, or potential future consequences, they will be responsive to vivid factors in the present behaviors space, such as the excitement of speeding, the demonstration of skill and independence, and the admiration from peers" (Zimbardo et al. 1997, p. 1008).

Zimbardo et al. (1997) tested this hypothesis by involving six separate samples of college students who completed the ZTPI and a questionnaire related to health risks. Specifically, they used five questions related to risk taking in (a) driving, car racing, and speeding, (b) biking, and (c) driving under the influence of alcohol. Participants responded how frequently they engaged in each of the behaviors by using a 5-point scale, and a standardized average of these ratings was used as a compound measure of "risky driving."

Zimbardo et al. (1997) found that participants who were more present-oriented reported more risky driving behaviors in that the pooled correlation between risky driving and the present subscale was highly significant ($r=0.29$, $p<.01$). However, the expected negative correlation between future-oriented time perspective and frequency of risky driving was low ($r=-.08$), but significant ($p<.01$, $N=1{,}662$). Zimbardo et al. (1997) concluded that "future time perspective is not as important as a predictor variable in risky driving as is present time perspective" (p. 1010). They also suggested that Future and Present time perspectives independent predictors of risky driving in that both partial correlations and multiple regression analysis indicated that present time perspective was a better predictor of risky driving than was Future time perspective.

These findings support the hypothesis that time perspective is systematically related to risk taking (see also Keough et al. 1999). However, it should be noted that their findings were based on subjective assessment of risky driving, rather than actual risk-taking behavior. In other words, individuals with past temporal orientation may consider themselves as less risk aversive than future-oriented individuals, but these metacognitive judgments do not necessarily translate to actual risk behavior.

To extend past work, Carelli (2012) examined the relationship between time perspective and actual risk taking behavior in adolescents and young adults. Following the study of Zimbardo et al. (1997), the primary hypothesis of the study was that future orientation would be related to risk taking. Although the Future scale was only weakly related to self-reported risky driving in Zimbardo et al. (1997), a number of studies suggest a close link between Future TP and measures of risk-related behavior, including sensation seeking and impulse control (see Boyd and Zimbardo 2005, for overviews). Furthermore, considering the findings of Carelli et al. (2011), we expected that the Future Positive and Future Negative scales of the Swedish version of the ZTPI (referred to as S-ZTPI) would have selective effects on risk taking. Carelli (2012) believed that one reason for the pattern of results reported by Zimbardo et al. (1997) is that the Future scale of the original ZTPI includes both Future negative and Future Positive items. It is reasonable to assume that these two individuals with Future Positive orientation are more risk aversive than individuals with a more negative view of the future.

To test these hypotheses, adolescents and young adults completed the Swedish version of the ZTPI (S-ZTPI) and a risk-taking task, developed and validated by Figner et al. (2009; see also Weber and Johnson 2009). In this Columbia Card Task (CCT), participants turn over a series of gain and loss cards. Each gain increases the total payoff while the risk of losing increases as more cards are turned over. The hot version of the CCT is a form a dynamic risk taking task, which is assumed to trigger affective decision processes by gradually increasing the risk of losing when additional cards are turned over and feedback of the outcome is given instantly. The cold version of the task is assumed trigger more deliberative decision processes. As the primary focus of the study was on affective decision processes, only the hot version of the CCT was used.

A related aim of the study was to examine individual differences in time orientation in relation to executive control functions. As most executive control functions are future-oriented in that they refer to planning, coordination and updating of goal-directed activities, it is reasonable to assume that individuals with well-developed frontal/executive functions are more future-oriented (and risk aversive) than individual with less efficient control functions. To test this hypothesis, developmental changes in two measures of executive functioning (n-back and connections, which are two commonly used tasks of working memory(WM) updating) were related to each participant's profile of time perspective, as measured by the S-ZTPI. Specifically, participants of the study were adolescents between 14 and 18 years of age and young adult (university students) between 19 and 29 years of age. The former individuals participated in a longitudinal study on memory development, in which they completed two test sessions: First time, when they were between 8 and 12 years (T1) and 4 years later when they were between 12 and 16(T2; see Forman et al. 2011, for details). The present study was completed about 2 years after T2, and the T1 and T2 measures of executive functioning were used as predictors of time perspective

(2 and 6 years later). Following the reasoning outlined above, it was hypothesized that participants with good performance in the executive functioning tasks would be more future-oriented than participants with less efficient control functions.

The findings of the study were consistent with these hypotheses in that risk taking, measured in terms of CCT scores, was selectively related to temporal orientation with a negative correlation between CCT and Future Positive scale ($r = -.34$, $p < .05$). This result suggests that future-oriented were more risk aversive than participants with a less future-oriented time perspective. The correlations with the remaining S-ZTPI scores, including those of the Future Negative and Present Fatalistic scales, were not significant. It should also be noted that this pattern of results was observed both in adolescents and young adults. This is consistent with earlier work on temporal orientation and sensation seeking (e.g., Lennings et al. 1998).

The second main finding of the study was that working memory development was a strong predictor of temporal orientation. Children who had efficient updating functions, as measured by the n-back and matrix monitoring tasks, showed high scores on the Future Positive scale of the S-ZTPI. Specifically, the correlation was highly significant with at T2 ($r = -.48$, $p < .01$), suggesting that children with low performance in the two updating tasks during the second session (2 years earlier) turned more cards in the CCT task than children with more efficient WM functions. A similar association was observed for the T1 data ($r = -.34$, $p < .08$). Although this correlation was not significant (possibly due to the sample size), it suggests that WM performance in early school-age predicts temporal orientation more than 6 years later in adolescence.

One reasonable interpretation of these findings is that executive/working memory functions are intimately related to planning and future-oriented cognitive activities, and that children with efficient updating functions can maintain and complete more complex goal-directed plans than children with less efficient cognitive control functions. It is also reasonable to assume that individual and developmental differences in working memory functions mediate scholastic achievement, and that children's success and failure in these and related activities also affect their attitudes and beliefs about the future. However, it should be emphasized that this interpretation reflects an association between working memory development and temporal orientation, rather than a causal relation. Although it is reasonable to argue that working memory and related higher cognitive functions have causal effects on temporal biases, a possibility also exists that differences in time perspective affect individual and developmental differences in higher cognitive functions (e. g., that future-oriented children plan and think ahead more than less future-oriented children and these differences also stimulate and train working memory and related executive functions).

Taken together, these findings suggest that systematic differences in adolescents' time perspective predict their actual behavior in a dynamic risk-taking task. The present findings also suggest a close link between the personality-oriented construct of temporal perspective and higher cognitive functions, including working memory updating and response inhibition.

Time Perspective and Meta-cognition

The term meta-cognition is used to denote "cognition of cognition" (Flavell 1979). It is very complex construct with many facets making difficult the distinction between monitoring and control and the sitting of the line between manifestations of the monitoring function, namely meta-cognitive knowledge and experience (Mitchell and Johnson 2000). Generally, meta-cognition is a model of cognition, which acts at meta-level and its related to the object – world through the monitoring and control functions (Efklides 2006). The three facets of meta-cognition are following: knowledge, skills, and experiences.

Meta-cognitive knowledge is declarative knowledge about cognition, which we derive from long-term memory. The importance of meta-cognitive knowledge (task, strategies, goals) is that it provides a framework of understanding one's as well as the other's cognition and this guides the interpretation of situational data so that proper control decision are made.

Meta-cognitive skills – or use of strategies – is procedural knowledge. They are manifestations of the control function. The important problem for the application of meta-cognitive skills is how does the subject know when he/she needs to apply skills. Meta-cognitive experiences (feelings, judgments) are products of the monitoring of good functioning and inform the person about a feature of cognitive processing.

According to some researchers, our perception of time is important factor determining controlling and planning our actions in time (Kozhevnikov 2007). Thus it is possible that time orientation influences our meta-cognition. Therefore, it seems reasonable to ask what are the relationships between Zimbardo's construct and various meta-cognitive aspects. In a recent project, Ledzińska (in preparation) tried to answer this question. At the beginning, the author took into account two widely known concepts from the meta-cognition area. First one described meta-cognitive skills within Cantwell's theory emphasizing the self-control and self-regulation dimension of learning (Cantwell 1998; Czerniawska and Cantwell 2003). It distinguishes two types of strategic control of learning: adaptive control and non-adaptive control. What differentiates them is the ability (or the lack of it) of adapting the utilized memory strategies to the situational context which is comprised of, among others, the type of information being received and the goal and intention of learning. Non-adaptive control assumes two forms: irresolute and flexible behavior.

The second concept used in Ledzinska's studies was meta-cognitive knowledge. In particular, the author considered Wells (1995; Wells and Matthews 1994) theory. In this paradigm, one may distinguish five aspects: (1) cognitive confidence – confidence regarding one's attention and memory (2) positive beliefs about worrying, (3) cognitive self-consciousness – a tendency to concentrate on actual stream of thoughts, (4) negative beliefs about thoughts that are uncontrollable and danger, (5) need for control – individual's tendency to control own thoughts.

Table 3 Correlations between SFQ, MCQ and ZTPI scales

Scales	Past Negative	Past Positive	Present Hedonistic	Present Fatalistic	Future
Adaptative control (SFQ)	0.01	0.17	0.04	0.22	0.40**
Inflexible control (SFQ)	0.21*	0.15	0.38**	−0.16	0.24*
Irresolute control (SFQ)	0.17	0.03	0.34**	0.04	−0.09
Positive beliefs (MCQ)	0.18	0.08	0.27*	0.05	0.19
Negative beliefs (MCQ)	0.38**	0.06	0.15	0.04	0.01
Cognitive confidence (MCQ)	0.17	−0.75	0.19	−0.12	0.13
Need for control (MCQ)	0.13	−0.05	0.09	0.06	0.16
Self- consciousness (MCQ)	0.23*	0.09	0.11	0.14	0.07

*$p<0.05$, **$p<0.01$

In the empirical evaluation of the project, 100 young adults (50 female and 50 male) took part. Three measures were used: a short version of Zimbardo Time Perspective Inventory, Strategic Flexibility Questionnaire (SFQ) in the Polish adaptation (Czerniawska and Cantwell 2003) – gives an image of strategic control of learning in Cantwell's framework, and Metacognitions Questionnaire (MCQ) (Wells et al. 2004) in the Polish adaptation (see Dragan and Dragan 2011; Dragan et al. 2011). The results of the study are presented in Table 3.

Three time perspectives tended to correlate with meta-cognitive skills and knowledge. The future orientation was positively associated with adaptive and inflexible control from Cantwell questionnaire. It is in line with previous investigation suggesting more adaptive behavior of people taking Future time perspective but that also may be less flexible in their plans (Zimbardo and Boyd 2008). Present hedonistic scale correlated positively with inflexible and at the same time with irresolute control, which is in agreement with the definition of this TP dimension (Zimbardo and Boyd 2008). Finally, negative evaluation of past time was related to maladaptive meta-cognition with respect to negative beliefs about thoughts that are uncontrollable and danger as well as self-consciousness, which means dysfunctional concentration on actual stream of thoughts.

Further, Ledzińska tried to determine the relationship between time perspective and a form of meta-cognitive experience. In particular, she was interested how the experience of information stress is associated with preferred time perspective. The former construct was described by Ledzińska (2007; Mongay and Ledzińska 2011). The notion of information stress arose due to cultural and civilization changes and is connected to the new phenomenon of global communication (Stiglitz 2004). Informational stress is a form of psychological stress in which the stressor is an excess of information (Ledzińska 2001). It occurs when an individual experiences a surge of information, that is, when the amount of available signals in the environment exceeds the capabilities of reception an processing. We are dealing with a great intensification in the contemporary world of the said phenomenon which is also referred to as overload or cognitive overload syndrome. This is caused by intense technical development the results of which is an unprecedented progress in the realm of communication (Rheinghold 1985). The global flow of a colossal amount of information can cause a feeling of disorientation, chaos, helplessness in cognitively immature persons (Bertman 1998). They may not be able to cope with the selection, ordering, integrating of massive portions of data received each day. On the side, we notice an increase of data flow (surge, flood), on the other, a person's limited capacity of receiving and processing the data. It is no wonder then, that many people are experiencing information stress, particularly those that are studying and working.

In this study, the same group of subjects took part as in previous one. They were administered with Zimbardo Time Perspective Inventory and The Intensity of Information Stress Questionnaire by Ledzińska. The latter is a diagnostic instrument of subjective experiences connected with life in conditions of excess information and quick pace of transfer. Ledzinska found, that Past Negative and Present Fatalistic TPs are positively correlated with the total score of information stress, while Past Positive is negatively related to information stress.

The results suggested, that the Past Negative and Present Fatalistic orientations intensify the experience of information overflow. Perhaps, people with high level of Present Fatalistic time perspective tend to often experience stress and negative affect and which results in their poorer intellectual performance, e.g. in intelligence test as was presented in this chapter above.

Future perspective is usually regarded as more adaptive (Zimbardo and Boyd 2008), and in our study it was not adversely correlated with information stress scales as one may expect from previous investigations (de Bilde et al. 2011). Interestingly, Past Positive orientation helps people to deal with information stress, at least as it comes to information output. It seems that time interpretation in terms of affect – either positive or negative – is related with meta-cognitive experiences.

Conclusions

We examined the cognitive processes in time perspective. First, we found that Present Fatalistic TP is negatively related to intelligence, and that future-oriented individuals tend to have higher general abilities. Further, we showed that that risk taking was selectively related to temporal orientation. Specifically, risk-taking as measured by the CCT task, was negatively correlated with the Future Positive scale of the S-ZTPI. Another finding discussed here was that working memory development was a strong predictor of temporal orientation. Children who had efficient working memory updating functions in early school age showed high scores on the Future Positive scale of the S-ZTPI when they were adolescents. Finally, time perspectives tended to correlate with meta-cognitive skills, knowledge and experiences, suggesting that time perspective may be regarded as a form (or, a consequence) of meta-cognitive processes.

References

Ackerman, P., & Heggestad, E. (1997). Intelligence, personality, and interests: Evidence for overlapping traits. *Psychological Bulletin, 121*, 219–245.

Austin, E. J., Deary, I. J., Whiteman, M. C., Fowkes, F. G. R., Pedersen, N., Rabitt, P., Bent, N., & McInnes, L. (2002). Relationships between ability and personality: Does intelligence contribute positively to personal and social adjustment? *Personality and Individual Differences, 32*, 1391–1411.

Bertman, S. (1998). *Hyperculture. The human cost of speed.* London: Praeger.

Boyd, J. N., & Zimbardo, P. G. (2005). Time perspective, health and risk taking. In A. Strathman & J. Joireman (Eds.), *Understanding behavior in the context of time.* Mahwah: Lawrence Erlbaum Associates Publishers.

Cantwell, R. H. (1998). The development of beliefs about learning from mid- to late- adolescence. *Educational Psychology, 18*, 27–39.

Carelli, M. G. (2012). *Time perspective on adolescent risk taking and working memory development.* Manuscript submitted for publication.

Carelli, M. G., Wiberg, B., & Wiberg, M. (2011). Development and construct validation of the Swedish Zimbardo Time Perspective Inventory (S-ZTPI). *European Journal of Psychological Assessment, 27*, 220–227.

Conway, A. R., Kane, M. J., & Engle, R. W. (2003). Working memory capacity and its relation to general intelligence. *Trends in Cognitive Sciences, 7*, 547–552.

Czerniawska, E., & Cantwell, R. H. (2003). Strategic control of learning: A polish replication of the Strategic Flexibility Questionnaire, *Kwartalnik Pedagogiczny* [Education Quarterly], *1–2*, 161–175.

de Bilde, J., Vansteenkiste, M., & Lens, W. (2011). Understanding the association between future time perspective and self-regulated learning through the lens of self-determination theory. *Learning and Instruction, 21*(3), 332–344.

Dragan, M., & Dragan, W. Ł. (2011). Właściwości psychometryczne polskiej wersji The Metacognitions Questionnaire – 30 [Psychometric properties of the Polish version of The Metacognitions Questionnaire – 30]. *Psychiatria Polska* [Polish Psychiatry], *4*, 545–553.

Dragan, M., Dragan, W. Ł., Kononowicz, T., & Wells, A. (2011). On the relationship between temperament, metacognition and anxiety: Independent and mediated effects. *Anxiety, Stress and Coping, 25*, 1–13.

Dweck, C. S. (1999). *Self-theories: Their role in motivation, personality, and development.* Philadelphia: Psychology Press.

Efklides, A. (2006). Metacognition and affect: What can metacognitive experiences tell us about the learning process? *Educational Research Review, 1*, 3–14.

Eysenck, H. J. (1967). *The biological basis of personality.* Thomas: Springfield.

Figner, B., Weber, E. U., Mackinlay, R. J., & Wilkening, F. (2009). Affective and deliberative processes in risky choice: Age differences in risk taking in the Columbia Card Task. *Journal of Experimental Psychology Learning Memory and Cognition, 35*, 709–730.

Flavell, J. H. (1979). Metacognition and cognitive monitoring: A new era of cognitive inquiry. *American Psychologist, 34*, 906–911.

Forman, H., Mäntylä, T., & Carelli, M. G. (2011). Time keeping and working memory development in early adolescence: A 4-year follow-up. *Journal of Experimental Child Psychology, 108*, 170–179.

Gottfredson, L. S. (1997). Why g matters: The complexity of everyday life. *Intelligence, 24*, 79–132.

Hong, Y., Chiu, C., & Dweck, C. S. (1995). Implicit theories of intelligence: Reconsidering the role of confidence in achievement motivation. In M. H. Kernis (Ed.), *Efficacy, agency, and self-esteem* (pp. 197–216). New York: Plenum Press.

Keough, K. A., Zimbardo, P. G., & Boyd, J. N. (1999). Who's smoking, drinking, and using drugs? Time perspective as a predictor of substance use. *Basic and Applied Social Psychology, 21*, 149–164.

Kozhevnikov, M. (2007). Cognitive styles in the context of modern psychology: Toward an integrated framework of cognitive style. *Psychological Bulletin, 133*, 464–481.

Ledzińska, M. (2001). Człowiek współczesny wobec nadprodukcji informacji, czyli o informacyjnym stresie [A contemporary person in an overproduction of information, i.e. information stress]. In W. Ciarkowska, & A. Matczak (Eds.), *Różnice indywidualne: wybrane badania inspirowane Regulacyjną Teorią Temperamentu Profesora Jana Strelaua* [Individual differences: Selected tests inspired by Professor Jan Strelau's Regulatory Theory of Temperament]. Warsaw: Interdyscyplinarne Centrum Genetyki Zachowania Uniwersytetu Warszawskiego.

Ledzińska, M. (2007). *The role of the individual's intelligence in the area information overflow.* Poster presented on the 12th Biennial conference European Association for Research on Learning and Instruction, 28 August – 1 September, 2007, Budapest, Hungary.

Ledzińska, M. (in preparation). *Time perspective and meta-cognition.*

Lennings, C. J., Burns, A. M., & Cooney, G. (1998). Profiles of time perspective and personality: Developmental considerations. *The Journal of Psychology Interdisciplinary and Applied, 132*, 629–641.

Matthews, G., Deary, I., & Whiteman, A. (2009). *Personality traits.* Cambridge: Cambridge University Press.

Matthews, G., Warm, J. S., Reinerman, L. E., Langheim, L. K., & Saxby, D. J. (2010). Task engagement, attention and executive control. In A. Gruszka, G. Matthews, & B. Szymura (Eds.), *Handbook of individual differences in cognition: Attention, memory and executive control* (pp. 205–230). New York: Springer.

Mitchell, K., & Johnson, M. K. (2000). Source monitoring: Attributing mental experience. In F. I. M. Craik (Ed.), *The oxford handbook of memory* (pp. 179–195). Oxford: Oxford University Press.

Mitchell, R. L. C., & Phillips, L. H. (2007). The psychological, neurochemical and functional neuroanatomical mediators of the effects of positive and negative mood on executive functions. *Neuropsychologia, 45*, 617–629.

Mongay, J., & Ledzińska, M. (2011). On reducing the detrimental information flood in the use internet. In W. W. Lamanauskas (Ed.), *Problems of psychology in the 21st century* (pp. 84–95). Siauliai: Scientia Educologica.

Raven, J. C., Court, J. H., & Raven, J. (1983). *Manual for Raven's progressive matrices and vocabulary scales. Section 4: Advanced Progressive Matrices.* London: H. K. Lewis.

Rheinghold, H. (1985). *Tool for thought: The people and ideas behind the next computer revolution.* New York: Simon & Schuster.

Stiglitz, E. (2004). *Globalizacja* [Globalization]. Warszawa: Wydawnictwo Naukowe PWN.

Stolarski, M., Bitner, J., & Zimbardo, P. G. (2011). Time perspective, emotional intelligence and discounting of delayed awards. *Time and Society, 20*, 346–363.

Weber, E. U., & Johnson, E. J. (2009). Mindful judgment and decision making. *Annual Review of Psychology, 60*, 53–85.

Wells, A. (1995). Metacognition and worry: A cognitive model of generalised anxiety disorder. *Behavioural and Cognitive Psychotherapy, 23*, 301–320.

Wells, A., & Cartwright-Hatton, S. (2004). A short form of the meta-cognitions questionnaire: Properties of the MCQ 30. *Behaviour Research and Therapy, 42*, 385–396.

Wells, A., & Matthews, G. (1994). *Attention and emotion: A clinical perspective.* Hove: Lawrence Erlbaum Associates.

Zajenkowski, M. (2013). Energetic arousal and language: Predictions from the computational theory of quantifiers processing. *Human Factors, 55*, 924–934.

Zhang, J. W., & Howell, R. T. (2011). Do time perspectives predict unique variance in life satisfaction beyond personality traits? *Personality and Individual Differences, 50*(8), 1261–1266.

Zajenkowski, M., & Stolarski, M. (in preparation). *Intelligence and time perspective.*

Zajenkowski, M., Goryńska, E., & Winiewski, M. (2012). Variability of the relationship between personality and mood. *Personality and Individual Differences, 52*, 858–861.
Zhang, J. W., Howell, R. T., & Bowerman, T. (2013a). Validating a brief measure of the Zimbardo Time Perspective Inventory. *Time and Society, 22*, 391–409.
Zhang, J. W., Howell, R. T., & Stolarski, M. (2013b). Comparing three methods to measure a balanced time perspective: The relationship between a balanced time perspective and subjective well-being. *Journal of Happiness Studies, 14*, 169–184.
Zimbardo, P. G., & Boyd, J. N. (1999). Putting time in perspective: A valid, reliable individual-differences metric. *Journal of Personality and Social Psychology, 77*, 1271–1288.
Zimbardo, P. G., & Boyd, J. N. (2008). *The time paradox*. New York: Free Press.
Zimbardo, P. G., & Maslach, C. (1992). Cognitive effects of biased time perspective. *International Journal of Psychology, 27*, 167.
Zimbardo, P. G., Keough, K. A., & Boyd, J. N. (1997). Present time perspective as a predictor of risky driving. *Personality and Individual Differences, 23*, 1007–1023.

Differences in Time Perspective Predict Differences in Future Simulations

Kathleen M. Arnold and Karl K. Szpunar

As outlined in various chapters of this volume, Future time perspective, or the degree to which one approaches life events with the future in mind, represents a highly adaptive individual difference characteristic. For instance, people who allow potential future implications to influence their decisions and behavior tend to be better off in terms of numerous variables related to personal health and adjustment (Henson et al. 2006). Nonetheless, relatively little remains known about how, in terms of cognitive mechanisms (see chapter "Cognitive Processes in Time Perspective" by Zajenkowski et al., this volume), future orientation gives rise to such personal and interpersonal benefits. In this chapter, we consider the possible relation between Future time perspective and episodic future thinking, the capacity to simulate events that may one day come to pass in the personal future (Atance and O'Neill 2001; Szpunar 2010). First, we present a brief overview of episodic future thinking and its relation to various other forms of future thinking. Second, we review the central defining feature of episodic future thinking, namely, autonoetic consciousness – the sense of pre-experiencing that accompanies mental simulations of the future (Tulving 1985). In doing so, we highlight the close relation of episodic future thinking to episodic memory, the capacity to remember or re-experience personal memories (Szpunar and Tulving 2009; Tulving 1983, 2002, 2005). Third, we focus on recent research demonstrating a close relation between Future time perspective and episodic future thinking, particularly in the context of autonoetic consciousness. Finally, we discuss the possible implications of elucidating the relation

K.M. Arnold (✉)
Department of Psychology and Neuroscience, Duke University,
Durham, NC, USA
e-mail: kathleen.arnold@duke.edu

K.K. Szpunar
Department of Psychology and Center for Brain Science, Harvard University,
Cambridge, MA, USA
e-mail: szpunar@wjh.harvard.edu

M. Stolarski et al. (eds.), *Time Perspective Theory; Review, Research and Application: Essays in Honor of Philip G. Zimbardo*, DOI 10.1007/978-3-319-07368-2_17,

of Future time perspective to autonoetic consciousness and related cognitive variables.

Episodic Future Thinking and Other Future-Oriented Cognitions

Episodic future thinking represents a highly *specific* and *flexible* future-oriented cognition. Episodic future thinking is *specific* in that it involves thinking about specific experiences that might one day come to pass in the future (Szpunar 2010). For instance, whenever someone imagines how their significant other will react to a gift they plan to give at dinner, how their business meeting will go tomorrow, or how much they will enjoy going to a baseball game with their best friend next week, they are engaging in episodic future thinking. This is to be distinguished from more general thoughts about the future that are not necessarily tied to specific events, such as worrying about how the bills will be paid next month, next summer's vacation, or retirement (Atance and O'Neill 2001; Klein et al. 2002). Of course, thoughts about more general events, such as next summer's vacation, may give rise to more specific simulations (e.g., relaxing on the beach), but they are not required.

By the same token, it is important to distinguish episodic future thinking from other distinct, but related, forms of future-oriented cognition. Here, we will focus specifically on prospective memory and planning. Prospective memory represents the capacity to remember to carry out intentions at some point in the future (Kliegel et al. 2008). For instance, people exercise their capacity of prospective memory whenever they remember to take food out of the oven after a certain amount of time has passed or to give a message to a coworker next time they run into that person. Importantly, there exist various forms of prospective memory; the two most widely studied being time- and event-based prospective memory. Time-based prospective memory involves remembering to do something at a specific time (e.g., taking food out of the oven), whereas event-based prospective memory involves remembering to do something when another event takes place (e.g., running into a coworker). With regard to the relation of episodic future thinking to prospective memory, episodic future thinking involves simulating a specific future occurrence, whereas prospective memory involves remembering to carry out an intention. Importantly, the generation of an intention (e.g., I need to pick up bread on the way home) does not necessitate the engagement of episodic future thinking (e.g., imagining the drive home and stopping into the local grocery store). Nonetheless, there is some evidence suggesting that engaging in episodic future thinking can increase the likelihood that prospective intentions will be carried out (e.g., Brewer and Marsh 2010; but see McDaniel et al. 2008). As was the case with the distinction between specific episodic future thoughts and more general thoughts about the future, episodic future thinking can be co-opted in the service of generating future intentions, but the two processes are distinct from one another (Szpunar and Tulving 2011).

Along these lines, it is also important to distinguish episodic future thinking from the concept of planning. Planning represents a multifaceted cognitive process that can involve various levels of abstraction (Hayes-Roth and Hayes-Roth 1979). For instance, when planning a summer vacation, one must consider general features such as where and when they will be going and more specific features such as weather forecasts and appropriate attire. Interestingly, as was the case with prospective memory, the more complex process of planning may also co-opt episodic future thinking in the service of devising better plans (Burgess et al. 2005; Szpunar and Tulving 2011). For instance, one might imagine what they would feel like bringing one outfit over another in order to make a more informed decision about their vacation wardrobe. Nonetheless, episodic future thinking and planning represent distinct cognitive processes.

In sum, episodic future thinking represents a cognitive process that is distinct from other forms of future-oriented cognition and one that can be used in various ways to improve future outcomes (e.g., realizing future intentions, making sounder plans). In the next section, we focus our attention on what is specifically known about episodic future thinking and why, perhaps paradoxically, it is more difficult to distinguish episodic future thinking from memory.

Episodic Future Thinking and Memory

Future event simulation has long been the focus of intense psychological inquiry within the fields of social (Wilson and Gilbert 2005) and clinical (Holmes and Mathews 2010) psychology. More recently, however, cognitive psychologists have begun to examine how this mental feat is accomplished. That is, how does our brain/mind construct simulations of the personal future?

The impetus for understanding the cognitive processes that give rise to episodic future thinking can be traced back to an early study by Tulving (1985) who observed an interesting dissociation between episodic and semantic memory in an amnesic patient, K.C., who had sustained a diffuse pattern of brain damage following a motorcycle accident. Specifically, although patient K.C. retained considerable knowledge about his past (e.g., knowing where his family typically vacationed in the summer; semantic memory), he was unable to remember or re-experience any details about any specific events from his past (e.g., he could not remember the details of any specific family vacation; episodic memory). Importantly, patient K.C. was also unable to imagine any event that might happen in his personal future, which prompted Tulving (1985) to hypothesize that *knowing* about the past or future and mentally *re-/pre-experiencing* specific personal events in the past or future likely reflected the functioning of distinct conscious states, namely, noetic and autonoetic consciousness. Patient K.C. lacked autonoetic consciousness. That is, although patient K.C. knew about the past and future, he was unable to mentally project himself backward or forward into any events that had happened or might happen in his personal past and future.

Over the past decade, there has been a steady accumulation of evidence consistent with Tulving's (1985) original observation. For instance, various other amnesic patients have been identified who, like patient K.C., are characterized by an inability to remember the personal past or imagine the personal future (e.g., Hassabis et al. 2007; Klein et al. 2002). Moreover, various other populations that are characterized by impaired episodic memory, such as people with Alzheimer's disease (e.g., Addis et al. 2009), people with mild cognitive impairment (Gamboz et al. 2010), and healthy older adults (Addis et al. 2008), have also been shown to possess concurrent impairments of future event simulation. Along the same lines, children below the age of 5 years, who are unable to remember specific details about their personal past, also have difficulty formulating detailed plans about their personal future (Atance 2008). Finally, functional brain imaging studies have demonstrated considerable overlap in the brain systems that are involved in remembering the past and simulating the future (Addis et al. 2007; Szpunar et al. 2007). Together, these lines of research converge on Tulving's (1985) hypothesis that memory and future thinking are closely linked to one another.

Although there are various aspects of memory and future thinking that overlap with one another (e.g., simulations of future events tend to be constructed on the basis of similar details drawn from memory; Schacter and Addis 2007), we will focus the remainder of our discussion on the concept of autonoetic consciousness. Specifically, we will focus on the sense of re- or pre-experiencing the past and future that typically accompanies memory and future thinking. This sense of mentally experiencing a past or future event is the hallmark of the subjective experience that accompanies autonoetic consciousness. We ask whether this sense of mental time travel (i.e., feeling as though one has mentally traveled backward or forward in time so that it feels as if one is currently experiencing the past/future event) is somehow related to Future time perspective. For instance, do people who approach life's events with the future in mind have a more intense experience of mentally traveling to those future points in time? Might such a relation predict how likely simulations of the future are to subsequently influence present behavior?

Time Perspective and Autonoetic Consciousness

Despite the potential importance of a relation between Future time perspective and autonoetic consciousness, few studies have examined a possible connection between these two concepts. In a relevant study, D'Argembeau et al. (2010) examined this relation in the context of a large-scale individual difference study that included multiple kinds of future- and past-oriented tasks as well as multiple individual difference measures. The authors were interested in what component processes (e.g., working memory, visual-spatial ability, relational processing) are involved in the ability to envision the future and remember the past. Because of this broad aim, the study had limited power to determine the relation between any two variables (such as Future time perspective and autonoetic consciousness). Each participant imagined only one future event and remembered only one past event. Individual differences in autonoetic consciousness were based on only one rating: participants' sense of pre- or re-experiencing the future and past while imagining/remembering these events. There was no significant relation between Future time perspective and autonoetic consciousness for either past or future events. However, the data did demonstrate a relation between Future time perspective and the number of sensory details that were generated while imagining future events (but not past events). The authors interpreted this finding as supporting the hypothesis that future orientation is in some way related to the subjective experience of mentally traveling through time to pre-experience future events.

More recently, Arnold et al. (2011) reported a more focused study on the relation between time perspective and autonoetic consciousness. In this study, participants remembered ten past events and imagined ten future events. For each event, they rated the memory or future event on several dimensions including two indicators of autonoetic consciousness: the degree to which they felt as though they were pre- or re-experiencing the event and the degree to which they felt as though they were mentally time traveling forward or backward to the event. By including two measures of autonoetic consciousness and ten trials for each temporal direction, this study provided a more reliable indicator of individual differences in autonoetic consciousness. Further, participants completed the entire Zimbardo Time Perspective Inventory (ZTPI), which allowed the investigators to examine the relation between autonoetic consciousness and all five ZTPI subscales: Future, Past-Negative, Past-Positive, Present-Hedonistic, and Present-Fatalistic (Zimbardo and Boyd 1999).

There was a significant positive relation between future orientation and autonoetic consciousness, and this relation was consistent for both remembering the past and imagining the future. That is, on average, the more future oriented the ZTPI scale indicated a participant was, the stronger that participant's reported autonoetic experience when both remembering the past and imagining the future. The consistency of this relation across temporal directions provides further support for Tulving's (1985) idea that autonoetic consciousness underlies the ability to mentally project oneself both forward and backward through time.

Further, a positive relation between future orientation and autonoetic experience has several important implications. For instance, the relation could suggest a possible reason why some people are more inclined to think about the future when making decisions; people who more vividly experience future events may be more likely to take into account future consequences. Conversely, the tendency to be future oriented may cause people to have more vivid autonoetic experiences; those who spend more time thinking about the future may have better developed abilities to mentally time travel. In the final section of this chapter, we discuss these and other possible implications in more detail.

Notably, the future-oriented scale was not the only ZTPI subscale to predict autonoetic experience in this study (Arnold et al. 2011). People who rated higher on the Present-Hedonistic subscale also tended to report more vivid autonoetic experiences for both past and future events. This is a curious finding given that the Future and Present-Hedonistic subscales were negatively correlated with each other. That is, those who were more Present-Hedonistic oriented tended to be less future oriented and vice versa. How high ratings on both of these seemingly opposing subscales can predict more vivid autonoetic experiences is unclear. Perhaps those who naturally have more vivid autonoetic experiences tend to become either future oriented or Present-Hedonistic oriented depending on other yet-to-be identified personality characteristics and/or personal experiences.

Alternatively, perhaps the personality characteristics that tend to make someone more future oriented and those that tend to make someone more Present-Hedonistic oriented both result in more vivid autonoetic experiences but for different reasons. For instance, a vivid sense of pre-/re-living may result mainly from cognitive processes (e.g., tendency to carefully think through possible scenarios) in people who are more future oriented but result mainly from emotional processes in people who are more Present-Hedonistic oriented. This latter idea is expanded upon in the next section.

The negative correlation between the Future and Present-Hedonistic subscales does more than present a challenge for interpreting these findings; it also indicates that suppression effects may be present. That is, the relation between future orientation and autonoetic consciousness may only emerge when the Present-Hedonistic subscale is included in the model (and vice versa). This may explain why, in contradiction to Arnold et al.'s (2011) findings, D'Argembeau et al. (2010) did not find a correlation between Future time perspective and vividness of autonoetic experiences; they did not include the Present-Hedonistic subscale in their study. The Present-Hedonistic subscale has been found to suppress the relation between the Future subscale and at least one other dependent variable (energetic arousal; Stolarski et al. in press). This result exemplifies the importance of including the entire ZTPI scale when looking for relations between time perspectives and other personality characteristics or behaviors.

Other Individual Differences Related to Autonoetic Consciousness

Time perspective is not the only individual difference related to autonoetic consciousness. Although not many studies have examined individual differences in autonoetic consciousness, those that have suggest that emotions play an important role in the ability to pre- and re-experience events (D'Argembeau and Van der Linden 2006; Rubin and Siegler 2004). In particular, having a tendency to be emotionally expressive seems to be related to having stronger autonoetic experiences.

In a study on the phenomenology of autobiographical memories, Rubin and Siegler (2004) investigated the role of individual differences in personality, as measured by the NEO Personality Inventory (Costa and McCrae 1992). They investigated how personality differences may affect various autobiographical memory components, including autonoetic consciousness. The personality facet that was most predictive of stronger autonoetic experiences was openness to feelings. That is, people who were more open to expressing and experiencing their own inner feelings and emotions tended to report stronger feelings of both re-experiencing and mentally time traveling back to past events. Openness to feelings was also predictive of other phenomenological characteristics including having more visual and auditory details and having a greater belief in the accuracy of the memory. These findings are in line with other research showing that emotional suppression, or inhibiting the expression of emotional impulses, is associated with poorer memory (Richards and Gross 2000). The authors argued that openness to feelings can be viewed as the antithesis of emotional suppression.

D'Argembeau and Van der Linden (2006) extended this finding into episodic future thinking. They found that habitual use of emotional suppression was predictive of lower reported feelings of autonoetic experiences when both remembering the past and imagining the future. Further, they found that higher levels of emotional suppression were related to lower ratings in many other phenomenological qualities including visual details and spatial context and that these decreases were very similar for both past and future events. Together, these studies suggest that those who have a tendency to be more open to and expressive with feelings in the present also tend to have more expressive autonoetic experiences when mentally time traveling backward and forward in subjective time.

The relation between expressive emotions and autonoetic consciousness may help explain the relation between Present-Hedonistic orientation and autonoetic consciousness. People who score high on the Present-Hedonistic scale tend to be less emotionally stable, more extraverted, and more impulsive than average (Zimbardo and Boyd 1999; Zhang and Howell 2011). Together, these traits indicate a high degree of emotional expressiveness among those who are Present-Hedonistic oriented, which could be driving their vivid sense of mental time travel.

Other individual difference studies on autonoetic consciousness have found that sensitivity both to one's own and to others' experiences is related to having stronger autonoetic experiences. D'Argembeau et al. (2010) found that higher scores on a scale of self-consciousness, or the tendency to focus on one's own inner experiences, were predictive of stronger feelings of pre-experiencing future events. The authors interpreted this finding to suggest that the ability to represent one's own mental states underlies an ability to mentally time travel to future events. Interestingly, they did not find a connection between self-consciousness and reported feelings of re-experiencing past events.

In contrast to the finding that focusing on oneself is associated with autonoetic consciousness, Quoidbach et al. (2008) found that a tendency to relate to and empathize with others is related to having stronger autonoetic experiences. In their study, participants who scored higher on a scale of cooperativeness, a measure of the degree to which one identifies with and accepts others, reported greater feelings of both re-experiencing past events and pre-experiencing future events. The authors suggest that this finding is related to nonverbal communication. Cooperativeness is part of a social dimension of personality, which includes nonverbal communication, and therefore, they argue that people who are high on this dimension have more sensorial representations of events, which leads to greater feelings of re-/pre-experiencing. It should be noted that Quoidbach et al. did not find the previously reported relation between openness to feelings and autonoetic consciousness. However, this study had a limited sample size (N=35), which limits the power to find individual differences.

Implications

Perhaps the most important conclusion that can be made from the research summarized in this chapter is also the most straightforward: there are individual differences in the degree to which healthy adults experience autonoetic consciousness. Moreover, these differences seem to be consistent across temporal directions. Factors related to individual differences in autonoetic consciousness tend to be related to the experience of mentally time traveling both into the past and into the future (with the possible exception of self-consciousness; D'Argembeau et al. 2010). These findings suggest that autonoetic consciousness underlies both episodic memory and episodic future thought, two concepts that play a vital role in many aspects of human life. Therefore, individual differences in autonoetic consciousness may have wide-reaching implications.

As discussed in the previous sections, multiple factors have been associated with individual differences in autonoetic consciousness (Future time perspective, Present-Hedonistic time perspective, openness to feelings, self-consciousness, and cooperativeness). Of these factors, Future time perspective is particularly intriguing because it has been previously associated with healthy life choices and behaviors. This raises the question of whether or not individual differences in autonoetic consciousness are themselves associated with healthy life choices and behaviors. This has not been directly tested, and so any discussion about such a relation is purely speculative. However, given the variety and importance of healthy behaviors associated with Future time perspective, understanding what role autonoetic consciousness may play could give important insights into increasing positive outcomes in individuals. For instance, do individual differences in autonoetic consciousness mediate the relation between Future time perspective and healthy behaviors? That is, does the degree to which one feels as though he or she is pre-experiencing imagined future events influence one's behaviors, and, if so, does this explain the relation between Future time perspective and healthy choices?

To understand the relations between Future time perspective, autonoetic consciousness, and healthy life choices, other questions must first be answered. For instance, the directionality of the relation between autonoetic consciousness and Future time perspective needs to be established. Do more vivid autonoetic experiences lead to individuals becoming more future oriented, or does being more future oriented lead to more vivid autonoetic experiences? If the former is true, perhaps greater feelings of pre-living cause people to empathize more with their future self (and perhaps others; cf. Quoidbach et al. 2009) and therefore consider the future more carefully in their present lives. If the latter is true, perhaps those who are more future oriented have more practice imagining future events and therefore have a more developed autonoetic consciousness. Alternatively, a third variable may mediate the relation between these two variables in which case there may not be a direct causal link between differences in future orientation and autonoetic consciousness.

Another important question is stability of individual differences in autonoetic consciousness. Are differences in autonoetic experiences stable throughout the lifespan, or do they fluctuate? Is mental time travel an ability that develops throughout childhood and becomes stable in adults, or does it continually change and develop even into adulthood? If it does fluctuate, is it a skill that can benefit from directed training? For instance, if research establishes a causal link between the vividness of autonoetic experiences and healthy life choices, can an intervention be made such that people can learn to have more vivid autonoetic experiences, which in turn can lead to making better decisions?

Developing more vivid autonoetic experiences may also aid other future-oriented cognitions. As was discussed earlier, engaging in episodic future thought can increase the likelihood of completing prospective memory intentions (Brewer and Marsh 2010) and can aid in the development of better planning (Burgess et al. 2005; Szpunar and Tulving 2011). Individual differences in autonoetic experiences may impact the influence of episodic future thought on these successful outcomes. If individuals who have more vivid autonoetic experiences can better capitalize on their imagined futures, interventions could aid these and other future-oriented cognitions.

Conclusions

Individual differences in Future time perspective predict individual differences in the intensity of one's autonoetic experiences (Arnold et al. 2011). This relation holds true for autonoetic experiences when both remembering the past and imagining the future, providing further evidence that autonoetic consciousness underlies both types of mental time travel. More importantly, this finding suggests the way in which one experiences mental simulation may affect one's behaviors and life choices. Being highly future oriented has been associated with many positive behaviors. Do autonoetic experiences mediate this relation? Does vividly experiencing mental time travel cause people to be more future oriented? Does being highly future oriented cause people to have more intense autonoetic experiences? Answers to these questions could provide both theoretical insights into the role of autonoetic consciousness in daily life and practical implications for encouraging positive life choices.

However, the relation between autonoetic experiences and positive choices may not be straightforward. Present-hedonistic time perspective, an orientation that has been associated with more risky behaviors (Henson et al. 2006), was also associated with vivid autonoetic experiences (Arnold et al. 2011). These seemingly contradictory results suggest that having a vivid autonoetic experience is not sufficient for increasing one's positive behaviors. The way in which those vivid autonoetic experiences emerge (i.e., through cognitive, thoughtful processes vs. through emotional, impulsive processes) or the way in which the experiences are interpreted may mediate a relation between autonoetic experiences and behavior.

Also noteworthy is the lack of relation between both past time perspectives and autonoetic experiences. Arnold et al. (2011) found no correlation between ratings on the past orientation subscales and the vividness with which one felt as though they were re-living or mentally time traveling back to the past event. Questions on these subscales include measures of how frequently one thinks about the past (e.g., "I often think of what I should have done differently in my life.") and how much pleasure one gets out of replaying the past (e.g., "It gives me pleasure to think about my past"; Zimbardo and Boyd 1999). The lack of relation suggests that the vividness with which one experiences past events does not necessarily influence the frequency with which one chooses to think about those past events nor the emotional impact of thinking about those events.

Individual differences other than time perspective, such as openness to feelings, are also related to the way in which one experiences mental time travel (D'Argembeau and Van der Linden 2006; Rubin and Siegler 2004). Like Future time perspective, the relation between these factors and autonoetic consciousness appears to be bidirectional. That is, individual differences in autonoetic experiences tend to be similar when mentally time traveling into both the past and the future. This symmetry indicates that mental simulation is one general ability that can be used in both temporal directions (for discussion relating to possible temporal functions, see Schacter et al. 2012).

Tulving (1985) first proposed autonoetic consciousness after observing parallel deficits in an amnesic patient who could not simulate past or future. The more recent findings discussed in this chapter demonstrate that even in young, healthy adults, there is variation in the extent to which mental simulation is "experienced." Moving forward, research that can elucidate the nature of autonoetic consciousness (for relevant discussion, see Klein 2013), individual differences in autonoetic consciousness, and what impact those individual differences may have on daily life will be of considerable interest.

References

Addis, D. R., Wong, A. T., & Schacter, D. L. (2007). Remembering the past and imagining the future: Common and distinct neural substrates during event construction and elaboration. *Neuropsychologia, 45*, 1363.

Addis, D. R., Wong, A. T., & Schacter, D. L. (2008). Age-related changes in the episodic simulation of future events. *Psychological Science, 19*, 33–41.

Addis, D. R., Sacchetti, D. C., Ally, B. A., Budson, A. E., & Schacter, D. L. (2009). Episodic simulation of future events is impaired in mild Alzheimer's disease. *Neuropsychologia, 47*, 2660–2671.

Arnold, K. M., McDermott, K. B., & Szpunar, K. K. (2011). Individual differences in time perspective predict autonoetic experience. *Consciousness and Cognition, 20*, 712–719.

Atance, C. M. (2008). Future thinking in young children. *Current Directions in Psychological Science, 17*, 295–298.

Atance, C. M., & O'Neill, D. K. (2001). Episodic future thinking. *Trends in Cognitive Sciences, 5*, 533–539.

Brewer, G. A., & Marsh, R. L. (2010). On the role of episodic future simulation in encoding of prospective memories. *Cognitive Neuroscience, 1*, 81–88.

Burgess, P., Simons, J., Coates, L., & Channon, S. (2005). The search for specific planning processes. In R. Morris & G. Ward (Eds.), *The cognitive psychology of planning* (pp. 199–223). New York: Psychology Press.

Costa, P. T., & McCrae, R. R. (1992). Normal personality assessment in clinical practice: The NEO Personality Inventory. *Psychological Assessment, 4*, 5.

D'Argembeau, A., & Van der Linden, M. (2006). Individual differences in the phenomenology of mental time travel: The effect of vivid visual imagery and emotion regulation strategies. *Consciousness and Cognition, 15*, 342–350.

D'Argembeau, A., Ortoleva, C., Jumentier, S., & Van der Linden, M. (2010). Component processes underlying future thinking. *Memory & Cognition, 38*, 809–819.

Gamboz, N., De Vito, S., Brandimonte, M. A., Pappalardo, S., Galeone, F., Iavarone, A., & Sala, S. D. (2010). Episodic future thinking in amnesic mild cognitive impairment. *Neuropsychologia, 48*, 2091–2097.

Hassabis, D., Kumaran, D., Vann, S. D., & Maguire, E. A. (2007). Patients with hippocampal amnesia cannot imagine new experiences. *Proceedings of the National Academy of Sciences, 104*, 1726–1731.

Hayes-Roth, B., & Hayes-Roth, F. (1979). A cognitive model of planning. *Cognitive Science, 3*, 275–310.

Henson, J. M., Carey, M. P., Carey, K. B., & Maisto, S. A. (2006). Associations among health behaviors and time perspective in young adults: Model testing with boot-strapping replication. *Journal of Behavioral Medicine, 29*, 127–137.

Holmes, E. A., & Mathews, A. (2010). Mental imagery in emotion and emotional disorders. *Clinical Psychology Review, 30*, 349–362.

Klein, S. B. (2013). Making the case that episodic recollection is attributable to operations occurring at retrieval rather than to content stored in a dedicated subsystem of long-term memory. *Frontiers in Behavioral Neuroscience, 7*, Article 3.

Klein, S. B., Loftus, J., & Kihlstrom, J. F. (2002). Memory and temporal experience: The effects of episodic memory loss on an amnesic patient's ability to remember the past and imagine the future. *Social Cognition, 20*, 353–379.

Kliegel, M., McDaniel, M. A., & Einstein, G. O. (2008). *Prospective memory: Cognitive, neuroscience, developmental, and applied perspectives*. New York: Taylor & Francis Group, LLC.

McDaniel, M. A., Howard, D. C., & Butler, K. M. (2008). Implementation intentions facilitate prospective memory under high attention demands. *Memory & Cognition, 36*, 716–724.

Quoidbach, J., Hansenne, M., & Mottet, C. (2008). Personality and mental time travel: A differential approach to autonoetic consciousness. *Consciousness and Cognition, 17*, 1082–1092.

Quoidbach, J., Wood, A. M., & Hansenne, M. (2009). Back to the future: The effect of daily practice of mental time travel into the future on happiness and anxiety. *The Journal of Positive Psychology, 4*, 349–355.

Richards, J. M., & Gross, J. J. (2000). Emotion regulation and memory: The cognitive costs of keeping one's cool. *Journal of Personality and Social Psychology, 79*, 410–424.

Rubin, D. C., & Siegler, I. C. (2004). Facets of personality and the phenomenology of autobiographical memory. *Applied Cognitive Psychology, 18*, 913–930.

Schacter, D. L., & Addis, D. R. (2007). On the constructive episodic simulation of past and future events. *Behavioral and Brain Sciences, 30*, 331–332.

Schacter, D. L., Addis, D. R., Hassabis, D., Martin, V. C., Spreng, R. N., & Szpunar, K. K. (2012). The future of memory: Remembering, imagining, and the brain. *Neuron, 76*, 677–694.

Stolarski, M., Matthews, G., Postek, S., Zimbardo, P. G., & Bitner, J. (in press). How we feel is a matter of time: Relationships between time perspectives and mood. *Journal of Happiness Studies*.

Szpunar, K. K. (2010). Episodic future thought: An emerging concept. *Perspectives on Psychological Science, 5*, 142–162.

Szpunar, K. K., & Tulving, E. (2009). Episodic memory. *Scholarpedia, 4*, 3332.

Szpunar, K. K., & Tulving, E. (2011). Varieties of future experience. In M. Bar (Ed.), *Predictions in the brain: Using our past to generate a future* (pp. 3–12). New York: Oxford University Press.

Szpunar, K. K., Watson, J. M., & McDermott, K. B. (2007). Neural substrates of envisioning the future. *Proceedings of the National Academy of Sciences, 104*, 642–647.

Tulving, E. (1983). *Elements of episodic memory*. New York: Clarendon.

Tulving, E. (1985). Memory and consciousness. *Canadian Psychology, 26*, 1–12.

Tulving, E. (2002). Episodic memory: From mind to brain. *Annual Review of Psychology, 53*, 1–25.

Tulving, E. (2005). Episodic memory and autonoesis: Uniquely human? In H. S. Terrace & J. Metcalfe (Eds.), *The missing link in cognition: Origins of self-reflective consciousness* (pp. 3–56). New York: Oxford University Press.

Wilson, T. D., & Gilbert, D. T. (2005). Affective forecasting: Knowing what to want. *Current Directions in Psychological Science, 14*, 131–134.

Zhang, J. W., & Howell, R. T. (2011). Do time perspectives predict unique variance in life satisfaction beyond personality traits? *Personality and Individual Differences, 50*, 1261–1266.

Zimbardo, P. G., & Boyd, J. N. (1999). Putting time in perspective: A valid, reliable individual-differences metric. *Journal of Personality and Social Psychology, 77*, 1271–1288.

Emotional Processes in Development and Dynamics of Individual Time Perspective

Gerald Matthews and Maciej Stolarski

Introduction

The link between time perspective (TP) and emotional experience is now well established. How we typically see the past, present, and future appears to shape our immediate moods, general sense of well-being, and even vulnerability to emotional disorder (chapter "Time Perspectives and Subjective Well-being: A Dual Pathway Framework" by Cunningham et al., this volume; Zimbardo and Boyd 2008; Zimbardo et al. 2012). For example, habitually seeing the past in a negative light may color immediate emotional experience. Indeed, Aristotle emphasized an overwhelming interdependence between attitudes toward time and emotions. In *The Art of Rhetoric*, he defined emotion as a kind of pain or discomfort which is related to an upcoming danger. He argued that distant events do not arouse anxiety – we are all aware of our mortality, but death only terrifies when it seems near in time. A similar view comes from modern work; the sense of an imminent, "looming" danger may be central to neurotic anxiety (Riskind and Williams 2006).

According to cognitive theory, emotional responses are shaped by appraisal processes (Scherer 2001), which, in turn, are influenced by stable self-beliefs maintained in long-term memory (Wells and Matthews 2006). For example, a student who encodes himself/herself as perpetually failing on tests will tend to appraise an upcoming test as threatening, based on the self-belief. Personality traits, including habitual TP, are associated with stable self-beliefs. Thus, negative beliefs about the past, a salient feature of TP, are likely to bias appraisal in the here and now, generating negative mood (Boniwell et al. 2010).

G. Matthews (✉)
Institute for Simulation and Training, University of Central Florida, Orlando, FL, USA
e-mail: gmatthew@ist.ucf.edu

M. Stolarski
Faculty of Psychology, University of Warsaw, Stawki Str. 5/7, 00-183 Warsaw, Poland
e-mail: mstolarski@psych.uw.edu.pl

M. Stolarski et al. (eds.), *Time Perspective Theory; Review, Research and Application: Essays in Honor of Philip G. Zimbardo*, DOI 10.1007/978-3-319-07368-2_18,

However, there is more to emotional experience than the immediate appraisal of isolated events. The flow of emotional experience itself exists in time as a dynamic process (Lazarus 1999). Emotion change is driven not just by changing external events but by internal self-regulative processes. We may make short-term "on-line" adjustments to the processes generating emotion in response to a discrete event, such as suppressing emotions we would prefer not to display to others (Gross and Thompson 2007). Over longer time periods we reflect on our emotions and develop new regulative strategies. For example, the student who comes to realize that his/her anxiety reaction to a simple test was disproportionate may make a point of self-reassurance prior to the next test.

In this chapter, we will build on research on TP, emotion, and well-being to address the possible role of TP in emotion regulation. For example, depression often involves a focus on the past, in ruminating on past, self-referent causes of emotional distress (Nolen-Hoeksema 1991): e.g., "I have always been a loser." Negative views of the past are likely to encourage such ruminations. Conversely, positive TPs may lead to more constructive reflections that promote positive emotions. There may be a link between a positive past perspective and "emotional intelligence" (EI), a trait referring to a variety of emotional competencies that promote understanding of emotion (Matthews et al. 2002; Mayer et al. 2000). These competencies may include abilities to use past emotional experiences constructively in regulating immediate mood.

This chapter is structured as follows. First, we will outline a conceptual model of TP, emotion, and emotion regulation. Second, we will elaborate on Zimbardo and Boyd's (1999, 2008) multiple dimensions of TP and their relevance to emotional processes. Third, we will explore the possible role of TP in promoting effective emotion regulation, as an element of emotional intelligence (EI), and how dysfunctional or "unbalanced" TP may contribute to vulnerability to emotional disorder. We will conclude with a summary of the role of TP in emotion regulation and its wider significance for understanding individual differences in the explicit and implicit processes that mediate between TP and emotional experience.

Conceptualizing Time Perspective and Emotion

Individuals differ in their habitual TP (Zimbardo and Boyd 2008). While momentary time orientation depends on a variety of factors, people show consistent tendencies toward dwelling on the past, living in the present moment, or anticipating the future. As an element of personality, Zimbardo and Boyd (1999, 2008) see TP as being shaped primarily by social and cultural influences, although biologically based temperamental influences may also play a role.

Studies of personality development suggest how sociocultural factors may shape TP. McAdams (2001) emphasizes the importance of the "life story" for personality. Each person builds an evolving narrative that gives meaning to life; such narratives necessarily require interpretation of past events and future projections. In terms of social cognitive theories of personality stability (Matthews et al. 2000; Robinson and Sedikides 2009), personal perspectives on time are incorporated into the self-schema (or schemas) that shapes experience and governs action. For example, people who suffered abuse as a child might see those events as central to who they are as adults. Thorne and Nam (2009) describe some relevant developmental processes in the construction of personal narratives, including how the person makes sense of difficult or negative past life events. Mothers instruct children on the causes of their emotions, how the emotion should be expressed, and how emotions may be resolved (depending on culture, social class, and gender). Similarly, development of emotional aspect of TPs may be partially influenced by attachment patterns, with secure attachment facilitating Past Positive, Present Hedonistic, and Future perspectives and low attachment predicting Past Negative TP (Laghi et al. 2009).

Identifying dispositional TPs with the narrative self-schema leaves open whether TP is a cognitive or emotional construct. Should past TPs be identified with a set of propositions about the past or the vivid reexperiencing of past feeling states (cf., Strack et al. 1985)? Standard cognitive theories of emotion, such as appraisal theory (Scherer 2001), see cognitive evaluation processes as the primary causal influence on emotional experience, with subjective experience as a by-product of appraisal. Lennings (1996) defines TP as "a cognitive operation that implies both an emotional reaction to imagined time zones (such as future, present or past) and a preference for locating action in some temporal zone" (p. 72). TP might influence specific appraisal processes such as top-down reinstatement (Clore and Ortony 2000), which refers to assessment of a situation by matching it to previous experiences (schematically encoded). That is, the emotional meaning of an event is derived by matching stimulus features of the current event to a corresponding prototype in memory. Typically, top-down reinstatement allows fast recognition of the personal significance of an event based on prior experience. However, it can elicit inappropriate emotions; Clore and Ortony (2000) cite the case of a Vietnam veteran for whom the lush foliage of a hothouse reinstated the fear of jungle warfare. Individual differences in TP might reflect either content factors – availability of relevant positive and negative prototype events – or process factors like ease of accessing prototypes. By contrast, cognitive analyses of emotion may miss the point by reducing emotions to cold rationalizations: cognitive processes and emotions may reflect separate neural or psychological systems (Zajonc 1984). Recent work on EI has followed Pascal's dictum that "The heart has reasons that reason cannot know." Perhaps TP relates not to schema-driven analyses, but to the emotion system driving insistent past recollections, the thrills of pleasure in the here and now, and the vivid experience of anticipated emotion. There are significant theoretical objections to assigning cognition and emotion to separate systems (Lazarus 1999; Matthews et al. 2002), and top-down reinstatement can generate vivid emotions through unconscious cognitive processing (Clore and Ortony 2000). However, the relationship between TP and immediate emotional experience should not be neglected, given that several TP dimensions have an emotional valence. Gruber et al. (2012) even describe Zimbardo Time Perspective Inventory (ZTPI) as an indicator of *emotional* TP.

Time Perspectives and Emotional Processes

Zimbardo and Boyd (1999) realized that people differ in characteristic TP, just as we might say colloquially that someone lives for the moment or is buried in the past. In this sense, TP is defined as "…the often non-conscious personal attitude that each of us holds towards time and the process whereby the continual flow of existence is bundled into time categories that help to give order, coherence, and meaning to our lives" (Zimbardo and Boyd 2008, p. 51). They identified five separate dimensions of TP. Identification and measurement of these dimensions via the Zimbardo Time Perspective Inventory (ZTPI) has been crucial for research on TP and emotion. The dimensions are as follows:

- *Past negative (PN)*: A generally negative, aversive view of the past, which may generate painful memories. It may develop through exposure of actual unpleasant or even traumatic events, through negative reconstruction of neutral or benign events, or via both processes.
- *Past positive (PP)*: A warm, sentimental attitude toward the past that may produce pleasant reminiscences. As with PN, it may reflect memories of actual events or positive reevaluation of neutral or negative events.
- *Present hedonistic (PH)*: A hedonistic attitude toward life, with high impulsivity and little concern for future consequences of one's actions. On the one hand, PH is associated with energy and *joie de vivre*; on the other with risk-taking and irresponsibility.
- *Present fatalistic (PF)*: Beliefs that the path of life is determined by chance rather than personal striving, so that there is little point in planning for the future. PF combines external locus of control (Peterson 1991) with apathy and resignation to the whims of fate.
- *Future (F)*: A general orientation toward planning for the future, with behavior dominated by striving for future goals and rewards. It reflects a conscientious but perhaps rather puritanical disposition.

Although Zimbardo and Boyd (1999) emphasized the social-cultural basis for TP, it is likely that biologically based temperamental factors also play a role (Stolarski et al. 2013a). Such factors include positive emotionality, negative emotionality, and effortful control (Rothbart et al. 2009). A fairly large-scale FFM study (Zhang and Howell 2011) confirmed that neuroticism (negative emotionality) correlated especially with higher PN and to a lesser degree with PF and low PH. Correlates of extraversion (positive emotionality) included higher PP and PH and lower PN, whereas conscientiousness (effortful control) was substantially correlated with F and to a lesser extent with lower PN and PF. Various traits associated with impulsivity and risk-taking also correlate with higher PH and lower F (Zimbardo and Boyd 1999).

However, there is more to TP than temperament. Zhang and Howell (2011) showed that the ZTPI scales explained substantial variance in well-being over and above the FFM: PP, PN, and PH were all independently significant predictors in a regression analysis. Indeed, when analyzed separately, the ZTPI explained more variance in well-being (33.5 %) than the FFM (24.2 %). Furthermore, relationships between personality and emotion reflect not only temperament but also individual differences in appraisal and coping (Matthews et al. 2006, 2009), as well as mood regulation processes (Lischetzke and Eid 2006). Different aspects of TP may be variously associated with vivid, immediate emotional experiences (or recollection of past experiences) or with a more "pallid" and distanced analysis of emotive events (Strack et al. 1985). The ZTPI dimensions that predict well-being most strongly (PP, PN, PH) may connect with vivid experience, whereas PF and F may be related more to strategic regulation of emotion. For example, the person high in F may be motivated to prevent negative experiences through careful planning and anticipation of threat.

Thus, understanding the emotional correlates of TP requires attention to underlying mechanisms and processes, which may be of various kinds. With this principle in mind, we will next outline research findings on the five ZPTI dimensions.

Past Time Perspectives

Past experiences are often considered as the basis of our identity, and influential movements in psychology ranging from psychoanalysis to behaviorism have emphasized the importance of early learning for personality development, albeit from very different theoretical standpoints. However, memories of the past are constructed at encoding and reconstructed at retrieval and so are not exact copies of the actual experience. Reconstructions of the past can be positive or negative, whatever the nature of the event. Zimbardo (in Zimbardo and Boyd 2008, pp. 71–73) recalls a grim experience as a 5-year-old, being quarantined with whooping cough and double pneumonia in a hospital ward filled with suffering and dying children. He describes how he transformed this experience by reframing it positively, as one in which he learned strategies for self-reliance and enduring hardship. Zimbardo and Boyd (2008) claim that one's subjective attitude toward past experiences is more important than the objective nature of life experiences.

Past TPs influence present emotional functioning, but it is important to distinguish PN and PP factors. Intuition might suggest that positive and negative past TPs should be opposed traits. In fact, factor analysis revealed two independent, only weakly correlated factors (e.g., Zimbardo and Boyd (1999) report a correlation of −.26). Some people may have strongly valenced past TPs, others may not develop any strong orientations to the past, whereas still others reveal emotionally ambivalent attitude toward past, scoring high on both past dimensions. Similarly, positive and negative affects represent separate psychological systems, which may sometimes be co-activated (Watson 2000).

Past TPs consequently reveal relationships with subjective well-being (chapter "Time Perspectives and Subjective Well-being: A Dual Pathway Framework" by Cunningham, et al., this volume). Relationships of TPs with various measures of life satisfaction reflect their emotional valence: PN is negatively related to well-being (usually at −.40 to −.50 level), while PP reveals opposite correlations (slightly weaker: .30 to .40). PN is the strongest correlate of well-being across all the studies, and it may be implicated in traumatic stress also (Holman and Silver 1998).

Stolarski et al. (2013b) have shown that the pattern of results is similar for currently experienced mood. In their study, PN was positively related to tension and negatively to energy and hedonic tone. Opposite relationships were obtained for PP. Moreover, past TPs proved significantly related to recalled mood, when mood was assessed on two separate days. PN was associated with higher recalled tension and lower energy and hedonic tone. However, in this case, recall was accurate rather than produced by a bias in memory. By contrast, individuals higher in PP tended to report higher levels of energy than they actually experienced, suggesting a reconstructive bias.

Studies of autobiographical memory may illuminate the role of TP in emotion. Courage and Howe (2010) point out that autobiographical memories are closely related to the "cognitive self" that begins to emerge at around 2 years old, as an organized, "objectified" set of self-beliefs. The cognitive self interacts dynamically with autobiographical memory in that the current self-concept (or "working self") reconstructs past memories and the past reconstructs the self (Conway and Pleydell-Price 2000). Broadly, stronger past TPs might signal the dominance of the latter process, i.e., retrieval of past autobiographical memory powerfully shapes the person's sense of who they are currently. Theories of autobiographical memory (e.g., Conway and Pleydell-Price 2000; Conway et al. 2004) are elaborate and beyond the scope of this chapter. For example, both autobiographical memory and the conceptual self encode multiple types of information, memory retrieval may be explicit or implicit, and emotion may enhance or block retrieval in different circumstances. We will merely pick out some features of autobiographical memory relevant to TP, at the cost of considerably simplifying the models to which we refer.

According to Conway et al. (2004), there is a fundamental tension between two functions of memory, "adaptive correspondence" and "self-coherence." The former refers to the need to keep accurate records of sensory experience in order to accomplish the action sequences necessary for goal attainment. Even relatively simple goals like boiling an egg required detailed, veridical episodic memory. Self-coherence refers to the need to maintain a consistent, conceptually rich, and comprehensible understanding of oneself, a function that may require neglect or reconstruction of those personal experiences that do not fit the schema.

TP may intrude at several points of the processing supporting adaptive correspondence and self-coherence. The working self functions in part by accessing relevant memories of plans for goal attainment from a knowledge base associated with current goals (Conway and Pleydell-Price 2000). These include what Conway et al. (2004) call self-defining memories, i.e., those of personally important goal transitions (most simply, success or failure). Significant goal transitions are typically accompanied by appropriate emotion. Especially salient memories may constitute turning points in life (Pillemer et al. 1996); perhaps Zimbardo's memory of the quarantine ward is of this kind. A strong past TP might be associated with the availability or accessibility of self-defining memories or with limitations in the capacity of the working self to generate novel solutions to familiar challenges. The near independence of PN and PP (Zhang and Howell 2011) suggests separate representations of positive and negative memories. Conway et al. (2004) argue that retrieval of emotionally intense memories may disrupt the balance between adaptive correspondence and self-coherence functions, producing a merging of present and remembered experience. Individuals with strong past TPs (perhaps PN especially) may be especially vulnerable to such disruptive effects.

Self-coherence – i.e., developing continuity in sense of self – is a key function of autobiographical memory (Olivares 2012). Processes such as self-verification and uncertainty reduction build and maintain self-continuity, but may distort veridical recall (Conway et al. 2004). Indeed, depressed individuals may preferentially recall negative information about the self in order to maintain a coherent self-schema (Swann 1997). A strong past TP may be associated with stronger motivations of this kind, with potentially damaging consequences in the case of PN. Conversely, PP might be associated with greater self-enhancement motives. Zimbardo and Boyd (2008) also cite evidence that PP is related to higher family involvement, consonant with the social bonding function of autobiographical memory (Olivares 2012). Grounding the self in positive memories of the family may promote well-being.

Present Time Perspectives

It is tempting, but ultimately misleading, to define a present TP as an absence of past or future orientation. We might see the present-oriented person as stimulus-driven and prone to neglect both the self-defining memories described in the last section and efforts at future planning. Such a definition captures the impulsivity characteristic of present TP (Zimbardo and Boyd 1999, 2008) but has other shortcomings. Impulsive behaviors may still be influenced by self-regulation and (conscious or unconscious) beliefs about the appropriateness of the impulsive act (Matthews et al. 2000, 2002). Seemingly spontaneous emotion may also be a consequence of memories of the past or projecting the future. In addition, the two present dimensions of the ZTPI, PH and PF, are systematically related to past orientation. In Zhang and Howell's (2011) large data set, PH correlated at .22 with PP, and PF correlated at .48 with PN. Both present-oriented dimensions showed modest negative correlations with F, supporting the idea that an absence of future planning contributes to present TPs.

Zimbardo and Boyd (1999) described two present TPs, each of which is robustly emotionally loaded. In fact, PH and PF have some attributes in common. Zimbardo and Boyd (2008) see both TPs as being associated with emotional instability, aggression, depression, as well as behavioral expressions of present orientation such as risk-taking, novelty-seeking, and poor impulse control. Zimbardo and Boyd (2008) suggest that difficult socioeconomic circumstances, in which trying to plan for the future seems pointless, may contribute to present orientation (see chapter

"Precariousness as a Time Horizon: How Poverty and Social Insecurity Shape Individuals' Time Perspectives" by Fieulaine & Apostolidis, this volume).

In other respects, PH and PF are differentiated in relation to emotion. Present fatalistic TP corresponds to a helpless, hopeless attitude toward life and future (Zimbardo and Boyd 1999). It is related to negative emotions (Stolarski et al. 2013b), low self-esteem (Zimbardo and Boyd 1999), and decreased well-being (Boniwell et al. 2010; Zhang et al. 2013). This emotional profile may result from external locus of control and, in general, learned helplessness. It may seem paradoxical that PF relates to negative emotion, given that the fatalist expresses a sense of resignation and lack of concern about the future. PF may then represent a style of coping with emotional disturbance. Perhaps acceptance of one's unhappiness works to some degree in distancing the self from negative emotions, but the strategy seems generally ineffective.

Present hedonism is a rather harder nut to crack if we seek for its emotional correlates or consequences. Present hedonists are energetic and impulsive sensation and novelty seekers (Zimbardo and Boyd 1999). They strive for intense pleasure and excitement, which leads them to such behaviors as risky driving (Zimbardo et al. 1997), substance use (Keough et al. 1999), or risky sexual behaviors (Henson et al. 2006). However, according to meta-analysis (Stolarski et al. 2012), PH explains less than 2.9 % of variance in well-being. Moreover, present hedonists are more prone to mania (Gruber et al. 2012); they are more aggressive and depressive and less emotionally stable and display lower impulse control. Zimbardo and Boyd (2008) summarize the typical emotions of hedonists by stating that they have more energy, but also greater depression and emotional instability (consistent with bipolar tendencies). By contrast, Stolarski et al. (2013b) found that individuals high in PH reported higher energy, but also lower tension and higher hedonic tone.

We have two comments on the seemingly contradictory findings. First, the snapshots of affective correlates of PH available from standard cross-sectional studies may not do justice to the role of the trait in the dynamics of emotion. Those in PH may enjoy hedonistic activities but also suffer an emotional "hangover" later on (and perhaps a literal hangover on occasion also). Similarly, the social context may be important. A hedonistic orientation may not be emotionally damaging for those living freewheeling, unstructured lives (including some university students), but may clash with adult career and family responsibilities.

Second, the emotional impact of hedonism may be moderated by other elements of TP. Stolarski and colleagues (2012) found that happiness is predicted by significant interactions between the present hedonistic and future-oriented TPs. Specifically, individuals with both present hedonistic and future-oriented TPs experienced the highest levels of well-being. Maximum happiness necessitates both an appreciation for pleasure seeking and an ability to delay gratification. Excessive focus on the future to the exclusion of the present may stifle spontaneous enjoyment of life.

Although not represented in the standard ZTPI, Zimbardo and Boyd (2008) draw attention to a third perspective, the present holistic perspective, which supports superior affective functioning. Consistent with Eastern philosophies, this perspective emphasizes the mindful awareness of the present, surrendering past preoccupations and ceasing to worry about the future. Such an orientation may be a fruitful direction for future research, especially as Drake et al. (2008) found that both PH and PF were negatively associated with mindfulness.

Future Time Perspective(s)

Future TP is a fundamental dimension, momentous for personal development, creating the basis for delay of gratification processes (Husman and Lens 1999; Nuttin 1985). Future perspective allows people to overcome immediate hedonic drives and impulses and helps to give value to more distant but also more important goals. It may be a metacognitive process of emotional regulation that keeps hedonic striving on healthy and responsible tracks. In fact, F is only weakly related to higher well-being (Zhang et al. 2013), suggesting that its role in emotion may be more strategic than experiential. The aforementioned study of mood (Stolarski et al. 2013b) found that F is a dispositional predictor of energy, which reflects motivation to act, but it is not related to hedonic tone. The affective benefits of F may in part reflect more adaptive coping with stressors. The relationship between coping and TP has been rather neglected, which is surprising given that the contemporary transactional theory of stress (Lazarus 1999) emphasizes the temporally dynamic nature of stressful encounters. However, some conceptual and empirical links between coping and TP can be established.

A simple model of coping differentiates task-focused (or problem-focused), emotion-focused, and avoidant strategies (Endler and Parker 1990). Task-focused coping entails developing an organized plan of action to deal with the issue at hand, implying strategizing for the future. By contrast, emotion focus does not correspond to a clear TP – it could involve reflecting on both past and future – and avoidance seems geared toward preventing present discomfort. Although the effectiveness of the different coping strategies depends on the nature of the challenge faced by the person, task focus appears to be broadly the most successful strategy, especially when the person has some power to influence events (Endler and Parker 1990). F may be associated with greater – or more effective – use of task-focused coping, contributing to lower stress and higher well-being. Supporting this prediction, Epel et al. (1999) found that homeless individuals high in F were more likely than others to engage in proactive search for housing and to engage in task-focused activities like enrolling in school. A recent study using a Greek sample showed that high F was related to greater proactive coping, a construct similar to task focus (Anagnostopoulos and Griva 2012). High F may also protect against stress resulting from disease, given that this TP may relate to greater participation in preventive medical checkups such as breast cancer screening (D'Alessio et al. 2003; Zimbardo and Boyd 2008). Traits overlapping with F, especially conscientiousness, also seem to confer greater resilience to stress: task-focused coping mediates effects of conscientiousness on positive emotions (Matthews et al. 2006). High F may exert a similar influence on affective well-being.

Another perspective concerns the different types of coping that may be appropriate as an event unfolds in time (McGrath and Tschan 2004). These authors describe five temporal stages relevant to understanding coping with a disastrous event such as a flood: preventive coping (performed long before: e.g., building flood defenses), anticipatory coping (soon before: e.g., evacuation from a low-lying area), dynamic coping (present: e.g., climbing to the top of a flooded building), reactive coping (soon after: e.g., finding temporary accommodation), and residual coping (long after: e.g., renewing flood insurance). Future work on TP and coping might productively address temporal dynamics. We might expect Future TP to relate to preventive and anticipatory coping, present orientations to dynamic coping, and past orientations to residual coping.

A final issue is that Zimbardo and Boyd (1999), as well as other Future TP researchers (see Zaleski 1994), do not distinguish between positive and negative views of future, rather opposing it to present orientation. However, there are different points of view. Worrell and Mello (2007) first suggested a six-factor structure of TP, dividing future into two dimensions. A similar psychometric operationalization within the Zimbardo theory came from Carelli et al. (2011). The authors describe future negative dimension as related to concerns and anxiety, whereas future positive is expressed in hope and expectation. Both dimensions have a motivational character, but whereas in the former the motivation comes from fear of numerous threats, in the latter it results from strive to realize one's potential through taking advantage from forthcoming opportunities. These orientations are represented by two motives: approach and avoidance. Naturally, approach motives tend to be associated with positive emotions and avoidance motives with negative emotions, depending also on the specific motive involved (e.g., performance or mastery goals: Huang 2011).

Time Perspective and Competence in Emotion Regulation

We have seen how all five of the Zimbardo and Boyd (1999, 2008) TPs contribute to emotion regulation, although not necessarily adaptively. TPs may influence both vivid, emotionally charged regulative processes, such as retrieval of memories of life-changing events, and strategic regulative processes, such as coping with stress, whose effects on emotional experience may be indirect. Research also illustrates how emotion regulation may operate over varying timespans, from the immediate challenges posed by events to the person's lifelong personal narrative (McGrath and Tschan 2004; Thorne and Nam 2009). Indeed, older age may systematically change TP as the person adjusts, often adaptively, to shrinking future horizons (Carstensen et al. 1999).

Thus far, studies of TP have rarely connected directly with the emerging psychology of emotion regulation (e.g., Gross and Thompson 2007), which differentiates various specific strategies used by people to influence emotion (with more focus on shorter rather than longer timespans). Emotion regulation implies monitoring of emotional state, providing a target for emotion regulation efforts, and deploying strategies to attain the target emotion. Both monitoring (i.e., self-appraisal) and strategy choice may be influenced by TP. Often such regulation is conscious and voluntary. However, habitual styles of emotion regulation may become proceduralized and thus somewhat automatic and inaccessible to consciousness, especially in the case of the dysfunctional strategies used by individuals with emotional disorders (Wells and Matthews 2006). We will consider the application of TP research to two focal issues in emotion regulation: emotional competency and emotional disorder.

As discussed above, well-being tends to correlate positively with PP and F and negatively with PN and PF, whereas PH is associated with diverse affective outcomes. Zimbardo and Boyd (1999) also emphasized the importance of a balanced TP. The differing challenges of life call for differing TPs, so that people will benefit from the capacity to shift perspective according to the current context. Even if PP and F are predominantly beneficial, it may sometimes be advantageous to recall past failures (PN) or to give up on an intractable problem (PF). An extreme bias toward any single TP may block access to other perspectives when they are in fact appropriate. A balanced TP thus represents the optimum configuration of the various TPs, broadly defined as low (but not zero) PN and PF, as well as moderate to high scores on PP, PH, and F (Zimbardo and Boyd 1999). Zhang et al. (2013) compared various metrics for estimating balanced TP from the ZTPI and confirmed that balance was positively associated with various facets of well-being.

If there is an optimum profile of TPs, it may contribute to some overall competence in emotion regulation. The new construct of EI (Matthews et al. 2002; Mayer et al. 2000) is broadly defined as an array of aptitudes, competencies, and skills in identifying, understanding, and managing emotion. The emotionally intelligent person should benefit both from competency in monitoring emotional state and in choosing regulative strategies for attaining a target emotion (Salovey et al. 1995). Indeed, Salovey et al.'s (1995) account of mood regulation strategies includes facets for both clarity of thinking about one's emotions and mood repair.

Stolarski et al. (2011) pointed out some conceptual similarities between TP and EI. As in accounts of TP, Salovey et al. (2002) distinguished experiential ("hot") and strategic ("cold") elements of EI. In their four-branch model of EI, emotion perception and assimilation of emotion into thought are considered experiential, and emotion understanding and management are strategic. Stolarski et al. collected data on the ZTPI (Zimbardo and Boyd 1999) and a test of EI developed for use with Polish samples. Their findings illustrate how TP and EI may be connected at both experiential and strategic levels.

Past TPs are often experiential (as they are based on our past experiences), but they remain under influence of cognitive interpretations and strategies for retrieval from memory. Hence, past TPs should be related to both forms of EI. Consistent with expectation, Stolarski et al. (2011) found that overall EI was positively associated with PP and negatively correlated with PN. Furthermore, the two past TPs correlated significantly with both experiential and strategic branches of EI. Turning to present TP, there was no association between PH and EI. PH might be expected to be positively related to experiential EI (i.e., more openness toward emotional experiences) but negatively to strategic (i.e., poorer regulation), but these predictions were not confirmed. A sharper focus on mood regulation in rewarding and exciting contexts may be needed here. By contrast, PF was the strongest correlate of overall low EI (both strategic and experiential EI branches). Fatalism may encourage both impoverished emotional experience and poorer strategic regulation of emotion, perhaps reflecting an external locus of control.

High F was expected to confer the affective benefits of strategic regulation but proved to be unrelated to EI, possibly because Polish culture inclines toward negative conceptions of the future. The distinction between Future Negative and Future Positive TPs advocated by Carelli et al. (2011) may be worth developing in further studies. Stolarski et al. (2011) also found that a measure of balanced TP correlated at .31 with overall EI and correlated significantly with all four branches.

Stolarski et al.'s (2011) study confirms that TP may impinge on overall emotional competency, including both its experiential and strategic aspects. It remains an open question whether competency shapes TP or vice versa (or some more complex interaction). However, individual differences in mood regulation cannot be studied only from a dispositional perspective. Indeed, studies of EI have been criticized for neglecting the role of situational factors in emotional competence (Matthews et al. 2002). A next step for research is to examine how dimensions of TP influence emotion regulation within specific laboratory and real settings. Contextual factors such as the relevance of past experience, the availability of opportunistic rewards, and the predictability and controllability of future events may all moderate the impact of TP on mood-regulative processes.

Time Perspective and Dysfunctional Emotion Regulation

Certain TPs, especially PN and PF, tend to accompany reduced emotional competence, although that is not to say they are maladaptive in all circumstances. In this section, we consider the clinical perspective on dysfunctional TPs, drawing especially on recent studies of trauma, as well as other relevant emotional disorders.

Obviously, memories of the past are central to the stress ensuing from exposure to traumatic events and posttraumatic stress disorder (PTSD). Indeed, vividly reexperiencing the event (e.g., flashbacks) comprises one of the three core symptom clusters of the disorder (along with avoidance and hyperarousal symptoms). When memories of the trauma dominate current existence, the person may experience an especially malign form of Past Negative TP. Cognitive theories of trauma (e.g., Feeny and Foa 2006) are broadly consistent with this view. PTSD reflects difficulties in assimilating trauma memories into the person's preexisting schemas for the self and the world. Recovery from trauma requires the person to construct and organize a personal narrative that can be integrated into these broader schemas or, in Conway et al.'s (2004) terminology, repairing self-coherence.

TPs are potentially relevant both to the onset of PTSD, remembering that only some individuals exposed to trauma develop persistent clinically significant symptoms, and to recovery. Naively, it might seem that high PN would increase vulnerability to PTSD, but this may not be the case. Feeny and Foa (2006) argue that it is actually rigidity of schematized beliefs that is the vulnerability factor, suggesting that the critical TP issue is whether high PP and PN imply rigid beliefs about the past, an issue that remains to be investigated. The issues for recovery may be somewhat different. Here, there is evidence that past TP may be a crucial factor in coping with trauma. Holman and Silver (1998) showed that when traumatized individuals become stuck in their prior traumatic experience, reported symptoms of trauma remain elevated long after the experience has passed. Moreover, their results suggest that people who are able to maintain a future orientation in the aftermath of trauma are less likely to experience elevated distress over time; an opposite pattern was observed for present orientation scores. In terms of cognitive theory (Feeny and Foa 2006), we may speculate that a future orientation facilitates the strategic restructuring of memory requisite for recovery, such as accommodating the memories of the event within a forward-looking personal narrative.

Time Perspective Therapy (Zimbardo et al. 2012; see also chapter "Time Perspective Therapy: Transforming Zimbardo's Temporal Theory Into Clinical Practice" by Sword et al., this volume) is a promising example of applying TP theory to facilitating recovery from PTSD. This therapeutic approach is based on the idea of balanced time perspective (see chapter "Assessing Temporal Harmony: The Issue of a Balanced Time Perspective" by Stolarski et al., this volume) and focuses on (1) reconstruction of the past toward its positive interpretation, (2) facilitation of the competence to enjoy present life pleasures, and, above all, (3) building one's future plans and goals constructively (the latter ability is severely impaired in PTSD syndrome). The therapy revealed an impressive effectiveness (Sword et al. 2014), showing that TP theory provides a useful framework for therapeutic interventions in emotional disorders.

Another relevant dynamic process is the perseverative negative self-referent thinking prevalent in many emotional disorders (Wells and Matthews 2006). This style of thinking is described as rumination when backward-looking (e.g., brooding on past failures) and worry when forward-looking (toward future threats). Rumination is seen as characteristic of depression and worry of Generalized Anxiety Disorder (GAD), although neither process is exclusive to these conditions. We might expect that PN would facilitate rumination and negative future orientation would encourage worry. In addition, a "looming" cognitive style in which future threats are seen as imminent has been implicated across the spectrum of anxiety disorders (Riskind and Williams 2005), representing a maladaptive Future TP. Many maladaptive forms of thinking represent metacognitions, i.e., beliefs about one's mental experiences and strategies for controlling thoughts and imagery (Wells and Matthews 2006). Linking TPs to dysfunctional metacognitions may be a fruitful avenue for future research. In a pilot study, Ledzińska (in preparation) showed that PN and PH time perspectives are positively related to maladaptive metacognitive beliefs (at .34 and .25 level, respectively) measured with MCQ-30 questionnaire. Perhaps excessive rumination on past failures represents beliefs that it is important to dwell on such memories; worry may in part be driven by beliefs that worrying about the future is an effective strategy to forestall the feared event (Wells and Matthews 2006).

The clinical application of research on TP and emotional dynamics is new but promising. Certain aspects of TP may disrupt both accurate monitoring of mental state (e.g., overestimating the importance of an intrusive memory) and effective mood regulation (e.g., excessive worry about future dangers). Although beyond the scope of this chapter, we have described briefly how TP theory may provide a framework for therapeutic interventions in emotional disorders (Sword et al. 2014; Zimbardo et al. 2012).

Conclusion

Emotions unfold in time so it is no surprise that TPs may shape emotional experience and regulation. Dispositional TPs may be conceptualized as fairly stable, but not immutable, elements of personality shaped in childhood by socialization processes (and perhaps also influenced by temperament). The majority of research in this field has been directed toward establishing links between the different TPs identified by Zimbardo and Boyd (1999, 2008) and affective outcomes such as well-being (see chapter "Time Perspectives and Subjective Well-being: A Dual Pathway Framework" by Cunningham et al., this volume). We have seen that all five TPs are associated with characteristic patterns of emotional functioning, varying in whether they are experiential or strategic in nature. One task for the future is to map how TPs relate to specific emotions and feeling states. Basing on the nature of particular TPs, as well on the research on their correlates (e.g., Zimbardo and Boyd 1999; Carelli et al. 2011), we might suppose that anxiety and worry are the core of FN, whereas regret, sadness, and pain constitute PN. FP could be defined as hope, curiosity, and positive expectancy, whereas PP might consist of nostalgia, fond reminiscence, and tenderness. Finally, PF manifests in feeling of helplessness and passivity, while high levels of PH refers to specific pleasures such as lust and euphoria.

It is important too to determine the underlying processes that mediate the effects of TPs on emotion. The contemporary cognitive theory of emotions suggests plausible – though insufficiently tested – explanations for the impact of TPs, including biases in cognitive appraisal, in the interplay between current self-concept and autobiographical memory and the use of working memory to anticipate future outcomes. A comprehensive cognitive-psychological account of TPs should accommodate both strategic processes, which are often explicit and implicit processes which, though closed to introspection, may still generate vivid and even overwhelming emotional experiences.

A deeper understanding of the role of TPs in emotion regulation may have both theoretical and practical benefits. As EI researchers (e.g., Salovey et al. 2002) have stressed, emotional competency is important in numerous real-life contexts: forming intimate relationships, succeeding at work, and finding personal fulfillment. Understanding the role of TPs in effective management of the emotional challenges of such central life goals may contribute to various branches of applied psychology. Conversely, dysfunctional styles of emotion regulation associated with maladaptive TPs may increase vulnerability to emotional disorder or slow recovery and response to therapy.

References

Anagnostopoulos, F., & Griva, F. (2012). Exploring time perspective in Greek young adults: Validation of the Zimbardo Time Perspective Inventory and relationships with mental health indicators. *Social Indicators Research, 106*, 41–59.

Boniwell, I., Osin, E., Linley, P. A., & Ivanchenko, G. V. (2010). A question of balance: Time perspective and well-being in British and Russian samples. *The Journal of Positive Psychology, 1*, 24–40.

Carelli, M. G., Wiberg, B., & Wiberg, M. (2011). Development and construct validation of the Swedish Zimbardo Time Perspective Inventory. *European Journal of Psychological Assessment, 27*, 220–227.

Carstensen, L. L., Isaacowitz, D. M., & Charles, S. T. (1999). Taking time seriously: A theory of socioemotional selectivity. *American Psychologist, 54*, 165–181.

Clore, G. L., & Ortony, A. (2000). Cognition in emotion: Always, sometimes, or never? In R. D. Lane & L. Nadel (Eds.), *Cognitive neuroscience of emotion* (pp. 24–61). New York: Oxford University Press.

Conway, M. A., & Pleydell-Price, C. W. (2000). The construction of autobiographical memories in the self-memory system. *Psychological Review, 107*, 261–288.

Conway, M. A., Singer, J. A., & Tagini, A. (2004). The self and autobiographical memory: Correspondence and coherence. *Social Cognition, 22*, 491–529.

Courage, M. L., & Howe, M. L. (2010). Autobiographical memory: Individual differences and developmental course. In A. Gruszka, G. Matthews, & B. Szymura (Eds.), *Handbook of individual differences in cognition: Attention, memory, and cognitive control* (pp. 403–417). New York: Springer.

D'Alessio, M., Guarino, A., de Pascalis, V., & Zimbardo, P. G. (2003). Testing Zimbardo's Stanford Time Perspective Inventory (STPI) – short form: An Italian study. *Time & Society, 12*, 333–347.

Drake, L., Duncan, E., Sutherland, F., Abernethy, C., & Henry, C. (2008). Time perspective and correlates of wellbeing. *Time & Society, 17*, 47–61.

Endler, N., & Parker, J. (1990). Multi dimensional assessment of coping: A critical review. *Journal of Personality and Social Psychology, 58*, 844–854.

Epel, E. S., Bandura, A., & Zimbardo, P. G. (1999). Escaping homelessness: The influences of self-efficacy and time perspective on coping with homelessness. *Journal of Applied Social Psychology, 29*, 575–596.

Feeny, N. C., & Foa, E. B. (2006). Cognitive vulnerability to PTSD. In L. B. Alloy & J. H. Riskind (Eds.), *Cognitive vulnerability to emotional disorders* (pp. 285–301). Mahwah: Lawrence Erlbaum.

Gross, J. J., & Thompson, R. A. (2007). Emotion regulation: Conceptual foundations. In J. J. Gross (Ed.), *Handbook of emotion regulation* (pp. 3–24). New York: Guilford Press.

Gruber, J., Cunningham, W. A., Kirkland, T., & Hay, A. C. (2012). Feeling stuck in the present? Mania proneness and history associated with present-oriented time perspective. *Emotion, 12*, 13–17.

Henson, J. M., Carey, M. P., Carey, K. B., & Maisto, S. A. (2006). Associations among health behaviors and time perspective in young adults: Model testing with boot-strapping replication. *Journal of Behavioral Medicine, 29*, 127–137.

Holman, E. A., & Silver, R. C. (1998). Getting" stuck" in the past: Temporal orientation and coping with trauma. *Journal of Personality and Social Psychology, 74*, 1146–1163.
Huang, C. (2011). Achievement goals and achievement emotions: A meta-analysis. *Educational Psychology Review, 23*, 359–388.
Husman, J., & Lens, W. (1999). The role of the future in student motivation. *Educational Psychologist, 34*, 113–125.
Keough, K. A., Zimbardo, P. G., & Boyd, J. N. (1999). Who's smoking, drinking, and using drugs? Time perspective as a predictor of substance use. *Basic and Applied Social Psychology, 21*, 149–164.
Laghi, F., D'Alessio, M., Pallini, S., & Baiocco, R. (2009). Attachment representations and time perspective in adolescence. *Social Indicators Research, 90*, 181–194.
Lazarus, R. S. (1999). *Stress and emotion: A new synthesis*. New York: Springer Publishing Company.
Ledzińska, M. (in preparation). *Time perspective and meta-cognition*.
Lennings, C. J. (1996). Self-efficacy and temporal orientation as predictors of treatment outcome in severely dependent alcoholics. *Alcoholism Treatment Quarterly, 14*, 71–79.
Lischetzke, T., & Eid, M. (2006). Why extraverts are happier than introverts: The role of mood regulation. *Journal of Personality, 74*, 1127–1162.
Matthews, G., Schwean, V. L., Campbell, S. E., Saklofske, D. H., & Mohamed, A. A. R. (2000). Personality, self-regulation and adaptation: A cognitive-social framework. In M. Boekarts, P. R. Pintrich, & M. Zeidner (Eds.), *Handbook of self-regulation* (pp. 171–207). New York: Academic.
Matthews, G., Zeidner, M., & Roberts, R. (2002). *Emotional intelligence: Science and myth*. Cambridge, MA: MIT Press.
Matthews, G., Emo, A. K., Funke, G., Zeidner, M., Roberts, R. D., Costa, P. T., Jr., & Schulze, R. (2006). Emotional intelligence, personality, and task-induced stress. *Journal of Experimental Psychology: Applied, 12*, 96–107.
Matthews, G., Deary, I. J., & Whiteman, M. C. (2009). *Personality traits* (3rd ed.). Cambridge: Cambridge University Press.
Mayer, J. D., Salovey, P., & Caruso, D. (2000). Models of emotional intelligence. In R. Sternberg (Ed.), *Handbook of intelligence* (pp. 92–117). San Francisco: Jossey-Bass.
McAdams, D. P. (2001). The psychology of life stories. *Review of General Psychology, 5*, 100–122.
McGrath, J. E., & Tschan, F. (2004). Time, stress, and coping processes. In J. E. McGrath & F. Tschan (Eds.), *Temporal matters in social psychology: Examining the role of time in the lives of groups and individuals* (pp. 69–98). Washington, DC: American Psychological Association.
Nolen-Hoeksema, S. (1991). Responses to depression and their effects on the duration of depressive episodes. *Journal of Abnormal Psychology, 100*, 569–582.
Nuttin, J. R. (1985). *Future time perspective and motivation: Theory and research method*. Hillsdale: Erlbaum.
Olivares, O. J. (2012). Meaning making, uncertainty reduction, and autobiographical memory: A replication and reinterpretation of the TALE questionnaire. *Psychology, 3*, 192–197.
Peterson, C. (1991). Meaning and measurement of explanatory style. *Psychological Inquiry, 2*, 1–10.
Pillemer, D. B., Picariello, M. L., Law, A., & Reichman, J. S. (1996). Memories of college: The importance of specific educational episodes. In D. C. Rubin (Ed.), *Remembering our past: Studies in autobiographical memory* (pp. 318–337). New York: Cambridge University Press.
Riskind, J. H., & Williams, N. L. (2005). The looming cognitive style and generalized anxiety disorder: Distinctive danger schemas and cognitive phenomenology. *Cognitive Therapy and Research, 29*, 7–27.
Riskind, J. H., & Williams, N. L. (2006). A unique vulnerability common to all anxiety disorders: The looming maladaptive style. In L. B. Alloy & J. H. Riskind (Eds.), *Cognitive vulnerability to emotional disorders* (pp. 175–206). Mahwah: Lawrence Erlbaum Associates Publishers.

Robinson, M. D., & Sedikides, C. (2009). Traits and the self: Toward an integration. In P. J. Corr & G. Matthews (Eds.), *Cambridge handbook of personality psychology* (pp. 457–472). Cambridge: Cambridge University Press.

Rothbart, M. K., Sheese, B. E., & Conradt, E. D. (2009). Childhood temperament. In P. J. Corr & G. Matthews (Eds.), *The Cambridge handbook of personality psychology* (pp. 177–190). Cambridge: Cambridge University Press.

Salovey, P., Mayer, J. D., Goldman, S., Turvey, C., & Palfai, T. (1995). Emotional attention, clarity, and repair: Exploring emotional intelligence using the Trait Meta-Mood Scale. In J. W. Pennebaker (Ed.), *Emotion, disclosure, and health* (pp. 125–154). Washington, DC: American Psychological Association.

Salovey, P., Mayer, J. D., & Caruso, D. (2002). The positive psychology of emotional intelligence. In C. R. Snyder & S. J. Lopez (Eds.), *Handbook of positive psychology* (pp. 159–171). New York: Oxford University Press.

Scherer, K. R. (2001). Appraisal considered as a process of multi-level sequential checking. In K. R. Scherer, A. Schorr, & T. Johnstone (Eds.), *Appraisal processes in emotion: Theory, methods, research* (pp. 90–120). New York/Oxford: Oxford University Press.

Stolarski, M., Bitner, J., & Zimbardo, P. G. (2011). Time perspective, emotional intelligence and discounting of delayed awards. *Time & Society, 20*, 346–363.

Stolarski, M., Zimbardo, P. G., Howell, R. T, & Zhang, J. W. (2012, September 5–8). *Looking for the bright side of life: How to shape your time perspective to become happier?* Paper presented at the 1st international conference on time perspective, Coimbra, Portugal.

Stolarski, M., Ledzińska, M., & Matthews, G. (2013a). Morning is tomorrow, evening is today: Relationships between chronotype and time perspective. *Biological Rhythm Research, 44*, 181–196.

Stolarski, M., Matthews, G., Postek, S., Zimbardo, P. G., & Bitner, J. (2013b). How we feel is a matter of time: Relationships between time perspectives and mood. *Journal of Happiness Studies*, 1–19. Advance online publication. doi:10.1007/s10902-013-9450-y.

Strack, F., Schwarz, N., & Gschneidinger, E. (1985). Happiness and reminiscing: The role of time perspective, affect, and mode of thinking. *Journal of Personality and Social Psychology, 49*, 1460–1469.

Swann, W. B., Jr. (1997). The trouble with change: Self-verification and allegiance to the self. *Psychological Science, 8*, 177–180.

Sword, R. M., Sword, R. K. M., Brunskill, S. R., & Zimbardo, P. G. (2014). Time perspective therapy: A new time-based metaphor therapy for PTSD. *Journal of Loss and Trauma, 19*, 197–201. doi:10.1080/15325024.2013.763632.

Thorne, A., & Nam, V. (2009). The storied construction of personality. Cognitive processes and models. In P. L. Corr & G. Matthews (Eds.), *Cambridge handbook of personality* (pp. 491–505). Cambridge: Cambridge University Press.

Watson, D. (2000). *Mood and temperament*. New York: Guilford Press.

Wells, A., & Matthews, G. (2006). Cognitive vulnerability to anxiety disorders: An integration. In L. B. Alloy & J. H. Riskind (Eds.), *Cognitive vulnerability to emotional disorders* (pp. 303–325). Hillsdale: Lawrence Erlbaum.

Worrell, F. C., & Mello, Z. R. (2007). The reliability and validity of Zimbardo time perspective inventory scores in academically talented adolescents. *Educational and Psychological Measurement, 67*, 487–504.

Zajonc, R. B. (1984). On the primacy of affect. *American Psychologist, 39*, 117–123.

Zaleski, Z. (Ed.). (1994). *Psychology of future orientation*. Lublin: Towarzystwo Naukowe KUL.

Zhang, J. W., & Howell, R. T. (2011). Do time perspectives predict unique variance in life satisfaction beyond personality traits? *Personality and Individual Differences, 50*, 1261–1266.

Zhang, J. W., Howell, R., & Stolarski, M. (2013). Comparing three methods to measure balanced time perspective: The relationship between balanced time perspective and subjective well-being. *Journal of Happiness Studies, 14*, 169–184.

Zimbardo, P. G., & Boyd, J. (1999). Putting time in perspective: A valid, reliable, individual differences metric. *Journal of Personality and Social Psychology, 77*, 1271–1288.
Zimbardo, P. G., & Boyd, J. (2008). *The time paradox: The new psychology of time that can change your life*. New York: Free Press.
Zimbardo, P. G., Keough, K. A., & Boyd, J. N. (1997). Present time perspective as a predictor of risky driving. *Personality and Individual Differences, 23*, 1007–1023.
Zimbardo, P. G., Sword, R. M., & Sword, R. K. M. (2012). *The time cure: Overcoming PTSD with the new psychology of time perspective therapy*. San Francisco: Jossey-Bass.

The Motivational Properties of Future Time Perspective Future Orientation: Different Approaches, Different Cultures

Rachel Seginer and Willy Lens

> Enekdu said, "Dear friend, quickly,
> Before another moment goes by.
> Kill Humbaba…
> Establish your fame, so that forever
> Men will speak of brave Gilgamesh…" (Mitchell 2004, p. 126).

The notion that the future – as represented in the present life space (Lewin 1931) – prompts behavior might be as old as human thinking. Centuries before psychology has become an area of scientific inquiry, the story of Gilgamesh drew on the motivational power of eternal fame for inducing risky behavior. As we follow from the story of Gilgamesh to the Book of Proverbs and leap from there to modern literature for adults and children alike, we find recurrent expressions – each reflecting its time, culture, and audience – of the effect of the future on present behavior. A Kenyan proverb says "treat the earth well; it was not given to you by your parents it was loaned to you by your children".

The founding fathers of contemporary conceptualizations of future thinking were Frank (1939), Israeli (1930, 1936) and Lewin (1939, 1942/1948). Although following different theoretical paths, their work shares three basic assumptions: the construction of the future and its behavior regulation take place in the present, it is *thematic* so that images of the future consist of different content, and the content may be personal or social, realistic or ideal, and reality-based or fantastic. Drawing on these early conjectures, we pursue the thematic approach emphasizing *content*,

Willy Lens (Deceased)

R. Seginer (✉)
Department of Counseling and Human Development, University of Haifa, Haifa, Israel
e-mail: rseginer@edu.haifa.ac.il

W. Lens
Department of Psychology, University of Leuven, Leuven, Belgium

Unit for Professional Training and Services in the Behavioral Sciences (UNIBS), University of the Free State, Bloemfontein, South Africa
e-mail: Willy.Lens@ppw.kuleuven.be

M. Stolarski et al. (eds.), *Time Perspective Theory; Review, Research and Application: Essays in Honor of Philip G. Zimbardo*, DOI 10.1007/978-3-319-07368-2_19,

focus mainly on the personal future, and follow Lewin's proposition that "regardless of whether the individual's picture of the future is correct or incorrect at a given time, this picture deeply affects the mood and the action of the individual at that time." (1942/1948, pp. 103–104).

The chapter consists of three parts. In the first and the second we present our two approaches: *Future time perspective* (FTP) (Lens) and *future orientation* (*FO*) (Seginer); particularly addressing their motivational properties. In the third part we align the two approaches and show their commonalities, complementarity, and weight for continued research.

The two approaches were developed independently, and draw on different psychological bodies of knowledge. The work of Lens since its beginning focused on motivation ("the future is motivation's space", Nuttin and Lens 1985, p. 39). Seginer – as a developmental psychologist studying adolescence – approached FO as "the self in the future" (Coleman et al. 1977), essential for understanding adolescent behavior and personality (Douvan and Adelson 1966). She extended her work to the motivational aspects of FO as she developed the three component model of FO.

Future Time Perspective: Extension and Content Matter

Time perspective (Nuttin and Lens 1985) consists of experiencing the psychological present and looking from the present to the individual's past and future. Thus, our psychological life space (Lewin 1935) is not restricted to the chronological present. Instead, the remembered past and the anticipated future are integrated into it. Depending on which of the three time periods is the most dominant part of their present life space, people are either past- present- or future-oriented (De Volder 1979; Seginer 2009). *Future time perspective (FTP)* refers to the integration of the anticipated future into the psychological present. Its two main characteristics are *extension* (i.e., how far into the chronological future one's psychological future reaches) and *content* (i.e., what does one anticipate in the future).

In line with earlier European scholars (Bergius 1957; Fraisse 1963; Guyau 1902; Lersch 1938; Lewin 1931, 1942), Nuttin viewed the psychological future as a motivational construct: "… the psychological future is not just a learning effect of the past, … the future is the time quality of the goal object; the future is our primary motivational space" (1964, p. 63). Thus, FTP is a cognitive-motivational personality construct: it develops in a motivational setting and has motivational consequences (de Bilde et al. 2011; Lens 1986; Nuttin and Lens 1985).

FTP and Goal Setting

Based on past experiences and other available information, people cognitively elaborate their needs, motives, cravings, desires and fears into specific motivational goals, behavioral plans and projects. Thus, the human need for *achievement* is translated into goals like "to be the first of the class". The need for *power* is transformed into a strong desire to become a national politician, and the need for *competence* into the aspiration to become a top brain surgeon. Each can be analyzed for its content and temporal localization, and each has motivational consequences.

Content

Our basic premise is that people do not anticipate an empty future. Instead, they cognitively foresee two kinds of prospective events: those they want to achieve ("to become a decent housefather") or avoid ("to be a playboy"). These events are the basis for goal setting. Using different terminology, several researchers share this view. Thus, following Markus and Nurius (1986) researchers have studied the ideal, real, and feared "possible selves" to indicate that anticipation of the future has individually relevant content. Seginer (2009) has described it as the *thematic approach*, assessed by hopes and fears. Other approaches conceptualize FTP as *athematic*. Notable among them are the work of Zimbardo and Boyd (1999; Boyd and Zimbardo 2005) and of Worrell et al. (2013) about attitudes toward the future (as one aspect of all three time zones). More recently Carelli et al. (2011; this volume) elaborated the Zimbardo-Boyd scale to assess FTP by distinguishing a positive and a negative FTP, analogous to Zimbardo-Boyd's Past-Positive and Past-Negative scales. Anticipating a predominantly positive or negative future implies that people at least implicitly consider pleasant and unpleasant future events (See also Worrell et al. 2013).

Temporal Localization

For Lewin (1931) extension of the psychological life-space was based on the temporal displacement of goals into the future. Drawing on Lewin, the second dimension of FTP pertains to its length: the more goals and fears are set in the more distant future the longer is the individual's FTP. Altogether, the FTP ranges from very short ("to have a drink") to very long ("to become a famous surgeon"). Thus, while the present temporal life space of people with a short FTP includes only the very near future, that of people with a long FTP includes also goals in the distant future. Moreover, these people have no problem striving for events or action-outcomes in the distant future.

One may even formulate goals for the afterlife ("I hope our children stay good friends after we die"). To assess it, Boyd and Zimbardo (1997; Zimbardo and Boyd 2009) developed the transcendental time perspective scale.

Temporal Localization and Delay of Gratification

Conceptualization of FTP as goal setting in the near or distant future has much in common with the delay of gratification construct (Mischel 1974, 1981). Setting goals in the near or distant future is like choosing between a smaller immediate reward and a higher value delayed reward. Nonetheless, the two approaches differ in two ways.

One is *time span*. Mischel's children had to wait for a maximum of 20 min while important life goals are situated in the distant future. The second is *passivity* vs. *activity*. In Mischel's experiment the children *wait*ed passively to receive the preferred reward while one has to *work* to achieve goals. Moreover, for Mischel, waiting is frustrating whereas pursuing a distant goal may involve the achievement of rewarding subgoals, or be gratifying by itself. Thus, one can simultaneously pursue future goals and enjoy the present (Lens 2006).

Motivational Effects of FTP

Extension and content of FTP have motivational consequences. Each is discussed separately.

Extension of FTP

Extension of FTP is positively related to motivation: overall, people with a longer FTP have higher motivation. Underlying it is the negative correlation between FTP extension (length) and prospective psychological distance (Gjesme 1982, 1996; Lens 1996). Ten years is psychologically closer for people with long FTP than with short FTP (Lens and Moreas 1994). This has two implications. One is that the longer their FTP, the easier it is for people to see the instrumentality of present actions for future outcomes, anticipate the future implications of present actions, and thus set their plans and projects in the more distant future. The *utility* or *instrumental value* of present actions for distant goals increases with longer FTP.

Drawing on *expectancy x value theories of motivation* (Feather 1982; Eccles and Wigfield 2002) it was expected and found that perceived instrumentality is positively related to motivation (Creten et al. 2001; De Volder and Lens 1982; Husman and Lens 1999; Husman and Shell 2008; Lens and Decruyenaere 1991; Kover and Worrell 2010; Miller et al. 1999). The second implication draws on the conceptualization of FTP as an individual disposition to ascribe higher valence to goals, even if more remote in time. Thus, although the anticipated value of a goal decreases the more delayed it is (Rachlin 1995), for people with a longer FTP (whose psychological distance towards a future goal is shorter), the anticipated value of the future goal decreases less steeply.

To summarize, FTP has a cognitive and a dynamic components (De Volder and Lens 1982). The cognitive component refers to the capacity to anticipate events and behavioral outcomes in the (distant) future. The dynamic component refers to the incentive value of delayed goals: it decreases (because of the delay) less for people with a longer FTP.

Content of FTP Matters

Content may relate to multiple meanings. In the FTP conceptualization, content pertains to the motivational qualities of future goals as specifically indicated by intrinsic and extrinsic goals and motivation (Deci and Ryan 2000; Lens and Vansteenkiste 2006)

Intrinsic vs. Extrinsic Motivation

When one asks students why they study or go to school, future goals are among their important reasons. They want to succeed in the exams, go to college, become a plumber, hairdresser or a psychiatrist. Such future goals create *extrinsic motivation. Extrinsic motivation* means that one is motivated to achieve an outcome of an activity that is not inherently related to that activity as such. The activity is instrumental for achieving something outside it. *Intrinsic motivation* means that one is doing something because one enjoys doing it. The behavior itself is the goal: the behavior is *auto-telic*.

Many of our daily activities are both intrinsically and extrinsically motivated (e.g., studying a course on motivation is interesting but also helps passing the exam). Hence, plausibly, the total strength of motivation can be increased by increasing one or both components. Parents, teachers and employers frequently use extrinsic rewards and future outcomes to enhance student or workers' motivation. Most of us are familiar with the (good) advice "Do your best at school, it is so important for your future".

But – and more so in educational psychology than in organizational psychology – extrinsic motivation is of lower quality than intrinsic motivation, and may even undermine intrinsic motivation (Deci 1975; Lepper and Greene 1978; Pintrich and Schunk 2002). Consequently, motivating students by emphasizing future goals contingent on academic success may interfere with high quality intrinsic motivation and result in a lower quality motivation.

Autonomous Versus Controlled Motivation and Intrinsic Versus Extrinsic Goals

Based on empirical results showing that different types of extrinsic motivation differ in the quality of their outcomes, Self-Determination Theory (SDT; Deci and Ryan 2000, 2002; Vansteenkiste et al. 2006) has elaborated its conceptualization so that it now consists of *autonomous* and *controlled* motivation and *intrinsic* and *extrinsic* goals. Based on many empirical studies, SDT proposes that autonomous motivation has more adaptive outcomes than controlled motivation and that pursuing intrinsic goals is better than pursuing extrinsic goals. Future goals are sources of extrinsic motivation, but their quality (i.e., their (mal)adaptive consequences for learning and well-being) depends on their *content (intrinsic* versus *extrinsic) and on the motivation (autonomous* versus *controlled) for pursuing them.* Pursuing intrinsic rather than extrinsic future goals and being prompted by autonomous and not by controlled motivation is more adaptive for optimal functioning and well-being.

The "What" of Goal Pursuit

SDT makes a distinction between two types of goal contents: intrinsic versus extrinsic goals. Examples of *intrinsic goals* are self-development, physical fitness, competence, community contributions, affiliation, and altruism. Examples of extrinsic goals are financial success, power, status, physical attractiveness. Much empirical evidence shows that striving for intrinsic rather than extrinsic goals results in such positive outcomes as persistence, positive affect, satisfaction, adaptive learning strategies, and well-being (Kasser and Ryan 2001; Vansteenkiste et al. 2006, 2008). The reason being that intrinsic (future) goals satisfy (and extrinsic goals frustrate) the three innate basic psychological needs for *autonomy* (self-determination), *competence*, and *relatedness*.

The "Why" of Goal Pursuit

Intrinsic motivation is always *autonomous motivation*: its perceived locus of causality is internal (e.g., intrinsic interest, enjoyment, task-inherent satisfaction). However, *extrinsic motivation may also have qualities of autonomous motivation*. This is related to two types of goal regulation: identified and integrated. When a goal is perceived as personally important (e.g., to become a psychologist), the regulation of the goal pursuit is *identified regulation*. When the external reason or future goal is perceived as totally congruent with one's true self (e.g., studying medicine to join "doctors without borders") the regulation of the goal pursuit is integrated (*integrated regulation*). Altogether, autonomous motivation includes intrinsic motivation and future goals whose pursuit is characterized by *identified* or *integrated* behavior regulation.

Extrinsic motivation has the qualities of controlled *motivation* when regulation is external or introjected. Behavior done for achieving external goals or for totally external reasons (e.g., rewards, avoid punishment, imposed rules) is *externally regulated*. Behavior prompted by external reasons which are not accepted as personally important is pursued by *introjected regulation* (e.g., doing something to avoid feelings of guilt or shame).

In sum, future goals create instrumental *extrinsic* motivation. However, what really matters is their content and the reasons underlying their pursuit. It is more optimal to strive for goals that are autonomously motivating (than for externally motivated goals). Such goals are intrinsic goals and extrinsic goals whose regulation is identified or integrated. Extrinsic goals whose regulation is external or introjected (i.e., controlled) are less optimal.

Empirical Evidence

We finish this section by summarizing findings which validate SDT based propositions. Examining internal regulation, our findings showed that stressing the personally important consequences of present learning tasks enhanced task-orientation and decreased the less adaptive performance-orientation for students who were initially intrinsically or extrinsically motivated (Simons et al. 2000).

In two additional experiments, the effect of *intrinsic* vs. *extrinsic goals* was tested on physical education students learning the Tae Bo. In study I, the students participated in an experiment consisting of three induced conditions: intrinsic goals, extrinsic goals, and no future goals. Findings showed significant differences between the three conditions: students in the intrinsic goal condition scored higher on task- versus ego-involvement and level of performance. Moreover, the effect of goal content on academic performance was fully mediated by students' task-orientation (Vansteenkiste et al. 2007).

Study II included a fourth condition, consisting of "future content-free" (i.e., learning Tae Bo was very useful for their future, without an intrinsic or extrinsic goal). Findings showed no significant differences between the "no-future control condition" and the "future content-free condition". Participants in these two conditions scored significantly lower than those in the intrinsic goal condition but significantly higher than those in the extrinsic goal condition. Moreover, inducing these goals in an *autonomy-supportive*, rather than a controlling way, resulted in the same motivational and behavior benefits as future intrinsic goal framing (Vansteenkiste et al. 2004).

While these studies showed the stronger effect of intrinsic rather than extrinsic goals, the question still remained whether adding an extrinsic future goal to an intrinsic one would result in higher scores than intrinsic goals only. Contrary to predictions based on "expectancy x value" theories but in line with SDT, the intrinsic goal condition scored best, the extrinsic goal condition worst, and the double-goal condition fell in between (Vansteenkiste et al. 2004). Moreover, pursuing intrinsic goals is more adaptive, even in a context promoting extrinsic goals (Vansteenkiste et al. 2008). Finally, examining content similarity of present activity and future goal showed that *endogenous instrumentality* (i.e., high content similarity) yields a more adaptive motivational and behavioral pattern, and intrinsic future goals independently made the motivational and behavioral pattern even more conducive to optimal performance (Simons et al. 2003, 2004).

Concluding Remark

Stressing the motivational importance of FTP does not mean that past and present time perspectives are motivationally irrelevant. Past events will be remembered because of their affective or motivational importance (Nuttin and Lens 1985, p. 91). Positive and negative past perspectives may function respectively as positive and negative models for the future. Future goals are then based on past experiences. Past time perspectives can affect present and future perspectives (Stolarski et al. in press). Also Present-Hedonic and Present Fatalistic perspectives have of course immediate motivational implications. A present-hedonic orientation requires pursuing immediate hedonic pleasure. Being present oriented for fatalistic reasons will de-motivate people because such people are convinced that they have no control over their future (Potgieter et al. 2011).

Future Orientation: A Three-Component Model

The conceptualization of future orientation (FO) is based on three premises. One, FO consists of a subjective image about the future. Notably, it is not about predicting the future but about the *hopes* individuals have about the future and the *fears* they would like to avoid. Second, this image is thematic (Nuttin and Lens 1985); as individuals imagine the future they relate to events and experiences which can be grouped to life domains such as education, work, and family. Third, FO is a multi-dimensional construct. Like Nurmi's model (1991) it consists of three components.

The Three Component Model

The Starting Point

Work carried out on FO for many years by psychologists (Douvan and Adelson 1966; Gillespie and Allport 1955; Gjesme 1983; Mönks 1968; Nurmi 1991; Nuttin and Lens 1985; Poole and Cooney 1987; Raynor and Entin 1982; Seginer 1988; Trommsdorff and Lamm 1980) and sociologists (Cantril 1965) was uni-dimensional. It focused on the cognitive representation of the future, and like the FTP approach examined two questions: how far into the future individuals projected themselves (Lessing 1972) and set their goals (Nuttin and Lens 1985), and what themes were included in their constructed future.

Analyses showed that when asked about their hopes and fears (or concerns) about the future individuals list various prospective events and experiences (Nurmi

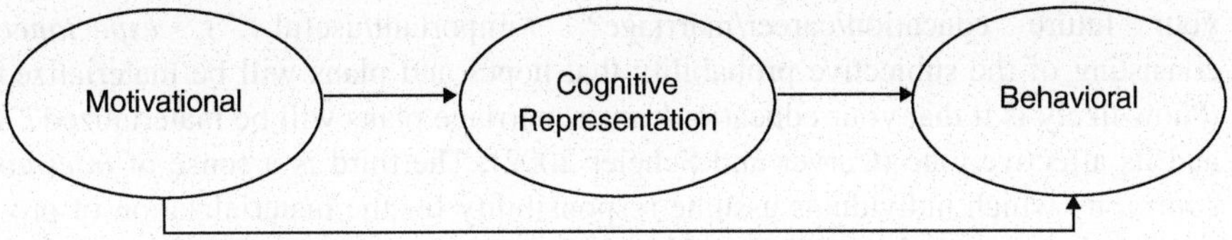

Fig. 1 The future orientation three-component model

1989; Seginer and Schlesinger 1998; Trommsdorff et al. 1979). Altogether, adolescents from different cultural settings include in their subjective future both common and culture-specific future life domains. They commonly relate to a core of three domains: education, work and career (competence domains), and marriage and family (relational domain) (Nurmi et al. 1995; Seginer 2008). The culture-specific life domains listed by adolescents pertain to leisure by Australians (Poole and Cooney 1987), property by Finns (Nurmi and Pulliainen 1991), Military service by Finn boys (Nurmi et al. 1995), Jewish girls and boys and Druze boys in Israel (Seginer and Halabi-Kheir 1998), and the community by Muslims in Israel (Seginer 1988).

Developing the Model

The narrowness of a theoretical construct consisting of only the cognitive representation of the future led Nurmi (1991) and Seginer (1995, 2009; Seginer et al. 1991, 2004) to construct multi-dimensional FO models. The present model expanded the FO uni-dimensional conceptualization. Taking the cognitive representation as its starting point, it was developed to answer two basic questions: what prompts thinking about the future (i.e., cognitive representation) and what are its outcomes.

Drawing on a basic premise that cognitive representation is induced by motivational forces and results in behavior, the expanded model consists of motivational, cognitive representation, and behavioral components. Together they form a multiple-step model in which the motivational component affects the cognitive and the behavioral components, and the cognitive component affects the behavioral component (see also Fig. 1). The components are theoretical and indicated by empirical variables described below. Moreover, the model applies to different life domains.

The Motivational Component

Guided by motivation theory (Atkinson 1964; Eccles and Wigfield 2002) and FO conceptualization (Nuttin and Lens 1985; Trommsdorff 1983), three variables indicate this component: the *value* of the prospective life domain ("how do you evaluate your future education/career/marriage?" "important/useful..."); *expectance* consisting of the subjective probability that hopes and plans will be materialized ("how likely is it that your education/career/marriage plans will be materialized?") and its affective tone (Carver and Scheier 2002). The third is a sense of *internal control* by which individuals assume responsibility for the materialization of prospective hopes and plans ("What effect will each of the factors listed below have on the realization of your plans about education/career/marriage?" "Personal ability/personal effort/self esteem...").

The Cognitive Representation Component

Underlying its conceptualization are two assumptions: (1) that future thinking consists of both hopes and fears ("Thinking about the future how often do you think hopefully/worry about each of the following issues?" "My education/career/marriage"), and (2) individuals differ in how often they think about various life domains ("How often do think about or plan your education/career/marriage?").

The Behavioral Component

Two variables indicate the behavioral component: exploration and commitment. *Exploration* relates to seeking information and advice regarding future options and testing if they fit personal abilities and values, social expectations and environmental circumstances (Lewin 1939) ("Which of the following things have you been doing now to get you closer to realizing your education/career/marriage plan?" "Talking to people/checking whether this education/career/marriage fits me..."). Commitment consists of the decision to pursue one option and results in "a sense of knowing where one is going" (Erikson 1968, p. 165) ("I have clear plans concerning my education/career/marriage"). Both add to the instrumentality of FO for the achievement of future hopes, goals, and plans.

Domain Specificity

Drawing on the proposition that "...time perspective ...cannot be conceived independently of its content..." (Nuttin and Lens 1985, p. 23), the three-component model is domain specific. Thus, the thematic approach initially used to describe the cognitive representation of the future also applies to the extended model, and has been tested on different life domains.

Empirical Evidence

Four questions have guided the empirical tests of the three component model. Together, they relate to the motivational power FO has to induce educational and developmental outcomes in interpersonal and socio-cultural context. However, although each question is stated separately, the analyses they have guided relate to some or all of them simultaneously. Specifically, the four questions ask (1) whether the multiple-step three-component model can be empirically estimated, (2) what is the effect of the model on developmental outcomes, (3) does it indicate domain specificity, so that testing the model and its outcomes for different life domains shows similar or different results, and (4) does context matter? Here we focus mainly on the cultural milieu. Obviously, context relates to additional indicators ranging from intrapersonal characteristics (personality, age, gender) to family and other aspects of the microsystem (Seginer 2009).

Research carried out in the last decade was conducted mainly with Jewish and Arab adolescents in Israel, but also with Israeli Jewish emerging adults and adults, and analyzed by structural equation modeling (SEM). These analyses show that applying it to competence (higher education, work and career) or relational (marriage and family) life domains, tested by itself or in relation to interpersonal relationships, the model has been empirically estimated. Three findings are especially pertinent here.

1. **The effect of the motivational component**. Across all our analyses (Seginer 2009; Seginer and Mahajna 2012a, b; Seginer and Shoyer 2012; Seginer et al. 2004) the motivational component has a positive effect on both the cognitive and the behavioral components of the model. Thus, whether its domain-specific content relates to education, work, or family, the value, expectance, and internal control – which are the empirical indicators of the motivational component – prompt two processes: thinking about the future (cognitive representation), and doing work toward the materialization of plans in that life domain (the behavioral component). This work consists of exploring future options and examining their suitability, and engaging in decision making (the behavioral component).
2. **FO prompts behavior**. FO – as conceptualized in terms of the three component model – has a positive effect on adolescents' academic achievement, the achieved identity of emerging adults (Seginer and Ablin 2012), and adults' adjustment to major life changes (Seginer 2009). Here, the focus is on academic achievement. Research carried out with high school students, including secular Jewish girls and boys, ultra orthodox Jewish girls (Seginer 2009), and Muslim girls and boys in Israel (Seginer and Mahajna 2012a, b) all show that when the three component model is tested on a *competence* domain (i.e., education, work and career), the effect of FO on school reported academic achievement is positive.
3. **Culture and gender moderate the FO-behavior link**. When the model applies to the *relational* domain (marriage and family) the results vary by cultural milieu and gender. Specifically, for non-observant Jewish girls and boys and for Muslim boys in Israel the effect of marriage and family on academic achievement is low

and non significant. For Muslim girls in Israel the effect is negative, and for the ultra-orthodox Jewish girls it is positive. The explanation draws on two considerations. One is extension into the future. As FTP research shows, all other things being equal, the closer in time the goal is the higher is its motivational effect. Muslim girls in Israel and ultra-orthodox Jewish girls marry younger than the other groups (Israel Central Bureau of Statistics 2011).

The second consideration relates to the meaning of marriage and family for each of these groups, and thus intertwined with the socio-cultural context. Jewish non-observant girls and boys and Muslim boys in Israel pursue competence domains goals and plans before those related to marriage and family, and high school grades are unrelated to marriage and family. For girls in the Jewish ultra-orthodox and Muslim societies in Israel, both religious societies, the meaning of marriage and family is strongly related to the norm of early marriage. However, the reality of married women and the responsibilities of mothers in these societies differ.

Muslim women take care of the household and bring up their children. Thus, the negative effect of marriage and family on academic achievement for Muslim girls in Israel indicates a twofold conflict between working towards hopes, goals and plans in the competence and the relational domains. One is to pursue an *emancipated path* by which higher education and possibly also career precede marriage. The other is to follow the *traditional path*: get married at an early age and give up higher education. Both are voiced in girls' narratives about the future (Seginer and Mahajna 2012b): "I hope to graduate from high school, go on with my university education and have no intention to get married before I get my degree and secure myself a good future", and "what happens in the future is that I will end up in the kitchen. I am getting married in the summer, so why should I worry about school".

In the Jewish ultra-orthodox society women's responsibility includes children's education and the family income, so that husbands devote themselves to religious learning. Thus, for them the competence and relational domains are positively related. The path to being good wives and mothers starts at school (Seginer 2010). This is expressed in a school's slogan "raising the Jewish mothers of tomorrow" (Fishkoff 2003, p. 246) and in the girls' narratives: "…I want to work hard and study to reach the goal [becoming school teacher] because education is also important for my future children", and "… to graduate from high school, get all necessary certificates (Matriculation, psychometric test) and then study toward an occupation that allows me to earn money and raise a family" (Dekel 2009).

Summary

The motivational properties of the three component model draw on two processes. One is inherent to the model and indicated by the paths from the motivational component to the cognitive and the behavioral motivational components. The second is indicated by the path from the behavioral component (in itself linked to the motivational component both directly and indirectly via the cognitive component) to academic achievement for high school students, achieved identity for emerging adults, and adjustment to major transition for adults (Seginer 2009). However, whereas the motivational power of the motivational component applies across different life domains (content), gender, age (adolescents and mothers alike) (Seginer and Shoyer 2012) and cultural milieu, the effect of FO on academic achievement is domain by culture specific.

Aligning the FTP and the FO Approaches

Originating from different psychological paradigms, the FTP and the FO approaches used different conceptualizations, terminologies, and research designs to study a similar question: factors promoting and obstructing the motivational effect of the psychological future on present behavior. They share an interest in learning and schooling. However, FTP research uses experimental designs and hence assesses contrived learning tasks and FO research uses field research and assesses school reported academic achievement. The aim of this concluding section is to bridge the two approaches and point out new questions based on their alignment. Seemingly, the two approaches differ on two major issues related to content: its meaning, and endogenous instrumentality (content similarity between goals and behavior).

The Meaning of Content

In the FTP approach the content of goals relates to their motivational properties whereas FO examines the motivational properties – as well as the cognitive representation and behavioral engagement – of future life domains such as education, career (competence domains) and marriage and family (relational domain). Particularly, FTP distinguishes between *intrinsic* and *extrinsic* goals and autonomous vs. controlled motivation whereas FO assesses the *extent* of intrinsic motivation, as indicated by the value (important/central to my life/enriching) attributed to the domain's hopes, goals and plans, and sense of internal of control attributed to their materialization.

Although by itself the subjective probability of materializing one's hopes, goals and plans (expectance) may apply to extrinsic and intrinsic goals, its commonality with the value and internal control indicators of the motivation component enhances its intrinsic properties. Aligning the two approaches prompts several questions. One addresses the advantages of intrinsic over extrinsic motivation in the FO three-component model, and the other relates to expanding the FTP research to additional competence and relational life domains.

Endogenous Instrumentality

FTP findings that content similarity between goals and behavior enhances the motivational power of goals have been supported by two FO studies in which Jewish adolescents (Seginer 2009) and emerging adults (Seginer and Ablin 2012) were tested. However, as research is carried out among adolescent girls growing up in religious settings such as the Jewish ultra-orthodox (Dekel 2009; Seginer 2009) and the Muslim society in Israel (Seginer and Mahajna 2012a), endogenous instrumentality becomes culture specific. Particularly, the cultural meaning attributed to marriage and family resulted in a significant negative effect of FO on academic achievement among Muslim girls (Seginer and Mahajna 2012a) and positive effect among Jewish ultra-orthodox girls (Seginer 2009). Aligning the two approaches, the effect of endogenous instrumentality in traditional settings may be examined by applying it to the FTP approach.

In sum, aligning the FTP and the FO approaches brings to the fore their unique contributions as well as their commonalities in describing and explaining the motivational relevance of the psychological future to present behavior. Thus, and together with the time perspective approach developed by Zimbardo and Boyd (1999; Boyd and Zimbardo 2005) and Worrell et al. (2013) they bring additional support to the proposition that "…the mental construct called the 'future' is the building site of constructive behavior and human progress" (Nuttin and Lens 1985, p. 40).

References

Atkinson, J. W. (1964). *An introduction to motivation*. Princeton: Van Nostrand.

Bergius, R. (1957). *Formen des Zukunfsterlebens [Types of experiencing the future]*. Munich: Johann Ambrosius Barth.

Boyd, J. N., & Zimbardo, P. G. (1997). Constructing time after death: The transcendental –future time perspective. *Time and Society, 6*, 5–24.

Boyd, J. N., & Zimbardo, P. G. (2005). Time perspective, health, and risk-taking. In A. Strathman & J. Joireman (Eds.), *Understanding behavior in the context of time: Theory, research, and applications* (pp. 85–107). Mahwah: Erlbaum.

Cantril, H. (1965). *The pattern of human concerns*. New Brunswick: Rutgers University Press.

Carelli, M. G., Wiberg, B., & Wiberg, M. (2011). Developmental and construct validation of the Swedish Zimbardo Time Perspective Inventory. *European Journal of Psychological Assessment, 27*, 220–227.

Carver, C. S., & Scheier, M. F. (2002). Optimism. In C. R. Snyder & S. J. Lopez (Eds.), *Handbook of positive psychology* (pp. 231–243). New York: Oxford University Press.

Coleman, J., Herzberg, J., & Morris, M. (1977). Identity in adolescence: Present and future self concepts. *Journal of Youth and Adolescence, 6*, 63–75.

Creten, H., Lens, W., & Simons, J. (2001). The role of perceived instrumentality in student motivation. In A. Efklides, J. Kuhl, & R. M. Sorrentino (Eds.), *Trends and prospects in motivation research* (pp. 37–45). Dordrecht: Kluwer Academic Publishers.

de Bilde, J., Vansteenkiste, M., & Lens, W. (2011). Understanding the association between future time perspective and self-regulated learning through the lens of self-determination theory. *Learning and Instruction, 21*, 332–344.

De Volder, M. (1979). Time orientation: A review. *Psychologica Belgica, 19*, 61–79.
De Volder, M., & Lens, W. (1982). Academic achievement and future time perspective as a cognitive-motivational concept. *Journal of Personality and Social Psychology, 42*, 566–571.
Deci, E. L. (1975). *Intrinsic motivation*. New York: Plenum.
Deci, E. L., & Ryan, R. M. (2000). The "What" and "Why" of goal pursuits: Human needs and the self-determination of behavior. *Psychological Inquiry, 11*, 227–268.
Deci, E. L., & Ryan, R. M. (2002). *Handbook of self-determination research*. Rochester: University of Rochester Press.
Dekel, S. (2009). *The world of ultra-orthodox girls: An ecological analysis of women's roles and future orientation*. Doctoral dissertation, University of Haifa, Israel.
Douvan, E., & Adelson, J. (1966). *The Adolescent experience*. New York: Wiley.
Eccles, J. S., & Wigfield, A. (2002). Motivational beliefs, values, and goals. *Annual Review of Psychology, 53*, 109–132.
Erikson, E. H. (1968). *Identity, youth and crisis*. New York: Norton.
Feather, N. T. (1982). *Expectations and actions: Expectancy-value models in psychology*. Hillsdale: Erlbaum.
Fishkoff, S. (2003). *The Rebbe's army: Inside the world of Habad-Lubavitch*. New York: Schocken Books.
Fraisse, P. (1963). *The psychology of time*. Westport: Greenwood.
Frank, L. K. (1939). Time perspectives. *Journal of Social Philosophy, 4*, 293–312.
Gillespie, J. M., & Allport, G. W. (1955). *Youth's outlook on the future; a cross-national study*. Garden City/New York: Doubleday.
Gjesme, T. (1982). Psychological goal distance: The lost dimension in achievement motivation research. In W. Hacker, W. Volpert, & M. von Cranach (Eds.), *Cognitive and motivational aspects of action* (pp. 86–98). Amsterdam: North Holland.
Gjesme, T. (1983). On the concept of future time orientation: Considerations of some functions' and measurements' implications. *International Journal of Psychology, 18*, 443–461.
Gjesme, T. (1996). Future-time orientation and motivation. In T. Gjesme & R. Nygard (Eds.), *Advances in motivation* (pp. 210–224). Oslo: Scandinavian University Press.
Guyau, J. M. (1902). *La genése de l'idée de temps* [The origin of the concept of time]. Paris: Alcan.
Husman, J., & Lens, W. (1999). The role of the future in student motivation. *Educational Psychologist, 34*, 113–125.
Husman, J., & Shell, D. F. (2008). Beliefs and perceptions about the future: A measurement of future time perspective. *Learning and Individual Differences, 18*, 166–175.
Israel Central Bureau of Statistics. (2011). *Women and men*. . (Hebrew): Central Bureau of Statistics.
Israeli, N. (1930). Some aspects of the social psychology of futurism. *Journal of Abnormal and Social Psychology, 25*, 121–132.
Israeli, N. (1936). The psychology of prediction: Judgments relating of the past and future. *Psychological Exchange, 4*, 129–132.
Kasser, T., & Ryan, R. M. (2001). Be careful what you wish for: Optimal functioning and the relative attainment of intrinsic and extrinsic goals. In P. Schmuck & K. M. Sheldon (Eds.), *Life goals and well-being: Towards a positive psychology of human striving* (pp. 116–131). Seattle: Hogrefe & Huber Publishers.
Kover, D. J., & Worrell, F. C. (2010). The influence of instrumentality beliefs on intrinsic motivation: A study of high-achieving adolescents. *Journal of Advanced Academics, 21*, 470–498.
Lens, W. (1986). Future time perspective: A cognitive-motivational concept. In D. R. Brown & J. Veroff (Eds.), *Frontiers of motivational psychology* (pp. 173–190). New York: Springer.
Lens, W. (1996, August 16–21). *Goal setting and future time perspective in student motivation*. Paper presented at the 26th international congress of psychology, Montreal (Abstracts, p. 404). *International Journal of Psychology, 27*, 337.
Lens, W. (2006). Future time perspective: A psychological approach. In Z. Uchnast (Ed.), *Psychology of time: Theoretical and empirical approaches* (pp. 51–64). Lublin: Wydawnictwo KUL.

Lens, W., & Decruyenaere, M. (1991). Motivation and demotivation in secondary education: Student characteristics. *Learning and Instruction, 1*, 145–159.
Lens, W., & Moreas, M. A. (1994). Future time perspective: An individual and a societal approach. In Z. Zaleski (Ed.), *Psychology of future orientation* (pp. 23–38). Lublin: Towarzystwo Naukowe KUL.
Lens, W., & Vansteenkiste, M. (2006). Motivation: About the "why" and "what for" of human behavior. In K. Pawlik & G. d'Ydewalle (Eds.), *Psychological concepts: An international historical perspective* (pp. 249–270). Hove: Psychology Press.
Lepper, M. R., & Greene, D. (1978). *The hidden costs of reward*. Hillsdale: Erlbaum.
Lersch, P. (1938). *Aufbau der Person [Construction of the person]*. Munich: Johann Ambrosius Barth.
Lessing, E. E. (1972). Extension of personal future time perspective, age and life satisfaction of children and adolescents. *Developmental Psychology, 6*, 457–468.
Lewin, K. (1931). An address given in February 1931 at a convention on problems of the Montessori Method. *Die Neue Erziehung, 2*, 99–103.
Lewin, K. (1935). *A dynamic theory of personality: Selected papers*. New York: McGraw-Hill.
Lewin, K. (1939). Field theory and experiment in social psychology. *American Journal of Sociology, 44*, 868–896.
Lewin, K. (1942/1948). Time perspective and morale. In K. Lewin (Ed.), *Resolving social conflict* (pp. 103–124). New York: Harper & Brothers Publishers.
Markus, H., & Nurius, P. (1986). Possible selves. *American Psychologist, 41*, 954–969.
Miller, R., DeBacker, T. K., & Greene, B. A. (1999). Perceived instrumentality and academics: The link to task valuing. *Journal of Instructional Psychology, 26*, 250–260.
Mischel, W. (1974). Processes in delay of gratification. In L. Berkowitz (Ed.), *Advances in experimental social psychology* (Vol. 7). New York: Academic.
Mischel, W. (1981). Objective and subjective rules for delay of gratification. In G. Ydewalle & W. Lens (Eds.), *Cognition in human motivation and learning* (pp. 33–58). Leuven/Hillsdale: Leuven University Press/Erlbaum.
Mitchell, S. (2004). *Gilgamesh: A new English version*. New York: Free Press.
Mönks, F. (1968). Future time perspective in adolescents. *Human Development, 11*, 107–123.
Nurmi, J. E. (1989). Development of orientation to the future during early adolescence: A four-year longitudinal study and two cross-sectional comparisons. *International Journal of Psychology, 24*, 195–214.
Nurmi, J. E. (1991). How do adolescents see their future? A review of the development of future orientation and planning. *Developmental Review, 11*, 1–59.
Nurmi, J. E., & Pulliainen, H. (1991). The changing parent–child relationship, self-esteem, and intelligence as determinants of orientation to the future during early adolescence. *Journal of Adolescence, 14*, 35–51.
Nurmi, J.-E., Seginer, R., & Poole, M. (1995). Searching for the future in different environments: A comparison of Australian, Finnish and Israeli adolescents' future orientation, explorations and commitments. In P. Noack, M. Hofer, & J. Youniss (Eds.), *Psychological responses to social change: Human development in changing environments* (pp. 219-238). Berlin: De Gruyter.
Nuttin, J. (1964). The future time perspective in human motivation and learning. In *Proceedings of the 17th international congress of psychology* (pp. 60–82). Amsterdam: North-Holland.
Nuttin, J., & Lens, W. (1985). *Future time perspective and motivation: Theory and research method*. Leuven/Belgium/Hillsdale: Leuven University Press/Erlbaum.
Pintrich, P. R., & Schunk, D. H. (2002). *Motivation in education: Theory, research, and applications*. Upper Saddle River: Prentice Hall.
Poole, M. E., & Cooney, G. H. (1987). Orientation to the future: A comparison of adolescents in Australia and Singapore. *Journal of Youth and Adolescence, 16*, 129–151.
Potgieter, J. C., Heyns, P. M., & Lens, W. (2011). The time perspective of the Alzheimer caregiver. *Dementia, 54*, 321–333.

Rachlin, H. (1995). Self-control: Beyond commitment. *Behavioral and Brain Sciences, 18*, 109–159.

Raynor, J. O., & Entin, E. E. (1982). *Motivation, career striving, and aging*. New York: Hemisphere.

Seginer, R. (1988). Adolescents facing the future: Cultural and socio-political perspectives. *Youth and Society, 19*, 314–333.

Seginer, R. (1995). The hopes and fears of anticipated adulthood: Adolescent future orientation in cross-cultural context. In G. Trommsdorff (Hsg.), *Kinderheit und Jugend im Kulturvergleich* (pp. 225–247). Weinheim: Juventa.

Seginer, R. (2008). Future orientation in times of threat and challenge: How resilient adolescents construct their future. *International Journal of Behavioral Development, 32*, 272–282.

Seginer, R. (2009). *Future orientation: Developmental and ecological perspectives*. New York: Springer.

Seginer, R. (2010, May). Adolescent girls' future orientation in the context of two cultural religious settings in Israel: Muslim and Jewish. Paper presented in the Jacobs Foundation Conference *The role of values and religion in youth development: A culture-informed perspective* (G. Trommsdorff and X. Chen, conveners). Schlos Marbach, Germany.

Seginer, R., & Ablin, E. (2012). *Future orientation and achieved identity in emerging adulthood: A longitudinal analysis*.

Seginer, R., & Halabi-Kheir, H. (1998). Adolescent passage to adulthood: Future orientation in the context of culture, age, and gender. *International Journal of Intercultural relations, 22*, 309–328.

Seginer, R., & Mahajna, S. (2012a). With God's help: The future orientation of Palestinian girls in Israel growing up Muslim. In G. Trommsdorff & X. Chen (Eds.), *Values, religion, and culture in adolescent development* (pp. 253–270). New York: Cambridge University Press.

Seginer, R., & Mahajna, S. (2012b, July). From high school to adulthood: The future orientation of Muslim adolescent girls and boys in Israel. In C. Cooper & R. Seginer (Chairpersons). *Transition from adolescence to early adulthood in three multicultural societies: Navigating cultures, immigration, and gender*. Symposium conducted at the 22nd biennial meeting of the International Society for the Study of Behavioral Development. Edmonton, Alberta, Canada.

Seginer, R., & Schlesinger, R. (1998). Adolescents' future orientation in time and place: The case of the Israeli kibbutz. *International Journal of Behavioral Development, 22*, 151–167.

Seginer, R., & Shoyer, S. (2012). How mothers affect adolescents' future orientation: A two source analysis. *Japanese Psychological Research, 54*, 310–320.

Seginer, R., Nurmi, J.-E., & Poole, M. (1991). *Adolescent future orientation in cross-cultural perspectives*. Paper presented in the 11th meeting of International Society for the Study of Behavioral Development. Minneapolis, MN.

Seginer, R., Vermulst, A., & Shoyer, S. (2004). The indirect link between perceived parenting and adolescent future orientation: A multiple-step analysis. *International Journal of Behavioral Development, 28*, 365–378.

Simons, J., Dewitte, S., & Lens, W. (2000). Wanting to have versus wanting to be: The effect of perceived instrumentality on goal orientation. *British Journal of Psychology, 91*, 335–351.

Simons, J., Dewitte, S., & Lens, W. (2003). "Don't do it for me, do it for yourself". Stressing the personal relevance enhances motivation in physical education. *Journal of Sport and Exercise Psychology, 25*, 145–160.

Simons, J., Vansteenkiste, M., Lens, W., & Lacante, M. (2004). Placing motivation and future time perspective theory in a temporal perspective. *Educational Psychology Review, 16*, 121–139.

Stolarski, M., Matthews, G., Postek, S., Zimbardo, P. G., & Bitner, J. (in press). How we feel is a matter of time: Relationships between time perspectives and mood. *Journal of Happiness Studies*.

Trommsdorff, G. (1983). Future orientation and socialization. *International Journal of Psychology, 18*, 381–406.

Trommsdorff, G., & Lamm, H. (1980). Future orientation of institutionalized and noninstitutionalized delinquents and nondelinquents. *European Journal of Social Psychology, 10*, 247–278.

Trommsdorff, G., Lamm, H., & Schmidt, R. W. (1979). A longitudinal study of adolescents' future orientation (time perspective). *Journal of Youth and Adolescence, 8*, 131–147.

Vansteenkiste, M., Simons, J., Soenens, B., & Lens, W. (2004a). How to become a persevering exerciser? Providing a clear, future intrinsic goal in an autonomy supportive way. *Journal of Sports and Exercise Psychology, 26*, 232–249.

Vansteenkiste, M., Simons, J., Lens, W., Soenens, B., Matos, L., & Lacante, M. (2004b). Less is sometimes more: Goal-content matters. *Journal of Educational Psychology, 96*, 755–764.

Vansteenkiste, M., Lens, W., & Deci, E. L. (2006). Intrinsic versus extrinsic goal contents in self-determination theory: Another look at the quality of academic motivation. *Educational Psychologist, 41*, 19–31.

Vansteenkiste, M., Matos, L., Lens, W., & Soenens, B. (2007). Understanding the impact of intrinsic versus extrinsic goal framing on exercise performance: The conflicting role of task and ego involvement. *Psychology of Sport and Exercise, 8*, 771–794.

Vansteenkiste, M., Soenens, B., & Duriez, B. (2008a). Presenting a positive alternative to materialistic strivings and the thin-ideal: Understanding the effects of extrinsic relative to intrinsic goal pursuit. In S. J. Lopez (Ed.), *Positive psychology: Exploring the best in people* (Vol. 4, pp. 57–86). Westport: Greenwood Publishing Company.

Vansteenkiste, M., Timmermans, T., Lens, W., Soenens, B., & Van den Broeck, A. (2008b). Does extrinsic goal framing enhance extrinsic goal-oriented individuals' learning and performance? An experimental test of the match-perspective vs. self-determination theory. *Journal of Educational Psychology, 100*, 387–397.

Worrell, F. C., Mello, Z., & Buhl, M. (2013). Introducing English and German versions of the adolescent time attitude scale. *Assessment, 20*, 496–510.

Zimbardo, P., & Boyd, J. N. (1999). Putting time in perspective: A valid, reliable, individual-differences metric. *Journal of Personality and Social Psychology, 77*, 1271–1288.

Zimbardo, P., & Boyd, J. (2009). *The time paradox: The new psychology of time that will change your life*. New York: Free Press.

More Time to Procrastinators: The Role of Time Perspective

Juan Francisco Díaz-Morales and Joseph R. Ferrari

People in Western cultures adopt "usually" long-term educational, financial, and health goals, engaging in planned activities and, in general, that are future oriented (Schmuck and Sheldon 2001). These activities are related to many positive consequences, such as higher socio-economic status, superior academic achievement, less sensation seeking, and fewer health risk behaviour (Zimbardo and Boyd 1999). On the contrary, the lack of engagement in planned or future oriented behaviours is associated with negative consequences. Most likely, one negative consequence related to poor future planned behaviour is *chronic procrastination,* the purposive and frequent delay in beginning or completing a task to the point of experiencing subjective discomfort (Ferrari et al. 1995). People who procrastinate do not work on-task and as a result, "feel bad" (anxiety, regret) from their delaying tactics. Procrastination may include substantial impairment in personal, academic, and occupational functioning (Ferrari 2010). People who are procrastinators are often viewed (even by other procrastinators) as bad, harmful or foolish in nature (Ferrari and Patel 2004; Ferrari and Pychyl 2012; Van Eerde 2003). Research has shown that procrastination can result in poor academic performance, experiencing negative emotions such as shame and guilt about oneself, depression, and negative health behaviors, such as delaying seeking care for health problems (Steel 2007; Sirois et al. 2003).

Procrastination is also typically viewed as being volitional; that is, it involves the voluntary choice of one behavior or task over other competing options, and, second, although the concept of procrastination remains closely related to meeting

J.F. Díaz-Morales (✉)
Individual Differences and Work Department, Faculty of Psychology,
Complutense University of Madrid, Madrid, Spain
e-mail: juanfcodiaz@psi.ucm.es

J.R. Ferrari
DePaul University of Chicago, Chicago, IL, USA
e-mail: jferrari@depaul.edu

M. Stolarski et al. (eds.), *Time Perspective Theory; Review, Research and Application: Essays in Honor of Philip G. Zimbardo*, DOI 10.1007/978-3-319-07368-2_20,

deadlines within a specific timeframe, studies have also demonstrated that chronic procrastination is related to a number of affective, behavioral, and cognitive characteristics reflecting more than inefficient time management (Ferrari and Pychyl 2000).

Although procrastination, or putting off until tomorrow what one should do today, is a phenomenon well-known for thousands of years, it is only recently that systematic research was conducted with respect to its manifestations, causes, consequences, and cures (Schouwenburg et al. 2004). The first scientific studies date only from the mid 1980s (Lay 1986), and the first scholarly book summarizing research results in the area dates to 1995 (Ferrari et al. 1995). Next, three relevant contributions were realized: one special issue in the *Journal of Social Behavior and Personality* (Ferrari and Pychyl 2000), a book about academic procrastination (Schouwenburg et al. 2004), and the recent Ferrari's book (Ferrari 2010), which reviewed for popular use more than 25 years of research about the causes, consequences and cures on this topic.

Procrastination typically is defined as a voluntary delay of an individual's intended action toward some task despite foreseeable negative consequences and a potentially overall worse outcome (Ferrari 2010). But, what do we know about this complex tendency? What is the relationship between procrastination and time perspective? In this chapter we present the principal characteristics notes of procrastination (concept and definition, measure and some correlates) and the results of recent research related to procrastination and Time Perspective (TP).

The Nature of Procrastination

The term procrastination come from the Latin procrastinates, which literally means "forward tomorrow" and it has been defined as purposively delaying an intended course of action to the point of experiencing subjective discomfort (Ferrari et al. 1995). Definitions of procrastination have included similar items: time delay and discomfort or wrong with this behavior. For instance, Solomon and Rothblum (1984) suggested that because definitions of procrastination stress both behavioral delay and psychological distress, the degree of procrastination and the degree to which it presents a problem should be considered together. From this point of view, procrastination has been defined as an irrational tendency to delay tasks that should be completed (Lay 1986), as the unnecessary delaying of activities that one ultimately intends to complete, especially when done to the point of creating emotional discomfort (Lay and Schouwenburg 1993). Schouwenburg et al. (2004) suggested that procrastination referred to as postponing of tasks is inferred from the behavioral manifestations including lack of promptness either in intention or behavior, whereas Steel (2007) consider procrastination as "voluntarily delay an intended course of action despite expecting to be worse off for the delay".

One cognitive process related to the voluntary delay of start/completing tasks or the poor realization of action–intention program has been *indecision*, or decisional procrastination. Indecision may drive chronic behavioral procrastinators to create excuses to justify why they do not focus on a target behavior. If you are a procrastinator, the delay seems logical and justifiable; however from an external point of view is irrational and can damage other people's perception of you (Ferrari 2010). According to the theory of planned behavior (Ajzen 1991) attitudes are not strong predictors of what people doing, but they predict intention. Subsequently, behavioral intention is the best predictor of behavior, a much better predictor of an action that simply one's attitude is. Lay (1986) claimed that procrastination is a function of the behavioral intention-behavior gap: procrastinators fail to move forward with their intentions. When people fail to "mind the gap" and not realize their goals, they could made different logical raisons such as excuses or regrets and also self-sabotage actions or rebellions against others (Ferrari 1991a, 2010; Ferrari and Pychyl 2000).

Obviously, individuals who see themselves as procrastinators often wish to reduce it by setting realistic goals and deadlines in order to complete tasks in a reasonable time frame, which always is underestimated (Ariely and Wertenbroch 2002). Non-procrastinators, in contrast, are individuals who perform most tasks in a timely manner. Studies indicated that chronic procrastination is related to a variety of personality variables, including low states of self-confidence and self-esteem (Ferrari and Díaz-Morales 2007b) and high states of depression, neurosis, self-awareness, social anxiety, forgetfulness, disorganization, non-competitiveness, dysfunctional impulsivity, behavioral rigidity, and lack of energy (Burka and Yuen 1983; Ferrari et al. 1995; Ferrari and Pychyl 2000). Procrastination has been linked to two main personality traits, high neuroticism and low conscientiousness, specifically low self-discipline (Schouwenburg and Lay 1995). Also, procrastination has been characterized by a personality style profile of inaction and accommodation to circumstances created by others (motivational aims), avoidance tangible and concrete information and preference by symbolic and unknown ideas (cognitive style), and unconventional/dissenting and seeking social stimulation (behavioral disposition) (Díaz-Morales et al. 2008a).

Usually, people procrastinate as a way to avoid certain outcomes and situations (Haghbin et al. 2012). Also, procrastinators say that they procrastinate because it gives them a "thrill," thinking that waiting until the last minute might seem adaptive and functional, although research has showed that they are wrong in their belief that they work best under pressure (Ferrari 2001). Recent research, however, proposed that the positive thrill experience reported by some procrastinators for waiting actually may be state anxiety mislabeled to avoid confronting the delay (Simpson and Pychyl 2009). Placing procrastination among related concepts, Schouwenburg et al. (2004) considered procrastination as a concept clustering of related traits: trait procrastination, weak impulse control, lack of persistence, lack of work discipline, lack of time management skill, and the inability to work methodically (see also Díaz-Morales et al. 2006a).

Procrastination, therefore, appears as a complex phenomenon integrates cognitive, emotional and behavioral aspects, plus the temporal component that indicated the deadline to do the task (Ferrari 2010; Ferrari et al. 1995). Steel (2007) argued that procrastination is reflected in the equation $E \times V/\Gamma D$, where E = expectancy or likelihood of an outcome occurring, V = value or desirability of an outcome, Γ = sensitivity to time delays, and D = the time until a rewarding stimulus becomes available. According to this function, a pattern of temporal discounting characterizes procrastination, wherein the value of distant, large rewards is downplayed relative to more immediately available, smaller rewards. Using this conceptualization is suggested that procrastinators are less future oriented and more oriented to present. We return to this issue and discuss this idea later in this chapter.

Prevalence of Procrastination

Research over the past 25 years has shown that procrastination is a common problem in the general population and reflective of a maladaptive style to life. *Everyone procrastinates, but not everyone is a procrastinator.* This sentence, included as headline inside the Ferrari's book, reflects the difference between delaying an action, something that all people realize in some occasion, and postponing the task which must be done (see Ferrari 2010). If one delays to gather more information or postpones a decision because he or she needs to do something important before the target act, then theses strategies are not procrastination.

Procrastination affects virtually everyone to some degree. It involves knowing that a task must be performed, yet intentionally failing to motivate oneself to carry out the task within the desired time frame (Ackerman and Gross 2005). When procrastination is a chronic behavior, becomes a maladaptive lifestyle. As many as 20–25 % of normal, healthy adult men and women, were classified as *chronic procrastinators,* individuals who engage in a needless delay of relevant and timely tasks across situations and settings. One series of trans-cultural studies showed that in Australia, Peru, Spain, United Kingdom (UK), United States (US) and Venezuela, the prevalence of chronic procrastinators is around 15–20 % of people (Ferrari et al. 2004, 2007; Harriott and Ferrari 1996). Although the tendency toward delaying the start of completing of tasks is common among adults living in six countries, consistent with previous literature reviews (Van Eerde 2003), large and significant country effects emerged between countries when raw procrastination scores was examined: UK reported significantly higher chronic procrastination compared to adults from Peru, US, Spain, and Australia with the lowest reported tendencies among adults from Venezuela.

In general, studies showed that prevalence of procrastination is similar to men and women. Most studies found no significant difference by *sex*, although Van Eerde's (2003) meta-analysis stated that tendency to procrastinate was more common among the male than female participants. However, sex/gender variables hasn't been considered until recently and it would be interesting to research how everyday or quotidian tasks associate to one of the two genders are related to procrastination (Özer et al. 2009). Regarding *occupation*, white-collar workers and professional employees tend to demonstrate higher levels of procrastination than blue-collar workers and unskilled employees (Díaz-Morales et al. 2006b; Hammer and Ferrari 2002).

Finally, regarding *age*, some studies showed a significant negative correlation between procrastination and age among adults (Ferrari et al. 2005; Hammer and Ferrari 2002), indicating that procrastination moderately decreases with age (i.e. $r = -0.27$, Díaz-Morales et al. 2008a; $r = -0.19$, Gupta et al. 2012). No difference has been found related to *level of studies*. It is important consider the age of samples includes in procrastination studies, because usually procrastination has been frequently studied among undergraduates and scarcely studied among adults (Díaz-Morales et al. 2006a).

Also, people may procrastinate in one life area, but not in other areas. An example of situational procrastination is *academic procrastination*. It is different from chronic or everyday procrastination. *Academic procrastination* among students is defined as the delay in studying or completing academic assignments (Solomon and Rothblum 1984). It has been estimated that procrastination is prevalent in about 70 % of college students on academic tasks such as studying, registering form classes, completing reading assignments, or keeping appointments with professors. In-depth analysis of academic procrastination may be found in other sources (see Ferrari 2010; Schowenburg et al. 2004).

Measure of Procrastination

During the 1990s of past siècle, several experimental or quasi-experimental studies were realized in real situations (see Ferrari et al. 1995). For example, in the workplace, employees were confronted with tasks in which they are either likely to fail (Lay 1990; Van Eerde 2003) or tasks that have open-ended deadlines (Ferrari 1992). Among students a common behavioral index of procrastination was the time of submitted course assignments relative to assignment due dates. Students who scored higher on procrastination were more likely to postpone submission of assignments than were students who scored lower on procrastination scale (Digdon and Howell 2008).

At present, several reliable and valid measures of chronic procrastination have been identified (see Ferrari et al. 1995, for actual items and psychometric properties of most chronic and academic self-report procrastination measures). Among adults the most frequently used scales has been the *General Procrastination* scale (GP; Lay 1986), the *Adult Inventory of Procrastination* (AIP; McCown et al. 1989), or the *Decisional Procrastination scale* (DP; Mann 1982). Among students, frequently used has been the *Procrastination Assessment Scale -Student* (PASS; Solomon and Rothblum 1984), the *Aitken Procrastination Inventory* (API; Aitken 1982), and the *Tuckman Procrastination Scale* (TPS; Tuckman 1991).

Procrastination scales by adults have been validated in different cultural contexts (Ferrari et al. 1995, 2009; Díaz-Morales et al. 2006a; Mariani and Ferrari 2012). Lay's *General Procrastination* scale (GP, Lay 1986) measure dilatory behavior across different situations related to personality variables such as low self-control, rebelliousness, and extraversion. It is composed by 20 items such as "*I am continually saying I'll do it tomorrow"* and "*When preparing to go out, I am seldom caught doing something at the last minute*". The GP scores on this scale have been related to external attributes or excuses for delays (Ferrari 1993) and poor performance when environmental stressors existed that heightened arousal at task deadlines (Ferrari 2001). Researchers typically found the scale to have a single factor structure (Ferrari et al. 2005; Díaz-Morales et al. 2006a), although in Italian sample two factors has been identified (Mariani and Ferrari 2012). The *Adult Inventory of Procrastination* (*AIP*; McCown et al. 1989) measures chronic tendency to postpone tasks in various situations. It examines procrastination motivated by fears (e.g., success or failure), avoidance of disclosure of skill inabilities, and insecurities of performance (Ferrari 1991b). The AIP is composed of 15 items such as "*I am not very good at meeting deadlines*" and "*I don't get things done on time*". It is a global measure of frequent procrastination examining a variety of tasks in order to deflect potential disclosure of perceived inabilities and incompetence (Ferrari 1993) and self-relevant information about one's skills and competence (Ferrari 1991b). Two factors were extracted from a Spanish sample of adults, labeled *lack of punctuality* and *lack of planning* (Díaz-Morales et al. 2006a), and among Turkish adult sample named *positive aspects of avoidance* and *negative aspects of avoidance* (Ferrari et al. 2009), whereas among Italian adult samples the AIP was considered as one-dimensional (Mariani and Ferrari 2012).

Whereas *GP* and *AIP* scales were developed to assess the frequency with which people postpone performing everyday behavioural tasks or activities, a more cognitive measure of procrastination (indecision) is evaluate by *Decisional Procrastination Scale* (DP, Mann 1982), described as the purposive delay in making decisions within some specific time frame (Effert and Ferrari 1989). It is a reliable and valid measure composes by five items such as *"I delay making decisions until it is too late"* or *"I put off making decisions"*.

Procrastination has been viewed both as a single trait dimension and as a complex trait composed of several component antecedents (Ferrari et al. 1995; Ferrari and Pychyl 2000). In this way, procrastination started to be analyzed from a multidimensional point of view. The logic was to analyze what is the dimensionality of more frequently procrastination scales. When factorial structure of the three combined scales was realized among Spanish adults by first time, four reliable components were identified (Díaz-Morales et al. 2006a). They may reflect four essential elements of trait procrastination that are conceptuality-relevant: *dilatory behaviors*, a summary of the predisposition to manifest intention behavior gaps; *indecision*, putting off making a decision within some specific time frame; *lack of punctuality*, such as an inability to work diligently on a task to meet its deadline; and *lack of planning*, a lack of self-discipline to stay focused on a target task. The principal component, *dilatory behaviors*, configures the most "pure" component of procrastination because give count of the shared variance of the three scales of procrastination (Díaz-Morales et al. 2006a).

Subsequently, Steel (2010) replicated a similar psychometric study with these three scales among English speakers and found three similar factors: *general procrastination, rushing and appointment keeping*, and *promptness and doing tasks immediately*. Finally, Mariani and Ferrari (2012) tested different structure models using the same scales of procrastination. Not surprisingly, many different measures have been proposed to measures this needless and irrational delay, but from the beginning of research on procrastination, only recently the dimensionality of these scales has become to be analyzed.

Procrastination and Psychological Time

Time perspective (TP), an individuals' understanding of one's psychological past, present, and future, may be fundamental to understand human behaviour. The cognitive abilities to "travel through time" using one's memory to move into the past or the imagination for the future may be considered to be a uniquely human capability (Sunddendorf and Corballis 1997). Past research has related either past, present or future orientations to psychological constructs such as well-being, optimism, controllability, self-direction or achievement motivation, and their effects to selected outcome behaviours (Zaleski 1994). The conceptualisation of how the perspective of future influences the self-regulation of behaviour has been stated from different theoretical approaches such as future possible selves (Markus and Nurius 1986), consideration of future consequences (Strathman et al. 1994), and anxiety of future (Zaleski 1996).

Time is constant: it does not fly! There are 24 h in a day, every day for 365 days a year. Time moves constantly. We can't simply say, "time fly", we must fly with it to take in all of the gusto and joy that life has to offer (Ferrari 2010). This implies, for example, that employees who organize their time in an effective manner will be perceived to be of greater value by employers, by virtue of the fact that they make a greater contribution to organizational efficiency. Procrastinators, in contrast, lead to increased employer costs by taking more time than necessary to complete requisite tasks. Deadlines play an important role in determining schedules for completing tasks and in guiding and focusing plans for action.

Although shown to be associated to affective, behavioral, and cognitive characteristics reflecting more than inefficient time management (Ferrari et al. 1995; Ferrari and Pychyl 2000), the concept of procrastination remains closely related to meeting deadlines within a specific timeframe. The existence of the approaching deadline may be, in itself, an important factor. However, procrastination is a cognitive-behavioral problem that is complex and has many intertwined roots. It is not merely a problem of time management.

Despite the obvious importance of time to procrastination, little research has examined this important relationship although the temporal component seems to be a key defining concept of procrastination. For instance, research indicated that chronic procrastinators compared to non-procrastinators spend less preparation time on tasks that were likely to succeeded and more time on projects likely to fail (Lay 1990; Lay et al. 1989), tended to underestimate the overall time required to complete a task (McCown et al. 1987), spend less time searching for information needed to complete tasks (Ferrari and Dovidio 2000), started academics task (e.g. studying for exams) at the last minute (Lay and Burns 1991; Pychyl et al. 2000a), and are more "present-oriented" (Blatt and Quinlan 1967, in Ferrari et al. 1995).

Vodanovich and Seib (1997) indicated that individuals with a heightened tendency to procrastinate reported difficulties in structuring their time and viewed their use of time as less personally meaningful than non-procrastinators. Others empirical studies on time management and procrastination found negative correlations (Lay 1992), and Lay and Schouwenburg (1993) hypothesized that time management was a mediator of the relation between procrastination and dilatory behavior. In a work-related context, Van Eerde (2003) showed that time management training increases the ability to manage time and decreases rates of preoccupation and procrastination.

Because procrastination is viewed as wasting time, time perspective has been studied in relation to procrastination. Chronic procrastinators prefer short-term activities (Ferrari and Emmons 1995; Lasane and Jones 2000; Pychyl et al. 2000a) avoiding or dismissing future goals in favor of reducing present tension (Baumeister 1997; Ferrari 2001) or seeking more immediate rewards (Pychyl et al. 2000b). In this way, chronic procrastinators look for immediate pleasurable rewards in the present time (Steel 2007). Time perspective represents an individual's way of relating to the psychological concepts of past, present, and future. Individuals use past, present, and future frames in encoding, storing, and recalling experienced events and in forming expectations, goals, and imaginative views (Boyd and Zimbardo 2005). Procrastination is conceptually representative of self-regulatory failure (Ferrari 2001) and consequently disables individuals from guiding their goal-directed activities across changing circumstances and over time (Karoly 1993).

Researchers demonstrated that dilatory behavior related stronger to a present orientation in comparison with a future orientation. An emphasis on future time orientation requires a long-time perspective. A person with this orientation may need longer time for important decisions, especially when there are long delays along the course of action. To determine the extent to which procrastination is associated with Time Perspective (i.e. past, present and future), Specter and Ferrari (2000) found that chronic procrastination in making decisions and postponing the beginning or finishing of tasks, was negatively associated with a future orientation, positively associated with a past orientation, and not associated with a present time orientation. After controlling negative affect, Jackson et al. (2003) showed that academic procrastination among students had robust positive associations with a negative evaluation of the past, a fatalistic view of the present and negatively related to future. Also, these researchers found that low levels of structured and purposed time were related with high procrastination. Whereas Specter and Ferrari (2000) found that decisional procrastination were related to low future and high past orientation, Jackson et al. (2003) found that academic procrastination was related to low Future, high Present Fatalistic and Past-Negative. Clearly, in these two studies where two different scales of procrastination were used (decisional and academic procrastination), procrastination was related to low Future time perspective. Still, the common

Table 1 Zero-Order Correlations found in studies about relations between Procrastination Scales and Time Perspective (ZTPI)

Studies		Past-Negative	Past-Positive	Present-Hedonistic	Present-Fatalistic	Future
Specter and Ferrari (2000)	AIP					−0.45
Jackson et al. (2003)		0.39		0.31	0.57	−0.53
Ferrari and Díaz-Morales (2007a)	GP			0.14	0.28	−0.53
	AIP	0.13		0.20	0.31	−0.59
Díaz-Morales et al. (2008a, b)	AIP	0.13		0.20	0.31	−0.61
	DP	0.38	0.16		0.30	−0.47

Note: GP General Procrastination scale, *AIP* Adult Inventory of Procrastination, *DP* Decisional Procrastination scale

statement that procrastinators prefer immediate pleasurable rewards in the present time wasn't confirmed.

More recently, several studies found that procrastination correlates positively with fatalistic and/or hedonistic presents and negatively with future time orientations, using Zimbardo's *Time Perspective Inventory* (ZTPI) (Ferrari and Díaz-Morales 2007a; Díaz-Morales et al. 2008b; Digdon and Howell 2008).

Ferrari and Díaz-Morales (2007a) found significant zero-order correlations between two scales of procrastination (GP and AIP, respectively) and Time Perspective (TP) dimensions of Spanish version of ZTPI (Díaz-Morales 2006): negative correlation with future, and positive correlations with Present-Fatalistic and Present-Hedonistic TP. The positive relation to Past-Negative TP was significant to AIP but not to GP (see Table 1 for details). Moreover, when shared variance between both procrastination scales and age were controlled in a hierarchical regression model, scores on AIP scale (controlling GP and age) was negatively predicted by Present-Fatalistic TP, whereas scores on GP scale (controlling AIP and age) was positively predicted by present-hedonist TP, and negatively associated with Future TP.

The zero-order correlation profile indicated that as hedonistic as fatalistic view of the present were related to procrastination, similar to zero-order correlations showed by Jackson et al. (2003, p. 21). Results concerning the two procrastination scales in the hierarchical regression analysis were of interest. When the shared variance of each scale was controlled (plus age), AIP was related to fatalistic present TP, whereas GP was related to hedonistic present TP. As indicated the authors, perhaps, both procrastination scales measures different form of procrastination: more related to avoidance, the AIP, and more related to arousal, the GP. Recent findings have discussed about this conceptualization and more research is necessary (Steel 2010).

However, the relationship between AIP and Past-Negative, and the results of regression analysis where shared variance of both AIP and GP procrastinations scales and age were controlled, was one good raison to follow researching and to analyze if relationship between time perspective dimensions and procrastination were different when different procrastination scales were used. Moreover, as we indicated before, previous studies had found that high decisional procrastination was associate to low future, high past, and not associated to present time orientations (Specter and Ferrari 2000), whereas academic procrastination among students was associated to Past-Negative, Present-Fatalistic or negative view of the present, and negatively to Future time perspective (Jackson et al. 2003). What could explain theses apparent differences of time perspective profile of procrastinators? It could be possible that differences were because procrastination was measured by indecision scale (Specter and Ferrari 2000), a more cognitive form of procrastination, and by academic procrastination scale, a more situational form of procrastination (Jackson et al. 2003).

Following this line of reasoning, Díaz-Morales et al. (2008b) study analyzed the time perspective profile of procrastinators when behavioral and cognitive measures of procrastination were used. As behavioral measure of procrastination it was chose the *Adult Inventory Procrastination* (AIP, McCown et al. 1989) plus another measure related to time, more biological-behavioral, the morningness-eveningness orientation, evaluated by the *Composite Scale of Morningness* (CS, Smith et al. 1989). As typical cognitive measure of procrastination it was chose the *Decisional Procrastination Scale* (DP, Mann 1982). Despite the fact that both Morningness-Eveningness (M/E) and Time Perspective (TP) relate to the area of human temporal functioning their mutual relationships had poorly been investigated until recently (Díaz-Morales et al. 2008b). Moreover, given that people's ability to organize their day is at the core of the timing of many daily behaviors, it was assessed how procrastinators and indecisive individuals differed in their *time perspective* (i.e., their way of relating to the past, present, or future) and also in *morningness–eveningness* (i.e., their preference for specific times during the day to do task or feel best moment).

Behavioral procrastination (evaluated by AIP) was negatively related to future and positively related to Present-Fatalistic, Present-Hedonistic, and Past-Negative TP (see Table 1). The profile was identical to found previously in a similar Spanish adult sample (Ferrari and Díaz-Morales 2007a). Decisional procrastination (indecision) was negatively related to Future, and positively related to Present-Fatalist, Past-Negative, and Past-Positive TP, but was not related to Present-Hedonist TP (see Table 1).

These results are similar to Specter and Ferrari's (2000, p. 200) study, who evaluated indecision (zero-orders correlations coefficients of $r=-0.45$ with future, and $r=0.32$ with past time orientations of *Temporal Orientation Scale* by Jones et al. 1996) and similar to Jackson et al. (2003) who evaluated academic procrastination and found negative relation with future, and positive relations with Present-Fatalistic, Present-Hedonistic, and Past-Negative TP. The correlation with Past-Positive TP was not significant).

Recently, Gupta et al. (2012) using a shortened version of the ZTPI (15 items) found that procrastination was inversely predicted by Future and Past-Negative TP, and positively by Present-Fatalistic and Past-Positive TP. Although in the paper zero-order correlations was not indicated (only regression coefficients), and despite the differences between average age of samples and measures used, the results are similar to zero-order correlations found previously among the two referenced studies with Spanish adults (see Table 1): procrastination (AIP scale used in both studies) was negatively related with future, and positively related with Present-Fatalistic, Present-Hedonistic and Past-Negative TP (Ferrari and Díaz-Morales 2007a, and Díaz-Morales et al. 2008a, respectively). Past-Positive TP was not related to procrastination in any of two studies (0.01 and 0.01, respectively).

On other hand, procrastination (evaluated by AIP scale) was negatively related to morningness, whereas the negative correlation between indecision and morningness was not significant. Perhaps individual who procrastinates delayed their daily activities because they believed they performed best in the afternoon or evening. It seemed that among adult men and women, procrastination, but not indecision, related to being a night person. Procrastinators likely performed activities during the evening, specifically much later than most people (Ferrari et al. 1997; Hess et al. 2000).

It is well-know that procrastination negatively relates to conscientiousness, as people postpone necessary duties to protect their self-esteem (Schouwenburg and Lay 1995; Van Eerde 2003; Watson 2001). Therefore, it may be that the reason why evening individuals are not held in the same regard as morning people is their tendency to avoid certain obligations during the day, making them low in conscientiousness and likely to not conform to certain tasks that need immediate attention. Also, people high in morningness represent the best values and standards because they are more conscientious (Jackson and Gerard 1996) and have a dutiful or conformist personality style (Díaz-Morales 2007). The findings suggest that procrastination may mediate the relation between morningness-eveningness and a variety of maladaptive processes related to a low future and high present time orientations. Future oriented individuals exhibit various conscientious behaviors in regard to structuring time. They stress punctuality, wear watches and use agendas more often, and prefer regularity in their lives. Procrastinator people act with an opposite profile.

Other subsequent studies about procrastination have analyzed their relation to morningness-eveningness preference. Academic procrastination has been negatively related to M/E, point out that poor self-regulation is a salient characteristic of evening students (Digdon and Howell 2008). It is possible that self-regulation difficulties causes delayed sleep schedule causing the realization of task to the end of day, or that evening preference causes difficulties of self-regulation and the person would be out of sync with earlier schedules required by daytime commitments. Similar results has been found among Poland students sample remarking that probably morning people is predominately thinking in tomorrow, whereas evening people live in the present moment (Stolarski et al. 2013). Interestedly, self-control has also been proposed mediating the chronotype-time perspective relationships (Milfont and Schwarzenthal 2014).

Future-oriented people tend to carefully plan and organize their work activities, which is the opposite of procrastinators who show low persistence, work discipline, time management skills, and the ability to work methodically (Milgram and Tenne 2000). A present-focus orientation may relate to completing tasks as close to a deadline as possible. Such a strategy may energize the individual to work quickly especially if the task is unattractive or not challenging (Van Eerde 2003). An higher score on Present-Hedonistic TP is a characteristic of individuals what seek pleasure and enjoyment, have high levels of energy, and they lack emotional stability (Zimbardo and Boyd 1999), whereas an higher score on procrastination is typical of people who tend to be sensation seekers, focusing on pleasure in the moment as opposed to the completion of tasks that fail to provide high levels of sensation or pleasure (Steel 2007). Also, Present-Fatalistic individuals exhibit low levels of conscientiousness, depression, and high levels of emotional instability, which is related to task evasiveness and emotional instability of procrastinators (Dewitte and Schouwenburg 2002). The relations showed in some studies between procrastination and both Present-Hedonistic and Present-Fatalistic time orientations could be explained by the way to evaluate procrastination, the characteristic of the sample (students vs. adults), or even the cultural context.

However, both dimensions of Present, Hedonistic and Fatalistic, have logical relations with procrastination. Procrastinators could engage in pleasurable activities or make excuses to gain additional time for completing tasks, feeling bad and discomfort with the situation (Ferrari et al. 1995). Emphasis on past time orientation might enable a person to take a long-term perspective, avoid risks, and emphasize stability, whereas an emphasis on present time orientation might facilitate a person to live in the here and now focusing on short-term perspectives (Brislin and Kim 2003). Studies have shown that a motivational mechanism of procrastination may include neglecting previous experience, particularly failures (Buehler et al. 1997), which result in postponement of action motivated by an avoidance response. The relationship between indecision and both Past-Negative and Positive TP could be explained because indecisive individuals may be too preoccupied with reminiscing about both positive and negative past events, and this form of rumination may result in indecision (Janis and Mann 1977).

Some final limitations must be indicated, because when the comparison of different results obtained from different studies is realized trying to elucidate the relations between procrastination and time perspective, several aspect must been considered. First, demographics characteristics of the samples are not directly identical: age (students or adults) and nationality. Second, when time perspective dimensions are considered, usually a regression analysis is realized considering time dimensions as predictors and procrastination as criteria. However some studies included covariates (i.e. age, other procrastination or time scales) and the results of regression coefficients are not directly comparable. For this reason, zero-order correlations coefficients have been revised in this chapter. An third, the size effect of correlations coefficients was high to Future, moderated to Present time orientations and Past-Negative, and small to Present Hedonistic and Past Positive.

Conclusions: Is It About Time?

Procrastination refers to an irrational tendency to delay beginning and/or completing tasks that should be completed, feeling subjective discomfort. Procrastinators know they should perform and activity and may even want to do so but they fail to motivate themselves to initiate and finish activities within desired or expected time frames (Ferrari 2010). More than half of college students consider procrastination is a severe problem in their lives and about 15–20 % of the general populations of very different countries (Ferrari et al. 2007). Results of several studies indicated that people with cognitive (indecision) procrastination tendencies reported that they were focus less in the Future, more in Present Fatalistic and, at the same time, in Past-Positive and Past-Negative time perspective.

A plausible explanation for the relation to both, negative and positive, past orientations is that indecisive individuals may be too preoccupied with reminiscing about both positive and negative past events, and this form of rumination may result in indecision. On the other hand, people reported high behavioral procrastination claimed low Future and high Present-Fatalistic, Present-Hedonistic and Past-Negative time perspectives. The lack of Future TP was related to both tendencies to a fatalistic and hedonic view of the present. The resigned present and negative past are antecedents of a reduced motivation to plan ahead, congruent to a negative vision of the future. On other hand, focus on immediate pleasures and not in complicated plans to future, is also supported in some studies, suggesting that chronic procrastinators focus on present pleasures more than non-procrastinators. Past researches have noted that when procrastinators engage in pleasurable activities or make excuses to gain additional time for completing tasks, the also report increased guilt (Ferrari and Beck 1998). Finally, although research about counseling the procrastination has been compiled (Schouwenburg et al. 2004), from the recent findings about unbalanced or biased time perspective, procrastination could be treated (Boniwell and Zimbardo 2004). Also, the potential utility of Time Perspective Therapy proposed recently (Zimbardo et al. 2012) could be added in the research agenda for future. In consequence, it is possible that procrastinators experience the present with both hedonistic and fatalism terms and the correlational studies realized among undergraduates or adults, using different measures and in different age range, not provide sufficient discrimination power. As would say a typical procrastinator: more time is necessary to elucidate these complex but interesting relationship.

References

Ackerman, D., & Gross, B. L. (2005). My instructor made me do it: Task characteristics of procrastination. *Journal of Marketing Education, 27*, 5–13.

Aitken, M. E. (1982). *A personality profile of the college student procrastinator*. Doctoral dissertation, University of Pittsburgh, 1982). *Dissertation Abstracts International, 43*, 722.

Ajzen, I. (1991). The theory of planned behavior. *Organizational Behavior and Human Decision Processes, 50*, 179–211.

Ariely, D., & Wertenbroch, K. (2002). Procrastination, deadlines and performance: Self control by precommitment. *Psychological Science, 13*, 219–224.

Baumeister, R. F. (1997). Esteem threat, self-regulatory breakdown and emotional distress as factors in self-defeating behavior. *Reviews of General Psychology, 1*, 145–174.

Boniwell, I., & Zimbardo, P. G. (2004). Balancing one's time perspective in pursuit of optimal functioning. In P. A. Linley & S. Joseph (Eds.), *Positive psychology in practice*. Hoboken: Wiley.
Boyd, J. N., & Zimbardo, P. (2005). Time perspective, health, and risk taking. In A. Strathman & J. Joireman (Eds.), *Understanding behavior in the context of time* (pp. 85–10). Mahwah: LEA.
Brislin, R. W., & Kim, E. S. (2003). Cultural diversity in people's understanding and uses of time. *Applied Psychology, 52*, 363–382.
Buehler, R., Griffin, D., & McDonald, H. (1997). The role of motivated reasoning in optimistic time predictions. *Personality and Social Psychology Bulletin, 23*, 238–247.
Burka, J. B., & Yuen, L. M. (1983). *Procrastination: Why you do it and what to do about it*. Reading: Addison-Wesley.
Dewitte, S., & Schouwenburg, H. (2002). Procrastination, temptations, and incentives: The struggle between the present and the future in procrastinators and the punctual. *European Journal of Personality, 16*, 469–489.
Díaz-Morales, J. F. (2006). Estructura factorial y fiabilidad del Inventario de Perspectiva Temporal de Zimbardo [Factorial structure and reliability of Zimbardo Time Perspective Inventory]. *Psicothema, 18*, 565–571.
Díaz-Morales, J. F. (2007). Morning and evening-types: Exploring their personality styles. *Personality and Individual Differences, 43*, 769–778.
Díaz-Morales, J. F., Ferrari, J. R., Díaz, K., & Argumedo, D. (2006a). Factorial structure of three procrastination scales with Spanish adult population. *European Journal of Psychological Assessment, 22*, 132–137.
Díaz-Morales, J. F., Ferrari, J. R., Díaz, K., & Argumedo, D. (2006b). Procrastination and demographic characteristics in Spanish adults: Further evidence. *The Journal of Social Psychology, 146*, 629–633.
Díaz-Morales, J. F., Cohen, J., & Ferrari, J. R. (2008a). An integrated view of personality styles related to avoidant procrastination. *Personality and Individual Differences, 45*, 554–558.
Díaz-Morales, J. F., Ferrari, J. R., & Cohen, J. R. (2008b). Indecision and avoidant procrastination: The role of morningness-eveningness and time perspective in chronic delay lifestyles. *The Journal of General Psychology, 135*, 228–240.
Digdon, N. L., & Howell, A. J. (2008). College students who have an eveningness preference report lower self-control and greater procrastination. *Chronobiology International, 25*, 1029–1046.
Effert, B. R., & Ferrari, J. R. (1989). Decisional procrastination: Examining personality correlates. *Journal of Social Behavior and Personality, 4*, 151–161.
Ferrari, J. R. (1991a). Self-handicapping by procrastinators: Protecting social-esteem, self-esteem, or both? *Journal of Research in Personality, 25*, 245–261.
Ferrari, J. R. (1991b). A preference for a favorable public impression by procrastination: Selecting among cognitive and social tasks. *Personality and Individual Differences, 12*, 1233–1237.
Ferrari, J. R. (1992). Psychometric validation of two procrastination inventories for adults: Arousal and avoidance measures. *Journal of Psychopathology and Behavioral Assessment, 14*, 97–110.
Ferrari, J. R. (1993). Christmas and procrastination: Explaining lack of diligence at a "real-world" task deadline. *Personality and Individual Differences, 14*, 25–33.
Ferrari, J. R. (2001). Procrastination as self-regulation failure of performance: Effects of cognitive load, self-awareness, and time limits on "working best under pressure.". *European Journal of Personality, 15*, 391–406.
Ferrari, J. R. (2010). *Still procrastinating: The no regrets guide to getting it done*. Hoboken: John Wiley & Sons.
Ferrari, J. R., & Beck, B. L. (1998). Affective responses before and after fraudulent excuses by academic procrastinators. *Education, 118*, 529–538.
Ferrari, J. R., & Díaz-Morales, J. F. (2007a). Procrastination: Different time orientations reflect different motives. *Journal of Research in Personality, 41*, 707–714.
Ferrari, J. R., & Díaz-Morales, J. F. (2007b). Perceptions of self-concept and self-presentation by procrastinators: Further evidence. *The Spanish Journal of Psychology, 10*, 91–96.
Ferrari, J. R., & Dovidio, J. F. (2000). Examining behavioral processes in indecision: Decisional procrastination and decision-making style. *Journal of Research in Personality, 34*, 127–137.

Ferrari, J. R., & Emmons, R. (1995). Methods of procrastination and their relation to self-control and self-reinforcement: An exploratory study. *Journal of Social Behavior and Personality, 10*, 135–142.

Ferrari, J. R., & Patel, T. (2004). Social comparisons by procrastinators: Rating peers with similar and dissimilar delay tendencies. *Personality and Individual Differences, 37*, 1493–1501.

Ferrari, J. R., & Pychyl, T. A. (2000). *Procrastination: Current issues and new directions*. Corte Madre: Select Press.

Ferrari, J. R., & Pychyl, T. A. (2012). "If I wait, my partner will do it:" The role of conscientiousness as a potential mediator for academic procrastination and perceived social loafing. *North American Journal of Psychology, 14*, 13–24.

Ferrari, J. R., Johnson, J., & McCown, W. (1995). *Procrastination and task avoidance: Theory, research, and treatment*. New York: Plenum Press.

Ferrari, J. R., Harriott, J. S., Evans, L., Lecik-Michna, D. M., & Wenger, J. M. (1997). Exploring the time preferences of procrastinators: Night or day, which is the one? *European Journal of Personality, 11*, 187–196.

Ferrari, J. R., O'Callaghan, J., & Newbegin, I. (2004). Prevalence of procrastination in the United States, United Kingdom, and Australia: Arousal and avoidance delays among adults. *North American Journal of Psychology, 6*, 1–6.

Ferrari, J. R., Doroszko, E., & Joseph, N. (2005). Procrastination in corporate settings: Sex, status, and geographic comparisons of arousal and avoidance types. *Individual Differences Research, 3*, 140–149.

Ferrari, J. R., Díaz-Morales, J. F., O'Callaghan, J., Díaz, K., & Argumedo, D. (2007). Frequent behavioral delay tendencies by adults: International prevalence rates of chronic procrastination. *Journal of Cross-Cultural Psychology, 38*, 458–464.

Ferrari, J., Özer, B., & Demir, A. (2009). Chronic procrastination among Turkish adults: Exploring decisional, avoidant, and arousal styles. *The Journal of Social Psychology, 149*, 302–308.

Gupta, R., Hershey, D. A., & Gaur, J. (2012). Time perspective and procrastination in the workplace: An empirical investigation. *Current Psychology, 31*, 195–211.

Haghbin, M., McCaffrey, A., & Pychyl, T. A. (2012). The complexity of the relation between fear of failure and procrastination. *Journal of Rational-Emotive and Cognitive-Behavior Therapy, 30*, 249–263.

Hammer, C. A., & Ferrari, J. R. (2002). Differential incidence of procrastination between blue-and whitecollar workers. *Current Psychology, 21*, 333–338.

Harriott, J., & Ferrari, J. R. (1996). Prevalence of procrastination among samples of adults. *Psychological Reports, 78*, 611–616.

Hess, B., Sherman, M. F., & Goodmand, M. (2000). Eveningness predicts academic procrastination: The mediating role of neuroticism. *Journal of Social Behavior and Personality, 15*, 61–74.

Jackson, L. A., & Gerard, D. A. (1996). Diurnal types, the "big five" personality factors, and other personal characteristics. *Journal of Social Behavior & Personality, 11*, 273–284.

Jackson, T., Fritch, A., Nagasaka, T., & Pope, L. (2003). Procrastination and perceptions of past, present, and future. *Individual Differences Research, 1*, 17–28.

Janis, I. L., & Mann, L. (1977). *Decision making: A psychological analysis of conflict, choice, and commitment*. New York: Free Press.

Jones, J. M., Banicky, L., Lasane, T., & Pomare, M. (1996). *The temporal orientation scale*. Unpublished measure available from T. Lasane, Department of Psychology, St. Mary's College, St. Mary's City, MD

Karoly, P. (1993). Mechanisms of self-regulation: A system view. *Annual Review of Psychology, 44*, 23–52.

Lasane, T. P., & Jones, J. M. (2000). When socially-induced temporal myopia interferes with academic goal-setting. *Journal of Social Behavior and Personality, 15*, 75–86.

Lay, C. H. (1986). At last, my research on procrastination. *Journal of Research in Personality, 20*, 479–495.

Lay, C. H. (1990). Working to schedule on personal projects: An assessment of person-project characteristics and trait procrastination. *Journal of Social Behavior and Personality, 5*, 91–103.

Lay, C. (1992). Trait procrastination and the perception of person-task characteristics. *Journal of Social Behavior and Personality, 7*, 483–494.

Lay, C. H., & Burns, P. (1991). Intentions and behavior in studying for an examination: The role of trait procrastination and its interaction with optimism. *Journal of Social Behavior and Personality, 5*, 91–193.

Lay, C. H., & Schouwenburg, H. C. (1993). Trait procrastination, time management, and academic behavior. *Journal of Social Behavior and Personality, 8*, 647–662.

Lay, C. H., Edwards, J. M., Parker, J. D. A., & Endler, N. S. (1989). An assessment of appraisal, anxiety, coping, and procrastination during an examination period. *European Journal of Personality, 3*, 195–208.

Mann, L. (1982). Decision making questionnaire: Parts I and II. In J. R. Ferrari, J. L. Johnson, & W. McCown (Eds.), *Procrastination and task avoidance*. New York: Plenum Press.

Mariani, M. G., & Ferrari, J. R. (2012). Adult Inventory of Procrastination scale (AIP): A comparison of model with and Italian sample. *Testing, Psychometric, Methodology in Applied Psychology, 19*, 3–14.

Markus, H., & Nurius, P. (1986). Possible selves. *American Psychologist, 41*, 954–969.

McCown, W., Petzel, T., & Rupert, P. (1987). An experimental study of some hypothesized behaviors and personality variables of college student procrastinators. *Personality and Individual Differences, 8*, 781–786.

McCown, W., Johnson, J., & Petzel, T. (1989). Procrastination, a principal components analysis. *Personality and Individual Differences, 10*, 197–202.

Milfont, T. L., & Schwarzenthal, M. (2014). Explaining why larks are future-oriented and owls are present-oriented: Self-control mediates the chronotype-time perspective relationships. *Chronobiology International, 31*(4), 581–588.

Milgram, N., & Tenne, R. (2000). Personality correlates of decisional and task avoidant procrastination. *European Journal of Personality, 14*, 141–156.

Özer, B. U., Demir, A., & Ferrari, J. R. (2009). Exploring academic procrastination among Turkish students: Possible gender differences in prevalence and reasons. *The Journal of Social Psychology, 149*, 241–257.

Pychyl, T. A., Morin, R. W., & Salmon, B. R. (2000a). Procrastination and the planning fallacy: An examination of the study habits of university students. *Journal of Social Behavior and Personality, 15*, 135–150.

Pychyl, T. A., Lee, J. M., Thibodeau, R., & Blunt, A. (2000b). Five days of emotion: An experience sampling study of undergraduate student procrastination. *Journal of Social Behavior and Personality, 15*, 239–254.

Schmuck, P., y Sheldon, K. M. (2001). *Life goals and well-being*. Seattle: Hogrefe & Huber.

Schouwenburg, H. C., & Lay, C. H. (1995). Trait procrastination and the Big-Five factors of personality. *Personality and Individual Differences, 18*, 481–490.

Schouwenburg, H. C., Lay, C. H., Pychyl, T. A., & Ferrari, J. R. (2004). *Counseling the procrastinator in academic settings*. Washington, DC: American Psychological Association.

Simpson, W. K., & Pychyl, T. A. (2009). In search of the arousal procrastinator: An investigation of the relation between procrastination, arousal-based personality traits and beliefs about procrastination motivations. *Personality and Individual Differences, 47*, 906–911.

Sirois, F. M., Melia-Gordon, M. L., & Pychyl, T. (2003). "I'll look after my health, later": An investigation of procrastination and health. *Personality and Individual Differences, 35*, 1167–1184.

Smith, C. S., Reilly, T. C., & Midkiff, K. (1989). Evaluation of three circadian rhythm questionnaires with suggestions for an improved measure of morningness. *Journal of Applied Psychology, 74*, 728–738.

Solomon, L. J., & Rothblum, E. D. (1984). Academic procrastination: Frequency and cognitive-behavioral correlates. *Journal of Counseling Psychology, 31*, 503–509.

Specter, M. H., & Ferrari, J. R. (2000). Time orientations of procrastinators: Focusing on the past, present, or future? *Journal of Social Behavior and Personality, 15*, 197–202.

Steel, P. (2007). The nature of procrastination: A meta-analytic and theoretical review of quintessential self-regulatory failure. *Psychological Bulletin, 133*, 65–94.

Steel, P. (2010). Arousal, avoidant and decisional procrastinators: Do they exist? *Personality and Individual Differences, 48*, 926–934.

Stolarski, M., Ledzińska, M., & Matthews, G. (2013). Morning is tomorrow, evening is today: relationships between chronotype and time perspective. *Biological Rhythms Research, 44*, 181–196.

Strathman, A., Gleicher, F., Boninger, D. S., y Edwards, C. S. (1994). The consideration of future consequences: Weighing immediate and distant outcomes of behavior. *Journal of Personality and Social Psychology, 66*, 742–752.

Sunddendorf, T., y Corballis, M. C. (1997). Mental time travel and the evolution of the human mind. *Genetic, Social and General Psychology Monographs, 123*, 133–167.

Tuckman, B. (1991). The development and concurrent validity of the Procrastination Scale. *Educational Psychological Measurement, 5*, 473–480.

Van Eerde, W. (2003). A meta-analytically derived nomological network of procrastination. *Personality and Individual Differences, 35*, 1401–1418.

Vodanovich, S. J., & Seib, H. M. (1997). Relationship between time structure and procrastination. *Psychological Reports, 80*, 211–215.

Watson, D. C. (2001). Procrastination and the five-factor model: A facet level analysis. *Personality and Individual Differences, 30*, 149–158.

Zaleski, Z. (1994). *Psychology of future orientation*. Lublin: Lublin University Press.

Zaleski, Z. (1996). Future anxiety: Concept measurement and preliminary research. *Personality and Individual Differences, 21*, 165–174.

Zimbardo, P. G., & Boyd, N. (1999). Putting time in perspective: A valid, reliable, individual-differences metric. *Journal of Personality and Social Psychology, 17*, 1271–1288.

Zimbardo, P., Sword, R., & Sword, R. (2012). *The time cure: Overcoming PTSD with the new psychology of time perspective therapy*. San Francisco: Wiley.

Goals Need Time Perspective to Be Achieved

Zbigniew Zaleski and Aneta Przepiórka

Introduction

Within the scope of this book, we review theoretical assumptions and research outcomes concerning the link between time perspective and goal theory. The first section inspired by goal theory reviews research and is a form of synopsis of the progress made in this area. It is worthwhile posing the questions of what has been found in the area of goal-theory so far and whether at the beginning of the second decade of the twenty-first century we have anything new to add to the accumulated knowledge on the role of goals in human life. What has been found and confirmed in replication investigations is not necessarily new but gives strong support for previous findings.

Since the work of Bühler (1933), the literature on goal setting and their motivational function has grown substantially, in particular during the last three decades. Some authors describe the process of how goals are set (Heckhausen and Kuhl 1985), what relationships occur between proximal and distal goals (Raynor and Entin 1982) and how they motivate people to act (Locke and Latham 1984; Zaleski 1991). However, the main focus of goal psychology falls on their motivational aspects and their contribution to life satisfaction. It is not erroneous to repeat after Nuttin (1984) that it is often more important to people who they want to become or will become in the future than who they are now. What is also very promising is that goal psychology is being successfully implanted into many projects and practical programs for young entrepreneurs, managers, sportsmen, inventors, adventure teams or educators of highly gifted individuals as well as into weight control and drug addiction control programs. Thus, theory and confirmatory findings make this

Z. Zaleski (✉) • A. Przepiórka
Institute of Psychology, The John Paul II Catholic University of Lublin, Lublin, Poland
e-mail: zal@kul.pl; aneta.przepiorka@gmail.com

M. Stolarski et al. (eds.), *Time Perspective Theory; Review, Research and Application: Essays in Honor of Philip G. Zimbardo*, DOI 10.1007/978-3-319-07368-2_21,

knowledge useful. There seems to be no doubt that the title of a book by Locke and Latham (1984) – "Goal setting: A motivational technique that works!" – reflects the actual state of affairs.

Goals in a Lifespan Perspective

People's actions are driven by different needs, values and motives, but in the field literature, there is a popular view of the human being as *homo teleologicus*. The concept emphasizes intentional human nature, which expresses itself in making plans, setting goals, defining ways for their attainment and finally pursuing, and achieving them. McDougall (1911) underlined purpose in human behavior and perceived planning as a specifically human feature. People's actions are driven by different needs, values and motives.

The concept of goal itself has been conceived in many ways. Nuttin (1984) assumed that the goals are the result of cognitive processing of needs and thus they are *sui generis* motives little comparable to any other determinant of behavior. Goal is understood as an internal representation of the desired states, which guides action as well as affects, decisions, effort and persistence (Austin and Vancouver 1996). The authors distinguished the following dimensions of goals: (a) importance – commitment, (b) difficulty – level, (c) specificity – representation, (d) temporal range, (e) level of consciousness, and (f) connectedness – complexity (p. 343). Brunstein (1993) proposed three dimensions: commitment, attainability and progress. As a result of his longitudinal study done on 88 participants, he concluded that the attainment of a goal leads to greater well-being. Progress in achieving a goal was a mediator in the relationship between commitment, attainability and well-being.

Consensus on the issue of what kind of goals motivate us stronger – proximal or distal ones – has not as yet been reached. Future goals play an important role in motivation: helping to maintain a sufficient level of motivation even while one is facing failures, they help to concentrate on opportunities to improve or develop the situation in the future (Nuttin and Lens 1985). Proximal goals are more powerful incentives than distal ones in spheres such as weight control (Bandura and Simon 1977). On the other hand, Zaleski (1991) emphasized that desirable future states play a motivating role in difficult life conditions. In fact, the discrepancy between current and desired states includes a motivating aspect (Earley and Lituchy 1991). In other life spheres, distal goals may be stronger motives.

An increasing body of evidence argues that the content and hierarchy of goals change with age, depending on the stage of life. At the age of about 18–20 years, young people begin to formulate their potential selves mostly in relation to professional occupation, but these formulations may also include place of living, family status, nonprofessional competencies and standards of particular character (Nurmi 1991). It is often linked to the choice of educational track. People work on their life goals, sometimes writing them down and sometimes just thinking of them without wording them in an explicit way. Whatever form or shape goals are given, people know what they intend to do, who they want to become and what their life should be like.

In accordance with the theory of development, young people set more expansive goals, connected with power, acquisition, or possession, while middle aged persons undertake more actions aimed at contributing to the society: they want to hand something down to the next generation and to share their knowledge and experience with their offspring (Oleś 2011; Salmela-Aro et al. 1993).

Setting a goal is not a single decision step. Heckhausen and Kuhl (1985) proposed to view it as process from a wish to intentional actions. Setting a long-term goal is a matter of a complex decision process. This process can probably be characterized by some rationality rules proposed by the theory of decision, according to which decision involves calculation of the chance of reaching the final outcome. However, many other factors play no smaller role in each individual case, such as the hierarchy of needs, the system of values, the philosophy of life, *Zeitgeist* trends, family models, or social models (Bandura 1986). Even if only few of them come into play, the process of deciding on a distant personal goal requires plenty of cognitive work, analyses, comparisons, as well as evaluation of inner and outer resources. Most people come to a decision concerning what they want in life and set themselves realistic goals to achieve. However, due to encountered obstacles some persons never set any realistic goal and dwell on their wishes or imagined end states.

An interesting observation of the above-mentioned authors concerns the so-called "degenerated intentions," meaning intentions that for some reasons never lead to any action and never trigger any realization step. One desires something and sets it as an aim but lacks the means and resources to make it come true. In common parlance they are sometimes called "wishful thinking," which is not a very exceptional phenomenon. The expression suggests that a person wishes to have or become more than they can. Goal setting is a costly process and can sometimes be ineffective. However, when it successfully fulfills certain criteria, the goal becomes a useful guide and engine in life. Making a decision about one's goal and formulating intentions is compared to "crossing the Rubicon" (Heckhausen 1991). How does it function? Probably in many ways and some of them we can already describe.

The Motivational Function of Goals

Goals direct human action, stimulate people to greater effort, affect strategies for implementation (Locke et al. 1981) and are connected with motivation (Brett and Vandewalle 1999). The more important the goal, the stronger the motivation to achieve it (Heckhausen and Kuhl 1985).

Zaleski (1991) has enumerated different action dimensions in a goal-directed behavior. First, a goal *per se* enhances **effort** to work for it. It helps accumulate and concentrate strength and energy for starting and continuing activities. Similarly, it makes an actor more persistent in the endeavor towards the final state. **Persistence** is crucial, since many actions on the way bring no direct reward and the actor must wait for it until the final stage is achieved. Moreover, a goal helps **select significant information** for its attainment. A student who wants to prepare the diploma work will read the texts most suitable for the dissertation. Finally, a goal leads to search for and apply the optimal **action strategies** by organizing time and activities so as to maximize goal attainment.

As goal realization is extended in time, the work needs reinforcement; otherwise it may undergo inhibition. It is obvious is that each step brings us closer to the goal. In other words, each step enhances the probability of goal attainment. But this may not be enough to maintain a required level of repeated effort from day to day, from month to month. Subjective well-being would be endangered. What the goal does is to bring **emotional satisfaction** from a mere activity aiming at the desired standard (Zaleski 1991). Without this direct pleasure from doing something concrete it would be hard to return to repetitious actions in the longer run. There is a reciprocal feedback relationship: activity brings satisfaction and the satisfaction motivates activity. People report it when speaking about their goal-directed behaviors and psychologists or counselors should take this circular link into account when preparing a person for long-lasting work on a goal that requires extended effort.

So far, we have said what activity-related benefits a goal gives. But this is not the end of the story. A goal gives something more. When people work on something worthy for themselves or when they realize a commonly shared important value, their life acquires a special quality, which psychology calls **meaning in life** (e.g., Emmons 1986). This is so indeed. Those who strive for important goals feel that their life has meaning, that there is something to live for, that there is in them a will to live. Needless to say how powerful and important this feeling or awareness is. "The motor to live" would be an appropriate term for a personal goal; a person must live for something and must feel that his or her life has meaning. Within the self-regulation framework we would suggest that personal goals can be counterfactors and buffors for energy expiration for what is called self-depletion (Baumeister et al. 1998). Personal goals defend ego from getting tired and therefore passive.

According to humanistic psychology, humans are driven by their needs (Maslow 1943). Especially the need for self-realization is the focus of strivings for meaning in life, personal satisfaction and fulfillment. Engagement in important goals and the pursuit of important goals is related to the quality of life (Little and Chambers 2004). Similarly, Frankl (1959) indicated that time, values and goals are relevant to the experience of meaning in life. Goals determine self-esteem and meaning in life. This assumption has been confirmed especially in difficult and life-threatening situations such as labor camps in Siberia, when long-term objectives helped to survive and rise above the surrounding conditions, as was the case in Siberia or in Nazi labor camps (cf. Obuchowski 1995).

Within to the social cognitive perspective, goals direct human behavior to their attainment by regulating affective and cognitive processes depending on perceived self-efficacy (Bandura 1986). Those with higher self-efficacy strive more persistently to achieve challenging goals and visualize positive outcome of their actions, contrary to those with lower self-efficacy, who anticipate failure and put in less effort.

The characteristic feature of human action is a forethought, self-regulatory mechanism. In the pursuit of goals, we exert control upon our actions and predict their consequences. When facing difficult goals, it is easier to work towards them by dividing their attainment into subgoals that enhance self-efficacy and motivation (Stock and Cervone 1990). This method prevents discouragement. Being motivated intrinsically, we are more engaged in the task and more persistent when facing obstacles (Deci and Ryan 2000). Harré and Bullen (2010) applied Self-Determination Theory approach to two types of projects: educational and life projects. As a result, they concluded that integrity and competence played pivotal role in commitment to both types of projects in high school and university students. If students felt competent and if the activity was consistent with their values, the project was highly motivating for them.

The Link Between Goals and Time

Due to the fact that goals are by their nature related to time, it is impossible to explain or understand them without reference to the temporal dimension. The last 30 years of research and speculation on temporal dimensions of human psychological reality lead to some conclusions and predictions and stimulate new questions. Human beings live in time: looking into and "digging" in their memory of the **past**, when acting in the **present** and thinking about or planning their own **future** (Zimbardo and Boyd 2008). What do they do with these dimensions and how do they use them to make their lives satisfactory? First, the relationships among the three temporal dimensions must be set in such a way that there is consonance rather than destructive conflict within this temporal triangle. Therefore, there is the challenge of how much attention should be placed on each of these dimensions and to what extent each one should be salient in everyday life. Then there is the crucial decision of whom a person wants and intends to be. What should be the end of their efforts, struggles and invested energy? What should be the structure of time from setting a goal to its attainment? And finally, what coordinates and integrates the evaluation processes, affective states and overt action?

Temporal perspective plays a role as a regulator of human action; its impact on human activity, motivation and attitude toward time is widely recognized (Zaleski 1988, 1989). In a broader approach, Zimbardo and Boyd (1999) emphasize the important role of time in human life. Time is a kind of resource capital to use and having an adequate temporal perspective is conducive to purposeful activity. The authors describe time perspective as a psychological dimension that organizes personal experience within three time dimensions: the past, the present and the future. People have their yesterday, their today and their tomorrow. Let us now briefly focus on these temporal dimensions.

The past. In proverbs, stories, songs, diaries, books and notes one conserves registered events of the past, consisting of accomplishments, failures, as well as realized and "degenerated" intentions. The longer one lives the bigger this store grows. This store is fixed and only its perception and interpretation can be altered. Its content can be reinterpreted from the present or future perspective. Our simultaneous perception and evaluation of past events and actions performed in the already elapsed time may differ from how we see these events and actions now. What is more, they can be regarded in a particular way when conclusions are to be drawn for the future. Thus, our past can serve us as a treasury of experience in facing challenges to come. According to Zimbardo and Boyd (1999), a positive attitude to the past is linked with a sense of satisfaction, with higher self-esteem, lower anxiety, and a general friendly attitude. Such persons may also experience more social support and fewer conflicts. They cope better with stressful situations, which enhances their self-efficacy.

In the above sense, the past "exists" in our present and in our future. People refer to, compare, copy, or negate what they have done until now in order to be more efficient in their tomorrow. We can firmly state that our past is, if not necessary, then at least very useful for future endeavors (cf. Zimbardo and Boyd 2008).

Like a geologist, one digs in the personal memory store to pull out the experiences from which to draw inspiration, advice, or critical judgment of what to undertake now and where to invest energy and resources. This usage is not automatic or simple copying of things of the past. They are reinterpreted in many ways, reanalyzed, and reconstructed before use is made of them in the construction of future goals. To be fruitful, this process requires applying the cognitive processes of analysis, synthesis, and evaluation as well as comparison with scenarios of other successful and unsuccessful people, the ability to draw the most crucial experiences from memory and to rank them on a usefulness scale (Thiebaut 1998) Then another ability comes into play: one must incorporate or appropriately include the selected elements into a presently constructed goal and its realization plan. Also the experiences of others can be useful.

People have their life stories, and it is possible to benefit from them when one is allowed to get familiar with them. Vicarious learning (see Bandura 1986) is an adequate way to benefit from the experience of others. When it comes to making use of others' life "stories," we may have a hard time making a scrutiny because each scenario is very individual and we do not have full access to all the personal and environmental factors. However, it is advisable to listen to people's reports and their personal "register" of what they have done or how they perceived events and their own actions at a given time in the past and compared to how they perceive these events and actions now, in retrospect. What can be crucial is their evaluation of those events from a distance in time. Read or listened to, these life reports can be of value for a person's future plans. In sum, without our past it would not be easy to build our future.

The present. Fraisse (1957) used the term "presentist" in an almost scornful way to refer to those who focus their life on the "here and now" (*hic et nunc*). This description is justified, but only in the case of individuals who refuse to refer to and recall their past as well as escape from thinking and planning what they should do next week, next month, or next year and who they should become.

In our opinion, the present is crucial because all our actions take place in the present temporal space. We write, study, build or paint NOW, aware of our activity and the elapsing time until a finishing point such as noon, a break, weekend, or holidays. This present is a hard fact, although its conception and management may differ from person to person. First, the temporal dimension of the term "now" or "at present" is peculiar and not clearly defined. For some people, it can be a pretty limited period counted in minutes or hours. For others, this notion can cover several days, the current week, or a month. We do not know the reason for such a discrepancy but it should be taken into account in analyzing personal time structure. Perhaps for the first group time flies fast and they "chase" it like dogs running after an escaping hare. They may feel that everything is changing too fast. The second group may have a feeling of greater comfort in bringing some parts of their activity to an end because their present has a broader range.

Present activity is not an isolated unit but an element in a chain of actions being partly an effect of preceding steps and the foundation or even condition for the next steps to come. Feather and Bond (1994) speak of time structure as an important predictor of psychological well-being and adjustment. The connection of what has already happened with what is happening now and what will follow gives fluency to our work on the way to accomplishing something. There is a clear continuity in a person's efforts which builds their identity as the author of changes. Thanks to this, we can conceptualize activities, relate them to outside events, and write a diary on the one hand and a script for life on the other. Thus, although shorter than the other two dimensions, the present is crucial, since it is in the present that we realize our projects and, step by step, build our life through contingent activities (cf. Raynor and Entin 1982). Additionally, focus on the present gives enjoyment and energy to fulfill tasks (Sobol-Kwapińska 2009; Zimbardo and Boyd 1999).

The future. This temporal sphere differs from the previous dimensions in one particular feature: it is unknown. It can only be conceived of, thought of, imagined, projected, or partially anticipated (Timoszyk-Tomczak and Zaleski 2006). However, as in the case of the previous two dimensions, its chronological aspect should be described. The knowledge of average lifespan does not necessarily give any adequate ground to the cognitive evaluation of how long our future will be. One conceives of the future in terms of a year or somewhat more: a longer time extending this range is not included in thinking. Yet, the psychological nature of the future is very individual and differs from one person to another.

We can assume that people **should** think of the time when they will be 60 or 70 years old. But this is not necessarily the case. Some people in their twenties do not go so far; such an extended future does not preoccupy their minds. They preoccupy themselves with shorter periods, rather "easy" to think of, and perceive them in terms of content, events, places, and actions, but not necessarily in a temporal way. Students of psychology when asked to assign their short and long future are surprised to discover that what is a short perspective for one person is a long perspective for another. This, of course, concerns the time perspective measured in temporal units. The second important aspect is the content filling up this space. We call that simply **goals**, a term that is one of the most frequent in today's common language. The conception of entire future time perspective entails time space and goals to obtain. People conceive when, how, and where they accomplish their goals and put their intentions into reality. This strategy called *implementation intentions* makes them more committed to the goal and increases the chances of its attainment (see Gollwitzer and Oettingen 2013)

Zaleski et al. (2001) examined the relationship between FTP and subjective well-being. There were three factors extracted for FTP: preoccupation with present activities, possession of long-term goals, and plans for realizing long-term goals. The study, done on 306 high school students revealed that, in contrast with those who scored high on present preoccupation, those who scored high on long-term goals and plans for realizing long-term goals reported more meaningful life and higher social self-efficacy, were more persistent in obtaining goals, and suffered less from emotional distress and hopelessness. Przepiorka (2012) examined the relationship between attitude towards time and the presence of meaning in life. As a result, it was concluded that extended time perspective and better organized time perspective in terms of telicity, planning, detailness, and use of time was related to higher meaning in life. Positive time perception was also related to positive attitude towards one's life. It is optimal to have a balanced temporal structure embracing all three time dimensions. FTP facilitates achieving goals and positive past perspective reinforces a sense of identity. A study conducted on a group of 260 people confirmed the positive relationship between a balanced perspective, life satisfaction, and mindfulness (Drake et al. 2008).

Numerous studies have shown that psychological time – its perception – is influenced by emotional states (Strzałecki 2006, 2010), and the way we perceive time may translate into commitment to the goals, especially long term ones. In practice, with the increase of conviction that a goal can be achieved, the psychological time distance towards the accomplishment of this goal decreases. Distant goals that are likely to be achieved are more attractive to us; they are more challenging and we feel more committed to them.

Moreover, temporal orientation is an expression of personal commitment and focuses on one of the dimensions of time (Simons et al. 2004). Long-term future time perspective, in contrast to a short-term one, has a more positive impact on performance in academic tasks (De Volder and Lens 1982). Students with a long FTP are more persistent in their work for long-term objectives. Additionally, people with a long FTP can work harder for short term goals and derive more pleasure from this activity (Zaleski 1987, 1991). The extent of temporal perspective plays a motivational function, improves endurance, and prevents frustration.

Subjects with longer FTP have higher need for achievement and set themselves more ambitious goals. They are distinguished by the ability to postpone gratification and make internal attributions of educational and professional success (De Volder and Lens 1982). Some relationships were found between construing own future and personality dimensions. Timoszyk-Tomczak and Zaleski (2006) carried out a study on 239 high school and university students. Six strategies were identified, namely: (1) authority strategy based on other's advice and suggestions, (2) realistic strategy entails observations outer world, analysis of personal experience and one's own capabilities, (3) wishful strategy built on fantasy often does not reflect the reality,

(4) carpe diem strategy constitutes the negligence of the future and concentration solely on the present, (5) social pressure strategy is externally elaborated under the obligations of parents or other people, and (6) awaiting strategy stems from the belief that we do not have influence on our life. The term strategy refers to the personal conceptualization of one's own future that involves values, plans, goals, paths to achieve them, and self-definition. The most frequently used in that age group were authority, realistic, and wishful strategies. For instance, those young people who used more often realistic strategy for planning their future had long term goals, were high on achievement motivation, more optimistic, and had internal locus of control. Out of many personality traits, it was extraversion, anxiety and value system that appeared significant for elaborating future projects.

Goal Theory in Different Spheres of Life

The variety of personal goals can be theoretically unlimited, though there is a list of aims most frequently set, particularly by young people. Studies carried out among Americans (Zaleski 1991) as well as on Polish (Mądrzycki 2002) and Japanese samples (Tsuzuki 2012) show that these aims belong to such spheres as education, family, professional occupation, income, travel, religion, or personal hobbies. TP theory was also used for determining the predictors of leisure time activity (Blachnio et al. 2009). Those with short FTP spent more time on the Internet and were more engaged in social networking. There was a negative correlation between short FTP and participation in trainings or reading. Long FTP correlated positively with trainings, and negatively with watching series, playing computer games, and discussing on Internet forums. Those who spent their leisure time actively had more organized long FTP. Those people who managed their time had longer FTP higher hope for success. Another study (Blachnio and Przepiorka, in press), where the Zimbardo Time Perspective Inventory was used for analysis of determinants of leisure time activity among students, revealed that hedonistic present correlated positively with social activity, surfing in the Internet, and good time management. Positive past perspective correlated positively with surfing in the Internet and with gardening.

Political, economic, and social changes also inspire the elaboration of reality-related goals. One of them is the rising phenomenon of entrepreneurship, particularly in the post-communist countries. Not everybody in free market conditions decides to start their own company but many do so, and this issue deserves a psychological study.

Bluedorn and Denhardt (1988) present the overview of the research on the link between time and organizations. According to them time is closely linked to productivity and its good management helps to achieve the objectives of the company. In a similar vein, Bird and West (1997) emphasize that temporal perspective plays a vital role in entrepreneurship. The way a person experiences and perceives time translates into future performance. Identifying opportunities, time management, the creation of vision, the perception of problems, planning – all of these happen within time and are part of a temporal horizon. Time can be regarded as the energy that entrepreneurs use to develop their company. Time is also a resource that can be allocated into interesting and creative activity. Perception, anticipation, and the ability to assess present action give rise to the formation of intentions.

The studies that compared entrepreneurs with the unemployed or employees revealed that the former were more oriented to the future, set more goals, and were better at planning and managing their time (Strzałecki 2010; Wesołowska 2003). The groups also differed in the ability to pursue long-term tasks, the ability to achieve them, and the willingness to postpone gratification. Moreover, effective entrepreneurs were more resistant to obstacles and less likely to dwell on negative events or miss opportunities (Baron 2000), which may result from their forward-looking orientation.

Recently, Zimbardo and Boyd's (1999) conception of time perspective (TP) has been applied to entrepreneurship. In her study, Przepiorka (2010) investigated the relationship between TP and the intention to start a business. TP was measured using the Polish adaptation of the ZTPI method. Based on the strength of intention to start a business, two groups were compared – participants with high intention and those without intention, the so-called potential entrepreneurs. It was found that those who wanted to start their company were more future-oriented, scored higher on Present Hedonistic, lower on Present Fatalistic, and lower on negative past. In a recent study (Przepiorka, in revision) it was revealed that actual entrepreneurs were future-oriented and scored the lowest on fatalistic present. They put more effort, were more persistent in realizing their goals, and tended to be more satisfied with them. They scored higher on hope for success and were more action-oriented according to Kuhl's (1981) theory. Considering the limited nature of the energy the effective managing and its regulation may be a prerequisite for achieving goals. Self-regulation helps in overcoming conflict of motives and preserves from giving up on undertaken action (e.g. Baumeister and Vohs 2007). By that means we spare the energy what results in a better performance and higher goal-achievement. Self-regulation requires sufficient amount of energy to monitor action and to regulate behavior. As a result of meta analysis of 83 studies (Hagger et al. 2010) *ego* depletion has a number of deterioration effects on effort or self-control task, results in fatigue and negative affect. Effective self-regulation may enforce the success in entrepreneurship. As a future recommendation it would be interesting to analyze the relationship between time perspective, self-regulation (*ego* deplition/defense) and their effect on the achieving entrepreneurial goals.

The results mentioned above show how applicable is the theory of time perspective. It is related to our vocational as well as private goals. We want to stress that positive attitude toward time and extended future is characteristic for those who performed better and had better achievements. The same was true the same for the entrepreneurs and those who had higher intention to start their own company in the future. This positive attitude towards time may reduce the anxiety (Zaleski 1996) and helps in effective self-regulation.

Final Remarks

We tried to outline the relationship between goal-directed behavior and time perspective. The studies illustrate links between these constructs as well as present their place and role in a broader meaning of human action. We referred to classic conceptions of goals and goal theories as well as to more recent research on goals and time perspective and their application in different spheres of human life. It has been proved that the goals have regulatory effect on our action. As goals are located in temporal space from now, therefore humans use their cognitive capacity to conceive and elaborate their future time but also to use the records of their past experiences. Focused on the future, a human is located in three time perspectives. We refer to three temporal spheres. Beneficial is, if these three dimensions are well balanced as such a balance results in effective activity and life satisfaction. The Zimbardo Time Perspective Theory has been investigated with reference to entrepreneurship, leisure time activity and time management. This theory is useful in understanding human actions and their motives, which is of paramount importance in our conception of life. Some of the raised questions can already be provided with quite satisfactory answers whereas some others remain open for future theoretical analyses and empirical research. This approach has a promising future.

To conclude this overview of the role of the time perspective in goal-attainment we may indicate the positive effect of given time orientations on our behavior. Future time perspective motivates us to setting goals and facilitates achieving them. Positive past perspective reinforces a sense of identity. Concentration on the present gives us energy to pursue goals and to enjoy our life. There are still many areas where we may verify the role of time perspective especially in a cross-cultural comparison.

References

Austin, J. T., & Vancouver, J. B. (1996). Goal constructs in psychology: Process and content. *Psychological Bulletin, 120*, 338–375.

Bandura, A. (1986). *Social foundations of thought and action*. Englewood Cliffs: Prentice-Hall.

Bandura, A., & Simon, K. M. (1977). The role of proximal intentions in self-regulation of refractory behavior. *Cognitive Therapy and Research, 1*, 177–193.

Baron, R. A. (2000). Counterfactual thinking and venture formation: The potential effect of thinking about "what might have been". *Journal of Business Venturing, 15*, 79–92.

Baumeister, R. F., & Vohs, K. D. (2007). Self-regulation, ego depletion and motivation. *Social and Personality Psychology Compass, 1*(1), 115–128.

Baumeister, R. F., Bratslavsky, E., Muraven, M., & Tice, D. M. (1998). Ego depletion: Is the active self a limited resource? *Journal of Personality and Social Psychology, 74*, 1252–1265.

Bird, B. J., & West, G. P., III. (1997). Time and entrepreneurship. *Entrepreneurship: Theory and Practice, 22*, 1–13.

Blachnio, A., & Przepiorka, A. (in press). The Polish Leisure Time Activity Questionnaire (LTAQ). *Time & Society*.

Blachnio, A., Przepiorka, A., & Zaleski, Z. (2009). Aktywni wygrani. Przyszłościowa perspektywa czasowa i nadzieja na sukces w zarządzaniu wolnym czasem. In A. Blachnio (Ed.), *Globalizacja a jednostka* (pp. 178–191). Bydgoszcz: Wydawnictwo UKW.

Bluedorn, A. C., & Denhardt, R. B. (1988). Time and organizations. *Journal of Management, 14*(2), 299–320.
Brett, J. F., & VandeWalle, D. (1999). Goal orientation and goal content as predictors of performance in a training program. *Journal of Applied Psychology, 84*, 863–873.
Brunstein, J. C. (1993). Personal goals and subjective well-being: A longitudinal study. *Journal of Personality and Social Psychology, 65*(5), 1061–1070.
Bühler, C. (1933). *Der menschliche Lebenslauf als psychologisches Problem*. Leipzig: Hirzel.
De Volder, M., & Lens, W. (1982). Academic achievement and future time perspective as a cognitive-motivational concept. *Journal of Personality and Social Psychology, 42*, 566–571.
Deci, E. L., & Ryan, R. M. (2000). The 'what' and 'why' of goal pursuits: Human needs and the self- determination of behavior. *Psychological Inquiry, 11*, 227–268.
Drake, L., Duncan, E., Sutherland, F., Abernethy, C., & Henry, C. (2008). Time perspective and correlates of well-being. *Time & Society, 17*(1), 47–61.
Earley, C., & Lituchy, T. (1991). Delineating goal and efficacy effects: A test of three models. *Journal of Applied Psychology, 76*, 81–98.
Emmons, R. A. (1986). Personal strivings: An approach to personality and subjective wellbeing. *Journal of Personality and Social Psychology, 51*, 1058–1068.
Feather, N., & Bond, M. (1994). Structure and purpose in the use of time. In Z. Zaleski (Ed.), *Psychology of future orientation* (pp. 121–140). Lublin: Towarzystwo Naukowe KUL.
Fraisse, P. (1957). *Psychologie du temps*. Paris: Presses Universitaires de France.
Frankl, V. E. (1959). *Man's search for meaning: An introduction to logotherapy*. New York: Simon & Schuster.
Gollwitzer, P. M., & Oettingen, G. (2013). Implementation intentions. In M. Gellman & J. R. Turner (Eds.), *Encyclopedia of behavioral medicine* (Part 9, pp. 1043–1048). New York: Springer.
Hagger, M. S., Wood, C., Stiff, C., & Chatzisarantis, N. D. (2010). Ego depletion and the strength model of self-control: A meta-analysis. *Psychological Bulletin, 136*(4), 495–525.
Harré, N., & Bullen, P. (2010). Personal project commitment in adolescence: The role of relatedness, competence and integrity. *European Journal of Social Psychology, 40*(2), 235–251.
Heckhausen, H. (1991). *Motivation and action*. Berlin: Springer.
Heckhausen, H., & Kuhl, J. (1985). From wishes to action: The dead ends and short cuts on the long way to action. In M. Frese & J. Sabini (Eds.), *Goal directed behavior* (pp. 78–94). Hillsdale: Erlbaum.
Kuhl, J. (1981). Motivational and functional helplessness: The moderating effect of state vs. action orientation. *Journal of Personality and Social Psychology, 40*, 155–170.
Little, B. R., & Chambers, N. C. (2004). Personal project pursuit: On human doings and well-beings. In W. Cox & E. Klinger (Eds.), *Handbook of motivational counseling: Concepts, approaches and assessment* (pp. 65–82). New York: Wiley.
Locke, E. A., & Latham, G. P. (Eds.). (1984). *Goal setting: A motivational technique that works*. Englewood Cliffs: Prentice-Hall, Inc.
Locke, E. A., Shaw, K. N., Saari, L. M., & Latham, G. P. (1981). Goal setting and task performance: 1969–1980. *Psychological Bulletin, 90*, 125–152.
Mądrzycki, T. (2002). *Osobowość jako system tworzący i realizujący plany*. Gdańsk: Wydawnictwo Uniwersytetu Gdańskiego.
Maslow, A. H. (1943). A theory of human motivation. *Psychological Review, 50*(4), 370–396.
McDougall, W. (1911). *Body and mind: A history and a defense of animism*. London: Methuen.
Nurmi, J.-E. (1991). How do adolescents see their future? A review of the development of future orientation and planning. *Developmental Review, 11*, 1–59.
Nuttin, J. (1984). *Motivation, planning and action*. Hillsdale: Erlbaum.
Nuttin, J., & Lens, W. (1985). *Future time perspective and motivation*. Hillsdale: Erlbaum.
Obuchowski, K. (1995). *Przez galaktykę potrzeb: psychologia dążeń ludzkich*. Poznań: Zysk i S-ka Wydawnictwo.
Oleś, P. (2011). *Psychologia człowieka dorosłego. Ciągłość. Zmiana. Integracja*. Warszawa: PWN.

Przepiorka, A. M. (2010). *Time perspective, proactive personality, and the Intention of Starting a Business.* The paper presented at the XVth European Conference on Personality, Brno, Czech Republic, 20–24 July, 2012.

Przepiorka, A. (2012). The relationship between attitude towards time and the presence of meaning in life. *International Journal of Applied Psychology, 2*(3), 22–30.

Przepiorka, A. (in revision). What makes successful entrepreneurs different in temporal and goal-commitment dimensions? *Time & Society*.

Raynor, J., & Entin, E. (1982). Theory and research on future orientation and achievement motivation. In J. Raynor & E. Entin (Eds.), *Motivation, career striving, and aging* (pp. 13–82). Washington, DC: Hemisphere.

Salmela-Aro, K. K., Nurmi, J. E., Aro, A. A., Poppius, E. E., & Riste, J. J. (1993). Age differences in adults' personal projects. *Journal of Social Psychology, 133*(3), 415–417.

Simons, J., Vansteenkiste, M., Lens, W., & Lacante, M. (2004). Placing motivation and future time perspective theory in a temporal perspective. *Educational Psychology Review, 16*(2), 121–139.

Sobol-Kwapińska, M. (2009). Forms of present time orientation and satisfaction with life in the context of attitudes toward past and future. *Social Behavior and Personality, 37*(4), 433–440.

Stock, J., & Cervone, D. (1990). Proximal goal-setting and self-regulatory processes. *Cognitive Therapy and Research, 14*, 483–498.

Strzałecki, A. (2006). Psychological time and the subjective probability of attaining life goals. In Z. Uchnast (Ed.), *Psychology of time. Theoretical and empirical approaches* (pp. 79–96). Lublin: Wydawnictwo KUL.

Strzałecki, A. (2010). Twórczość i prawdopodobieństwo subiektywne osiągania celów życiowych a czas psychologiczny. In G. Sędek & S. Bedyńska (Eds.), *Życie na Czas Perspektywy Badawcze Postrzegania Czasu* (pp. 293–328). Warszawa: Wydawnictwo PWN.

Thiebaut, E. (1998). La perspective temporelle, un concept a la recherché dùne definition operationelle. *L'Année Psychologique, 98*, 101–125.

Timoszyk-Tomczak, C., & Zaleski, Z. (2006). Personality and construing one's own future. *Polish Psychological Bulletin, 37*(3), 172–184.

Tsuzuki, M. (2012). Dynamic changing process of hope in early adolescence: Analysis of individual differences during the transition from elementary school to junior high school. *Japanese Psychological Research, 54*(3), 253–262.

Wesołowska, E. (2003). *Psychologiczny portret prywatnego przedsiębiorcy*. Olsztyn: Wydawnictwo Uniwersytetu Warmińsko – Mazurskiego.

Zaleski, Z. (1987). Behavioral effects of self-set goals for different time ranges. *International Journal of Psychology, 22*, 17–38.

Zaleski, Z. (1988). Attributions and emotions related to future goal attainment. *Journal of Educational Psychology, 80*, 563–568.

Zaleski, Z. (1989). Przyszłościowa perspektywa czasowa jako wymiar "Ja". In A. Biela, Z. Uchnast, & T. Witkowski (Eds.), *Wykłady z psychologii w KUL 1986/87* (pp. 227–234). Lublin: RW KUL.

Zaleski, Z. (1991). *Psychologia zachowań celowych*. Warszawa: Państwowe Wydawnictwo Naukowe.

Zaleski, Z. (1996). Future anxiety: Concept, measurement and preliminary research. *Personality and Individual Differences, 21*, 165–174.

Zaleski, Z., Cycoń, A., & Kurc, A. (2001). Future time perspective and subjective well-being in adolescent samples. In P. Schmuck & K. Sheldon (Eds.), *Life goals and well-being: Towards a positive psychology of human striving* (pp. 58–67). Göttingen: Hogrefe & Huber.

Zimbardo, P. G., & Boyd, J. N. (1999). Putting time in perspective: A valid reliable individual differences metric. *Journal of Personality and Social Psychology, 77*, 1271–1288.

Zimbardo, P., & Boyd, J. (2008). *The time paradox: The new psychology of time that will change your life*. New York: Free Press.

Part IV
Non-clinical Applications of Time Perspective

Time Perspective as a Predictor of Healthy Behaviors and Disease-Mediating States

Peter A. Hall, Geoffrey T. Fong, and Genevieve Sansone

Time perspective has been defined as an individual difference variable reflecting temporal biases in thinking about the self and one's own actions. Those with a more future-oriented time perspective are thought to be more attentive to, and influenced by, long-term contingencies (costs vs. benefits) than those who are more present-oriented. Time perspective—and specifically future orientation—is hypothesized to be a causal factor in behaviors for which time matters, that is, for behaviors with cost and benefits that occur along different time frames (now vs. later; Zimbardo and Boyd 1999; Strathman et al. 1994; Fong and Hall 2003). Phil Zimbardo and his colleagues were the first to fully integrate the concept of time perspective into contemporary personality and social psychology research, and the *Zimbardo Time Perspective Inventory* (ZTPI) remains the most widely used self-report measure of time perspective by a wide margin. Other self-report measures of time perspective exist as well, including the *Consideration of Future Consequences Scale* (CFC; Strathman et al. 1994), the *Time Perspective Questionnaire* (TPQ; Fong and Hall 2003), and its behavior-specific counterparts (Hall et al. 2012b).

These measures are more circumscribed than the ZTPI in that they do not include a past orientation subscale (in the case of the CFC) and/or do not include subdivisions of future/present experience. However, they do focus on what is largely thought to be the most relevant dimension of time perspective for understanding health behavior: future orientation. In this chapter, we review some of our research on future orientation (measured using the TPQ) and health-related behaviors/outcomes.

P.A. Hall (✉)
Faculty of Applied Health Sciences, University of Waterloo, Waterloo, ON, Canada
e-mail: pahall@uwaterloo.ca

G.T. Fong • G. Sansone
Department of Psychology, University of Waterloo, Waterloo, ON, Canada
e-mail: gfong@uwaterloo.ca; gsansone@uwaterloo.ca

M. Stolarski et al. (eds.), *Time Perspective Theory; Review, Research and Application: Essays in Honor of Philip G. Zimbardo*, DOI 10.1007/978-3-319-07368-2_22,

Time Perspective and Health Behavior Performance

Many health behaviors are characterized by a disjunction between the time course of costs and benefits: health-protective behaviors such as exercise and healthy dietary behaviors have long-term benefits to appearance and well-being but subtle short-term costs (i.e., inconvenience, time cost). Despite the relatively minor nature of such costs, they are rendered disproportionately influential because of their temporal proximity (Loewenstein and Thaler 1989; Ainslie 2010). As such, attention to less visceral but ultimately more profound long-term contingencies (e.g., longer lifespan, more disability-free years) is a potentially important determinant of one's decision to engage in health-protective behaviors. Essentially the same dynamics are at play for health risk behaviors, such as substance use, unsafe driving practices, and sexual risk behaviors. In these cases, benefits are more proximal, rendering action more likely, despite the substantial costs over the long run.

Over the past two decades, many empirical investigations have examined the association between individual differences in time perspective and health-related behaviors (Adams 2009; Adams and Nettle 2009; Adams and White 2009; Daugherty and Brase 2010; Fieulaine and Martinez 2010; Hall and Fong 2003; Hall et al. 2012a; Heckman et al. 2009; Henson et al. 2006; Joireman et al. 2012; Keough et al. 1999; Kovač and Rise 2007; Orbell and Hagger 2006; Orbell and Kyriakaki 2008; Rappange et al. 2009; Rothspan and Read 1996; Strathman et al. 1994; Wills et al. 2001; Zimbardo and Boyd 1999; Zimbardo et al. 1997). In these studies, time perspective typically has some association with health behavior, normally in the direction of stronger future orientation (or less present orientation) predicting healthier behavioral trajectories.

Though most of the original studies examining this association between time perspective and health outcomes were small in sample size (prototypical of behavioral sciences research), some more recent studies have begun to examine such trends in large international datasets (prototypical of epidemiological research). For instance, the International Tobacco Control (ITC) Surveys are a set of international surveys that have been examining the association between time perspective and smoking behavior around the world over the past decade. Currently the ITC Project encompasses 23 countries, representative of half of the world's population of smokers (Fong et al. 2006). Although the data are just beginning to emerge regarding the time perspective construct, initial ITC findings regarding the relationship between smoking behavior and time perspective are promising. Two current studies have found that a more future-oriented time perspective is associated (cross-nationally) with lower likelihood of being a smoker (Sansone et al. 2012; Fig. 1), and among current smokers, a greater likelihood of making quit attempts prospectively (Hall et al. 2012b). In the latter investigation, time perspective was in fact a much better predictor of quit attempts than sensation-seeking, a construct that has a long history in smoking and personality research. A recent follow-up study confirmed that future-oriented time perspective predicts successful cessation and that the effects are attributable to the more faithful engagement in the quit cycle among

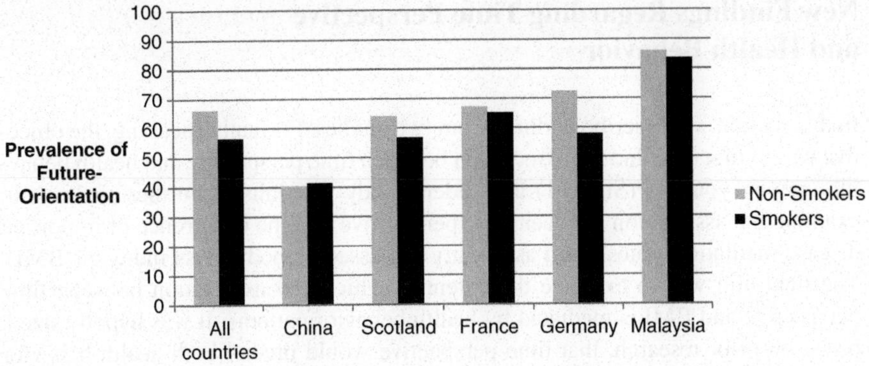

Fig. 1 Prevalence of future orientation by smoking status (From Sansone et al. 2012)

future-oriented smokers (Hall et al. 2014). Perhaps most encouraging about the ITC findings thus far is the fact that the predictive trends appear to hold across many countries of origin, which vary in ethnic milieu, culture, language, and wealth distribution (e.g., the United States, Canada, Australia, the United Kingdom, France, Germany, China, and Malaysia).

By now, the basic association between time perspective and health behaviors has been reasonably well established, and attention has turned to understanding time perspective as a mediator of social/contextual effects on behavior (e.g., Adams and White 2009) and to understanding the mechanism by which time perspective influences health behavior (e.g., Hall et al. 2012a; Joireman et al. 2012; Wills et al. 2001).

Time Perspective and Disease-Mediating States: Obesity

Given that the association between time perspective and health behavior is well documented, it is possible that time perspective also has a "downstream" influence on disease-mediating states such as obesity. It is further possible—given the established association between time perspective and health behavior—that time perspective may confer vulnerability to obesity via its influence on health behaviors. For example, those with a more future-oriented time perspective may engage in more physical activity and avoid consumption of fatty foods in part due to their concern about the eventual health consequences of failing to do so. Such behavioral tendencies in turn might eventually result in better body composition (i.e., BMI) toward mid- or later life, with enough passage of time for such behaviors to have a cumulative effect. At least one study has previously documented an association between time perspective and BMI (Adams and White 2009; Adams and Nettle 2009); however, to date no mediational analyses have been conducted in order to determine exactly *how* a future-oriented time perspective translates into lower BMI.

New Findings Regarding Time Perspective and Health Behavior

In this section, we describe findings from two studies. Formally speaking, the objective was to first examine the association between time perspective and health behaviors among younger (Study 1) and older (Study 2) adults. A further aim was to examine the association between time perspective and the occurrence of important disease-mediating states, such as obesity (assessed as body mass index, or BMI). The final aim was to examine the extent to which any association between time perspective and BMI is mediated by health behavior patterns. It was hypothesized, based on prior research, that time perspective would predict both health behavior patterns and BMI and that health behavior performance would mediate the relationship between time perspective and BMI. To test this hypothesis, in Study 1, we assessed time perspective in a sample of healthy younger adults and examined its association with an index of health behavior tendencies. In this study, we further examined the extent to which the association was independent of a more established construct (impulsivity) and how well the association holds for men versus women. Then, in Study 2, we examined the association between time perspective and BMI in a sample of middle-aged and older adults and conducted a mediational analysis to determine whether health behavior was partially responsible for this association.

Study 1

The first objective of Study 1 was to examine the extent to which time perspective predicts health behavior tendencies and whether the variability predicted is unique from that predicted by individual differences in impulsivity. A second objective was to examine the extent to which the strength of these associations differs significantly between males and females. It was hypothesized that time perspective scores would predict health behavior tendencies in all models and that the effects would be invariant by gender; for impulsivity, however, it was anticipated that the effects would be significantly stronger for males than females as has sometimes been found in prior studies. Participants were 357 undergraduates (99 males, 258 females) from an introductory psychology class, with a mean age of 19. All participants voluntarily completed the three measures used for the present study in partial fulfillment of their course requirements.

Our measure of time perspective was the *Time Perspective Questionnaire* (TPQ). The TPQ is a 13-item measure that is designed to assess individual differences in the tendency to consider short- versus long-term consequences of their own actions (Fong and Hall 2003). The TPQ presents respondents with a variety of items pertaining to orientation toward (and valuation of) short- versus long-term consequences of one's own actions; respondents are required to use a 7-point scale to indicate their level of endorsement of each item, where 1 = "disagree very strongly"

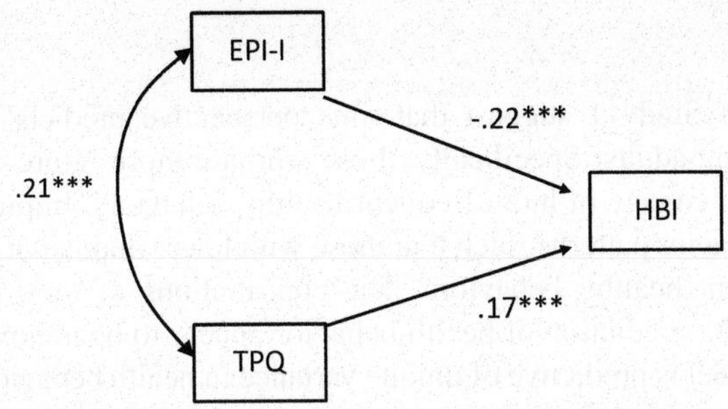

Fig. 2 Path model for health behavior as predicted by time perspective and impulsivity scores (N=357); EPI-I=Eysenck Personality Inventory Impulsivity scale; TPQ=Time Perspective Questionnaire; HBI=health behavior index; *** $p < .001$; $R^2 = .091$, $p < .001$

and 7="agree very strongly." To obtain a total TPQ score for each individual, scores on short-term items were reverse scored and averaged together with long-term items. Higher scores on the TPQ therefore reflect greater degrees of future-oriented thinking. For the current sample, Cronbach's alpha was .83, and item-total correlations ranged from .29 to .60 (M=.42). Impulsivity, on the other hand, was measured using the Impulsivity Scale of the Eysenck Personality Inventory (EPI-I)—a well-established measure in the personality research literature.

A global health behavior index was developed to measure individuals' tendency to engage in health-protective and health-damaging behavior across a wide variety of domains (i.e., alcohol consumption, condom use, dental hygiene, diet, and use of seat belts); participants were asked to indicate the frequency with which they engage in each behavior using a 1 to 7 response scale where 1="never" and 7="all the time." Scores on this measure were standardized and averaged together across domains to yield a single score to be used as an index of general health behavior, with higher scores reflecting healthier behavior patterns.

In order to test whether the power of the TPQ to predict health behaviors would be evident when controlling for impulsivity, a multiple regression analysis was conducted in which the TPQ and the EPI-I were entered as simultaneous predictors of health behavior index scores. In this analysis (Fig. 2), the TPQ emerged as a significant predictor of HBI scores after controlling for impulsivity (β=.17, p<.001). Impulsivity, as measured by the EPI-I, was also a significant predictor of HBI scores when controlling for TPQ scores (β=−.22, p<.001).

To test for gender differences in the predictive models, interaction terms were created between a dummy-coded gender variable and each of the two personality variables. The main effect variables were entered on the first step of a multiple regression analysis predicting HBI scores. Both product terms were entered on the second step, and the change in R^2 was calculated. The additional variance in HBI scores accounted for by the addition of the interaction terms was not statistically significant (R^2 change=.01, F (2, 351)=.31, p=.73), indicating that the predictive models did not vary significantly by gender.

Discussion

The findings of Study 1 suggest that time perspective predicts health behavior patterns in young adults. Specifically, those who are more future oriented in their thinking tend to engage in more frequent healthy behaviors. Impulsivity also predicts health behavior patterns, such that those with lower impulsivity tend to engage in more frequent healthy behaviors. The contributions of time perspective and impulsivity to the prediction of health behavior appear to be nonoverlapping, such that each construct is predictive of unique variance in health behavior when controlling for the other. This finding supports the argument that time perspective and impulsivity are conceptually distinct. Finally, it was found that –for the most part— the predictive models of health behavior did not vary significantly by gender.

Although this study was partially informative about the predictive power of time perspective for health behavior patterns in young adults, the age range was restricted and the target population comprised only university students. It is unknown how well time perspective would predict health behavior patterns in an older and more representative sample. In addition, we do not know to what extent time perspective might predict more downstream physiological states (e.g., obesity) that might arise from repeated unhealthy behavioral tendencies.

In Study 2, we examine these research questions in an adult population drawn from the community. We hypothesized that those with a more future-oriented time perspective would engage in healthier behavior patterns and have lower BMI than their more present-oriented counterparts.

We also hypothesized that health behavior patterns would mediate the association between time perspective and BMI.

Study 2

In Study 2, we examined the association between time perspective and one of the hypothesized downstream outcomes of health behavioral practices: body composition (operationalized as body mass index, or BMI). It was hypothesized that those with a more future-oriented time perspective would have lower BMI; that is, there would be a negative association between TPQ scores and BMI. Moreover, we hypothesized that health behavioral practices (specifically diet and exercise) would mediate the association between TPQ scores and BMI scores. We tested these hypotheses using a subsample of functionally mobile middle-aged and older adults ($M_{age}=54.59$) drawn from a larger community sample ($N=142$; Hall and Epp 2013); seven participants were excluded because English was not their first language leaving a final sample of 135.

Participants responded to advertisements for the study placed around the community inviting them to attend a lab session wherein they filled out questionnaires and were fitted with a triaxial accelerometer. Participants returned to the lab 1 week later and returned the accelerometer, after which the data was downloaded and analyzed. Participants wore the accelerometers for 7 days (5 days minimum) to assess average daily physical activity and completed a self-report measure of dietary behavior (see below for description). These two variables were standardized and combined into a single health behavior index (HBI) as in Study 1, with higher scores indicating more healthy behavioral practices. All three focal variables (time perspective, body mass index, and health behavior index) showed minor positive skewness and so were subjected to a square root transformation, which was successful in improving normality of the distributions.

To assess dietary behavior, participants completed the *National Cancer Institutes (NCI) Fat Screener*. This measure required the participants to respond to a number of items querying the frequency with which they make high- or low-fat choices for foods consumed during the previous month. The NCI has previously demonstrated adequate reliability and validity as a self-report measure of dietary behavior in adult samples (Thompson et al. 2004; Snyder et al. 2004). Scores on the NCI were reverse scored and then standardized for inclusion in the health behavior index, such that higher scores indicated higher levels of healthy dietary behavior (i.e., lower percentage calories from fat).

The health behavior index, in this case, was derived as a linear combination of the standardized physical activity (RT-3) and dietary behavior (NCI screener, reverse scored) measures. Higher scores on the HBI indicated higher levels of healthy behavior. Physical activity and diet were included in this version of the index because they are the two health behaviors that are most relevant for determining the chronic energy imbalance that leads to obesity (i.e., high BMI).

Finally, *time perspective* was again measured using the 13-item Time Perspective Questionnaire (TPQ; Fong and Hall 2003). This scale was administered at two time points separated by 1 week; the resulting scores were standardized and averaged together to yield an overall TPQ score. Both the first (Cronbach's alpha = .78) and second (Cronbach's alpha = .81) administrations showed strong internal consistency reliability. Scores from the two administrations of the TPQ were highly correlated with each other ($r = .79$, $p < .001$), indicating strong 1-week test-retest reliability.

Descriptive analyses indicated that participants were on average well educated, with 57.7 % having completed at least some university- or college-level training. The sample was predominantly female (74.1 %) and Caucasian (94.7 %). Though the majority of participants were within the normal weight range (43.7 %; BMI $\leq$ 25), 39.3 % were overweight (BMI > 25) and 17 % were obese (BMI $\geq$ 30). Average accelerometer counts per day ($M = 236{,}950$, $SD = 93{,}815$) and mean percent calories from fat ($M = 32.6$, $SD = 4.2$) were comparable to norms for adult community samples.

Zero-order correlations among the TPQ, HBI, and BMI were in the expected directions. TPQ scores were associated with HBI scores, such that a more future-oriented perspective was associated with better health behavioral practices ($r = .25$, $p = .01$). In addition, TPQ scores were negatively correlated with BMI; increased future-orientedness was associated with lower BMI ($r = -.16$, $p = .03$). Within the age range of the present sample (35–89, age was negatively associated with TPQ scores ($r = -.16$, $p = .03$) and HBI scores ($r = -.16$, $p < .05$) but not BMI ($r = .06$,

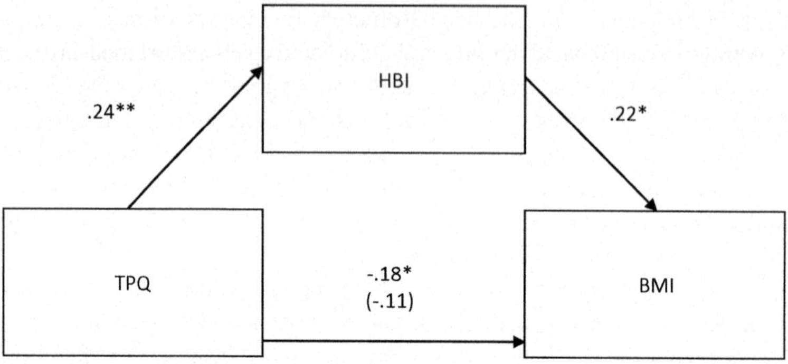

Note. $N = 135$; TPQ=Time Perspective Questionnaire; HBI=Health Behavior Index; * $p \leq .05$; ** $p \leq .01$; *** $p \leq .001$; control variables: age, gender.

Fig. 3 Mediational model for BMI

$p = .24$). Gender was not significantly associated with TPQ scores ($r = .04$, $p = .31$), HBI scores ($r = .02$, $p = .41$), or BMI ($r = -.05$, $p = .27$).

Mediational analyses were undertaken to examine the extent to which the association between TPQ scores and BMI can be explained by HBI scores. We conducted hierarchical linear regression analyses using the causal steps approach described by Baron and Kenny (1986); the results are summarized in Fig. 3. As predicted, TPQ scores predicted BMI; TPQ scores also predicted HBI scores, which in turn predicted BMI. Finally, the association between TPQ and BMI scores was attenuated when taking into account HBI; specifically, the TPQ-BMI association was reduced by 34 % when accounting for health behavior, rendering the original association no longer statistically significant ($\beta = -.11$, $t = -1.26$, $p = .21$).

In a set of descriptive analyses, we partitioned the sample according to TPQ score and examined the prevalence of obesity within each TPQ group. Figure 4 shows the proportion of individuals in low (−1 SD), moderate (M), and high (+1SD) TPQ categories who are obese, as defined by the $\text{BMI} \geq 30$ criterion. As can be seen in the figure, the prevalence of obesity among those in the most future-oriented group (13 %) was almost half that among those who were least future oriented (23 %; $p = .046$).

Finally, we examined the association between hypothesized exogenous variables (age, gender, SES, and its subcomponents) and TPQ scores, to identify potential determinants of individual differences in time perspective. We found that age ($r = -.15$, $p = .04$) was negatively associated with time perspective; occupational category ($r = .16$, $p = .03$) and income level ($r = .19$, $p = .02$) were positively associated with time perspective. As well education was marginally associated with TPQ scores ($r = .13$, $p = .07$). An overall index of SES comprising these three components was significantly associated with time perspective as well ($r = .19$, $p = .02$). Gender was not related to time perspective.

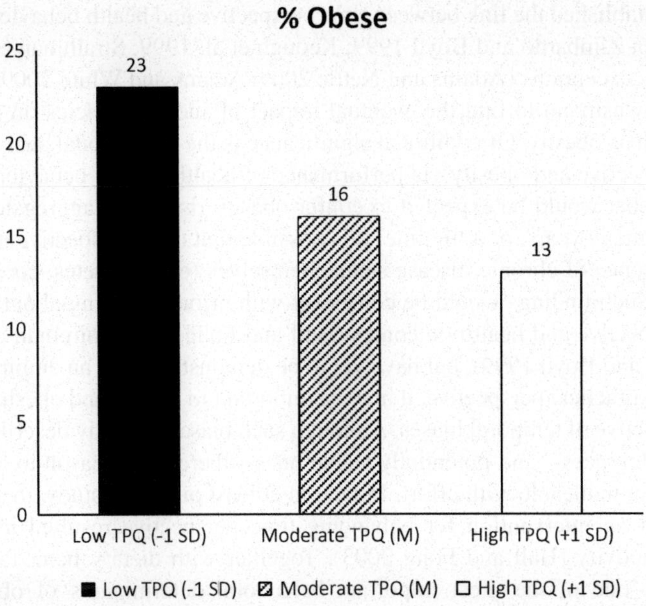

Fig. 4 Prevalence of obesity (BMI ≥ 30) as a function of TPQ category

General Discussion

Here we have presented the findings of two studies whose purpose was to examine the associations among time perspective, health behavior performance, and one important downstream manifestation of such behaviors: body composition (i.e., BMI). It was hypothesized that those with a more future-oriented time perspective would engage in more healthy behavioral practices than their more present-oriented counterparts, and these healthier practices would explain the predicted association between time perspective and body composition. To test this hypothesis, we conducted two studies, the first involving a sample of healthy undergraduate students (Study 1), and the second involving a sample of healthy middle-aged and older adults (Study 2). In Study 1, it was found that future orientation was positively associated with healthy behavioral practices in this younger sample. In Study 2, it was found that time perspective was associated with both healthier behavioral practices and negatively associated with BMI. Most importantly, however, there was evidence that healthy behavioral practices mediated the association between time perspective and BMI. That is, more future-oriented individuals had lower BMI, in part, because they engaged in healthier behavioral practices.

These findings are of potential interest from both a theoretical and a practical perspective. From a theoretical perspective, this study is among the first to link individual differences in time perspective with a pre-disease state that has important health implications (c.f. Adams and White 2009). Although prior studies have already established the link between time perspective and health behaviors (Henson et al. 2006; Zimbardo and Boyd 1999; Keough et al. 1999; Strathman et al. 1994), with a few exceptions (Adams and Nettle 2009; Adams and White 2009), few have looked downstream to find the eventual impact of such tendencies on pre-disease states such as obesity. Of additional significance is the mediational analysis linking time perspective and obesity via performance of health-related behaviors (exercise and diet) that would be expected to confer obesity risk when aggregated over the course of many years, or a lifetime. It is possible that time perspective may predict the occurrence of chronic disease states themselves (e.g., diabetes, coronary heart disease). Such findings would be consistent with prior theorizing about the role of time perspective and health outcomes (Hall and Fong 2007; Joireman et al. 2006; Zimbardo and Boyd 1999), but have yet to be demonstrated on an empirical level.

From a practical perspective, it may be important to understand obesity risk from the perspective of temporal biases. Although such biases are aptly described as individual differences—and potentially stable ones—there is no reason to believe that they are not malleable with effort. In fact, in at least one prior study, there was evidence that an intervention for enhancing time perspective resulted in increased physical activity (Hall and Fong 2003). Together with dietary behavior, physical activity is one of the most important behavioral determinants of obesity. Any approach to increasing activity and improving healthy dietary choice may benefit from a time perspective component.

Determinants of Time Perspective

Of secondary interest were the associations between exogenous (demographic) variables and time perspective. It was found that overall SES was positively associated with time perspective, such that those in higher SES strata had more future-oriented time perspectives than their lower SES counterparts. Examination of each of the individual SES subcomponents (education level, occupational category, and income) revealed similar patterns of association, with education having perhaps less influence than income and occupational category. The notion that SES is causally related to time perspective is intuitively appealing and supported by prior theorizing and empirical findings (e.g., Lamm et al. 1976; Nurmi 1992; Adams and White 2009).

The negative association between time perspective and age is also potentially interesting. The interpretation of this finding depends partially on the age composition for the sample, which in this case included only middle-aged and older adults. It is possible that the relationship between age and time perspective reverses when including younger participants. For example, children and adolescents may have relatively short-time horizons compared to young adults. In this way, it is possible that time horizon peaks in young adulthood, but decreases on either side of this developmental stage, for different reasons (i.e., lack of ability to envision the future vs. relatively less time left). This is also consistent with some approaches to time horizons and lifespan development (Carstensen et al. 1999; Charles and Carstensen 2010; Nurmi 1992).

Limitations and Strengths

There are several limitations of the current set of studies that bear some mention. First and foremost, the measures of health behavior in Study 1 were self-reported, as was the case for one of the components of the index measure used in Study 2. It is possible that those who are more future oriented are more likely to report engaging in behaviors that have relevance for the future, as they are more cognitively salient. Although we do not have specific reason to believe that this is the case here, we cannot rule out the possibility. However, the second component of the index measure used in Study 2 (accelerometer-assessed physical activity) was not self-report and so would not suffer from this particular bias. A second limitation of this study has to do with the cross-sectional nature of the data, which precludes causal inference about the impact of time perspective on health behavior or BMI. Experimental studies involving time perspective manipulations and observation of changes in health behavior would help to more conclusively examine the causal status of the observed association. Finally, although BMI is the most widely used measure of body composition, it is subject to several well-known limitations; as such, there may be additional error variance in the BMI measure as a result.

There are additionally some strengths of the current study. First, we were able to demonstrate the association between time perspective and health behavior in two separate samples (one undergraduate and one older community-based sample); the replicability of the effect enhances our confidence in the reliability of the finding. Second, we were able to demonstrate that the effect of time perspective on health behavior is potentially important, in that it may explain the association between time perspective and another important disease state: obesity. If these associations are causal in nature, we know that enhancing time perspective may be a good way of preventing obesity and that such effects may occur via alteration of health behavior patterns that we already know are linked to the development of the energy imbalance that generates excess body fat (low activity levels and high levels of fatty food consumption).

Future studies would benefit from examining the link between time perspective and health outcomes (behavioral and otherwise) using experimental designs. These would assist in determining the extent to which the association between time perspective is causal. In addition, efforts should be made to examine the extent to which time perspective predicts risk for and early onset of other disease states that have behavioral determinants or for which obesity is a precursor. Some prime examples of such chronic conditions include type 2 diabetes, cardiovascular disease, and stroke.

Conclusion

In two studies, we examined the association between time perspective and health behavior tendencies. In both studies—one involving undergraduate students (Study 1) and the other involving community dwelling adults (Study 2)—we found that a more future-oriented time perspective was associated with healthier behavioral tendencies. Study 2 additionally demonstrated that more future-oriented individuals had lower BMI and that the association between time perspective and BMI was mediated by health behavior. That is, more future-oriented individuals had lower BMI, and this association was accounted for by the tendency for more future-oriented individuals to engage in healthier behavioral patterns. These studies add to the growing body of findings implicating future orientation in the promotion and maintenance of healthy behavioral trajectories.

These findings reinforce the breadth of applicability of the time perspective construct within the health domain. New trends in health-related time perspective research include both larger-scale survey studies (e.g., Adams 2009; Hall et al. 2012b, 2014; Sansone et al. 2012) and increasing interest in the mechanistic factors underlying time perspective effects on health and behavior (Hall et al. 2012b). Likely the elucidation of mechanism will rely heavily on the building of bridges between experimental psychology and time perspective research. Examples of literature that exemplify this latter approach would be Yacoov Trope's work on temporal construal theory (Trope and Liberman 2003) and George Ainslie's work on the neurobiology of intertemporal bargaining (Ainslie 2013). If it is possible to successfully integrate experimental and epidemiological approaches to the investigation of time perspective, the horizon for Zimbardo's concepts in the domain of health promotion will be quite expansive indeed.

References

Adams, J. (2009). The role of time perspective in smoking cessation amongst older English adults. *Health Psychology, 28*, 529–534.

Adams, J., & Nettle, D. (2009). Time perspective, personality and smoking, body mass, and physical activity: An empirical study. *British Journal of Health Psychology, 14*, 83–105.

Adams, J., & White, M. (2009). Time perspective in socioeconomic inequalities in smoking and body mass index. *Health Psychology, 28*, 83–90.

Ainslie, G. (2010). *Picoeconomics: The strategic interaction of successive motivational states within the person*. Cambridge: Cambridge University Press.

Ainslie, G. (2013). Picoeconomics in neural and evolutionary contexts. In P. Hall (Ed.), *Social neuroscience in public health: Foundations for the science of chronic disease prevention*. New York: Springer.

Baron, R. M., & Kenny, D. A. (1986). The moderator-mediator variable distinction in social psychological research: Conceptual, strategic and statistical considerations. *Journal of Personality and Social Psychology, 51*, 1173–1182.

Carstensen, L. L., Isaacowitz, D. M., & Charles, S. T. (1999). Taking time seriously. A theory of socioemotional selectivity. *American Psychologist, 54*, 165–181.

Charles, S. T., & Carstensen, L. L. (2010). Social and emotional aging. *Annual Review of Psychology, 61*, 383–409.

Daugherty, J. R., & Brase, G. L. (2010). Taking time to be healthy: Predicting health behaviors with delay discounting and time perspective. *Personality and Individual Differences, 48*, 202–207.

Fieulaine, N., & Martinez, F. (2010). Time under control: Time perspective and desire for control in substance use. *Addictive Behaviors, 35*, 799–802.

Fong, G. T., & Hall, P. A. (2003). The importance of time perspective in predicting, understanding, and reducing health risk behaviors among adolescents. In D. Romer (Ed.), *Reducing adolescent risk: Toward an integrated approach*. Newbury Park: Sage.

Fong, G. T., Cummings, K. M., Borland, R., Hastings, G., Hyland, A., Giovino, G. A., Hammond, D., & Thompson, M. E. (2006). The conceptual framework of the International Tobacco Control (ITC) Policy Evaluation Project. *Tobacco Control, 15*, iii3–iii11.

Hall, P. A., & Epp, L. (2013). Does domain-specific time perspective predict accelerometer assessed physical activity? An examination of ecological moderators. *Journal of Sport and Exercise Psychology, 14*(1), 50–56.

Hall, P. A., & Fong, G. T. (2003). The effects of a brief time perspective intervention for increasing physical activity among young adults. *Psychology & Health, 18*, 685–706.

Hall, P. A., & Fong, G. T. (2007). The effects of a brief time perspective intervention for increasing physical activity among young adults. *Psychology & Health, 18*, 685–706.

Hall, P. A., Fong, G. T., & Cheng, C. (2012a). Time perspective and weight management behaviors in newly diagnosed Type 2 diabetes: A mediational analysis. *Journal of Behavioral Medicine, 35*, 569–580.

Hall, P. A., Fong, G. T., Yong, H. H., Sansone, G., Borland, R., & Siahpush, M. (2012b). Do time perspective and sensation-seeking predict quitting activity among smokers? Findings from the International Tobacco Control (ITC) Four Country Survey. *Addictive Behaviors, 37*, 1307–1313.

Hall, P. A., Fong, G. T., & Meng, G. (2014). Time perspective as a determinant of smoking cessation in four countries: Direct and intention-mediated effects from the International Tobacco Control (ITC) 4-Country Surveys. *Addictive Behaviors, 37*, 1307–1313.

Heckman, C. J., Wilson, D. B., & Ingersoll, K. S. (2009). The influence of appearance, health, and future orientations on tanning behavior. *American Journal of Health Behavior, 33*, 238–243.

Henson, J. M., Carey, M. P., Carey, K. B., & Maisto, S. A. (2006). Associations among health behaviors and time perspective in young adults: Model testing with boot-strapping replication. *Journal of Behavioral Medicine, 29*, 127–137.

Joireman, J., Strathman, A., & Balliet, D. (2006). Considering future consequences: An integrative model. In L. Sanna & E. Chang (Eds.), *Judgments over time: The interplay of thoughts, feelings, and behaviors* (pp. 82–99). Oxford: Oxford University Press.

Joireman, J., Shafer, M. J., Balliet, D., & Strathman, A. (2012). Promotion orientation explains why future oriented people exercise and eat healthy: Evidence from the two-factor consideration of future consequences-14 scale. *Personality & Social Psychology Bulletin, 38*, 1272–1287.

Keough, K. A., Zimbardo, P. G., & Boyd, J. N. (1999). Who's smoking, drinking, and using drugs? Time perspective as a predictor of substance use. *Basic and Applied Social Psychology, 21*, 149–164.

Kovač, V. B., & Rise, J. (2007). The relation between past behavior, intention, planning, and quitting smoking: The moderating effect of future orientation. *Journal of Applied Biobehavioral Research, 12*, 82–100.

Lamm, H., Schmidt, R. W., & Trommsdorff, G. (1976). Sex and social class as determinants of future orientation (time perspective) in adolescents. *Journal of Personality and Social Psychology, 34*, 317–326.

Loewenstein, G., & Thaler, R. (1989). Anomalies: Intertemporal choice. *Journal of Economic Perspectives, 3*, 181–193.

Nurmi, J. E. (1992). Age differences in adult life goals, concerns, and their temporal extension: A life course approach to future-oriented motivation. *International Journal of Behavioral Development, 15*, 487–508.

Orbell, S., & Hagger, M. (2006). Temporal framing and the decision to take part in type 2 diabetes screening: Effects of individual differences in consideration of future consequences. *Health Psychology, 25*, 537–548.
Orbell, S., & Kyriakaki, M. (2008). Temporal framing and persuasion to adopt preventive health behavior: Moderating effects of individual differences in consideration of future consequences on sunscreen use. *Health Psychology, 27*, 770–779.
Rappange, D. R., Brouwer, W. B. F., & Van Exel, N. J. A. (2009). Back to the consideration of the future consequences scale: Time to reconsider? *Journal of Social Psychology, 149*, 562–584.
Rothspan, S., & Read, S. J. (1996). Present versus future time perspective and HIV risk among heterosexual college students. *Health Psychology, 15*, 131–134.
Sansone, G., Fong, G. T., Hall, P. A., Guignard, R., Beck, F., Mons, U., Pötschke-Langer, M., Yong, H. H., Thompson, M., Omar, M., & Jiang, Y. (2012). *Time perspective as a predictor of smoking status: Findings from the International Tobacco Control (ITC) Surveys in Scotland, France, Germany, China, and Malaysia. BMC Public Health, 13*, 346.
Snyder, D. C., Sloane, R., Lobach, D., Lipkus, I., Clipp, E., Kraus, W. E., & Demark-Wahnefried, W. (2004). Agreement between a brief mailed screener and an in-depth telephone survey: Observations from the Fresh Start study. *Journal of the American Dietetic Association, 104*, 1593–1596.
Strathman, A., Gleicher, F., Boninger, D. S., & Edwards, C. S. (1994). The consideration of future consequences: Weighing immediate and distant outcomes of behavior. *Journal of Personality & Social Psychology, 66*, 742–752.
Thompson, F. E., Midthune, D., Subar, A. F., Kahle, L. L., Schatzkin, A., & Kipnis, V. (2004). Performance of a short tool to assess dietary intakes of fruits and vegetables, percentage energy from fat and fibre. *Public Health Nutrition, 7*, 1097–1105.
Trope, Y., & Liberman, N. (2003). Temporal construal. *Psychological Review, 110*, 403–421.
Wills, T. A., Sandy, J. M., & Yaeger, A. M. (2001). Time perspective and early-onset substance use: A model based on stress–coping theory. *Psychology of Addictive Behaviors, 15*, 118–125.
Zimbardo, P. G., & Boyd, J. N. (1999). Putting time in perspective: A valid, reliable individual-differences metric. *Journal of Personality & Social Psychology, 77*, 1271–1288.
Zimbardo, P. G., Keough, K. A., & Boyd, J. N. (1997). Present time perspective as a predictor of risky driving. *Personality & Individual Differences, 23*, 1007–1023.

Time Perspective in Consumer Behavior

Martina Klicperová-Baker, Jaroslav Košťál, and Jiří Vinopal

Introduction

The economic behavior is a field in which a proper time perspective is particularly important on the private as well as on the public levels. After all, these levels are related, and not just etymologically ("οἶκος" or "oikos" is the Greek word for a house or household). Importantly, economy is also closely linked to political culture and political conduct of citizens; economies and entitlements depend substantially on national policies.

One might wish consumers as well as economists (political economists in particular) would have both (a) the capacity for immediate improvisation whenever necessary and, simultaneously, (b) a prudent foresight, the ability to engage a long-term Future time perspective. Yet history documents our proneness to devastating *temporal faults and illusions*.

(a) On one hand, many keenly fall for the bait of *immediate gratification*. Suffering from a short attention span and overvaluing proximal gains, citizens fall prey to advertising practices (consumer advertising as well as political campaigning) which stress immediacy and ostentatiously disregard delays of gratification. Entrapment in the present time hurts our personal as well as state economies, not to mention sound political development.

(b) On the other hand, not just citizens but whole nations have been deceived by unsubstantiated, *false future visions*. Oppressive ideologies such as Nazism or

M. Klicperová-Baker (✉) • J. Košťál
Institute of Psychology, Academy of Sciences of the Czech Republic,
Praha, Czech Republic
e-mail: Klicperovabaker@gmail.com

J. Vinopal
Institute of Sociology, Academy of Sciences of the Czech Republic,
Praha, Czech Republic

M. Stolarski et al. (eds.), *Time Perspective Theory; Review, Research and Application: Essays in Honor of Philip G. Zimbardo*, DOI 10.1007/978-3-319-07368-2_23,

Communism manipulated populace by promises of the life of plenty and happiness in the future Utopia. By the same token, followers of religious fanatics are willing to sacrifice for a mirage of an exultant afterlife and gamblers invest whatever they do or do not have for an illusion of future riches. From both of the noted temporal extremes, the one focusing on the hedonistic present time seems to be the one more perilous for modern societies.

This chapter consists of three parts somewhat symbolically reflecting the past, present and future: a historical review, a current empirical probe and a parting thought about the role of the future.

The Historical Review—Conceptual and Empirical Research in Time and Economy

The phenomenon of time has been a traditional puzzle for philosophers, physicists, educators, anthropologists, and especially psychologists. It gained a particular momentum in the last third of the twentieth century. Since then, 'time perspective' and 'psychology of time' command high levels of interest that is well illustrated by the Google Ngram viewer which documents the usage of English language words and phrases across time.[1]

The 1960s are memorable for both theoretical and empirical accomplishments in the psychology of time. Paul Fraisse stands out among the early time researchers with his extensive monograph *The Psychology of Time* (1967). Yet, Fraisse's book is not remembered as well as an experiment which was conducted in the same period at Stanford University—'the marshmallow test.'

The marshmallow test stands out as an elegantly simple research situation assessing immediate or delayed gratification. Walter Mischel and his colleagues challenged 4-year old preschoolers to either help themselves to a tasty marshmallow or wait 15 min to double their reward. This simple situational test turned out to yield surprisingly consequential results and thus grew into a longitudinal project with multiple follow-up studies over 40 years (Mischel et al. 1972, 2011). The preschooler marshmallow test was able to predict mental, cognitive, and social health over the life course of the participants. The children who were able to resist temptation later received better grades in school, they were healthier, more stable in their relationships, and professionally more successful. The marshmallow experiment became a classic.

The significance of time perspective in the economic context was soon established. It gained formal recognition in 1981 when the *Journal of Consumer Research* (after publishing individual time-related studies—cf. Jacoby 1976) devoted to the phenomenon of time a special issue. An array of stimulating articles provided

[1] https://books.google.com/ngrams/

mostly insights into the time economy of households—the working time, discretionary time, measurement of travel time savings, the time use of working wives, married women volunteering, etc.

A seminal article was devoted to the cross-cultural perception of time. There, Graham (1981) elaborated the earlier findings which a cultural anthropologist Edward T. Hall described in his book *Silent Language* from 1959. Graham characterized various cultural time apperceptions such as: the linear-separable model usual in the Anglo culture which recognizes a linear axis with discrete segments of the past, present, and future; the circular-traditional model of Latino cultures according to which time is perceived as a cyclical pattern with repeated events; and the loosely understood present-oriented and procedural concept of time usual among societies such as American Indians (their traditional approach disregards the time duration and stresses the 'right procedure' instead). These different concepts have an obvious importance for economic practice, including purchase and post-purchase consumer behavior.

One of the articles of the special issue was more conceptual than others, almost encyclopedic. It was a study by Feldman and Hornik (1981). They captured time from various angles, starting with the economy of time (the price of time, time-budget decisions, the phenomenon of 'saving time', etc.) and they developed a cogent theoretical framework; they also renewed the attention to the concepts of monochronic and polychronic personality coined, again, by the anthropologist E. T. Hall (1966). Approaching time allocation from a consumer perspective, Feldman and Hornik scrutinized the components of time structure. They concluded the study with a consolidated time-use model which took into account both the meaning of time and individual lifestyle, i.e., timestyle (a concept they coined).

The timestyles, customary ways in which people perceive and use time, were further developed by Cotte et al. (2004). The authors recognized Feldman and Hornik's basic approach by which timestyle is derived from the choices of typical daily activities. Cotte et al. elaborated the main orientations (temporal, social, planning and polychronic dimensions). They also pointed out the variety of temporal features and situational frames. Thus, they poetically likened time to a threatening pressure cooker, to a map which gives direction, a feedback providing mirror, a river we are immersed in and, finally, to a feast—an opportunity to be enjoyed. All these epithets carry a significant meaning with respect to consumer behavior, its quality and intensity. Interestingly, their theory did not stress one of the most apparent economic association between time and money.

Time and Money

The relationship between time and money was a subject of a number of interesting studies: some directly focused on the relationship of value of both commodities in the production and managerial contexts (e.g. the effect of polychronicity on human performance studied by Kantrowicz et al. 2012) or the value of time and/or money in philantrophic behavior (e.g., donating and volunteering across Europe by Bauer et al. 2013). Among the most interesting studies from this area are studies of human freedom or poverty with respect to time and money, which are expressed by a single quantitative measure, the FDT—freely disposable time (Hobbes et al. 2011).

Bonke et al. (2009) followed the time and money analyses by a study of economic and leisure satisfaction, Mogilner (2010) added a humanistic interest in the importance of time with significant others for the pursuit of happiness, contrasting it to the working time. Doyle (2013) crowned the scrutiny of time and money trade-offs by respective mathematical models.

Satisfaction and feeling of happiness, crucial concepts in the research of economic behavior, were often studied with respect to consumption and spending to determine consumer satisfaction. Guven (2012) took an original perspective when he reversed the traditional research paradigm and tested to what degree happiness itself may influence consumption and saving. His conclusion from a research on a Dutch sample was unequivocal and would not surprise anyone who knows the relationship between depression and (over)eating: Guven (2012, p. 701) found that happier people save more and spend less, they have a lower marginal propensity to consume, they take more time for making decisions and have more control over expenditures; happier people expect a longer life and (accordingly) seem more concerned about the future than about the present day; they also expect less inflation in the future. A similar theme was tackled from yet another perspective by Zaleskiewicz et al. (2013) who demonstrated that saving money can buffer death anxiety, create a sense of control and constitute a more effective buffer than spending money.

While mechanisms of spending money have been relatively generously researched, processes of savings were studied less frequently. K.-E. Wärneryd (1999) helped to balance the process by his monograph *Psychology of Saving* devoted to psychology and economics (economics as the study of self-interest, pleasure, and pain) and to economic psychology. He analyzed saving (and also investing and herding) in an integrative, multilevel framework.

Assessing Time Perspective

The many insights into the diversity of meanings of time were soon logically followed by attempts to dissect time experience into concrete dimensions and quantify them. Some studies were inspired by practical problems (such as questions of the freely disposable time important for organizational psychology or assessing intergenerational relationships in social psychology—e.g., Peters and Bolkan 2009). Other measures were simply inspired by curiosity over the diverse nature of time meanings. Time inventories were administered to various samples, the results were factor analyzed and the resulting factors were interpreted in terms of respective time dimensions.

Thus, an early study by Calabresi and Cohen (1968) compared hundreds of college students with psychiatric patients; factor analysis was used to identify dimensions of Time Anxiety, Time Possessiveness, and Time Flexibility. Significant differences between patients and students were then found on all scales: the psychiatric patients scored higher than students on Time Anxiety and Time Possessiveness, and lower on the Time Flexibility dimension. The researchers interpreted the results in terms of psychology of personality and personality differences in attitudes toward time.

Gonzalez and Zimbardo (1985) succeeded in involving a wide body of readers of *Psychology Today* magazine into a time perspective survey. Their data yielded seven factors and demonstrated statistical differences among the social demographic groups which took part in the study. The Future time perspective stood up as crucial for personal achievement. Future was most prominent among the factors, four of seven factors were interpreted in terms of future.

The 1980s brought another noteworthy study of time perspective. Bond and Feather developed a Time Structure Questionnaire (TSQ) and obtained five factors which were significantly related to such phenomena as: sense of purpose in life, self-esteem, reported health, optimism, and efficient study habits (Bond and Feather 1988, p. 327).

Almost a quarter century after the *Psychology Today* study, Zimbardo along with J. Boyd followed-up his earlier research on time. In their study *Putting time in perspective: A valid, reliable individual-differences metric* they stressed that time had "the pervasive and powerful yet largely still unrecognized influence on much human behavior" (Zimbardo and Boyd 1999, p. 1271). In this study Zimbardo and Boyd described the time perspective biases and profiles, altogether five factors: Past-Negative, Past-Positive, Present Hedonistic, Present Fatalistic, and Future. Their theory of time was further elaborated and popularized by a popular book *The Time Paradox: The New Psychology of Time that Will Change Your Life* (2008) as well as by numerous presentations, among others, a popular TED talk (Zimbardo 2009).

Zimbardo's approach was seminal in several aspects. Perhaps most importantly, Zimbardo is a master in sharing and he made sure that the psychological knowledge and tools were 'given away to the public.' His theory was comprehensive and easy to apply (e.g., in mental hygiene to optimize the balance between the past, present, and future, or in clinical practice, as in rehabilitation of PTSD in veterans). Zimbardo's theory was also accompanied by a useful assessment tool—the ZTPI inventory, an inventory which soon gained a widespread popularity.

The useful technique and the charismatic mentor soon inspired scholars from all over the world to form an International Research Network on Time Perspective (http://www.timeperspective.net/). The network members translate ZTPI to national languages and conduct research. They frequently communicate and meet not just in their panels at psychological congresses but they also organize their own dedicated conferences. No wonder that such a stimulating environment enticed us to translating ZTPI into Czech and administering the ZTPI inventory to a representative sample in the Czech Republic.

An Empirical Probe in Time Perspective and Saving/Spending Behavior

A representative sample of the Czech Republic was administered the ZTPI inventory and inquiries about their financial behavior (saving habits and loan repayment). Additionally, the participants were asked about significant purchases from the current year and purchases planned for the next year.

The Czech Republic, a country in the heart of Europe, has restored the democratic political system at the end of the twentieth century (1989) and also returned to the market economy at that occasion. As attested by OECD (2013), the Czech Republic performs favorably in main measures of well-being and generally ranks close to the world average in the main topics of the *Better Life Index*. It thus can be considered a useful research example.

The older Czech generation experienced the frugal years of Nazi occupation during WWII followed by a Communist dictate of the Soviet Union and rigidly planned command economy. The younger generation though, as youth of the free world elsewhere, was socialized under the conditions of democracy and free market. Hence, the Czech population, as well as citizens of other free market economies, experienced their share of advertising seductions, temptations to travel (which in the past was strictly limited), a vast choice of brand name goods along with the enticement of lenders, banks and credit card companies. Thus, loans became a natural part of the consuming behavior.

A well established public opinion research agency, CVVM (the Center for Research of Public Opinion) affiliated with the Institute of Sociology of the Czech Academy of Sciences collected quality data representative of the whole Czech Republic. Data from 1,049 respondents aged 15–89 years were obtained by face to face interviews and with the pen & paper methodology; the field work was executed in early December 2003 as a part of a regular Omnibus assessment 'Our Society.' The full Zimbardo Time Perspective Inventory (ZTPI) questionnaire (56 items) was included in the battery with the usual 5-point response scale (from 1-definitely agree to 5-definitely disagree). The Czech versions of ZTPI underwent careful psychometric scrutiny with good results (Lukavská et al. 2011; Košťál et al. submitted).

Almost 71 % of participants (N = 738) answered all ZTPI questions in a valid way, assigning scores from 1 to 5 to respective questions. One item was omitted by 13 % (N = 139), 6 % respondents failed to answer two items and the remaining 10 % dropped three or more items. In addition to the ZTPI, several questions related to consumer behavior were asked, particularly about financial behavior (regular savings and payback of loans) as well as realized and anticipated purchasing behavior.

Financial Behavior

The survey of the Czech society revealed a high frequency of saving and a moderate occurrence of debt re-payment. The majority of participants (almost two thirds—62.2 %) asserted they put aside regular savings, about a third saved up to a

1,000 Czech crowns (CZK) and an additional quarter saved regularly within an interval of 1,001–5,000 CZK. That is a modest to fair level, considering the exchange ratio of the crown[2] and the monthly gross wages equaling 16,430 CZK.[3] Majority of participants stated they had no debts they would pay off. Only about one third of respondents (38.4 %) admitted they had a loan and their installments were most often between 1,000 and 5,000 CZK a month. Less than 3 % declined to answer the financial questions.

Purchases

The survey included questions on purchases of various costly commodities in the past year or anticipated in the future year (vacation abroad, home furnishing, an apartment, a car). Furnishing was defined as furniture, refrigerator, bathroom remodeling and the like.

The realized purchases of cars and apartments within the past year turned out rather rare and planned purchases of these items were exceptional and in single digit percents (only 4 % reported a purchase of an apartment and 8 % purchase of a car; anticipated purchases in the next year were also rare—4 % and 3 % respectively).

However, purchases of vacations or furnishings were fairly common: almost every other Czech (46 %) has bought furnishings and well over a quarter (29 %) vacationed abroad. About a third of respondents also anticipated such a purchase over the next year (35 % anticipated a purchase of furnishings and 31 % a purchase of vacations abroad).

Our further analyses focused on the most frequent activities, i.e. activities in which at least one third of respondents participated. These were: purchased furnishings, vacations abroad, and planned purchase of furnishings. We scrutinized their incidence with respect to the demographic variables and the time perspective dimensions.

The Spending and Saving Behavior and the Time Perspective

In accordance with the usual practice, we reduced the 56 ZTPI items to five variables, i.e., into two Past, two Present and one Future dimensions. Their main statistics are summarized in Table 1.

Data were then submitted to a series of multiple linear regressions (in case of financial behavior) and to logistic regression (in case of other types of consumer behavior data which had a dichotomic character). Our aim was to reveal the role of time perspective among other variables which we hypothesized would have the

[2] There were approximately 32 Czech crowns for one euro and 29 Czech crowns for one US dollar in 2003. http://www.penize.cz/kurzy-men/6596-euro; http://www.finance.cz/makrodata-eu/menove-ukazatele/statistiky/kurzy-czk/

[3] http://www.finance.cz/makrodata-eu/trh-prace/statistiky/mzda/

Table 1 Descriptive statistics of five dimensions of ZTPI

Dimension	N	Minimum	Maximum	Mean	SD
Past-Positive	976	16.67	100.0	61.26	13.66
Past-Negative	923	0.00	97.5	50.89	17.09
Present Hedonistic	941	13.33	100.0	55.27	15.63
Present Fatalistic	891	0.00	100.0	50.48	16.85
Future	929	15.38	100.0	60.84	12.71

Table 2 ZTPI dimensions and selected demographics relevant to financial behavior: results of linear regression (Beta significance)

	Savings	Loan payments
Variable	Beta	Beta
ZTPI—Future dimension	0.094*	0.084*
ZTPI—Present Fatalistic dimension		0.071*
Gender (male 1, female 2)		–0.125**
Age		–0.114*
Secondary vocational education w diploma		0.156**
Monthly household income	0.193***	
Living with a partner		0.082*
Household standard of living	0.161***	
Student or apprentice		–0.136*
Retiree		–0.129
Manager/employee	0.145**	
Multiple R	0.580	0.423
R-square	0.293	0.124
N	803	772

*≤0.05, **≤0.01, ***≤0.001

decisive impact. Thus, we expected income to play a crucial role for saving behavior yet we expected the time perspective to be also significantly involved. The equations as a whole were tested by ANOVA (linear regression) and CHI-square (logistic regression) and they were found significant.[4]

Saving behavior results are presented in the first part of Table 2. It was confirmed that the *Future time orientation contributed significantly to regular saving behavior*. The TP intervened within the economic conditions (such as the household income, standard of living and a managerial position at work) which played the major role for the amount of monthly savings. Furthermore, it can be safely assumed that some demographic variables (higher social and economic status) are also results of Future time orientation.

[4]The significance of the individual independent variables is tested at least twice, at first the equation is tested as a whole so that at least one predictor is significant, then each predictor is tested individually by *t*-test (multiple linear regression) and Wald's test (logistic regression).

Loan payments results are illustrated in the latter column of Table 2. Analysis of variables playing a major role in repaying loans also revealed a significant effect of time perspective. *Interestingly, two time dimensions were involved here: both the Future and the Present Fatalistic dimensions were significantly involved in the payback of loans*. Besides the time perspective, again, re-payment of loans was positively associated with demographic variables, namely: the male gender, a younger age, living in a household with a partner and achieving secondary vocational education with diploma. All socio-professional groups except being a student/apprentice or a retiree were also slightly associated with loan repayment.

We found strong relationship between financial behavior and predictors, i.e., ZTPI and socio-demographic categories. The multiple correlations for dependent savings and loans were .423 and .580, respectively. Adjusted R-square indicate percentage of explained variance by predictors.

Purchasing Behavior

Finally, we analyzed the purchasing behavior. Some categories of purchases were too infrequent to pass Hosmer-Lemeshow test, thus we concentrated on the more common activities, i.e., past purchases of furnishings and vacations and purchases of furnishings anticipated in the next year.

We focused on their relationship with time perspective and with various demographic indicators (levels of occupation, marital status, etc.). Table 3 (abridged for brevity) shows the selection of categories where significant relationships were found (significant Beta). Significant strong relationships (R-square: Cox-Snell/Nagelkerke) were also confirmed between predictors, i.e., between ZTPI and socio-demographic variables on one hand, and both past and anticipated purchases on the other.

Three out of five ZTPI dimensions played an important role in reported purchasing behavior which was confirmed by statistical evidence. With respect to the realized purchases, more frequent realized purchases of home furnishings were reported by those who were Future oriented. Conversely, participants with the Present Fatalistic orientation reported lower purchases of vacations in the past year.

Demographic variables indicated that purchasing vacations abroad was significantly more frequent among university/college graduates (who served as a statistical reference group) and less frequent among people with a lower level of secondary/vocational education. Respondents of every marital status except widowers were anticipating some new home furnishings in the coming year (married respondents in particular).

With respect to the anticipated purchase of furnishings, a moderate but significant ($p<.01$) relationship was found between not just one but two time orientations: *both the Future dimension and the Present Hedonistic dimension positively influenced anticipated purchases of home furnishings*. And understandably, a furnishing purchase was also more often anticipated by people who assessed their household standard of living as high.

Table 3 ZTPI dimensions and selected demographics relevant to financial behavior: results of linear regression (Beta significance)

	Vacations bought this year	Furnishings bought this year	Furnishings anticipated next year
Variable	Beta	Beta	Beta
ZTPI—Future dimension		0.018*	0.026**
ZTPI—Present Hedonistic dimension			0.028**
ZTPI—Present Fatalistic dimension	–0.016*		
Marital status—single			1.960*
Marital status—married			1.986**
Marital status—divorced			1.795*
Vocational education	−1.029*		
Secondary education w/o diploma	−1.491***		
Secondary vocational with diploma	−1.343***		
Secondary general with diploma			
Household standard of living			0.438*
R-square Cox-Snell/ Nagelkerke	0.245/0.348	0.168/0.225	0.220/0.296

*≤0.05, **≤0.01, ***≤0.001

Discussion of Results

Although financial behavior (savings and loan repayment) as well as substantial spending are primarily linked to the socio-economic status (we confirmed strong relationships especially with the increasing household income, household standard of living, higher occupational status, male gender and lower rather than higher age), the time perspective still demonstrated significant effects. In fact, *all ZTPI time dimensions played significant roles except the Past dimensions*, roles of which were not supported by evidence. Neither Past-Positive nor Past-Negative dimension produced important relationships.

The *Future orientation* was particularly prominent in the relationship to both financial behavior and to purchases. We observed that:

1. The Future oriented respondents saved significantly more than other respondents. That is not surprising as thanks to their ability to plan and achieve their goals, they also typically reach higher education and higher social economic status; saving money then is easier for them than for other groups.

2. The Future oriented not just saved more but also more often paid back their loans. (Only Present Fatalists were comparable with them in the loan repayment frequency). We could not analyze the amounts and reasons for the loans but one can assume that the Future oriented have the highest consumer ambitions and they are also the most likely and most welcome customers for any bank. Overall, the Future oriented appeared financially as the most active.
3. With regard to purchases, the Future oriented respondents were more likely than other groups of respondents to report past furnishings purchases, they were also very likely to anticipate furnishing purchases in the future.

The results of Future oriented participants fit well the Zimbardo time perspective theory. Future oriented people are generally recognized as more successful in academic achievement and in psychological health (Peetsma and van der Veen 2011; Barber et al. 2009; Zimbardo and Boyd 1999). Thus, the Future oriented people tend to get better education and obtain better paid positions and become most affluent. In a good example of a positive feedback, most affluent Future oriented people can more easily set aside greater resources for their future. Likewise, when evaluating the effect of time perspective and demographic categories on financial and consumer behavior, one has to keep in mind that such *demographic variables as high income and high status profession are also to a great degree a product of high Future time orientation.*

The *Present-Fatalists* stood out by their admittance of loan repayment activity while having no special tendency to savings or purchases, in fact, they showed a negative tendency to go on vacations abroad. Since Present Fatalism is generally linked to "absence of personal efficacy" (Zimbardo and Boyd 2008, p. 64), it is not surprising that Present Fatalists occasionally need to take a loan. In contrast to the Future oriented debtors, the Present Fatalists probably do not have much to show for their debts. Rather than an aid with a valuable investment, their loan may be a relief in the situation of financial constraints. One may assume that the Future oriented might use loans for a house or a car payment while the Present Fatalists may more likely borrow cash for daily expenses. However, the reasons for loans at this point are only a speculation; a deeper analysis of the loans would be needed and our data do not allow it.

Present Hedonism is very much defined by enjoyment of life and impulsive purchases. One would hypothesize that hedonists do not save money but they might be particularly tempted to apply for loans to satisfy their impulses; on the other hand, they may have the hardest time to qualify for a loan as they typically represent the youngest strata with the least purchasing power.

That situation has reflected in our survey: the hedonists did not score high in either saving or loan payments. Yet, they were high in anticipating their future purchases. In fact, the Present Hedonists were competitive in the planning of furnishings with the Future oriented respondents. However, the realism of the plans of the Future oriented participants was partially verified by their alleged realized furnishing purchases during the current year. In contrast, the Present Hedonists appear more like dreamers who only imagine what they might buy.

Parting Thoughts on the Cautionary Trends Disregarding Future

Homo Psychologicus

The importance of psychology for explaining economic phenomena has been recognized for at least half a century now. Katona (1963, 1975), among others, argued that subjective, psychological conditions rather than objective ones determine economic behavior. On a similar note, Starr more recently (2007, p. 215) pointed out that in the economic research "Homo psychologicus is in many respects a significant improvement over the much criticized homo economicus." However, psychology is not always used on behalf of the customers and in defense of the vulnerable in the business interaction (the young, the elderly, and the handicapped). Psychological sciences are too often used in economy and in politics against the citizen interests. While Taylorism helped us to be more productive, it did not necessarily help us to be more humanistic. Does the future belong to the "destructive, present-oriented capitalism practiced by Enron" (Zimbardo and Boyd 2008, p. 272)?

Time as a Commodity

Time, the most precious of all resources, has also become a commodity. After all, it is widely believed that 'time is money,' and in reality, one can often buy (or sell) vacation time and the quality time with friends and family (cf. Nickols and Fox 1983). However, instead of using or taming time, we are becoming its slaves. The overworked on one hand and the precariat or unemployed workers on the other hand bear a witness.

Time poverty is a new concept relevant to discretionary time and to un/freedom (Goodin et al. 2008). If the current world suffers too often from the plague of inequality, discrimination in the use of time (and especially the quality time with loved ones) seems to be the most painful (cf. *Time poverty: The unequal distribution of temporal autonomy,* a review by Whillans 2011).

Immediate Gratification in Economy and Politics

This chapter has mentioned the marshmallow test, the simple experiment of the ability to delay gratification for a future return. This model situation often comes to mind when one notices the shortsighted policies of most of the modern societies. Instead of being aware of future trends and investing into the social capital and environment, the focus is on a short-sighted and unrealistic economic growth. Not surprisingly, our era tends to be labeled as 'the age of greed' (Madrick 2011; Mason 2009; Kodas 2009) and the young generation is sometimes called 'the Generation Me' (Twenge 2006). We are, indeed, becoming the *Temporary Society* as Bennis and Slater foresaw in 1968.

The economic calendars shrunk from the long-term visions to the proximal earnings quarters; likewise, our democratic political system partitioned our era to short election cycles. Politicians seem to preferentially address (and misinform) what is now euphemistically called "a low information voter," i.e., a voter with a limited memory, short attention span, misconceptions, and black & white thinking without nuances. The advertisers appear to ignore a rational, Future-oriented shopper. Instead, they seem to talk consumers down, stressing their vanity, lower needs and immediate gratification.

Economic Models Targeting the Young and Immature

Better yet for the businesses, rather than to infantilize adult consumers, why not to focus on the immature adults right away and bring them up to the industry's liking? After all, the immature consumers command a surprisingly high spending power of parents and grandparents. Thus, the food industry creates addiction of children to sugar and fat and the cigarette producers target the youngest populations to instill a long term nicotine dependence. The film and gaming industries profit from the aggressive tendencies in boys, fashion and cosmetic retailers use social inclinations of girls and prey on their vanity. Arredondo et al. (2009), among others, drew attention to the brand loyalty of children as young as 4–8 years when it comes to fast or healthy food. Graham (2001) pointed out the exploitation of "tweenies" and "kidults" (aged between 9 and 14) who are brand-oriented, technically savvy, who have attitude, lifestyle and demand things immediately. The youth is painfully aware how their social status depends on wearing top brand outfits and flashing the newest electronic gadgets. A growing body of knowledge proves the effects of shopping malls on teenagers and their identity formation (e.g., Cotrau 2008; Spilkova and Radova 2011). The youth, as a fifth column in their families, take over the advertising job, persuading and swaying their families to otherwise unlikely purchases of candy, fast food, toys, phone and internet service providers and cars with best video system on board.

The next logical step is to free the children from the parental control altogether and let them be the deciders: banks started to advertise credit cards to minors so they can circumvent their parents altogether.[5] The times when banks gladly offered free

[5] *Consumer Reports* (2007) alerts parents to the bank practices and to scary recruiting techniques targeting minors. Consumer Reports also warns against "hefty activation, maintenance and dormancy fees" along with painful overdraft and decline charges; at the same time it cautions against a practice which entices children with spending bonuses. Kiplinger's contributor Bodnar (2007)

saving accounts to children are gone. A reputable link (Wikihow 2014) advises parents to "instruct your child to apply for a small ($500) loan that he or she repays right away" in order to build a positive credit report and obtain one's own credit card. Many feel that there is an obvious ethical problem when children are encouraged to borrow before they even have real earnings.

The Marshmallow Pyramid Scheme

The world production is still increasing, consumer goods and services are available (although not necessarily affordable) to a growing number of households. More than ever, this is due to the fact that the production facilities have been moved to the third world. The global penetration of consumer goods can thus be symbolized by a "flying geese pattern" (Matsuyama 2002).

At the same time, the countries of the first and former second world are nearing the point of consumer saturation, their high purchasing levels seem to be maintained mainly by means of a decline in savings and by an increase of personal and national debt.[6] And thus, the individuals and the populace at large tend to borrow and spend, succumbing to the seduction of the present-day consume with little regard for future pay backs—financial or environmental.

The psychology of time has accumulated plenty of knowledge which can help people to optimize their time perspectives and assist them to live more fulfilling lives. Maturity and happiness seem to be the best protectors against reckless spending and defense against draining precious responses. *Until then, we are all failing the marshmallow test.*

Acknowledgment This project was partially supported by the Institute of Psychology, Academy of Sciences of the Czech Republic—RVO 68081740. The authors are grateful to the Center of the Research of Public Opinion (CVVM) at the Institute of Sociology, Academy of Sciences of the Czech Republic for enabling this study and to its director, Dr. Martin Buchtík, for general support and assistance.

---

warns that "Although the cards are billed as money-management tools, their main purpose is to make it easier for kids to spend money, especially online." Both Consumer Reports and Kiplinger quote the new advertising line by UPside card: 'Now buy online without asking your parents.'

[6] Dobrescu et al. (2012) point out a common trend—a dramatic decline in national savings over time. "France and Italy, for example, saved over 23 % and 19 % of national income in 1970, but only 9 % and 4 % in 2008; the U.S. saved around 11 % in 1970, but only 1 % in 2008." Lusardi et al. (2001) point out that the widely reported personal saving rate in the United States has dropped from double digits to below zero.

References

Arredondo, E., Castaneda, D., Elder, J. P., Slymen, D., & Dozier, D. (2009). Brand name logo recognition of fast food and healthy food among children. *Journal of Community Health, 34*, 73–78.

Barber, L. K., Munz, D. C., Bagsby, P. G., & Grawitch, M. J. (2009). When does time perspective matter? Self-control as a moderator between time perspective and academic achievement. *Personality and Individual Differences, 46*, 250–253.

Bauer, T. K., Bredtmann, J., & Schmidt, C. M. (2013). Time vs. money: The supply of voluntary labor and charitable donations across Europe. *European Journal of Political Economy, 32*, 80–94.

Bodnar, J. (2007). *Prepaid debit cards encourage spending*. http://www.kiplinger.com/article/credit/T016-C002-S001-prepaid-debit-cards-encourage-spending.html#jrW4fJ7ZYlZ6OiD9.99. Accessed 4 Feb 2014.

Bond, M. J., & Feather, N. T. (1988). Some correlates of structure and purpose in the use of time. *Journal of Personality and Social Psychology, 55*, 321–329.

Bonke, J., Deding, M., & Lausten, M. (2009). Time and money. *Journal of Happiness Studies, 10*(2), 113–131.

Calabresi, R., & Cohen, J. (1968). Personality and time attitudes. *Journal of Abnormal Psychology, 73*, 431–439.

Consumer Reports. (2007). Teen cards send mixed message. *Consumer Reports Money Adviser, 4*(3), 12.

Cotrau, D. (2008). Malls and the holy trinity of teens: Pleasure, leisure, and consumption in Transylvania. *Journal for the Study of Religions and Ideologies, 7*, 3–19.

Cotte, J., Ratneshwar, S., & Mick, D. G. (2004). The times of their lives: Phenomenological and metaphorical characteristics of consumer timestyles. *Journal of Consumer Research, 31*, 333–345.

Dobrescu, L. I., Kotlikoff, L. J., & Motta, A. (2012). Why aren't developed countries saving? *European Economic Review, 56*, 1261–1275.

Doyle, J. R. (2013). Survey of time preference, delay discounting models. *Judgment and Decision Making, 8*, 116–135.

Feldman, L. P., & Hornik, J. (1981). The use of time, the integrated conceptual model. *Journal of Consumer Research, 7*, 407–419.

Fraisse, P. (1967). *Psychologie du temps*. Paris: Presses universitaires de France.

Gonzalez, A., & Zimbardo, P. G. (1985, March). Time in perspective. *Psychology Today,* 20–26.

Goodin, R. E., Rice, J. M., Parpo, A., & Eriksson, L. (Eds.). (2008). *Discretionary time: A new measure of freedom*. Cambridge: Cambridge University Press.

Graham, R. J. (1981). The role of perception of time in consumer research. *Journal of Consumer Research, 7*, 335–342.

Graham, S. (2001). *Tweenies: Immature consumers with serious spending power*. http://www.mycustomer.com/topic/technology/tweenies-immature-consumers-serious-spending-power. Accessed 10 Feb 2014.

Guven, C. (2012). Reversing the question: Does happiness affect consumption and savings behavior? *Journal of Economic Psychology, 33*, 701–717.

Hall, E. T. (1959). *The silent language*. New York: Anchor Books.

Hall, E. T. (1966). *The hidden dimension*. New York: Anchor Books.

Hobbes, M., De Groot, W. T., & Sarkhel, S. (2011). Freely disposable time: A time and money integrated measure of poverty and freedom. *World Development, 39*, 2055–2068.

Jacoby, J. (1976). Time and consumer behavior: An interdisciplinary overview. *Journal of Consumer Research, 2*, 320–339.

Kantrowicz, T. M., Grelle, D. M., Beaty, J. C., & Wolf, M. B. (2012). Time is money: Polychronicity as a predictor of performance across job levels. *Human Performance, 25*, 114–137.
Katona, G. (1963). The relationship between psychology and economics. In S. Koch (Ed.), *Psychology: A study of a science* (pp. 639–676). New York: McGraw-Hill.
Katona, G. (1975). *Psychological economics*. New York: Elsevier.
Kodas, M. (2009). *High crimes: The fate of Everest in an age of greed*. New York: Hyperion.
Košťál, J., Klicperová-Baker, M., Lukavská, K., & Lukavský, J. (submitted). Short version of the Zimbardo Time Perspective Inventory (ZTPI-short) verified with nationally representative samples with and without an added Future Negative scale.
Lukavská, K., Klicperová-Baker, M., Lukavský, J., & Zimbardo, P. (2011). ZTPI—Zimbardův dotazník časové perspektivy [Zimbardo's Questionnaire of Time Perspective]. *Československá psychologie, 55*, 356–373 (in Czech).
Lusardi, A., Skinner, J., & Venti, S. (2001). Saving puzzles and saving policies in the United States. *Oxford Review of Economic Policy, 17*, 95–115.
Madrick, J. (2011). *Age of greed: The triumph of finance and the decline of America, 1970 to the present*. New York: Knopf.
Mason, P. (2009). *Meltdown: The end of the age of greed*. London: Verso.
Matsuyama, K. (2002). The rise of mass consumption societies. *Journal of Political Economy, 110*, 1035–1070.
Mischel, W., Ebbesen, E. B., & Zeiss, A. R. (1972). Cognitive and attentional mechanisms in delay of gratification. *Journal of Personality and Social Psychology, 21*, 204–218.
Mischel, W., Ayduk, O., Berman, M. G., Casey, B. J., Gotlib, I. H., Jonides, J., Kross, E., Teslovich, T., Wilson, N. L., Zayas, V., & Shoda, Y. (2011). 'Willpower' over the life span: Decomposing self-regulation. *Social Cognitive and Affective Neuroscience, 6*, 252–256.
Mogilner, C. (2010). The pursuit of happiness: Time, money, and social connection. *Psychological Science, 21*, 1348–1354.
Nickols, S. Y., & Fox, K. D. (1983). Buying time and saving time: Strategies for managing household production. *Journal of Consumer Research, 10*, 197–208.
OECD. (2013). *Better Life Index*. http://www.oecdbetterlifeindex.org/countries/czech-republic/. Accessed 3 May 2013.
Peetsma, T., & van der Veen, I. (2011). Relations between the development of future time perspective in three life domains, investment in learning, and academic achievement. *Learning and Instruction, 21*, 481–494.
Peters, C. L., & Bolkan, C. R. (2009). Measuring meaningful time experiences in intergenerational relationships. *Michigan Family Review, 13*, 21–31.
Spilkova, J., Radova, L. (2011). The formation of identity in teenage mall microculture: A case study of teenagers in Czech malls. *Sociologický časopis* [Czech Sociological Review], *47*, 565–586.
Starr, M. A. (2007). Saving, spending, and self-control: cognition versus consumer culture. *Review of Radical Political Economics, 39*, 214–229.
Twenge, J. M. (2006). *Generation me: Why today's young Americans are more confident, assertive, entitled—And more miserable than ever before*. New York: Free Press.
Wärneryd, K.-E. (1999). *The psychology of saving: A study on economic psychology*. Northampton: Edward Elgar Publishing Ltd.
Whillans, J. (2011). Review of books: Time poverty: The unequal distribution of temporal autonomy. *Time and Society, 20*, 137–140.
Wikihow. (2014). *How to get a visa credit card for your kid*. http://www.wikihow.com/Get-a-Visa-Credit-Card-for-Your-Kid. Accessed 1 Feb 2014.
Zaleskiewicz, T., Gasiorowska, A., & Kesebir, P. (2013). Saving can save from death anxiety: Mortality salience and financial decision-making. *PLoS One, 8*, e79407. doi:10.1371/journal.pone.0079407.

Zimbardo, P. (2009). *Ted talk on time*. http://blog.ted.com/2009/06/22/philip_zimbardo/. Accessed 8 Feb 2014.

Zimbardo, P. G., & Boyd, J. N. (1999). Putting time in perspective: A valid, reliable, individual-differences metric. *Journal of Personality and Social Psychology, 77*, 1271–1288.

Zimbardo, P. G., & Boyd, J. N. (2008). *The time paradox: The new psychology of time that will change your life*. New York: Basic Books.

Understanding Environmental Issues with Temporal Lenses: Issues of Temporality and Individual Differences

Taciano L. Milfont and Christophe Demarque

Introduction

A notable series of environmental incidents happened in recent years, including the Three Miles Island nuclear accident in the USA, the Bhopal gas tragedy in India and the Amoco Cadiz oil spill in France, and the Fukushima nuclear disaster in Japan. Common to these events are how they occur suddenly and brutally and also their immediate visible consequences to nature at large as well as many individuals. Although immediate and visible consequences are characteristic of environmental disasters, the negative consequences of many environmental problems are much more delayed. Additionally, humans are unable to perceive all signs of global environmental changes, which Pawlik (1991) referred to as the 'low signal-to-noise ratio of global change'. Signals of global environmental changes are often weak (both in terms of physical, perceptive signals and in terms of temporality), and sensory and memory mechanisms are unable to discern them as they are below the common thresholds of discernability.

Some environmental problems are also easier to notice than others because they have stronger physical signs and/or lower temporal delay. For example, it is easier to notice deforestation and air and water pollution than global climate change. Thus, most environmental problems are less easily perceptible due to our senses' limitations (e.g. nuclear radiation, greenhouse effect) and exhibit long-delayed effects or evolve too slowly to be perceived (Moser 2009). Moreover, as mentioned by Niemeijer and de Groot (2008), environmental processes are complex and do not

T.L. Milfont (✉)
School of Psychology and Centre for Applied Cross-Cultural Research,
Victoria University of Wellington, Wellington, New Zealand
e-mail: taciano.milfont@vuw.ac.nz

C. Demarque
Department of Social, Work and Organizational Psychology,
University of Toulouse Le Mirail, Toulouse, France

M. Stolarski et al. (eds.), *Time Perspective Theory; Review, Research and Application: Essays in Honor of Philip G. Zimbardo*, DOI 10.1007/978-3-319-07368-2_24,

obey unidirectional causal chains. For instance, the impact of the loss of biodiversity or global warming is not always directly related to humans. According to these authors, we are dealing with complex interrelated factors and it would be more relevant to speak about causal networks, which are often difficult to perceive.

Clearly, the physical signs and temporal delays inherent of environmental problems can hinder their perception and understanding and resulting concern towards them. This chapter focuses on the notion of temporality and is organised in two main sections. In the first section, we will further discuss aspects of temporality underlying environmental problems. It will be argued that environmental problems have temporal delays: problems we are facing now are a result of past behaviour and our current behaviours will have future environmental consequences. A brief overview of the recognition that intertemporal decision-making is necessary in fostering environmental sustainability will also be provided. Stemming from this assessment, the second and main section of this chapter focuses on individual differences in time perspective and their influence on pro-environmental attitudes and behaviours. Extant research using Zimbardo Time Perspective Inventory as well as other measures to capture time perspective and relate it to environmental issues will be reviewed. Suggestions for new research perspectives and conclusions are presented in the last section of this chapter.

The Temporality of Environmental Issues

As outlined above, most environmental problems present long-delayed effects or evolve too slowly to be perceived. There is a great temporal delay between human actions and their perceptible influence on environmental systems (i.e. cause–effect gradient; Pawlik 1991), which means that the environmental consequences of our behaviours go beyond a single generation. The maladaptive human behaviour of previous generations is responsible for many of the current environmental problems, while the maladaptive behaviours of today will have consequences not only for us but also for several generations to come. To illustrate, the consequences of climate change will be felt by plants, animals and humans for at least the next thousand years (Collins et al. 2007). Conversely, investment in courses of action to adapt and reduce risks from climate change would have to be done by the current generation, while the main effects of such actions would only benefit the future generations.

Actually, the temporal dimension of environmental issues has been at the heart of debates from the early stages of environmentalist movements. In particular, the necessity of taking into account long-term consequences of our behaviours appeared with the development, during the twentieth century, of new technologies with beneficial effects on the short term but more uncertain ones in the long term. When Rachel Carson published *Silent Spring* in 1962, one of the founding acts of environmentalism in the United States, Carson insisted on the fact that a massive use of dichlorodiphenyltrichloroethane (DDT), even if it could momentarily eliminate many pests, would lead to the development of long-term resistances and provoke a rise of mortality and reproduction disorders among birds. Similar questioning arises with nuclear energy: producing electricity with low carbon dioxide emissions but generating waste with an extremely long-life span that we do not know how to treat efficiently.

Recognition of the temporality of environmental issues is also evident in the discussion of sustainability. As defined in the Brundtland Report in 1987, sustainable development should meet the needs of the present generations without compromising the ability of future generations to meet their own needs. Sustainable development is intrinsically situated in the long run and thus focuses on the adoption of anticipatory behaviours on the principle of a consideration of our behaviours' consequences and of future generations' needs in the present. Thereby, environmental sustainability implies a focus on intertemporal decision-making because such decisions imply trade-offs between current and future rewards.

A temporal dilemma thus underlies environmental problems and pro-environmental behaviours are generally characterised by short-term costs and long-term benefits, as emphasised by Platt's (1973) work on social traps (see also Joireman 2005; Milfont and Gouveia 2006). In parallel, addressing environmental issues involves the management of limited resources which could simultaneously lead to a social dilemma. Indeed, according to Hardin, in his seminal 1968 article *The Tragedy of the Commons*, in such dilemmas individuals will try to maximise their personal profit over collective interests. It is in this way that environmental problems entail two distinct yet related conflicts: a social conflict between individual and collective interests and a temporal conflict between short-term and long-term interests.

With this in mind, Van Lange and Joireman (2008) proposed a review on how individual differences in social and temporal orientations could impact decision-making in social dilemmas. Most often, prosocial (altruistic, cooperative and egalitarian) and/or future-oriented people act in the interest of the collective. However, the authors mentioned possible paradoxical effects under certain conditions. For instance, Strathman et al. (1994) observed that future-oriented individuals were more likely to support an environmentally harmful action, off-shore oil drilling, when it carried short-term costs (oil seepage and diversion of research funds from alternative sources of energy) and long-term benefits (reduction in dependence on nuclear power and reduction of gas and oil prices).

In this section, we have reviewed some concepts and empirical evidence indicating the temporal nature of environmental issues. Besides this temporality underlying environmental issues, we mentioned that individual differences on time perspective are also important. Indeed, in light of this temporal aspect of environmental problems, we could intuitively expect time perspective (and especially Future time perspective) to be a relevant variable for studying individuals' perceptions of and engagement with the environment. In other words, people's capacity for and interest in thinking long term would influence decision-making regarding conflicting short- and long-term interests. The next section addresses more precisely this question.

Individual Differences in Time Perspective and Environmental Problems

There are strong individual differences in time perspective that influence behaviours. Based on their different relative view of the future, recollections of the past and present exigencies, individuals preferentially overemphasise the past, present or future, and this contributes to the decisions they make (Karniol and Ross 1996; Zimbardo and Boyd 2008). Other chapters in this volume provide a more throughout revision of this literature. Here we only provide a brief overview of individual differences in time perspective and focus on how these time perspective differences can help us understand apathy or engagement towards environmental problems.

Broadly speaking, individuals who adopt a past time perspective tend to have highly meaningful mental representations of the past, and engage in reflective, contemplative reconstructions of past experiences, which can be warm and sentimental but also entail reconstructive experiences of unpleasant or traumatic events. Present time perspective lies between the abstract, psychological reconstructions of the past and anticipated future, entailing a focus on concrete and empirically centred representations of present events. Future time perspective is characterised by planning and the achievement of future goals and entails meaningful mental representations of future events that pull individuals to behave in accordance with these representations (Karniol and Ross 1996; Zimbardo and Boyd 1999, 2008).

Three main scales are available to study individual differences in time perspective. The Consideration of Future Consequences (CFC) Scale determines individuals' tendencies to focus on the future or immediate consequences of their acts using 12 items (Strathman et al. 1994) or 14 items (Joireman et al. 2012). The Zimbardo Time Perspective Inventory (ZTPI; Zimbardo and Boyd 1999) covers five time frames (Past Positive and Negative, Present Hedonistic and Fatalistic and Future) using 56 items. The Temporal Focus Scale (TFS; Shipp et al. 2009) measures the extent to which individuals pay attention to perceptions of the past, present and future using 12 items. Studies have provided support for the psychometric properties of these measures and have also shown that they are related (e.g. Milfont and Schwarzenthal 2014; Shipp et al. 2009), but only the CFC and ZTPI have been consistently used in relation to pro-environmental engagement.

Concerning the ZTPI, research has shown a positive correlation between the future dimension of the scale, environmental attitudes (Milfont and Gouveia 2006) and water conservation practices (Corral-Verdugo et al. 2006; Corral-Verdugo and Pinheiro 2006). These findings suggest that greater future orientation is associated with higher pro-environmental engagement. No systematic associations have been observed for past and/or present. However, as expected due to the negative association between Present and Future time perspective, studies have also reported negative correlations between present time perspective and both environmental preservation (Milfont and Gouveia 2006) and water conservation behaviour (Corral-Verdugo et al. 2006).

The majority of studies have used the CFC Scale, with very consistent results. Individuals focusing on the future consequences of their current behaviours show stronger pro-environmental attitudes (Strathman et al. 1994). Moreover, CFC is linked with a diversity of 'green' behaviours (or behavioural intentions) (Joireman et al. 2001), including the use of public transportation (Joireman et al. 2004), involvement in pro-environmental activism (Joireman et al. 2001) or recycling (Lindsay and Strathman 1997; Ebreo and Vining 2001).

A recent meta-analytical summary of this literature (involving 19 independent samples and 6,301 participants from seven countries) showed that Future time perspective has a stronger influence on pro-environmental attitudes and behaviours than a combined score of past–present perspective (Milfont et al. 2012b). This study also showed that the association between Future time perspective and pro-environmental behaviours was stronger than the association for attitudes.

A number of recent experimental studies support these correlations (e.g. Arnocky et al. 2014; Kortenkamp and Moore 2006; Pahl and Bauer 2011; Rabinovich et al. 2010). For example, Kortenkamp and Moore (2006) investigated factors affecting temporal dilemmas in two resource dilemma tasks. They specifically examined whether varying time and uncertainty would influence participants' willingness to cooperate to reduce resource consumption and avoid resource depletion. Results showed that participants were more likely to cooperate to reduce resource use when the effects of resource depletion were immediate and when they were less uncertain. High future orientation together with pro-environmental attitudes also led to more cooperation and less temporal discounting.

In another experimental study, Pahl and Bauer (2011) examined the effects of perspective taking, or imagining oneself in someone else's position, on environmental engagement. Participants were allocated to three groups, with two groups shown a slideshow resembling the year 2105 containing the imagery of potential environmental degradation. The slideshow was accompanied by the voice of a woman describing the toll that environmental degradation has taken on her life. One group was asked to take her perspective by imagining they were in her position, while the second experimental group was asked to objectively evaluate the presented facts. The third, control group did not view the slideshow. The outcome measures were the time participants spent at an information stand on environmental issues and the number of brochures taken. Participants who had viewed the slideshow and were asked to engage in perspective taking spent significantly more time at the information stand and took significantly more brochures on environmental issues than those who were asked to evaluate the facts objectively or those who did not see the slideshow. Although it is unclear whether the psychological mechanism underlying these group differences are primarily a result of an increase in empathy or future thinking (or a combination of both), this research suggests that taking the perspective of another human being living in the distant future who is suffering from the environmental damages caused by current behaviour could encourage greater environmental engagement in the present.

Another recent study has extended past research in two substantial ways (Arnocky et al. 2014). Following recent developments in the field, the authors examined the efficacy of a two-factor model of consideration of future consequences (i.e. CFC-Future and CFC-Immediate) in understanding environmentally sustainable attitudes. They found that the immediate CFC factor was negatively related to pro-environmental measures, while the correlation for the future CFC factor was nonsignificant. In a second study, the authors made future consideration salient (by using a prime technique to implicitly activate future thinking) and examined the effect on pro-environmental measures. As expected, activating future thinking increased environmental concerns and behaviours, and the prime effect was mediated by decreased concerns with the *immediate* consequences of actions (and not by increased concerns with the *future* consequences of actions). These results indicate the importance of measuring both present and Future time perspective when understanding their influence on environmental engagement.

Contextual Influences on the Relations Between Time Perspective and Environmental Problems

Zimbardo and Boyd (1999) called attention to the Lewinian postulate considering time perspective as a construct determined by inter-individual differences, relatively stable a priori, and also by characteristics of the context. Thus, it is important to place an emphasis on the contextualised dimension of time perspective, in order to better comprehend the complexity of the psychosocial dynamics involved. Hence, the study of pro-environmental behaviours should not only take into account time perspective but also consider contextual factors (see, e.g. Cialdini 2003; Keizer et al. 2008).

An inspection of the literature reveals that many studies on time perspective have actually focused on interactions, assuming that time perspective is a moderator of the impact of some other factors within the individual (e.g. perceived environmental consequences; Joireman et al. (2004)) or a feature of the situation that has been manipulated (e.g. the framing of environmental messages; Strathman et al. 1994). Time perspective determines the way we comprehend a situation or an event, and as such it is interesting to look at how the context influences the effect of time perspective on the individuals' actions or perceptions. As it is suggested by Van Lange and Joireman (2008), we have to recognise both the stability and plasticity of people's temporal (and social) orientations across time and situations. For these authors, individuals are predisposed towards a temporal orientation, but the probability that this orientation may be activated will differ according to the situation. Indeed, it is well established that the weight of psychosocial factors in the setting up of pro-environmental behaviours varies in relation to the weight of contextual factors (Steg and Vlek 2009). As postulated by the ABC model (Guagnano et al. 1995), for example, behaviour (B) is a product of the interaction between personal-sphere attitudinal variables (A)—including norms, beliefs and values—and contextual factors (C).

Psychological variables will not predict behaviour in contexts where action is either extremely difficult or extremely easy (Stern 2000). In this topic, Guagnano and colleagues (1995) observed that components of the norm-activation model did not predict recycling behaviour when action was favoured by context (i.e. when households were equipped with plastic bins provided by the local authorities).

These empirical findings and theoretical considerations suggest that if time perspective offers a cognitive frame influencing individuals' behaviours and decision-making, it seems important to examine the potential moderating role that the context could play in this relationship. That was the aim of a study by Demarque et al. (2013), who examined the influence of external situations on the relationship between CFC and a pro-environmental behaviour to test whether the ABC model could be extended to the consideration of future consequences. Using the same reasoning as for attitudinal variables, they tested whether external conditions could moderate the relationship between CFC and decision-making. External conditions were conceived as 'all external sources of support or opposition to behavior, whether physical, financial, legal, or social' (Guagnano et al. 1995, p. 702). While most studies have focused on physical conditions, this conceptualization of external conditions also includes social influence as another way to investigate the situational strength.

In their study, Demarque et al. (2013) examined three types of communication situations with differing support for the pro-environmental behaviour (contributing to an environmentalist association): no communication, persuasive communication and commitment-based communication (committing to perform an inexpensive act before the reading of the persuasive message). The main result was an interaction effect between CFC and the communication situation, which suggests that the social context moderates the effect of CFC on decision-making, as the effect of CFC was significant only in the intermediate situation of persuasive communication. In line with the ABC model, the link between CFC and decision-making was weakest when external conditions were 'extreme' (no communication and commitment-based communication) and was strongest when contextual influences were moderate (persuasive communication). Thus, the effect of CFC on decision-making was moderated by the more or less favouring nature of the situation in which participants were placed.

What for Tomorrow? Future Research Directions and Possible Applications

On the whole, the reviewed results provide evidence for the relevance of time perspective in the environmental domain. However, many theoretical and empirical issues remain concerning the influence of situational variables and the involved psychological processes. We would like to suggest here some lines of future research, both on practical, theoretical and methodological levels.

First, the associations between time perspective and measures of pro-environmental orientations are expected to be weak for both past and present time perspective dimensions. However, this observation must be put into perspective considering the small number of studies conducted so far. The past and present dimensions should be further considered in subsequent research, as it seems obvious that they could play a role in the understanding of environmental issues. Chawla (1999) showed, for instance, that environmentalism is partly determined by positive emotional experiences with nature during childhood and also by the family structure.

One of the difficulties induced by the temporal nature of environmental issues is the level of effort required for an individual to create a link between a given behaviour and its consequences. This point is central in an applied perspective, as Stern (2005) reminds us that ‘People who do not see connections between their behavior and such consequences or who believe that their actions are so insignificant in the scheme of things as not to matter will not be motivated to act by an internalized sense of obligation’ (p. 788).

With this in mind, how could we make people more sensitive to the future consequences of their behaviours? A study by Hall and Fong (2003) already evidenced that an intervention enhancing long-term thinking about physical activity could increase subsequent physical activity among young adults. Similarly, the work by Arnocky and colleagues (2014) showed that inducing future thinking increased pro-environmental intentions. Both studies examined the influenced of long-term thinking on subsequent behaviour or intention, but not the change of time perspective itself. In this topic, a recent study showed that a commitment-based communication procedure could momentarily increase participants’ CFC scores (Demarque et al. 2012). Specifically, the CFC score of a group comprising 37 participants increased one week after a commitment-based communication intervention, a difference not observed in a persuasive communication intervention. Even if the observed difference was not particularly large, the result encourages us to consider that time perspective could be influenced directly by a socially influential situation, which is a stimulating possibility for the field of environmental education and awareness of environmental issues, as well as other applied fields. To be more efficient, this kind of behavioural incentive requires a better theoretical comprehension of the involved processes.

Another avenue for future studies is to combine different aspects of psychological time when examining environmental issues. It has been argued that psychological time has three major aspects (Block 1990): time duration (persistence of events or the interval between events), time succession (sequential occurrence of events as reflected by their temporal order) and time perspective (a person’s experiences and conceptions of past, present and future time). As reviewed in this chapter, most studies have so far focused only on time perspective without considering the other aspects of psychological time. A recent study has shown that time perspective can modulate subtle cognitive aspects of time succession (Nowack et al. 2013), which might have repercussions for the way individuals understand the sequential consequences of their actions on the environment. Other studies have examined the associations between time perspective and chronotype—individual differences in circadian preferences that characterise morning types and evening types (e.g. Milfont and Schwarzenthal 2014).

Theoretical advances also have to be made, such as the link with *construal level theory* (for reviews, see Trope and Liberman 2003; Liberman and Trope 2008). According to this theory, the greater the temporal distance of an event, the more it will be susceptible to be represented by a few abstract characteristics which convey its perceived essential qualities (high-level representation). In contrast, the shorter the distance is, the more the event will be represented with concrete terms and with secondary details (low-level representation). Thereby, each individual is able to give several meanings to the same event. For instance, 'make a gesture for the environment' may mean 'turn off appliances when not in use' if this action is planned for tomorrow; but if it is planned for next year, it will more likely mean 'think about future generations'. Moreover, the greater the temporal distance, or in other words the further away an event is in time, the more high-level representations will influence our behavioural intentions.

Recent studies have linked psychological distance to environmental issues (e.g. Evans et al. 2014; Milfont et al. 2011; Schultz et al. 2014; Spence et al. 2012). For Milfont (2010), psychological distance could put a considerable curb on the setting up of behaviours restricting climate change. In this view, we should decrease this distance in order to ease pro-environmental action. This idea is congruent with goal setting theory (Locke and Latham 1990) in which the setting of specific and detailed goals (that we could consider as low-level constructs) should increase the probability of action. However, the processes seem more complex. Some researchers (Trope and Liberman 2011) suggest that goal attainment will be more likely if the goal matches with the construal level. For instance, Eyal et al. (2009) showed that feasibility concerns (referring to low-level constructs) predicted behavioural intention in the near future, whereas variables such as values (referring to high-level constructs) predicted behavioural intention in the distant future. Rabinovich and colleagues' (2010) work supports this idea. Considering environmental behaviours as future oriented, their results showed that focusing individuals on a distant-future perspective increased attitude–behaviour consistency. More precisely, they measured participants' attitudes in a first phase. A week later, participants described their country's environmental situation, either in a month (short-term time perspective) or in 10 years (long-term time perspective), after which pro-environmental intentions were measured. The strongest link between attitudes and intentions was observed in the second condition (long term). These results highlight the importance of concordance between the construal level and the goal to reach.

In a nutshell, construal levels refer to temporal representations of an action or an event, whereas time perspective reflects an individual general disposition. A future research objective would be to know how inter-individual differences in time perspective influence these representations and, consequently, pro-environmental decision-making.

Another theoretical advance resides in the study of 'environmental generativity' (Milfont et al. 2012a; Milfont and Sibley 2011) or 'legacy motive' (Fox et al. 2010). Basically, having children or an exposure to death priming might activate intergenerational generosity, because individuals want to gain a sense of purpose in life, to guarantee environmental quality for their offspring and to make an impact that will live on after death. For instance, Wade-Benzoni et al. (2012) found that participants who had read an article about an aircraft accident said they would give more money to a future-oriented charity than to a present-oriented one. Environmental generativity, or the legacy motive, is interesting for us because it allows for a sidestepping of the gap between present action and future consequences. A possible research question would be: Do individual differences in time perspective moderate the efficacy of the legacy motive and its effects on decision-making?

We would also like to draw attention to the normative dimension of time perspective. Indeed, a future orientation is generally associated in the literature with the setting up of 'optimal' behaviours, which are often linked in Western countries to a personal and/or social accomplishment (Lasane and O'Donnell 2005). Moreover, Zimbardo et al. (1997) described future-oriented individuals as those who 'generally follow convention and social norms, generally doing what is good, right and proper' (p. 1020). This might explain in part the associations between responsibility and environmental issues, but also questions what is expressed by participants when answering time perspective scales: Are we measuring Future time perspective (proper) or normative orientation? Recent research (Guignard et al. 2014) has addressed this question using a socio-cognitive approach to social norms (Dubois 2003). To illustrate, results from one experiment showed that Future time perspective was higher for participants in a pro-normative self-presentation condition compared to both counter-normative and control conditions. This recent line of research suggests the normativity of Future time perspective.

Conclusion

There is no denying that we are facing serious environmental problems, ranging from loss of biodiversity and species extinction to climate change. Environmental problems are anthropogenic issues, and their effects pose real threats for human living conditions and ecosystems. This chapter considered the temporality of environmental problems and focused on the influence of individual differences on time perspective as another important variable in understanding pro-environmental engagement or the complete lack thereof. Environmental problems entail both a social conflict (between individual and collective interests) and a temporal conflict (between short-term and long-term interests), and Future time perspective seems to have clear implications for the fostering of environmental sustainability.

References

Arnocky, S., Milfont, T. L., & Nicol, J. (2014). Time perspective and sustainable behaviour: Evidence for the distinction between consideration of immediate and future consequences. *Environment and Behavior, 46*, 556–582.

Block, R. A. (1990). Models of psychological time. In R. A. Block (Ed.), *Cognitive models of psychological time* (pp. 1–35). Hillsdale, NJ: Erlbaum.

Carson, R. (1962). *Silent spring*. Boston: Houghton-Mifflin.

Chawla, L. (1999). Life paths into effective environmental action. *The Journal of Environmental Education, 31*(1), 15–26.

Cialdini, R. B. (2003). Crafting normative messages to protect the environment. *Current Directions in Psychological Science, 12*, 105–109.

Collins, W., Colman, R., Haywood, J., Manning, M. R., & Mote, P. (2007). The physical science behind climate change. *Scientific American, 297*, 64–71.

Corral-Verdugo, V., & Pinheiro, J. Q. (2006). Sustainability, future orientation and water conservation. *European Review of Applied Psychology, 56*, 191–198.

Corral-Verdugo, V., Fraijo-Sing, B., & Pinheiro, J. Q. (2006). Sustainable behavior and time perspective: Present, past, and future orientations and their relationship with water conservation behavior. *Interamerican Journal of Psychology, 40*, 139–147.

Demarque, C., Apostolidis, T., & Joule, R. V. (2012). Does binding communication increase consideration of future consequences and decision making facing a pro-environmental behavior? In S. Kabisch, A. Kunath, P. Schweizer-Ries, & A. Steinführer (Eds.), *Vulnerability, risks, and complexity: Impacts of global change on human habitats* (pp. 221–229). Göttingen: Hogrefe.

Demarque, C., Apostolidis, T., & Joule, R. V. (2013). Consideration of future consequences and pro-environmental decision making in the context of persuasion and binding commitment. *Journal of Environmental Psychology, 36*, 214–220.

Dubois, N. (Ed.). (2003). *A sociocognitive approach to social norms*. London: Routledge.

Ebreo, A., & Vining, J. (2001). How similar are recycling and waste reduction? Future orientation and reasons for reducing waste as predictors of self-reported behavior. *Environment and Behavior, 33*, 424–448.

Evans, L., Milfont, T. L., & Lawrence, J. (2014). Considering local adaptation increases willingness to mitigate. *Global Environmental Change, 25*, 69–75.

Eyal, T., Sagristano, M. D., Trope, Y., Liberman, N., & Chaiken, S. (2009). When values matter: Expressing values in behavioral intentions for the near vs. distant future. *Journal of Experimental Social Psychology, 45*, 35–43.

Fox, M., Tost, L. P., & Wade-Benzoni, K. A. (2010). The legacy motive: A catalyst for sustainable decision making in organizations. *Business Ethics Quarterly, 20*, 153–185.

Guagnano, G. A., Stern, P. C., & Dietz, T. (1995). Influences on attitude-behavior relationships: A natural experiment with curbside recycling. *Environment and Behavior, 27*, 699–718.

Guignard, S., Apostolidis, T., & Demarque, C. (2014). Discussing normative features of future time perspective construct: Renewing with the Lewinian approach from a sociocognitive perspective. *New Ideas in Psychology, 35*, 1–10.

Hall, P. A., & Fong, G. T. (2003). The effects of a brief time perspective intervention for increasing physical activity among young adults. *Psychology and Health, 18*, 685–706.

Hardin, G. (1968). The tragedy of the commons. *Science, 162*(3859), 1243–1248.

Joireman, J. A. (2005). Environmental problems as social dilemmas: The temporal dimension. In A. Strathman & J. Joireman (Eds.), *Understanding behavior in the context of time* (pp. 289–304). Mahwah: Erlbaum.

Joireman, J. A., Lasane, T. P., Bennett, J., Richards, D., & Solaimani, S. (2001). Integrating social value orientation and the consideration of future consequences within the extended norm activation model of proenvironmental behavior. *British Journal of Social Psychology, 40*, 133–155.

Joireman, J. A., Van Lange, P. A. M., & Van Vugt, M. (2004). Who cares about the environmental impact of cars? Those with an eye toward the future. *Environment and Behavior, 36*, 187–206.

Joireman, J., Shaffer, M. J., Balliet, D., & Strathman, A. (2012). Promotion orientation explains why future-oriented people exercise and eat healthy: Evidence from the two-factor consideration of future consequences-14 scale. *Personality and Social Psychology Bulletin, 38*, 1272–1287.

Karniol, R., & Ross, M. (1996). The motivational impact of temporal focus: Thinking about the future and the past. *Annual Review of Psychology, 47*, 593–620.

Keizer, K., Lindenberg, S., & Steg, L. (2008). The spreading of disorder. *Science, 322*, 1681–1685.

Kortenkamp, K. V., & Moore, C. F. (2006). Time, uncertainty, and individual differences in decisions to cooperate in resource dilemmas. *Personality and Social Psychology Bulletin, 32*, 603–615.

Lasane, T. P., & O'Donnell, D. A. (2005). Time orientation measurement: A conceptual approach. In A. Strathman & J. Joireman (Eds.), *Understanding behavior in the context of time* (pp. 11–30). Mahwah: Erlbaum.

Liberman, N., & Trope, Y. (2008). The psychology of transcending the here and now. *Science, 322*, 1201–1205.

Lindsay, J. J., & Strathman, A. (1997). Predictors of recycling behavior: An application of a modified health belief model. *Journal of Applied Social Psychology, 27*, 1799–1823.

Locke, E. A., & Latham, G. P. (1990). *A theory of goal setting & task performance*. Englewood Cliffs: Prentice-Hall Inc.

Milfont, T. L. (2010). Global warming, climate change and human psychology. In V. Corral-Verdugo, C. H. García-Cadena, & M. Frías-Arment (Eds.), *Psychological approaches to sustainability: Current trends in theory, research and practice* (pp. 19–42). New York: Nova Science.

Milfont, T. L., & Gouveia, V. V. (2006). Time perspective and values: An exploratory study of their relations to environmental attitudes. *Journal of Environmental Psychology, 26*, 72–82.

Milfont, T. L., & Schwarzenthal, M. (2014). Explaining why larks are future-oriented and owls are present-oriented: Self-control mediates the chronotype-time perspective relationships. *Chronobiology International, 31*, 581–588.

Milfont, T. L., & Sibley, C. G. (2011). Exploring the concept of environmental generativity. *International Journal of Hispanic Psychology, 4*, 21–30.

Milfont, T. L., Abrahamse, W., & McCarthy, N. (2011). Spatial and temporal biases in assessments of environmental conditions in New Zealand. *New Zealand Journal of Psychology, 40*, 56–67.

Milfont, T. L., Harré, N., Sibley, C. G., & Duckitt, J. (2012a). The climate change dilemma: Examining the association between parental status and political party support. *Journal of Applied Social Psychology, 42*, 2386–2410.

Milfont, T. L., Wilson, J., & Diniz, P. K. C. (2012b). Time perspective and environmental engagement: A meta-analysis. *International Journal of Psychology, 46*, 209–218.

Moser, G. (2009). *Psychologie environnementale: Les relations homme-environnement [Environmental psychology: Man-environment relations]*. Bruxelles: De Boeck.

Niemeijer, D., & de Groot, R. S. (2008). Framing environmental indicators: Moving from causal chains to causal networks. *Environment, Development and Sustainability, 10*, 89–106.

Nowack, K., Milfont, T. L., & van der Meer, E. (2013). Future versus present: Time perspective and pupillary response in a relatedness judgment task investigating temporal event knowledge. *International Journal of Psychophysiology, 87*, 173–182.

Pahl, S., & Bauer, J. (2011). Overcoming the distance: Perspective taking with future humans improves environmental engagement. *Environment and Behaviour, 20*, 1–15.

Pawlik, K. (1991). The psychology of global environmental change: Some basic data and an agenda for cooperative international research. *International Journal of Psychology, 26*, 547–563.

Platt, J. (1973). Social traps. *American Psychologist, 28*, 641–651.

Rabinovich, A., Morton, T., & Postmes, T. (2010). Time perspective and attitude-behaviour consistency in future-oriented behaviours. *British Journal of Social Psychology, 44*, 69–89.

Schultz, P. W., Milfont, T. L., Chance, R. C., Tronu, G., Luís, S., Ando, K., et al. (2014). Cross-cultural evidence for spatial bias in beliefs about the severity of environmental problems. *Environment and Behavior, 46*, 267–302.

Shipp, A. J., Edwards, J. R., & Lambert, L. S. (2009). Conceptualization and measurement of temporal focus: The subjective experience of the past, present, and future. *Organizational Behavior and Human Decision Processes, 110*, 1–22.

Spence, A., Poortinga, W., & Pidgeon, N. F. (2012). The psychological distance of climate change. *Risk Analysis, 32*, 957–972.

Steg, L., & Vlek, C. (2009). Encouraging pro-environmental behaviour: An integrative review and research agenda. *Journal of Environmental Psychology, 29*, 309–317.

Stern, P. C. (2000). Toward a coherent theory of environmentally significant behaviour. *Journal of Social Issues, 56*(3), 407–424.

Stern, P. C. (2005). Understanding individuals' environmentally significant behavior. *Environmental Law Reporter, 35*(11), 785–790.

Strathman, A., Gleicher, F., Boninger, D. S., & Edwards, C. S. (1994). The consideration of future consequences: Weighing immediate and distant outcomes of behavior. *Journal of Personality and Social Psychology, 66*, 742–752.

Trope, Y., & Liberman, N. (2003). Temporal construal. *Psychological Review, 110*, 403–421.

Trope, Y., & Liberman, N. (2011). Construal level theory. In P. A. M. Van Lange, A. W. Kruglanski, & E. T. Higgins (Eds.), *Handbook of theories of social psychology: Volume One* (pp. 118–134). London: Sage.

Van Lange, P. A., & Joireman, J. A. (2008). How we can promote behavior that serves all of us in the future. *Social Issues and Policy Review, 2*, 127–157.

Wade-Benzoni, K. A., Tost, L. P., Hernandez, M., & Larrick, R. P. (2012). It's only a matter of time: Intergenerational beneficence as a death anxiety buffer. *Psychological Science, 23*, 704–709.

Zimbardo, P. G., & Boyd, J. N. (1999). Putting time in perspective: A valid, reliable individual-differences metric. *Journal of Personality and Social Psychology, 77*, 1271–1288.

Zimbardo, P. G., & Boyd, J. N. (2008). *The time paradox: The new psychology of time that will change your life*. New York: Free Press.

Zimbardo, P. G., Keough, K. A., & Boyd, J. N. (1997). Present time perspective as a predictor of risky driving. *Personality and Individual Differences, 23*, 1007–1023.

Time and the Misfits: Temporal Framing and Priming in Persuasive Communication

Frédéric Martinez and Nicolas Fieulaine

As repeatedly evidenced in various chapters of this book, time perspective is a core concept and a crucial underlying factor to understand a wide range of individuals' attitudes and behaviors. The view people maintain on their past, present and future, their orientation and attitudes towards the various time frames, and the extent to which they consider the long- and short-term consequences of their behaviors are dispositional constructs that has been revealed as predictive of why people engage-or not-in sustainable behaviors (e.g. chapter "Understanding Environmental Issues with Temporal Lenses: Issues of Temporality and Individual Differences" by Milfont and Demarque, this volume; Boyd and Zimbardo 2005). This kind of behavior is broadly defined as behaviors having positive or non-impairing consequences for the self, others, societies, animals or the environment. Hence, consideration for future consequences or Future time perspective was evidenced as an important determinant of lower health risk-taking, greater environmental concerns and behaviors, and higher rates of preventive behaviors (Strathman and Joireman 2005). This relation is typically explained by the temporal dilemma, carried by many of our daily choices and behaviors, between short term and long-term costs and benefits (Van Lange and Joireman 2008), and by the "social traps" (Platt 1973) in which short-term consequences are positive but long-term consequences are negative. Exercise, sorting garbage, contributions to social goods, smoking cessation, schoolwork, and so on are behaviors that are costly for the present, but beneficial in the future (Dawes 1980; Hendrickx et al. 2001). When considering the future beyond the present, one is able to resist temptations or to accept constraints and efforts to achieve future benefits (Mischel et al. 1989). On the contrary, when people are, for various reasons, chronically focused on the present without taking into

Funding for this study was partially provided by IReSP/INPeS Grant 083/07-DAS.

F. Martinez (✉) • N. Fieulaine
Groupe de Recherche en Psychologie Sociale, Institut de Psychologie,
Université de Lyon, 69600 Bron, France
e-mail: frederic.martinez@univ-lyon2.fr

M. Stolarski et al. (eds.), *Time Perspective Theory; Review, Research and Application: Essays in Honor of Philip G. Zimbardo*, DOI 10.1007/978-3-319-07368-2_25,

account the future consequences, they are more likely to take risks for their health (substance use, risky driving, no condom use…, see Boyd and Zimbardo 2005) and therefore less likely to engage in sustainable behaviors. In the context of Zimbardo and Boyd's Time Perspective Theory (1999), many studies have evidenced this relation between Future time perspective and health or pro-environmental behaviors (e.g. Milfont et al. 2012; Henson et al. 2006). Hence, previous research has shown that future-oriented individuals are more concerned with potential negative future consequences and are more likely to take protective measures that will minimize future health risks. Present-oriented individuals are generally less concerned with potential future risks (Strathman et al. 1994). In the area of pro-environmental behaviors, Lindsay and Strathman (1997) reported that participants scoring higher on the consideration of future consequences scale (Strathman et al. 1994) are more likely to engage in consumer behavior that benefits the environment (see also Milfont and Demarque, this volume). Joireman et al. (2001) found that individuals scoring high in CFC reported more willingness to fund improvement in public transit. According to these studies, the consideration of future consequences made people more convinced of and affected by the long terms benefits of sustainable behaviors and more likely to contribute to public goods (Kortenkamp and Moore 2006). Another recent study by Joireman et al. (2004) indicated that higher scores in CFC correlated with preference for commuting to work by public transportation instead of by car (see also Van Lange et al. 2013). In sum, even if long-term future orientation may have paradoxical effects (Van Lange and Joireman 2008; Apostolidis et al. 2006a) and taking into account that other individuals' orientations (e.g. social orientations and values) may interact with temporal ones, this body of research strongly support the typical assumption that future orientation and consideration for delayed consequences beyond immediate ones are related to sustainable behaviors.

The Time Frame of Sustainability Promotion

If health, pro-environmental, and more generally *sustainable* behaviors are future-oriented ones, it seems to be obvious that public communication or advertisement aiming at promoting this kind of behaviors appear itself as future-oriented. In line with it, we must protect our environment for the well-being of future generations, and we have to stop smoking or to make exercise to avoid coronary diseases in the future. As a consequence, communications aiming to promote sustainable concerns or behaviors deeply shaped by the temporal frame they use to be persuasive, and previous studies demonstrated that the impact of individuals' future orientation in decisions related to temporal dilemmas is particularly true when the long-term consequences of a behavioral option are more salient (e.g. Joireman et al. 2004). Hence, messages should be (and actually are generally) temporally framed as oriented towards future, and this frame is a key determinant of how people perceive, interpret, construe the promoted concern or behavior, and finally of how and if people will engage in consequent action.

In persuasive and media communication, a frame is a central organizing idea, a point of view on an issue or object, emphasizing one or several aspects among others, and by this way defining what is relevant, what the situation is about, and what is the essence of the issue (Goffman 1974; Nelson et al. 1997; Levin et al. 1998; Borah 2011). Framing communication corresponds to the selection of "some aspects of a perceived reality and make them more salient in a communicating text, in such a way as to promote a particular problem definition, causal interpretation, moral evaluation, and/or treatment recommendation" (Entman 1993, p. 53). Framing effects are "more concerned with how issues or other objects (people, groups, organizations, countries, etc.) are depicted in the media than with which issues or objects are more or less prominently reported" and "are concerned with ways of thinking rather than objects of thinking" (Weaver 2007, pp. 145–146). Framing effect is namely the measurable impact of the selection of one frame or another on how individuals organize and use the information and on decision-making. Considerable research has examined the role played by message framing in persuasion processes, especially in health-related communications (e.g. Rothman and Salovey 1997). This body of research demonstrates that small changes in the presentation of an option choice can produce somewhat surprisingly large changes in attitudes, intentions and subsequent behaviors (for a review, see Chong and Druckman 2007; Gallagher and Updegraff 2012). Typically considered in experimental psychology through its "equivalency effects" (different but logically equivalent, phrases; whereas *issue* framing involve differences in the content and nature of options; Druckman 2001), message framing has been related to a wide range of dimensions along which message can vary. The most well-known is certainly the distinction made by Kahneman and Tversky between choices options of gains versus losses in their Prospect Theory (Kahneman and Tversky 1979; Tversky and Kahneman 1981). Their postulate is that decision makers organize information relevant to choice options in terms of potential gains (i.e., benefits) or potential losses (i.e., costs) as compared to a reference point (e.g., one's present status health status). In this context, message framing refers to the emphasis in the message on the positive or negative consequences of adopting or failing to adopt a particular behavior (Rothman and Salovey 1997). In relation to health behaviors, for instance sensitivity to recommendation for detection or preventive behaviors is impacted by how recommendations are framed. Whereas loss-framed messages were showed to increase positive attitudes towards, and intention to perform detection behaviors such as cholesterol testing (Maheswaran and Meyers-Levy 1990), HIV testing (Kalichman and Coley 1995), breast self-examination (Meyerowitz and Chaiken 1987) and skin cancer self-examination (Block and Keller 1995), people are more likely to perform health prevention behaviors such as the use of condoms (Kiene et al. 2005) and smoking cessation (Wonj and McMurray 2002), after they are presented with a gain-framed message. Since these early statements of Prospect Theory, various framing effects were observed in relation with different psychological perspectives trough which people may construe objects, build motivation or make decisions (Levin et al. 1998).

How Framing Operates? The Frame and the Fit

Framing thus appeared as an easy and effective approach to message tailoring and a well-established strategy to increase the persuasive impact of campaigns promoting sustainable behaviors. Beyond this main effect, considerable evidence suggests that this impact is under the dependence of individuals' or group's chronic tendencies and orientations. Hence, individuals will be more influenced by messages that are compatible with their mind-set (e.g., Clary et al. 1994; Petty et al. 2000) or their culture (e.g., Han and Shavitt 1994; Briley and Aaker 2006). This functional relation between communication content and individuals' dispositions, needs, and attitudes was particularly evidenced in the context of regulatory focus theory (Higgins 1997). According to it, all goal-directed behavior is regulated by two distinct basic motivational strategies. One strategy emphasizes the pursuit of gains (or the avoidance of nongains) and aspirations toward ideals, is termed *promotion focus*; the other emphasizes the avoidance of losses (or the pursuit of nonlosses) and the fulfillment of obligations, is termed *prevention focus*. Individuals are guided by these two fundamental goals and the related motives underlie the choices and decision people make. Each of these two motivational orientations corresponds to different strategy to achieve goals, but also to chronic and relatively stable individual (Crowe and Higgins 1997) and cultural (Lee et al. 2000) orientation. The concept of regulatory *fit* (Higgins 2000, 2005) address the possible interactions between chronic (cultural and individual) and situational (context-relevant) orientations, and postulates that people "feel right" and are more engaged in a task when they pursue a goal in a manner that sustains their chronic orientation. Under regulatory fit context, people have an "it just feels right" experience, which may be transferred to subsequent judgments (Camacho et al. 2003). As an example, participants give the same coffee mug a higher price when the strategy they use to acquire the mug fit their regulatory orientation (Higgins et al. 2003). In the persuasive communication framework it was evidenced that matching individuals regulatory focus and the orientation of a goal presented in a message increases the effectiveness of a persuasive appeal (Cesario et al. 2004; Lee and Aaker 2004; Cesario et al. 2007). As an example, Cesario et al. (2004) created a persuasive message advocating a new after-school program for grade-school children. In one condition, the description of program was designed to correspond to a promotion focus (advance children's education and support more children to succeed) and to a prevention focus in a second condition (secure children's education and prevent more children from failing). The effectiveness of the persuasive appeal increased when the message was congruent to individuals' chronic orientation. Research suggested multiple mechanisms that lead to increased persuasion when regulatory fit occurs (Cesario et al. 2007; Higgins et al. 2010). A primary mechanism is that recipients of a message that fits their chronic orientation have a feeling right experience, and that feeling is used as information to make congruent inferences related to the message (value transferred from the fit to the information; Higgins 2000). A second potential mechanism is that fit increases the strength of engagement in the message processing activity, and therefore intensifies persuasion. Individuals presented with a message frame that fit their chronic regulatory focus perceived the information to be easier to process (Lee and Labroo 2004) and the advocated cause more believable and worthy of pursuit (Cesario et al. 2004).

Beyond the classical effect of framing information in a positive or negative light (or emphasizing benefits vs. costs) on judgment and decision-making, and even if the fit effect apply with a preferred manner to self-regulatory systems, they are broad concepts that may apply to any dimension of a message that can match personal characteristic and by this way increase the persuasive impact of the message.

Among these other potential dimensions, time is not surprisingly the one we are interested in. Some studies (Orbell and Hagger 2006; Orbell and Kyriakaki 2008; Orbell et al. 2004) have shown that not only the gains vs. losses frame is important in persuasive communication, but also the *temporal frame* in which costs and benefits are perceived. Previous studies, even if not followed by many others, underlined the importance of how information is framed on the temporal dimension (temporal framing, Strathman et al. 1994; Lo et al. 2012). The same behavior may have consequence in the short and the long term future, some of them positive, other negative, and it depend not only on the decision of the actor to focus on one or the other, but also on the message to put the emphasize on one or the other time perspective. Several studies demonstrated that also the *temporal distance* of presented consequences of a promoted behavior make this behavior subjectively more proximal or more distal, this appearance leading to strong differences in how people construe, interpret and build decisions and action following a message (Chandran and Menon 2004; McElroy and Mascari 2007; Förster et al. 2004). Following the strongly supported statements of the Construal Level Theory (CLT, Trope and Liberman 2003; chapter "From Time Perspective to Psychological Distance (and Back)" by Maglio et al., this volume) various authors explored how temporal distance through which an event is presented can influence the decision making process (Liberman and Trope 1998, 2003; Mogilner et al. 2008; Dshemuchadse et al. 2013). Despite relying on different theoretical backgrounds, other studies highlighted how crucial is to take into consideration not only the temporal frame of the message, but also the persons' time perspective, to assess the efficacy and the potential counter effects of temporally framed communications (Strathman et al. 1994; Kees 2011; Demarque et al. 2012).

Temporal Fit and Temporal Misfit

The most convincing studies on this topic were conducted by Orbell and colleagues at University of Essex, UK (Orbell and Hagger 2006; Orbell and Kyriakaki 2008; Orbell et al. 2004; Kees 2011). They tested if, and how, individual differences in time perspective (consideration of future consequences, Strathman et al. 1994) influence the impact of a temporally framed persuasive communication. In these studies, individual differences in CFC were measured, and the time frame in which a message posits the occurrence of positive and negative consequences of a promoted behavior is manipulated. Although equivalent consequences of a given health protective behavior are presented (colorectal cancer screening, Orbell et al. 2004; Sunscreen use, Orbell and Kyriakaki 2008, Diabetes screening, Orbell and Hagger 2006), in one time frame negative consequences are presented as short term and the positive consequences as long term, and conversely in a second time frame (short term positive consequences and long term negative consequences). Findings from surveys and experimental studies revealed that high CFC individuals (1) were generally more sensitive to health communications; (2) have greater intentions to engage in healthy behavior when the long-term consequences are positive and the short-term consequences are negative. In contrast, lower CFC individuals indicated greater intentions when positive outcomes were presented as immediate and negative outcomes as delayed in the future. These findings confirmed the strong effect temporal framing of persuasive communication might have on individuals' sensitivity, depending on their time orientation. From Orbell et al. findings, but also relying on Kees (2011) study, it also appear that the persuasive impact of communications is lowered in low CFC audience when messages are framed as future-oriented. Of greater concern is the fact that in present oriented (or with low future orientation) audience, when benefits are presented as occurring in the future and the costs immediately, individuals develop a more negative attitude, and have lower intentions than in all other conditions. Highly future-oriented individuals remain partially convinced by the persuasive communication, mainly due to their greater sensitivity in general, but also because they are less discouraged by the unfit of message's temporal frame. In conclusion, not only messages are more persuasive when their temporal frame is matched with dispositional time perspective of the target audience, but there is a higher sensibility to a temporal mismatch in present-oriented people.

The Big Issue: How and for Whom Campaigns may be Ineffective?

When one knows that present-oriented people are those who are the most at risk to engage in unsustainable behaviors, we are dealing here with a big issue. Unfortunately, in contrast with these findings or without any knowledge of them, a great part of the public propaganda and of our everyday conversations, when promoting sustainable behaviors or concerns for sustainability, are temporally framed by emphasizing the long term benefits of short term costly behaviors ("It takes time to sort garbage, but it is for the future of next generations"; "it is hard to stop smoking but very beneficial for future health"; "you may feel difficult to respect the classwork, but it is the condition for future success", and so on…). But do this kind of persuasive communications achieve their goals? Do they change attitudes, or induce behavior? From the findings presented here, it seems that their temporal frame (largely unquestioned) may make this messages inefficient for - and sometimes rejected by - people who are more sensitive to short term consequences and not to long-term ones. And here is the points: (1) present-focused people are the most at risk of unhealthy behaviors (Adams and White 2009; Daugherty and Brase 2010; Henson et al. 2006) and (2) socioeconomically deprived people are more susceptible to be stuck in the present (for a review, see chapter "Precariousness as a Time Horizon: How Poverty and Social Insecurity Shape Individuals' Time Perspectives" by Fieulaine and Apostolidis, this volume). One may intuitively conclude that health communication, if presented in a future frame, can be not only ineffective, but may also contribute to maintain or reinforce social inequalities in health. Elaborated by and for future-oriented people (as a default option), future-framed persuasive communications are, by their very nature, potential *negative nudges* for the most deprived, and therefore for the most important target audience. This was confirmed by Fieulaine and Martinez (2010) in a prospective study conducted during a campaign promoting seasonal influenza vaccination in France. We collected data in a community sample of 161 people, aged 65 and over who received an invitation to vaccinate themselves and a voucher to reach for a free flu shot at the officine, sent by the national health insurance. Time perspective (Zimbardo Time perspective Inventory, Zimbardo and Boyd 1999), attitudes, perceived control and perceived norms towards influenza vaccination (planned behavior measures, following Ajzen 2002), and past behaviors were assessed by a self-questionnaire at the first wave. At the second wave, two months later, exposure to the promotion campaign (number of exposition to the message, channels of information, recall of information…) and behavior (taking a flu shot this year, or not) were assessed by explicit and implicit measures for the former, and with multi-items measure for the latter. There was 93.8 % of the sample at the follow-up, and among them, 35 % were not yet vaccinated. As determinant of vaccination behavior, Present-Hedonistic TP was a negative predictor of being vaccinate at the follow-up (OR = .47; 95 % CI: .13–.93; p = .05), whereas Present-Fatalistic TP was positively related to vaccination behavior (OR = 2.08; 95 % CI: 1.08–4.03; p = .02; all regression controlled for age, sex and planned behavior measures). If these findings are important in demonstrating a direct and independent relation of TP to vaccination behavior, they are particularly illustrative of the issue considered in this chapter. In fact, if present-hedonistically oriented individuals were less vaccinated than others, it may be partly due to the information they were exposed to. A test of an interaction effect between PHTP and exposure to the campaign on the evolution of intention between the two waves (intention at the end of the campaign – intention at the beginning), made appear a significant result (using the Baron and Kenny approach to moderation effects, see Baron and Kenny 1986): when splitting the non-vaccinated group between high and low orientation towards PHTP (median split), and plotting the relation of exposure to the campaign, we could interpret that not only the campaign had almost no impact for the low PHTP group, but it had a negative impact on the intention of the high PHTP group (see Fig. 1). Hence, one can conclude that vaccination promotion campaign lead to dissuade present-oriented people to vaccinate themselves, especially as the messages promoting vaccination are for a large part future-oriented.

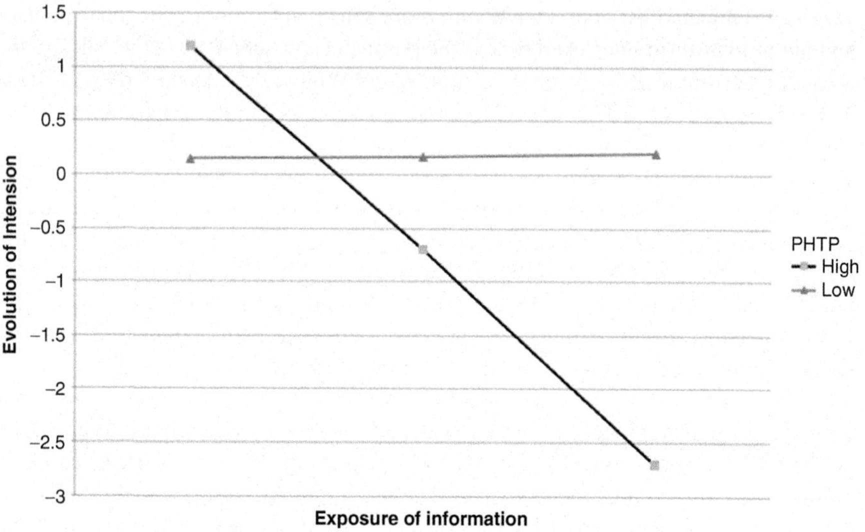

Fig. 1 Interaction effect of the exposure to vaccination promotion campaign on Intention for high and low present-oriented groups

Following these disturbing results, what solutions time perspective research can suggest to policy makers, health promotion practitioners, and media campaigns developers to deal with the differential impact of health communications in relation to individual time orientation?

A first option is to tailor communication in order to fit the messages temporal frame to the target people time perspectives. So, it seems necessary to build communications with arguments that emphasize short-term benefits given that present-focused people are the most at risk for risky and lack of preventive or sustainable behaviors. Hence, framing a persuasive message in proximal positive terms can have a persuasive impact on consumers who have difficulties in considering the future consequences of their actual behaviors without adversely affecting consumers who do typically take into account the future consequences of their behaviors (Chandran and Menon 2004). But there are strong limitations. First, it may be in many cases difficult to find some (reliable) short-term benefits of behaviors that are objectively costly in the present and beneficial only in the long term future (do think about the short term benefits of sorting garbage or cancer screening!). Most important in our view is the fact that if communications are temporally framed according to individuals' time perspective (on the basis of the group), they can sustain and develop these time perspectives. A tailored communication, adjusted for present-oriented people, by maintaining a present-focused atmosphere, can contribute to perpetuate a biased time perspective in particular groups and therefore to contribute to future problems.

A second possibility is to enhance long-term thinking or future mind-set through individual or group training. For example, Hall and Fong evidenced that a training program designed to enhance long-term thinking can promote initiation and maintenance of a preventive behavior (Exercise; cf. Hall and Fong 2003). Other interventions related to planning, mental contrasting or anticipated regret are also designed to alter individuals' time perspective in a way that favors the adoption of recommended behaviors (Loewenstein et al. 2003; Teuscher and Mitchell 2011). Even very powerful, such interventions are costly, difficult to generalize, and irrelevant for mass-media campaigns.

Beyond Individuals and Messages: A "Situationist" View on Time Perspective in Persuasive Communication

A third possibility is to create an adequate context to make recipients more sensitive and therefore communication more persuasive. In the context of regulatory fit theory, some studies showed that fit may be activated "incidentally", i.e. activated separately from the context of the task of interest. Hence, beyond recipients' chronic orientation and the framing of a message, regulatory fit can be induced independently to the persuasive message and this prior fit impacts subsequent message processing and persuasive impact (cf. Cesario et al. 2004, 2007). Freitas and Higgins (2002) developed a technique to induce either regulatory fit or nonfit. This technique consists of asking participants to first list either a current hope or aspiration (promotion focus induction) or a current duty or obligation (prevention focus induction). Then, participants must list either some strategies they could use to make sure everything goes right (eager means induction) or some strategies they could use to avoid anything that could go wrong (vigilant means induction). The regulatory fit or unfit conditions consisted of engaging congruent or non-congruent subsequent task. Results of Cesario et al. (2004) reveal that participants in the regulatory fit condition have higher intentions to perform a behavior consonant with the topic of the communication than participants in the regulatory nonfit condition after a same persuasive message. The induction of regulatory fit *outside* of the persuasion context itself indicates that fit can be induced by the situational induction of individuals' motivational orientation. This kind of induction to test causal relations of fit to decisions, intentions or (less often) behaviors, was applied to psychological time in relation with time perspective (Zimbardo et al. 1971), representation of time (Richmond et al. 2012), or construal level (Förster et al. 2004, study 5). In our view, this incidental technique of persuasion contrasts with intervention designed to train and develop a specific or non-biased time orientation, like in Hall and Fong (2003) study. In incidental source technique, the rationale do not rely on the objective to change in a durable manner the individuals' orientation, but to emphasize, make more relevant or salient a particular orientation. This kind of situational induction implies the addition of a third source of fit or match beyond the message frame and the target audience disposition, namely the situational (or contextual) time.

Then, it appear possible in a persuasive communication, to prime the context in which a message is delivered, in order to make this context congruent with the message frame or the individuals' orientation, or both. Can this priming effect overcome the low persuasive impact of future oriented messages for present oriented individuals? This is what Fieulaine and Martinez (2012b) have tested in a recent study. They explored whether the induction of a temporal context immediately prior the diffusion of a persuasive message could buffer the influence of individuals' time orientation. Hypothesis was that present-oriented participants, weakly influenced by a message focused on the future, would become more sensitive to the same message after the induction of a fit effect by a contextual induction. We tested this hypothesis in relation to a behavior with strong evidence of being related to time perspective, cannabis use. Hence, in recent correlational study, Fieulaine and Martinez (2010) showed that Present Hedonistic (positively) and Future time perspective (negatively) were significantly related to a composite score of substance use (see also Apostolidis et al. 2006a, b). This was confirmed (Fieulaine and Martinez 2012a) using a prospective design in a larger sample showing that PHTP is positively (and FTP negatively) related to attitudes, subjective norm and perceived control favoring cannabis use, and to subsequent behavior. In another study (Martinez and Fieulaine 2010), the persuasive impact of temporally framed communications promoting information seeking on excessive cannabis use was evidenced as moderated by individuals' time perspective.

To test for the potential effect of contextual fit, the study was designed as experimental, using a real-world health promotion message, promoting information seeking on excessive cannabis use. This message, as many others in mass-media campaigns, was focused on the long-term consequences of excessive cannabis use. In a first step, participants were invited to fill in the CFC scale (Strathman et al. 1994) to assess their individual time orientation (the questionnaire was introduced as unrelated to the study they were invited for). Then, and prior to the diffusion of the message, presenting the study timelines and objectives as short-term or long-term focused (without any induction for the control group) in the welcome address by the experimenter made the situational induction of a temporal context. Then, participants were invited to listen cautiously a health promotion message presented by a research assistant introduced as a health educator. Finally, participants gave their evaluation through measures of message reception (attitudes, willingness to perform the promoted, recall of risks evoked). 155 students from University of Lyon participated in the study (37 men et 118 women, 18–30 years old, $M_{age} = 20{,}36$) and were randomly affected to the three experimental groups: without induction ($N = 52$), Present-oriented induction ($N = 51$), and Future-oriented induction ($N = 52$). Check for randomization made appear no significant differences between groups on the measures of CFC and prior substance use. As a manipulation check, study was considered as more important for the immediate present in the present induction condition, and more important for the future in the future induction condition. Each group was divided in two groups of low- and high-CFC subjects using a median split on the mean scores on CFC. One-way (control group) and two-way (experimental conditions) ANOVAs were conducted using induction (none, present, future) and CFC (low vs. high) as independent variable and attitudes, intentions and number of recalled risks as dependent variables.

Results

Without any induction of a temporal context (control condition), results showed that high CFC subjects report greater intention to perform the promoted behavior than low CFC subjects (Fig. 2; F (1,47=3,94; p=.05) following the presentation of the message emphasizing the long-term risks of excessive cannabis use as well as long-term benefits of seeking information about cannabis.

This result is in line with previous studies on the greater sensibility to health communications in individuals with high scores on CFC, particularly when these communications are future-oriented (Orbell et al. 2004; Kees 2011). In order to test for the potential buffering effect of the temporal context induction, we performed 2 (context: present of future) X 2 (CFC: high or low) ANOVAs on dependent variables. Results showed a significant interaction effect for the intention to perform the promoted behavior, the number of risks recalled, and willingness to diffuse the message to others. Figure 3 depicts this interaction for intention and clearly show that when putted in a context emphasizing the present (i.e. when study is temporally framed as focused on immediate issues), participants with lower consideration of future consequences became more sensitive to a future-oriented message than people scoring higher on CFC (F(1, 96)=9,88; p<.01).

Fig. 2 Intention to perform the promoted behavior for high and low CFC subjects

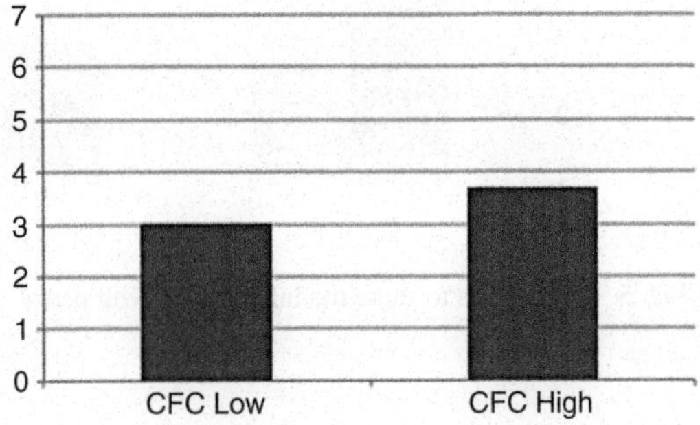

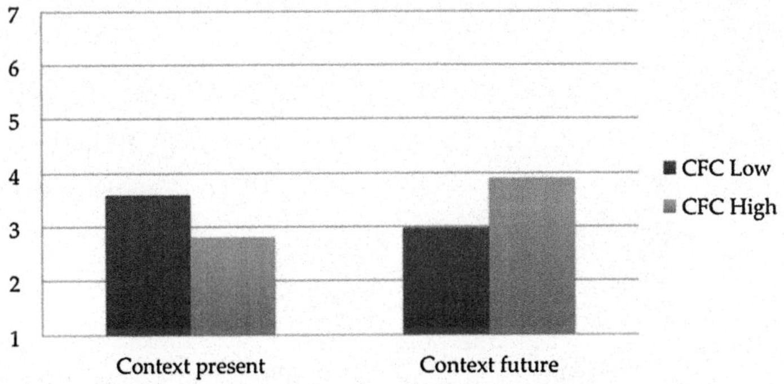

Fig. 3 Intention to perform the promoted behavior across experimental conditions

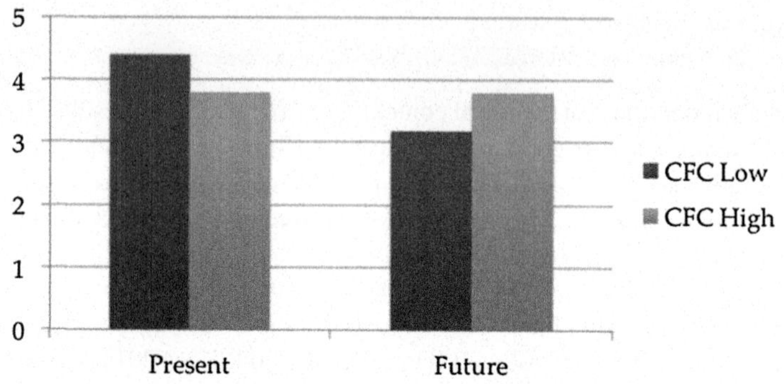

Fig. 4 Number of risks recalled by participants across experimental conditions

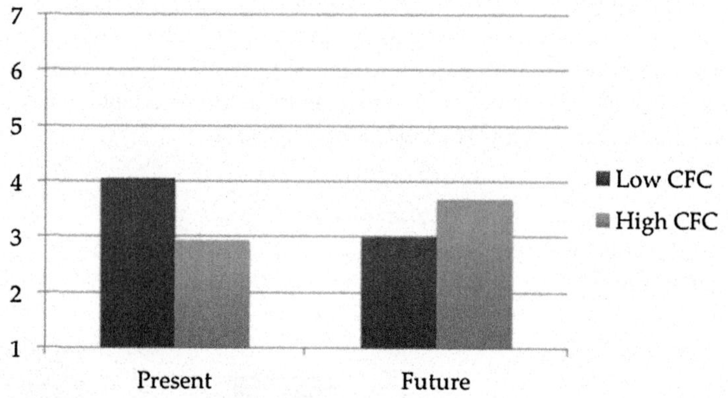

Fig. 5 Willingness to share the information with peers

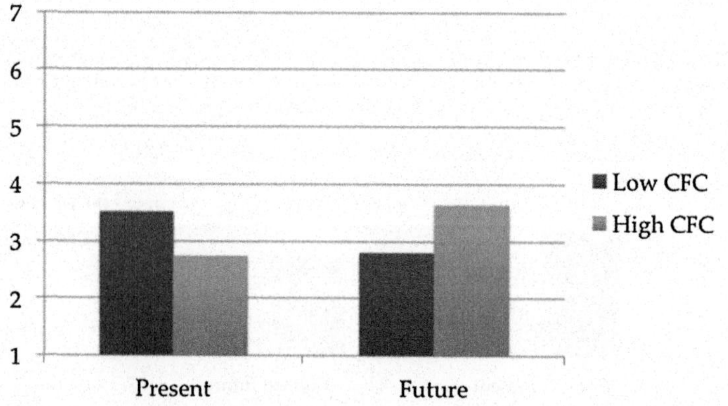

Fig. 6 Feelings of being involved in the situation

Hence, participants who were the less sensitive became the more sensitive to the same message when presented after an *incidental* emphasize on a *contextual* present time perspective. A same pattern of results appear for the number of risks recalled (Fig. 4; F (1, 97)=6,51; p=.01) and for the willingness to share the message with peers (Fig. 5; F(1, 96)=6,84; p=.01).

Interestingly, results showed that future-oriented people became less sensitive to the message when presented in a present-focused context. Potential mediators were observed, such as the feeling of involvement (Fig. 6; F(1, 96)=4,53; p=.03) or the easiness to understand. Hence, participants felt more involved and the future message was judged as easier to process when the context fits the individuals' dispositions, whenever the message unfit their personal time orientation.

The study was were replicated in a second student sample (N=376; with 60 subjects by conditions), and the contextual induction was also tested using a present-oriented message. Findings were in line with previous ones for future framed message, but no significant results were found with the present-oriented message largely because it was strongly rejected by participants and judged as unreliable.

Conclusions

Public media campaigns are deeply temporally framed, just as our everyday conversations. When talking about the future, we almost ever take it for granted that our counterpart will be sensitive to long term issues and consequences. In a real-world interpersonal interaction, one can be denied and then be able to reframe his/her argument to match it on other's expectations. But when it comes to public propaganda or mass media communication, there is no simple mean, until now, to immediately reframe a communication to fit the audience characteristics and to adjust the arguments to the target audience. Several studies provided evidence that temporal framing is a strong predictor of the persuasive impact of health communications (Orbell et al., op. cit.). Other studies, with different approaches, highlighted the impact of temporal framing of communications in other domains, such as political participation (Hakkyun et al. 2009), Public Policy (Lynch and Zauberman 2006) or environmental issues (Spence et al. 2012), and its potential effects on differential sensitivity according to audience's time orientation. In the health domain, it is particularly crucial to avoid making people insensitive to campaigns. If present-oriented people are not convinced by public health messages, this will not only make campaigns ineffective. Given that present-oriented people are the most at risk for unhealthy behaviors, and that a deprived socioeconomic status is strongly related to present time orientation (chapter "Precariousness as a Time Horizon: How Poverty and Social Insecurity Shape Individuals' Time Perspectives" by Fieulaine and Apostolidis, this volume), findings suggest that the effect of public health campaigns could be to increase or at least to maintain social inequalities in health. But individuals' time perspectives are not the sole dimensions to be considered when trying to tailor communication to make it more effective. Time horizon, defined as the unrelated temporal context in which a message is delivered, can overcome the buffering effect of individuals' time perspectives on the sensitivity to future-oriented persuasive communications. Therefore, these findings lead us to claim for a more holistic approach of psychological time, a "time landscape" model taking into account individuals' perspectives shaped by contextual situations, themselves located in a wider social space with particular time horizons. Our findings suggest that present-oriented people feel better in a situation where their temporality is accepted and valued, and that "feeling good" lead them to become sensitive to messages that are not matching their predominant time perspective. This effect has to be confirmed and developed by other studies, especially experiments aiming at establishing the "how" and the "why" of the observed results. Also, the role of time perspective in persuasive communication should be studied in the many other fields in which it may apply. How to make present-oriented people more concerned about ecological crisis, climate change, and sustainability? How long term issues could be considered in a time of crisis, when a growing number of people are living on a day-to-day basis? The (re)emerging research on psychological time and time perspective will be at the core center of the stakes societies will have to face in the coming decade. For sure, Phil Zimbardo's model of time perspective and the ZTPI will be very helpful to deal with future issues, at basic and applied levels.

References

Adams, J., & White, M. (2009). Time perspective in socioeconomic inequalities in smoking and body mass index. *Health Psychology, 28*(1), 83.

Ajzen, I. (2002, September). *Constructing a TpB questionnaire: Conceptual and methodological considerations*. Working paper, University of Massachusetts, Amherst. Available at http://www-unix.oit.umass.edu/~aizen/pdf7tpb.measurement.pdf

Apostolidis, T., Fieulaine, N., Simonin, L., & Rolland, G. (2006a). Cannabis use, time perspective and risk perception: Evidence of a moderating effect†. *Psychology and Health, 21*(5), 571–592.

Apostolidis, T., Fieulaine, N., & Soulé, F. (2006b). Future time perspective as predictor of cannabis use: Exploring the role of substance perception among French adolescents. *Addictive Behaviors, 31*(12), 2339–2343.

Baron, R. M., & Kenny, D. A. (1986). The moderator–mediator variable distinction in social psychological research: Conceptual, strategic, and statistical considerations. *Journal of Personality and Social Psychology, 51*(6), 1173.

Block, L. G., & Keller, P. A. (1995). When to accentuate the negative: The effects of perceived efficacy and message framing on intentions to perform a health-related behavior. *Journal of Marketing Research, 32*, 192–203.

Borah, P. (2011). Conceptual issues in framing theory: A systematic examination of a decade's literature. *Journal of Communication, 61*(2), 246–263.

Boyd, J. N., & Zimbardo, P. G. (2005). Time perspective, health, and risk taking. In A. Strathman & J. Joireman (Eds.), *Understanding behavior in the context of time: Theory, research, and applications* (pp. 85–107). Mahwah: Lawrence Erlbaum.

Briley, D. A., & Aaker, J. L. (2006). When does culture matter? Effects of personal knowledge on the correction of culture-based judgments. *Journal of Marketing Research, 43*, 395–408.

Camacho, C. J., Higgins, E. T., & Luger, L. (2003). Moral value transfer from regulatory fit: What feels right is right and what feels wrong is wrong. *Journal of Personality and Social Psychology, 84*, 498–510.

Cesario, J., Grant, H., & Higgins, E. T. (2004). Regulatory fit and persuasion: Transfer from "feeling right". *Journal of Personality and Social Psychology, 86*, 388–404.

Cesario, J., Higgins, E. T., & Scholer, A. A. (2007). Regulatory fit and persuasion: Basic principles and remaining questions. *Social and Personality Psychology Compass, 2*(1), 444–463.

Chandran, S., & Menon, G. (2004). When a day means more than a year: Effects of temporal framing on judgments of health risk. *Journal of Consumer Research, 31*, 375–389.

Chong, D., & Druckman, J. N. (2007). Framing theory. *Annual Review Political Science, 10*, 103–126.

Clary, E. G., Snyder, M., Ridge, R. D., Miene, P. K., & Haugen, J. A. (1994). Matching messages to motives in persuasion: A functional approach to promoting volunteerism. *Journal of Applied Social Psychology, 24*, 1129–1149.

Crowe, E., & Higgins, E. T. (1997). Regulatory focus and strategic inclinations: Promotion and prevention in decision-making. *Organizational Behavior and Human Decision Processes, 69*, 117–132.

Daugherty, J. R., & Brase, G. L. (2010). Taking time to be healthy: Predicting health behaviors with delay discounting and time perspective. *Personality and Individual Differences, 48*(2), 202–207.

Dawes, R. M. (1980). Social dilemmas. *Annual Review of Psychology, 31*, 169–193.

Demarque, C., Apostolidis, T., & Joule, R. V. (2012). Does binding communication increase consideration of future consequences and decision-making concerning pro- environmental behaviour? In S. Kabisch, A. Kunath, P. Schweizer-Ries, & A. Steinführer (Eds.), *Advances in people-environment studies* (Vulnerability, risks, and complexity: Impacts of global change on human habitats, Vol. 3, pp. 221–229). Göttingen: Hogrefe.

Druckman, J. N. (2001). The implications of framing effects for citizen competence. *Political Behavior, 23*, 225–56.

Dshemuchadse, M., Scherbaum, S., & Goschke, T. (2013). How decisions emerge: Action dynamics in intertemporal decision making. *Journal of Experimental Psychology. General, 142*(1), 93.

Entman, R. M. (1993). Framing: Toward clarification of a fractured paradigm. *Journal of Communication, 43*, 51–58.

Fieulaine, N., & Martinez, F. (2010). Time under control: Time perspective and desire for control in substance use. *Addictive Behaviors, 35*, 799–802.

Fieulaine, N., & Martinez, F. (2012a). About the fuels of self-regulation: Time perspective and desire for control in adolescents substance use. In F. Colombus (Ed.), *The psychology of self-regulation* (pp. 83–102). New York: Nova.

Fieulaine, N., & Martinez, F. (2012b). *Temporal context and individuals time orientation: The role of perspective fit in increasing health communication persuasiveness*. First international conference on time perspective, Coimbra, Portugal

Förster, J., Friedman, R. S., & Liberman, N. (2004). Temporal construal effects on abstract and concrete thinking: consequences for insight and creative cognition. *Journal of Personality and Social Psychology, 87*(2), 177.

Freitas, A. L., & Higgins, E. T. (2002). Enjoying goal-directed action: The role of regulatory fit. *Psychological Science, 13*, 1–6.

Gallagher, K. M., & Updegraff, J. A. (2012). Health message framing effects on attitudes, intentions, and behavior: a meta-analytic review. *Annals of Behavioral Medicine, 43*(1), 101–116.

Goffman, E. (1974). *Frame analysis: An essay on the organization of experience*. New York: Harper & Row.

Hall, P. A., & Fong, G. T. (2003). The effects of a brief time perspective intervention for increasing physical activity among university students. *Psychology and Health, 18*, 685–706.

Han, S., & Shavitt, S. (1994). Persuasion and culture: Advertising appeals in individualistic and collectivistic societies. *Journal of Experimental Social Psychology, 30*, 326–350.

Hendrickx, L., Poortinga, W., & van der Kooij, R. (2001). Temporal factors in resource dilemmas. *Acta Psychologica, 108*, 137–154.

Henson, J. M., Carey, K. B., Carey, M. P., & Maisto, S. A. (2006). Associations among health behaviors and time perspective in young adults: Model testing with boot-strapping replication. *Journal of Behavioral Medicine, 29*, 127–137.

Higgins, E. T. (1997). Beyond pleasure and pain. *American Psychologist, 52*, 1280–1300.

Hakkyun, K., Rao, A., & Lee, A. (2009). It's time to vote: Fit between construal level and temporal distance on political persuasion. *Journal of Consumer Research, 35*(6), 877–889.

Higgins, E. T. (2000). Making a good decision: Value from fit. *American Psychologist, 55*, 1217–1230.

Higgins, E. T. (2005). Value from regulatory fit. *Current Directions in Psychological Science, 14*, 209–213.

Higgins, E. T., Idson, L. C., Freitas, A. L., Spiegel, S., & Molden, D. C. (2003). Transfer of value from fit. *Journal of Personality and Social Psychology, 84*, 1140–1153.

Higgins, E. T., Cesario, J., Hagiwara, N., Spiegel, S., & Pittman, T. S. (2010). Increasing or decreasing interest in activities: The role of regulatory fit. *Journal of Personality and Social Psychology, 98*, 559–572.

Joireman, J. A., Van Lange, P. A. M., Van Vugt, M., Wood, A., Vander Leest, T., & Lambert, C. (2001). Structural solutions to social dilemmas: A field study on commuters' willingness to fund improvements in public transit. *Journal of Applied Social Psychology, 31*, 504–526.

Joireman, J., Van Lange, P. A. M., & Van Vugt, M. (2004). Who cares about the environmental impact of cars? Those with an eye toward the future. *Environment and Behavior, 36*, 187–206.

Kahneman, D., & Tversky, A. (1979). Prospect theory: An analysis of decision under risk. *Econometrica, 47*, 263–291.

Kalichman, S. C., & Coley, B. (1995). Context framing to enhance HIV-antibody- testing messages targeted to African American women. *Health Psychology, 14*, 247–254.

Kees, J. (2011). Advertising framing effects and consideration of future consequences. *Journal of Consumer Affairs, 45*(1), 7–32.

Kiene, S. M., Barta, W. D., Zelenski, J. M., & Cothran, D. L. (2005). Why are you bringing up condoms now? The effect of message content on framing effects of condom use messages. *Health Psychology, 24*, 321–326.

Kortenkamp, K. V., & Moore, C. F. (2006). Time, uncertainty, and individual differences in decisions to cooperate in resource dilemmas. *Personality and Social Psychology Bulletin, 32*(5), 603–615.

Lee, A. Y., & Aaker, J. L. (2004). Bringing the frame into focus: The influence of regulatory fit on processing fluency and persuasion. *Journal of Personality and Social Psychology, 86*(2), 205–218.

Lee, A. Y., & Labroo, A. (2004). Effects of conceptual and perceptual fluency on affective judgment. *Journal of Marketing Research, 41*, 151–165.

Lee, A. Y., Aaker, J. L., & Gardner, Y. L. (2000). The pleasures and pains of distinct self-construals: The role of interdependence in regulatory focus. *Journal of Personality and Social Psychology, 78*, 1122–1134.

Levin, I. P., Schneider, S. L., & Gaeth, G. J. (1998). All frames are not created equal: A typology and critical analysis of framing effects. *Organizational Behavior and Human Decision Processes, 76*(2), 149–188.

Liberman, N., & Trope, Y. (1998). The role of feasibility and desirability considerations in near and distant future decisions: A test of temporal construal theory. *Journal of Personality and Social Psychology, 75*, 5–18.

Liberman, N., & Trope, Y. (2003). Construal level theory of intertemporal judgment and decision. In G. Loewenstein, D. Read, & R. Baumeister (Eds.), *Time and decision: Economic and psychological perspectives on intertemporal choice* (pp. 245–276). New York: Russell Sage.

Lindsay, J. J., & Strathman, A. (1997). Predictors of recycling behavior: An application of a modified health belief model. *Journal of Applied Social Psychology, 27*, 1799–1823.

Lo, S. H., Smith, S. G., Taylor, M., Good, A., & von Wagner, C. (2012). The effect of temporal framing on behavioral intentions, expectations, and behavior: The case of healthy eating. *Journal of Applied Biobehavioral Research, 17*(3), 202–213.

Loewenstein, G. F., Read, D., & Baumeister, R. (2003). *Time and decision: Economic and psychological perspectives on intertemporal choice*. New York: Russell Sage.

Lynch, J. G., Jr., & Zauberman, G. (2006). When do you want it? Time, decisions, and public policy. *Journal of Public Policy and Marketing, 25*(2), 67–78.

Maheswaran, D., & Meyers-Levy, J. (1990). The influence of message framing and issue involvement. *Journal of Marketing Research, 27*, 361–367.

Martinez, F., & Fieulaine, N. (2010). For whom message framing is persuasive ? Investigation of goals and temporal framing effects on health information seeking. *International Congress of Applied Psychology*, Melbourne.

McElroy, T., & Mascari, D. (2007). When is it going to happen? How temporal distance influences processing for risky-choice framing tasks. *Social Cognition, 25*(4), 495–517.

Meyerowitz, B. E., & Chaiken, S. (1987). The effect of message framing on breast self-examination attitudes, intentions, and behavior. *Journal of Personality and Social Psychology, 52*, 500–510.

Milfont, T. L., Wilson, J., & Diniz, P. (2012). Time perspective and environmental engagement: A meta-analysis. *International Journal of Psychology, 47*(5), 325–334.

Mischel, W., Shoda, Y., & Rodriguez, M. L. (1989). Delay of gratification in children. *Science, 244*(4907), 933–938.

Mogilner, C., Aaker, J. L., & Pennington, G. L. (2008). Time will tell: The distant appeal of promotion and imminent appeal of prevention. *Journal of Consumer Research, 34*(5), 670–681.

Nelson, T. E., Oxley, Z. M., & Clawson, R. A. (1997). Toward a psychology of framing effects. *Political Behavior, 19*(3), 221–246.

Orbell, S., & Hagger, M. S. (2006). Temporal framing and the decision to take part in Type 2 diabetes screening: Effects of individual differences on persuasion. *Health Psychology, 25*, 537–548.

Orbell, S., & Kyriakaki, M. (2008). Temporal framing and persuasion to adopt preventive health behavior: Moderating effects of individual differences in consideration of future consequences on sunscreen use. *Health Psychology, 27*, 770–779.

Orbell, S., Perugini, M., & Rakow, T. (2004). Individual differences in sensitivity to health communications: Consideration of future consequences. *Health Psychology, 23*, 388–396.

Petty, R. E., Wheeler, S. C., & Bizer, G. Y. (2000). Attitude functions and persuasion: An elaboration likelihood approach to matched versus mismatched messages. In G. R. Maio & J. M. Olson (Eds.), *Why we evaluate: Functions of attitudes* (pp. 133–162). Mahwah: Erlbaum.

Platt, J. (1973). Social traps. *American Psychologist, 28*, 641–651.

Richmond, J., Clare Wilson, J., & Zinken, J. (2012). A feeling for the future: How does agency in time metaphors relate to feelings? *European Journal of Social Psychology, 42*(7), 813–823.

Rothman, A. J., & Salovey, P. (1997). Shaping perceptions to motivate behavior: The role of message framing. *Psychological Bulletin, 121*, 3–19.

Spence, A., Poortinga, W., & Pidgeon, N. (2012). The psychological distance of climate change. *Risk Analysis, 32*(6), 957–972.

Strathman, A., & Joireman, J. (Eds.). (2005). *Understanding behavior in the context of time: Theory, research, and application*. Mahwah: Lawrence Erlbaum.

Strathman, A., Gleicher, F., Boninger, D. S., & Edwards, C. S. (1994). The consideration of future consequences: Weighing immediate and distant outcomes of behavior. *Journal of Personality and Social Psychology, 66*, 742–752.

Teuscher, U., & Mitchell, S. (2011). Relation between time perspective and delay discounting: A literature review. *The Psychological Record, 61*, 613–632.

Trope, Y., & Liberman, N. (2003). Temporal construal. *Psychological Review, 110*, 403–421.

Tversky, A., & Kahneman, D. (1981). The framing of decisions and the psychology of choice. *Science, 211*, 453–458.

Van Lange, P. A. M., & Joireman, J. A. (2008). How can we promote behaviour that serves all of us in the future. *Social Issues and Policy Review, 2*, 127–157.

Van Lange, P. A., Joireman, J., Parks, C. D., & Van Dijk, E. (2013). The psychology of social dilemmas: A review. *Organizational Behavior and Human Decision Processes, 120*(2), 125–141.
Weaver, D. H. (2007). Thoughts on agenda setting, framing, and priming. *Journal of Communication, 57*(1), 142–147.
Wonj, C., & McMurray, N. E. (2002). Framing communication: Communicating the antismoking message effectively to all smokers. *Journal of Community Psychology, 30*, 433–447.
Zimbardo, P. G., & Boyd, J. N. (1999). Putting time in perspective: A valid, reliable individual differences metric. *Journal of Personality and Social Psychology, 77*, 1271–1288.
Zimbardo, P. G., Marshall, G., & Maslach, C. (1971). Liberating behavior from time-bound control: Expanding the present through hypnosis. *Journal of Applied Social Psychology, 1*(4), 305–323.

Time Perspectives and Subjective Well-Being: A Dual-Pathway Framework

Kerry F. Cunningham, Jia Wei Zhang, and Ryan T. Howell

Perhaps unique among all animals is the fact that humans have the capacity to travel backward and forward in time—to use the "specious present" (James 1890) both to relive past life events and to simulate the future (for a discussion see Suddendorf and Corballis 2007). This capacity to engage in mental time travel is essential for learning and planning. Without the capacity to review prior mistakes, learning would be impossible. Perhaps even more importantly, the ability to travel forward in time allows human beings to replace costly and potentially dangerous trial-and-error learning with less expensive and less risky mental experiments. However, while everyone engages in mental time travel, people vary in how much weight they assign to the various epochs (past, present, future) of their lives (Zimbardo and Boyd 1999). Some people appear to live in the past, ruminating on either the ecstasy (Past Positive) or the agony (Past Negative) of days gone by. Others seem to live only for the moment and have a devil-may-care (Present Hedonistic) or perhaps a God-only-knows (Present Fatalistic) approach to life. Meanwhile, others spend all of their time preparing for the future (future orientation) while assigning little value to the present moments.

Each of these time perspective can be adaptive and contribute to well-being depending upon one's life circumstances. For example, young adults contemplating long futures might be well advised to forego present indulgences in order to secure desirable future outcomes. Conversely, older adults may find solace near the end of life by dwelling on past accomplishments and joys, rather than pondering past mistakes. Ultimately, as Boniwell and colleagues (2010) have advised, the ideal is to have a balanced time perspective (BTP)—metering the influence of each time dimension and adjusting that balance to meet life's immediate and long-term

K.F. Cunningham (✉) • R.T. Howell
Department of Psychology, San Francisco State University, San Francisco, CA, USA
e-mail: kerryfc@gmail.com

J.W. Zhang
Department of Psychology, University of California, Berkeley, CA, USA

M. Stolarski et al. (eds.), *Time Perspective Theory; Review, Research and Application: Essays in Honor of Philip G. Zimbardo*, DOI 10.1007/978-3-319-07368-2_26,

demands. However, people often assign suboptimal weighting and valence to the individual time perspectives; this creates imbalances that have consequences for real-world attitudes and behaviors (Boniwell and Zimbardo 2004).

Time Perspective and Subjective Well-Being

The study of subjective well-being (SWB) is rapidly growing as we learn more about the predictors and benefits of happiness (see Lyubomirsky and Diener 2005 for a review). Many of the recent conceptions of SWB take into account the important role that perceptions of the past, present, and future play in people's well-being. For instance, the Temporal Satisfaction with Life Scale (Diener et al. 1999) measures how people evaluate their happiness in each of the three dimensions. Bryant (2003) likewise suggested that a person's SWB was comprised of their ability to reminisce about Past Positive events, to sustain or savor current positive events, and to anticipate Future Positive events. Another model (the time-sequential framework; Kim-Prieto et al. 2005) employs a time-based framework for understanding SWB. And, in fact, conceptions of time are the basis for Durayappah's 3P (the three P's refer to past, present, and prospect or future) model of SWB (Durayappah 2010). In the 3P model, SWB is the product of the habitual way in which a person evaluates their life in the past, the present, and prospect (future). Thus, according to the 3P model and others, time perspective should influence global evaluations of SWB. In the next section, we review the evidence connecting time perspectives to well-being.

The Past Negative and Past Positive

People with a Past Negative time perspective tend to look back on their lives with regret, ruminating on the bad things that have happened in the past. In sum, across time (Zimbardo and Boyd 1999; Zhang and Howell 2011) and cultures (Russian, British, American), people who are largely negative about the past are also unhappy and dissatisfied with life compared to their less Past Negative counterparts. People who tend to dwell on the negative events in their past are likely to experience more negative affect (*r*s between .38 and .56) and less positive affect (*r*s between −.21 and −.11) than people who do not dwell on the past (Zhang and Howell 2011; Zhang et al. 2013a, b). Likewise, Past Negative people enjoy less happiness ($r=-.45$, Boniwell et al. 2010) and satisfaction with life (SWLS; *r*s −.42 to −.59, Zhang and Howell 2011, 2013a, b). In contrast, people who look fondly on the past also report greater SWL ($r=.21$, Boniwell et al. 2010) and psychological need fulfillment (Zhang et al. 2013a). The relations between well-being measures and the Past Positive are weaker but consistent and between .15 and .44.

Present Hedonistic

People who are Present Hedonistic tend to have a live-for-the-moment attitude toward life. Interestingly, whether this attitude toward the moment proves to be adaptive or maladaptive seems to depend to a great extent on how this seize-the-day approach is modulated by a concern for the future. People who do live for the moment tend, in most cases, to enjoy life. Subjective happiness and SWL are consistently related with present hedonism (*r*s between .09 and .23). Hedonists also report experiencing more positive affect (*r*s .14–.27), being more energetic ($r=.27$; Zimbardo and Boyd 1999) and optimistic ($r=.20$, Boniwell et al. 2010), and feeling more vitality ($r=.31$; Zhang and Howell 2011). However, people who are more hedonistic also appear to be more aggressive and prone to depression (*r*s = .29 and .20; Zimbardo and Boyd 1999). These contradictory results suggest a dual pathway from which time perspective influences happiness, which we will describe later in this chapter.

Present Fatalistic

The extent to which people either assume agency in their own lives or instead believe that the events and circumstances of life are largely determined by powerful entities outside of their control (i.e., present fatalism) has a significant impact on well-being. Fatalists tend to be unhappy (*r*s = −.18, to −.23, Zhang and Howell 2011; Zhang et al. 2013a, b), less satisfied with life (*r*s = −.16 to −.39; Zhang and Howell 2011; Zhang et al. 2013a, b), less optimistic ($r=-.27$; Boniwell et al. 2010), and less energetic ($r=-.21$; Zimbardo and Boyd 1999) and have less vitality ($r=-.22$; Zhang et al. 2013a, b) than non-fatalists. Fatalists also appear to have a strong tendency to be more aggressive ($r=.39$; Zimbardo and Boyd 1999) and more depressed ($r=.37$; Zimbardo and Boyd 1999). Not surprisingly, people who do not believe they have much control on the present also tend to give little regard to the future (*r*s = −.29 to −.42; Zhang and Howell 2011; Zhang et al. 2013a, b).

Future

Of the five ZTPI time dimensions, the future time dimension is perhaps the least consistently associated with well-being measures. This may be somewhat surprising because as we shall see later in this chapter, the Future time perspective is associated with a variety of adaptive behaviors. Perhaps because their future orientation leads people to forego immediate pleasures, people who have a strong tendency to use the present moment to prepare for and ponder the future do not generally report being substantially happier than their less future-oriented peers (Boniwell et al. 2010; Zhang and Howell 2011; Zhang et al. 2013a, b). However, they do tend to experience somewhat more global satisfaction with life ($r = .14$ in Boniwell et al.'s Russian sample and $r = .15$ for Zhang & Howell's largely American sample; also see Zhang et al. 2013a, b). Compared to less future-oriented people, more future-oriented people are also less anxious and depressed ($rs = -.14$ and $-.19$, respectively; Zimbardo and Boyd 1999), are more optimistic ($r = .28$; Boniwell et al. 2010), and experience more positive as well as less negative affect (representative $rs = .24$ and $-.12$, respectively; Zhang et al. 2013a, b). As with the Present Hedonistic time perspective, these contradictory results suggest that the Future time perspective operates on well-being through two pathways.

Balanced Time Perspective

While most of the time perspective literature has focused on the relations of individual time perspective with measures of well-being, people do not simply have one time perspective. Instead, all people register somewhere on each of the five time perspectives. Therefore, as Zimbardo and colleagues have argued, it is the combination of these individual time perspective that truly informs behavior and attitudes (and in this case, well-being). Thus far, three methods for determining a balanced time perspective (BTP) have been proposed. Drake et al. 2008 proposed a BTP that is defined by low scores on Past Negative and Present Fatalistic and moderate to high scores on Past Positive, Present Hedonism, and Future. Boniwell et al. (2010) used a hierarchical cluster analysis to determine the time perspective groupings, while Stolarski et al. (2011) formulated a deviation from a balanced time perspective. Zhang et al. (2013a) compared these three methods and found that they are all related to psychological well-being (e.g., psychological need satisfaction, satisfaction with life, and subjective happiness). However, the deviation BTP method was the best predictor of SWB among the three methods. Thus, maintaining a healthy balance (e.g., low scores on Past Negative and Present Fatalistic and moderate to high scores on Past Positive, Present Hedonism) among the five time perspectives may be critical for psychological well-being.

A Dual-Pathway Framework

As the review above indicated, the associations between time perspective and well-being are generally strong and consistent, but the mechanism through which time perspective influences well-being has yet to be fully explored. Zhang and Howell (2011) examined the relative contributions of time perspective and personality to SWB and found that, not only does time perspective contribute unique variance to SWB, time perspective partially mediated the relationship between personality and SWB. In sum, the mediation models suggested that extraverts have an increased tendency to have a rosy view of their past (increased Past Positive) and a decreased tendency to have a negative view of the past (decreased Past Negative) while also tending to gravitate toward life's pleasures (increased Present Hedonism). The mediation models for the link between neuroticism and SWB showed that most of the negative association between neuroticism and life satisfaction was explained by neurotics' increased tendency to have a Past Negative time perspective (Zhang and Howell 2011).

Because time perspective mediated much of the relationship between personality and SWB, how—through what mechanisms—time perspective influences well-being remains an open question. Also, at least two time perspectives, the Present Hedonistic and Future, appear to have complex, sometimes contradictory relations with measures of well-being. Given that dual-pathway models have been successfully proposed to explain the correlations between personality traits and measures of well-being (see McCrae and John 1992, for a review), below we consider the evidence that suggests a dual-pathway model is a reasonable framework within which to view the relations between time perspective and well-being.

Top-Down and Bottom-Up

Life circumstances appear to account for about 10–15 % of the variance in well-being (Schimmack et al. 2002). Accordingly, the bottom-up (or instrumental) approach posits that individual differences (e.g., personality traits) impact those life circumstances through behavioral choices. In other words, some life situations and events are simply more conducive to well-being than others, and the choices people make are affected by their personality traits. Some decisions (e.g., to violently aggress as a means of settling an argument) can have both immediate and long-lasting effects on life circumstances (e.g., injuries, incarceration), which should then alter one's prospects for future happiness. Perhaps more subtly, some choices (e.g., eating a large bowl of ice cream after dinner each evening) may produce sensations of happiness in the present, while operating against happiness in the future (i.e., due to obesity, Type II diabetes, etc.).

On the other hand, the top-down (or direct) approach is generally regarded to be the more influential pathway, resulting from habitual cognitive processes (e.g., ruminating on past difficulties) and life satisfaction (Lucas and Baird 2004). Past research suggests that the cognitive processes by which individuals remember, experience, and anticipate the circumstances in their lives explain variance in life satisfaction (Lyubomirsky 2001). That is, when people judge their life satisfaction, they do so by reflecting on their *feelings* about their life circumstances (Schimmack et al. 2002). This suggests that the recollection, experience, and anticipation of life experiences are likely to be better predictors of SWB than the experiences or circumstances themselves. Hence, individual differences in the cognitive evaluation of one's past, present, and anticipated future may be the most direct mechanism by which time perspective leads to evaluations of well-being. We begin by presenting the evidence in support of the bottom-up pathway from time perspective to well-being.

The Bottom-Up (Indirect) Path

The evidence suggests that the Present and Future time perspectives influence well-being indirectly, through behaviors that influence life circumstances. Consider the example provided by visitors to the website, secretregrets.com. Secret regretters post heartfelt, often heartbreaking stories about the events and times of their lives that are particularly painful to ponder. One male visitor writes about his regret over indulging an impulse to experience the hedonistic pleasure of extramarital sex; he was found out and is now divorced from the love of his life. The circumstances of his life were dramatically altered by a choice he made. One may suppose that had he been less focused on fleeting pleasures (lower present hedonism) and perhaps more focused on the future consequences of his present actions (higher future), he may have acted differently.

Substantial evidence from the time perspective literature supports this supposition. For instance, more present-oriented (hedonism) female undergraduates are more sexually active and have more sexual partners (hence putting themselves at greater risk of contracting unwanted pregnancies and STDs) than those who are more future oriented (Rothspan and Read 1996). More evidence for an indirect path from time perspective to well-being is found in Stolarski et al. (2011), which assessed the relations between participants' time perspective, two emotional intelligence measures,[1] and reward discounting rate. They found that participants with a more balanced time perspective exhibited greater emotional intelligence as measured by two emotional intelligence constructs ($r=-.31$ and $-.46$ for criterion- and self-report-based measures, respectively) and were less prone to discounting future rewards in favor of short-term pleasures.

Also, Keough et al. (1999) found that the more present-oriented and less future-oriented participants were, the more likely they were to use substances and to do so more often and in greater quantities (*r*s with substance abuse were .37 and -.19 for a unitary present and a future orientation, respectively; Keough et al. 1999). Keough et al. (1999) also controlled for likely predictors of substance use (e.g., impulse control, ego control, conscientiousness, state-trait anxiety, and consideration of future consequences) and found that only ego control added variance above and beyond time perspective. In another study, more present-oriented students were found to engage in more risky driving, while being more future oriented reduced participants' likelihood of engaging in risky driving behaviors (Zimbardo et al. 1997). For both substance abuse and risky driving, the effect of present orientation was stronger than for future orientation, but each accounted for unique variance in substance abuse and risky driving. Hutton et al. (2001) found that the female prisoners they surveyed scored a full standard deviation higher on the present time perspective (hedonism) than a student sample and engaged in significantly more risky sexual behaviors. The prisoners' higher present

[1] The emotional intelligence measures were Polish-language versions of Mayer and Salovey's four-factor emotional intelligence model, one a criterion-based test and the other self-report.

time perspective, thus, might account for some of the variance in the behaviors that resulted in prison sentences (a life circumstance that is likely to reduce SWB).

The Present and Future time perspectives were also strongly related to the dispositional and behavioral characteristics of residents of a San Francisco homeless shelter (Epel et al. 1999). In this population, the more future-oriented residents had achieved longer tenures at their last job. Researchers also measured a number of behaviors believed to be related to the ultimate outcomes of finding stable work and housing. Not surprisingly, they found that more future and less present-oriented residents spent less time watching TV. Interestingly, a future orientation did not seem to influence how much time the men spent searching for a job or housing. More present-oriented men spent more time looking for housing but less time looking for a job.

The studies with prisoners and homeless shelter residents illustrated the influence of time perspective on behaviors that are likely to have both immediate and long-lasting impact on a persons' well-being. However, time perspective also contributes to patterns of behavior that may have a less dramatic, yet still important, impact on well-being. In one of the few studies that has demonstrated a link between a past time perspective and behavior, Shores and Scott (2007) found that a Past Negative time perspective was associated with lower desire to engage in physical fitness-related activities, while more future-oriented respondents were most likely to express an interest in physical fitness and learning-related activities. Both present time perspectives were associated with a lower desire for learning-related activities. Also, in their seminal 1999 paper, Zimbardo and Boyd found that more present-oriented students were more aggressive ($r_{\text{hedonism}} = .29$ and $r_{\text{fatalism}} = .39$) and reported more lying ($r_{\text{hedonism}} = .16$ and $r_{\text{fatalism}} = .17$).

Hence, it appears that time perspective may indirectly impact well-being by influencing the choices that people make—both immediately impactful ones such as the decision to take illicit narcotics, as well as more chronic "lifestyle choices," such as engaging in exercise and healthy eating.

The Top-Down Link

As described above, the top-down approach to well-being proposes that people's SWB is largely determined by the habitual way they reflect upon their feelings about the circumstances and events that comprise their lives (Schimmack et al. 2002), rather than the circumstances and events themselves. For example, when people assess their life satisfaction, they do so with reference to a consistent suite of data points—chiefly memories—and that these data points remain relatively constant over time. We suggest that because time perspective describes the way people habitually characterize their own life histories (as well as their prospects for the future), time perspective therefore constitutes an important source of what is chronically available to people when they assess their happiness. Hence, top-down models of well-being, such as the sustainable happiness model (Lyubomirsky and Diener 2005) propose that people can influence their well-being directly by managing the items that are chronically available in memory. By consciously savoring positive life experiences and reinterpreting negative events in a more positive light—by consciously becoming more Past Positive—people can have a direct and positive influence on their own well-being.

As an example of the reinterpreting strategy, consider the editors of *Good Old Days* magazine and its companion website, goodolddays.com. In their introductory "letter from the editors," Ken and Janice Tate describe one particularly good old day. As they recall it, the day was marked by oppressive heat and humidity, and much of the day was spent in a pickup truck that made them feel as if they were "riding a bronco rather than in a vehicle." The heat caused the truck's engine to boil over. But, perhaps owing to the torrential rain that began to fall, the truck cooled enough to run again, and the Tate's journey resumed (albeit haltingly because the truck had no windshield wipers to help see through the rain). Finally, after traversing a swollen stream with water lapping the doors of the truck and exhausted from their journey, the Tate's arrived at their soggy picnic—good old days, indeed! Crucially, however, for the day and their recollection of it, the picnic was topped off with a refreshing watermelon picked with pride from a nearby patch and shared with family. Through the auspices of the watermelon, Janice and Dan Tate recast the day, transforming it into one to be remembered fondly as an exemplar of how (much better) things used to be. Besides being an illustration of the peak-end rule (Fredrickson and Kahneman 1993), the Tate's recollection of that sweltering summer day typifies the way in which reinterpreting events from the past (taking a Past Positive view) can lead to positive affect in the present.

Indeed, while we have seen that the present time perspectives are more likely to bear strong relations with behavioral measures than the past time perspectives, the reverse is true when considering the relations of time perspective to well-being. When it comes to measures of well-being, the past time perspectives are stronger predictors than the present perspectives. For instance, people who are more Past Positive (habitually referring to positive events from their life) and less Past Negative (by reframing Past Negative events in a more positive light) experienced a more positive affective balance, as well as more subjective happiness and satisfaction with life (see both Boniwell et al. 2010; Zhang and Howell 2011). Indeed, women who experienced childhood incest were more likely to experience elevated psychological distress levels as adults but only if they were more past than future oriented. This was so even controlling for time elapsed since the incest and the women's tendency to ruminate. Similarly, Vietnam War combat veterans who tended to focus on the past were more likely to later experience psychological distress. The results remained even after controlling for the length and intensity of combat the soldiers had experienced and their tendency to ruminate (Holman and Silver 1998).

And as would be expected if past time perspectives had a more direct pathway to influence assessments of well-being than present time perspectives, the correlations between the past time perspectives and well-being are often nearly double those of the present time perspectives. For example, Zhang and Howell (2011) found correlations between the Past Positive and SWL between .36 and .52, whereas the correlations between present hedonism and SWL were between .10 and .24 in the same samples (Boniwell et al., found similar results in their 2010 study).

Consistent with findings that negative events and emotions are more powerful predictors of well-being than positive (Baumeister et al. 2001), the Past Negative is the stronger of the two past time perspectives for most outcome measures, including psychological need fulfillment ($r_{\text{past-negative}} = -.48$, $r_{\text{past-positive}} = .32$; Zhang and Howell 2011), mindfulness ($r_{\text{past-negative}} = -.42$, $r_{\text{past-positive}} = .21$; Drake et al. 2008), and purpose in life ($r_{\text{past-negative}} = -.46$, $r_{\text{past-positive}} = .25$; Boniwell et al. 2010).

Having chronically accessible positive memories also appears to be related to how one assesses both the present and the future. People who are Past Positive are also more optimistic ($r = .21$, Boniwell et al. 2010) and energetic ($r = .15$, Zimbardo and Boyd 1999) and less likely to be depressed ($r = -.17$, Zimbardo and Boyd 1999). However, the relations between the Past Positive and Present Fatalistic are not exceptionally strong, though consistently negative: people who take a rosy view of the past are also less fatalistic than others. The opposite pattern holds for the Past Negative ($r_{\text{optimism}} = -.27$, Boniwell et al. 2010; $r_{\text{energy}} = -.18$, Zimbardo and Boyd 1999; $r_{\text{depression}} = .59$, Zimbardo and Boyd 1999). In addition, people who are negative about the past are substantially less mindful ($r = -.49$, Drake et al. 2008). Given this evidence, we might hypothesize that there are significant differences between reminiscers and regretters in both their Past Positive and Past Negative time perspectives and that these differences would explain a substantial share of the variance in their satisfaction with life.

As we alluded to earlier, the present hedonist perspective appears to contribute both directly and indirectly to SWB. While it is associated with a variety of maladaptive behaviors as discussed above, present hedonism is also associated with positive affect and increased subjective happiness. As such, it appears that the pleasure-seeking nature of present hedonists may result in more pleasurable experiences but also may lead to behaviors that are ultimately maladaptive, such as risky driving, sex, and substance abuse.

The Future time perspective also appears to influence SWB directly, though its role appears less consistent than for the past dimensions. For example, many, though not all (see Boniwell et al. 2010), studies have demonstrated positive relations between the future dimension and measures of well-being. As noted earlier, people who are more future oriented tend to be more optimistic ($r = .28$, Boniwell et al. 2010), as well. In other words, people who tend to invest considerable energy in preparing for the future also tend to believe the future holds promise. However, they do this despite not being any more confident about their ability to achieve their goals (as measured by Schwarzer's generalized self-efficacy, $r = .04$, *ns*; Boniwell et al. 2010) or having greater self-esteem ($r = .13$, *ns*; Zimbardo and Boyd 1999) than people who do not devote as much energy to preparing for the future.[2] Also, Boniwell et al. (2010) found that future is the only time perspective not strongly

[2] Epel et al.'s (1999) study did find significant positive correlations between the Future time perspective and two measures of task-specific self-efficacy. The two specific self-efficacy measures concerned (a) finding a job ($r = .22$) and (b) finding housing ($r = .24$).

associated with the measure of actualized potential (MAP), a self-actualization measure. People who were Past Negative or Present Fatalistic were less actualized (*r*s = −.46 and −.17, respectively), while the Present Hedonistic and Past Positive were more so (*r*s = .45 and .31, respectively), but future orientation was uncorrelated with actualization. It may be that the future, like present hedonism, operates in both pathways simultaneously, such that people who are highly future-focused may miss out on opportunities to enjoy their life as it occurs in each passing moment. At the same time, they may create a more productive, fulfilling, and even comfortable life for themselves that improve their global well-being.

Finally, however, it may be that a future orientation is not a guarantor of present or future well-being because the Future time perspective may have a direct and negative impact on assessments of well-being. For instance, Americans who tended to think about and plan for the future experienced less psychological distress and more positive affect in the 3 years following the September 11, 2001 terrorist attacks. However, respondents who reported ruminating on their fears of potential future terrorist attacks experienced more distress (Holman and Silver 2005). Clearly, just as with thoughts of the past, the content of one's thoughts about the future may have a direct impact on well-being.

Conclusion and Future Directions

Across the numerous studies we have reviewed, we have seen that each of the time perspectives as well as composite measures of a balanced time perspective influences people's happiness. However, the two past time perspectives appear to exert a strong, direct influence on people's assessments of life satisfaction and subjective happiness, consistent with models such as the 3P model (Durayappah 2010) and the sustained happiness model (Lyubomirsky et al. 2009). Meanwhile, the present perspectives are more strongly correlated with behaviors that ultimately impact the life circumstances that account for an important share of people's subjective well-being. Both the Present Hedonistic and the Future time perspectives appear to operate powerfully in both pathways, perhaps contributing to well-being in conflicting ways at once.

The dual-pathway framework suggests a number of questions for future research. In the sections above, we speculate that the risky sexual behaviors, substance use, and incarceration, all of which have been linked to a strong present-oriented perspective, lead to lower subjective well-being. However, these links have yet to be examined empirically. Also, time perspective appears to be stable across time (Zimbardo and Boyd 1999). However, our data suggest that as people age, they become less Present Hedonistic. This begs the question of whether this decrease in hedonism a natural, biological process, or instead an artifact of decades of acculturation?

Some have suggested that time perspective is influenced by evolutionary developmental processes, akin to those addressed by life history theory (Kruger et al. 2008). Differences in life history strategies have been linked to many of the same maladaptive behaviors (e.g., substance abuse, risky sexual behavior; see Simpson et al. 2012) as the present time perspectives, suggesting the question of whether present hedonism and fatalism, for example, have a specific childhood etiology that can be characterized by instruments such as the Arizona Life History Battery.

Of the five dimensions of the ZTPI, the dimension with the least straightforward relationship with well-being appears to be the Future time perspective. Forthcoming research might investigate whether, and under what circumstances, the future perspective has a curvilinear relationship with measures of SWB. For example, as discussed above, it may be that the strongly future oriented engage in activities and behaviors that result in comfortable lives. However, might a person be too future oriented, such that they miss out on life's pleasures? Moreover, we have yet to investigate whether these long-held cognitive patterns are tractable. Are there interventions—perhaps such as mindfulness or gratitude interventions—that might mitigate maladaptive time balances?

Even more than personality, how people think about the epochs of life—their time perspective—plays a critical role in determining how happy people are (Zhang and Howell 2011). As the evidence we have reviewed suggests, time perspective appears to influence well-being through two pathways: (1) directly, through informing how people interpret the past and anticipate the future, and (2) indirectly, by influencing the behaviors that determine life circumstances. It is no wonder, then, that from time immemorial, novelists (e.g., Proust, *Remembrance of Things Past*), filmmakers (e.g., *Back to the Future*), philosophers (e.g., Heidegger, *Being and Time*), and physicists (e.g., Hawking, *A Brief History of Time*) have obsessed over the passage of time. The evidence reviewed above suggests that they were onto something.

References

Baumeister, R. F., Bratslavsky, E., Finkenauer, C., & Vohs, K. D. (2001). Bad is stronger than good. *Review of General Psychology, 5*(4), 323–370. doi:10.1037//1089-2680.5.4.323.

Boniwell, I., & Zimbardo, P. (2004). Balancing time perspective in pursuit of optimal functioning. In P. A. Linley & S. Joseph (Eds.), *Positive psychology in practice* (*Positive psychology in practice* pp. 165–180). Hoboken: Wiley.

Boniwell, I., Osin, E., Linley, P. A., & Ivanchenko, G. V. (2010). A question of balance: Time perspective and well-being in British and Russian samples. *The Journal of Positive Psychology, 5*(1), 24–40. doi:10.1080/17439760903271181.

Bryant, F. B. (2003). Savoring beliefs inventory (SBI): A scale for measuring beliefs about savoring. *Journal of Mental Health, 12*, 175–196.

Diener, E., Suh, E. M., Lucas, R. E., & Smith, H. L. (1999). Subjective well-being: Three decades of progress. *Psychological Bulletin, 125*(2), 276.

Drake, L., Duncan, E., Sutherland, F., Abernethy, C., & Henry, C. (2008). Time perspective and correlates of wellbeing. *Time and Society, 17*(1), 47–61. doi:10.1177/0961463X07086304.

Durayappah, A. (2010). The 3P model: A general theory of subjective well-being. *Journal of Happiness Studies, 12*, 681–716.

Epel, E. S., Bandura, A., & Zimbardo, P. G. (1999). Escaping homelessness: The influences of self-efficacy and time perspective on coping with homelessness. *Journal of Applied Social Psychology, 29*(3), 575–596.

Fredrickson, B. L., & Kahneman, D. (1993). Duration neglect in retrospective evaluations of affective episodes. *Journal of Personality and Social Psychology, 65*(1), 45–55.

Holman, E. A., & Silver, R. C. (1998). Getting "stuck" in the past: Temporal orientation and coping with trauma. *Journal of Personality and Social Psychology, 74*(5), 1146–1163.

Holman, E. A., & Silver, R. C. (2005). Future-oriented thinking and adjustment in a nationwide longitudinal study following the September 11th terrorist attacks. *Motivation and Emotion, 29*(4), 389–410.

Hutton, H., Treisman, G., & Hunt, W. (2001). HIV risk behaviors and their relationship to post-traumatic stress disorder among women prisoners. *Psychiatric Services, 52*(4), 508–513.

James, W. (1890). *The principles of psychology* (Vol. 1, 2). New York: Henry Holt.

Keough, K. A., Zimbardo, P., & Boyd, J. N. (1999). Who's smoking, drinking, and using drugs? Time perspective as a predictor of substance use. *Basic and Applied Social Psychology, 21*(2), 149–164.

Kim-Prieto, C., Diener, E., Tamir, M., Scollon, C., & Diener, M. (2005). Integrating the diverse definitions of happiness: A time-sequential framework of subjective well-being. *Journal of Happiness Studies, 6*(3), 261–300.

Kruger, D., Reischl, T., & Zimmerman, M. A. (2008). Time perspective as a mechanism for functional developmental adaptation. *Journal of Social, Evolutionary, and Cultural Psychology, 2*(1), 1–22. Retrieved from http://shell.newpaltz.edu/jsec/articles/volume2/issue1/Kruger2-1.pdf.

Lucas, R. E., & Baird, B. M. (2004). Extraversion and emotional reactivity. *Journal of Personality and Social Psychology, 86*(3), 473.

Lyubomirsky, S. (2001). Why are some people happier than others? The role of cognitive and motivational processes in well-being. *American Psychologist, 56*(3), 239.

Lyubomirsky, S., & Diener, E. (2005). The benefits of frequent positive affect: Does happiness lead to success? *Psychological Bulletin, 131*(6), 803–855. doi:10.1037/0033-2909.131.6.803.

Lyubomirsky, S., Dickerhoof, R., Boehm, J., & Sheldon, K. (2009). *Becoming happier takes both a will and a proper way: Two experimental longitudinal interventions to boost well-being (manuscript under review).*

McCrae, R., & John, O. P. (1992). An introduction to the five-factor model and its applications. *Journal of Personality, 60*(2), 175–215.

Rothspan, S., & Read, S. J. (1996). Present versus future time perspective and HIV risk among heterosexual college students. *Health Psychology, 15*(2), 131–134.

Schimmack, U., Diener, E., & Oishi, S. (2002). Life-satisfaction is a momentary judgment and a stable personality characteristic: The use of chronically accessible and stable sources. *Journal of Personality, 70*(3), 345–384.

Shores, K., & Scott, D. (2007). The relationship of individual time perspective and recreation experience preferences. *Journal of Leisure Research, 39*(1), 28–59.

Simpson, J., Griskevicius, V., Kuo, S., & Sung, S. (2012). Evolution, stress, and sensitive periods: The influence of unpredictability in early versus late childhood on sex and risky behavior. *Developmental Psychology* (in press).

Stolarski, M., Bitner, J., & Zimbardo, P. G. (2011). Time perspective, emotional intelligence and discounting of delayed awards. *Time & Society, 20*(3), 346–363.

Suddendorf, T., & Corballis, M. C. (2007). The evolution of foresight: What is mental time travel, and is it unique to humans? *Behavioral and Brain Sciences, 30*(03). doi:10.1017/S0140525X07001975.

Zhang, J. W., & Howell, R. T. (2011). Do time perspectives predict unique variance in life satisfaction beyond personality traits? *Personality and Individual Differences, 50*(8), 1261–1266. doi:10.1016/j.paid.2011.02.021.

Zhang, J. W., Howell, R. T., & Bowerman, T. (2013a). Validating a brief measure of the Zimbardo time perspective inventory. *Time and Society, 22*, 391–409.

Zhang, J. W., Howell, R. T., & Stolarski, M. (2013b). Comparing three methods to measure a balanced time perspective: The relationship between a balanced time perspective and subjective well-being. *Journal of Happiness Studies, 14*(1), 169–184.
Zimbardo, P. G., & Boyd, J. N. (1999). Putting time in perspective: A valid, reliable individual-differences metric. *Journal of Personality and Social Psychology, 77*(6), 1271–1288.
Zimbardo, P. G., Keough, K. A., & Boyd, J. N. (1997). Present time perspective as a predictor of risky driving. *Personality and Individual Differences, 23*(6), 1007–1023.

Part V
Clinical Applications of Time Perspective

Time Perspective and Social Relations: A Stress and Coping Perspective

E. Alison Holman

> *"I felt like time slowed down. Everything was in slow motion."* Laguna Beach resident following the October 27, 1993 firestorm
>
> *"It felt like forever…long enough to last a lifetime."* Jennifer Seeger, survivor of the Aurora, CO mass shooting July 20, 2012
>
> *"At times it feels like only yesterday, and at others it feels like many years have passed."* Nicole Hockley, mother of Dylan Hockley 6 year old boy killed at Sandy Hook Elementary School December 14, 2012

On the morning of December 14th, 2012, a 20-year old man killed his mother in bed, drove to Sandy Hook Elementary School in Newtown Connecticut and killed 6 adults and 20 six to seven year old children. Around midnight on July 20th, 2012, a man dressed as the Joker from the Batman series walked into a movie theater in Aurora, Colorado and opened fire killing 12, seriously injuring another 70 people. These events, like so many other traumatic, violent events that take place around the globe, made a few normally-short minutes seem like a lifetime to its survivors. Traumatic events like these peel away the façade of the future, urgently force people into the present moment, and expand current experience so that it fills conscious awareness. In so doing they interrupt the normal flow of experience that weaves the past, present, and future together into a fabric that anchors and supports personal identity. And, as is poignantly described by Ms. Seeger, this disruption creates perceptual distortions—the sense that time has stopped or slowed, and renders some vulnerable to becoming stuck in the traumatic experience long after it passes (Holman and Silver 1998).

Through the window of time we are able to see our life story unfold, build our identity, identify future ambitions, and feel proud of our success. It is with our sense of time that we connect who we have been with who we are and want to be. Without time our lives would consist of isolated, incoherent moments lacking the essential

E.A. Holman (✉)
Program in Nursing Science, University of California, Irvine, CA, USA
e-mail: aholman@uci.edu

M. Stolarski et al. (eds.), *Time Perspective Theory; Review, Research and Application: Essays in Honor of Philip G. Zimbardo*, DOI 10.1007/978-3-319-07368-2_27,

consciousness that makes us human. Indeed, the consequences of losing the continuity of one's own personal timeline following trauma can be quite serious—altered time perceptions contribute to peritraumatic dissociation, a component of acute stress disorder and predictor of posttraumatic stress disorder (PTSD) (American Psychiatric Association 2000).

Traumatic events, however, are not isolated, individual experiences—they do not occur in a "social vacuum" (Tait and Silver 1989). Like time, social relationships play a critical role in shaping who we are and how we respond to the world around us (Baumeister and Leary 1995). At the same time, our perceptual responses to negative life events are likely to influence, either directly or indirectly, how we engage with others. Indeed, much like the rose-colored glasses of the perennial optimist, our lens of time shapes our perceptions of, and behavior in, the social world around us.

A growing body of research addresses how time perceptions may influence our social world. Socioemotional Selectivity Theory (SST) (Carstensen et al. 1999; Lang and Carstensen 2002) proposes that in anticipation of an ending (e.g., graduation), our Future time perspective (TP) diminishes as we focus attention on our immediate emotional needs. This change encourages us to place priority on emotionally-satisfying social relationships in the present and decreases our interest in pursuing relationships that would advance future goals (as they are less important). These changes in TP can also support people to change their attitudes such that they become more willing to conform with social consensus when responding to persuasive messages (DeWall et al. 2006). Together this work suggests that when we move from an expansive future to focus predominantly our present circumstances, we choose to spend time with people more likely to satisfy our immediate socio-emotional goals (Carstensen et al. 1999; Trope and Liberman 2003).

But social relationships are not simply responsive to time perceptions—they may also help shape them. Social rejection promotes overestimation of time intervals as the present expands and the future shrinks away (Twenge et al. 2003). Past positive and negative TPs are associated with the nature/quality of family relationships (Goldberg and Maslach 1996; Holman and Zimbardo 2009), begging the question whether early life interactions with important people in our lives influence the nature and balance of our TP. When these experiences are characterized by interpersonal violence, survivors are more likely to report, and "get stuck" in a high Past Negative TP (Holman and Silver 1998). Clinical observations further suggest that such traumatic events can distort survivors' time perceptions so that they focus more on past events (e.g., as omens), or have a foreshortened sense of the future (Terr 1983). Other clinically-based research indicates that an imbalanced TP—that is, focusing predominantly on one TP to the exclusion of the others—may promote "desynchronized transactions" (p. 285) in social relationships that can foster interpersonal conflict (Melges 1982). A classic example of this would be a future-oriented parent telling the present-oriented child to forgo a chance to play with a treasured friend because s/he has to prepare for an important test. Such TP mismatches can wreak havoc on interpersonal relationships within families when they go unrecognized.

The clinical applications of these findings are many. Indeed, Zimbardo et al. (2012) recently published a book addressing the use of Zimbardo and Boyd's conceptualization of time perspective (Zimbardo and Boyd 2009) as a tool in therapy for individuals suffering from PTSD (Zimbardo et al. 2012). This book describes a therapeutic approach based upon Zimbardo's five time perspective constructs (Past Positive, Past Negative, Present Hedonist, Present Fatalist, and Future) and extends our original empirical work linking distortions in time perceptions/orientation to trauma response (Holman and Silver 1998) into the realm of time-based therapy. The success of this work reinforces our early assertion that changes in time perceptions/perspective are central components of coping with trauma (Holman and Silver 1998).

In sum, although TP and social relationships help shape our identities and guide our ability to make sense of the world around us, very little has been done to explore how they may jointly affect psychological functioning following exposure to traumatic life events. Given that trauma can distort our sense of time and elicit social responses that play a critical role in adaptation, these co-occurring responses make coping with trauma an ideal paradigm in which to study the TP-social relations connection. Indeed, it is not hard to imagine how traumatic life events could initiate a downward negative spiral in which a trauma-related focus on the past may increase risk for negative social interactions that only serve to reinforce the Past Negative TP, and potentially impede recovery. To my knowledge this type of reciprocal model has never been examined empirically.

Toward this end, this chapter describes findings from three studies examining the associations among time perspective, social relationships, and psychological adjustment. The purpose of these studies was to (a) explore how the quality of social relationships (support, conflict, etc.) and TP may work together to affect psychological well-being and (b) to investigate these dynamics in the context of coping with stress. The first study was a 3-month longitudinal study of undergraduates from three California universities. The second was a two-year longitudinal study conducted with residents of communities devastated by the 1993 Southern California firestorms. The third was a prospective longitudinal study conducted with a nationally representative sample of the American population following the September 11th, 2001 terrorist attacks. With these studies we see how time perspective and social relationships work together to affect well-being in general (study 1) and adjustment to stress over time (studies 2 & 3).

The Bay Area College Student Study

Time Perspective, Social Relationships, and Psychological Well-Being

We previously described important patterns linking TP and the characteristics of social networks and suggested that TP is a lens through which we perceive, understand, and function in the social world (Holman and Zimbardo 2009). We identified the importance of family ties for people with a Past TP (positive and negative) and how Future TP makes significant others highly salient in our lives. We now take those analyses a step further to examine how TP and social support from these important people are linked over time and their combined impact on overall well-being.

This three month longitudinal study, conducted in collaboration with Dr. Phil Zimbardo, included students from three universities serving very different segments of the population: Stanford University, College of San Mateo, and California State University, San Francisco. In the first wave (T1), 589 students completed an in-depth survey that included the following measures: (a) The Brief Symptom Inventory for psychological distress (Derogatis and Melisaratos 1983); (b) items modeled after previous research (Abbey et al. 1985; Norbeck et al. 1981) addressing the size/nature of respondents' social networks and general quality of social interactions (support, conflict, undermining) with spouse/significant other, family, close friends; (c) assessment of lifetime and recent (prior 6 months) stressful life events modeled after the Diagnostic Interview Schedule (Robins et al. 1981); (d) an assessment of social responses (support, conflict, undermining) to participants' attempts to cope with stress; and (e) the Zimbardo Time Perspective Inventory (ZTPI) . Three-months later, 352 of the original 387 respondents from two of the colleges who had participated in the first survey (91 % of respondents from the two colleges; 59.7 % of the full Time 1 sample) completed a similar survey with an assessment of stressors occurring in the previous 3 months. There were no significant changes in any of the TP dimensions between T1 and T2. Analyses to identify predictors of drop out suggest that younger students with high scores on T1 present hedonism were more likely to drop out between Time 1 and Time 2. No other time perspective scores were associated with drop out.

We then examined how time perspective and the quality of social relationships were associated with each other over time. Path modeling with mediational analyses was used with Sobel-Goodman tests to examine the proposed indirect effects. All analyses were adjusted for lifetime stress exposure. Figure 1a depicts findings showing that T1 familial social support contributes to increases in Past Positive TP 3 months later which is associated with both higher T2 support from family and lower T2 psychological distress: Indirect effect for T1 support to T2 support through increased T2 Past Positive TP was 15 % of total effect, $b=.10$, $z=4.16$, $p<.001$; indirect effect for T1 support to T2 distress through T2 Past Positive TP was 55 % of total effect, $b=-.06$, $z=-2.60$, $p=.009$. This suggests the possibility that a positive upward spiral occurs such that familial support boosts one's Past Positive TP which, in turn, contributes to increases in familial social support and lower distress over time. The importance of these findings for overall well-being is further highlighted by the fact that T2 Past Positive TP is associated not only with lower distress, but also with higher post-traumatic growth scores following stress ($pr[260]=.22$, $p<.001$) after adjusting for concurrent distress. Although we expected it, we did not find a comparable negative downward spiral linking Past Negative TP, social conflict, and distress.

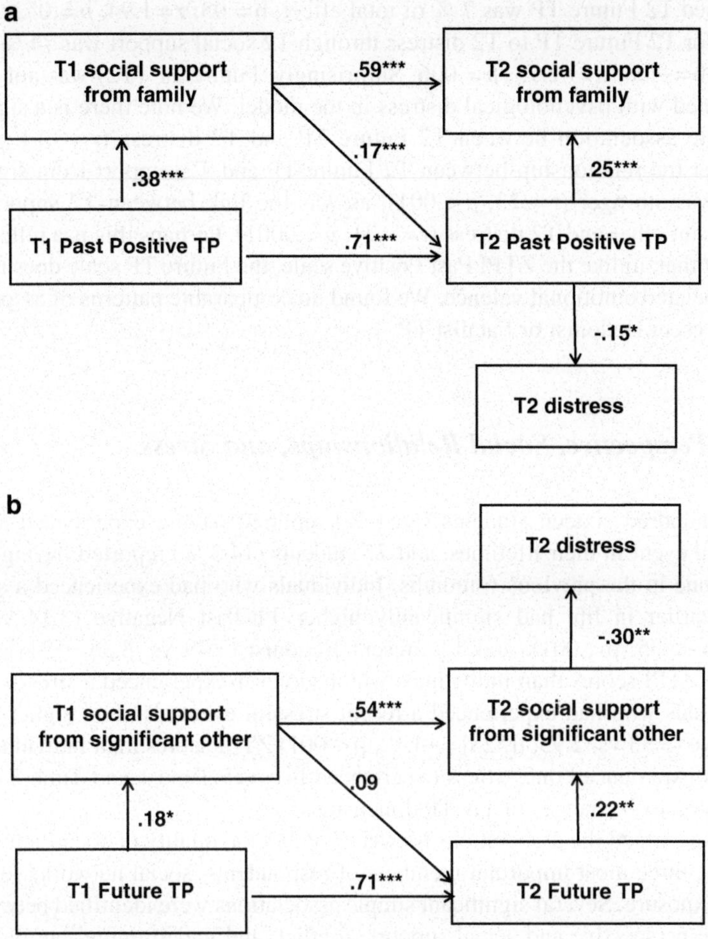

Fig. 1 (**a**) Early T1 support from family predicts subsequent T2 Past Positive time perspective which is associated with both higher T2 social support from family and lower Time 2 psychological distress. *$p<.05$, **$p<.01$, ***$p<.001$. (**b**) Early T1 support from significant other predicts subsequent T2 Future time perspective which is associated with higher T2 significant other support which, in turn, is associated with lower Time 2 psychological distress. *$p<.05$, **$p<.01$, ***$p<.001$

Similarly, Fig. 1b represents findings from a structural model demonstrating that T1 social support from a significant other contributes to increases in Future TP over time which is associated with increases in support from one's significant other that link to substantially lower psychological distress. Again we see what appears to be a positive upward spiral such that T1 support from significant others helps increase Future TP which encourages subsequent support that is tied to lower psychological distress: Indirect effect for T1 support to T2 support through increased T2 Future TP was 7 % of total effect, $b=.03$, $z=1.94$, $p=.052$; indirect effect for T2 Future TP to T2 distress through T2 social support was 74 % of total effect, $b=-.08$, $z=-2.73$, $p=.006$. Surprisingly, Future TP (T2) was not directly associated with psychological distress in the model. We note there is a significant bivariate association between T2 Future TP and T2 distress ($r=-.14$, $p=.02$); however the relationship between T2 Future TP and T2 support from significant other was stronger ($r=.23$, $p<.001$), as was the link between T2 support from significant other and T2 distress ($r=-.31$, $p<.0001$). Perhaps this is a reflection of the fact that, unlike the ZTPI Past Positive scale, the Future TP scale does not have an associated emotional valence. We found no comparable patterns of associations with Present Hedonist or Fatalist TP.

Time Perspective, Social Relationships, and Stress

Three hundred sixteen students (56.4 %) reported having experienced a highly stressful event in their lifetimes, and 77 students (14.3 %) reported having experienced one in the previous 6 months. Individuals who had experienced a stressful event earlier in life had significantly higher T1 Past Negative (3.14 vs. 2.83, $t[544]=-5.35$, $p<.001$), and T1 Present Hedonist (3.49 vs. 3.38, $t[544]=-2.32$, $p<.03$) ZTPI scores than individuals who had never experienced a stressful event. Individuals who had experienced a recent stressful event also had higher T1 Past Negative (3.33 vs. 2.95, $t[523]=-4.42$, $p<.001$) ZTPI scores than individuals who had not experienced one. Stress experienced between Time 1 and Time 2 was not associated with changes in any TP dimensions.

We examined the associations between TP and the quality of social interactions with the three most important members of respondents' social networks following stress exposure. Several significant simple associations were identified between T1/T2 time perspective and social support, conflict, and undermining, but only three remained significant after adjusting for current distress: T1 Past Positive TP was positively associated with T1 post-stress social support ($pr=0.31[142]$, $p<.001$) and negatively associated with T2 post-stress social conflict ($pr=-0.27[63]$, $p<.04$); and T1 Future TP was negatively associated with T2 post-stress social conflict ($pr=-0.28[63]$, $p<.03$).

Altogether, these preliminary data suggest that under normal circumstances, social relationships and TP may cyclically affect one another in a feed forward manner. Following stress, Past Positive and Future TPs were associated with higher concurrent stress-related social support and lower subsequent post-stress social conflict. As the three-month interval is a relatively short period of time, however, the sample of respondents who had experienced stress was small ($N=63$) making it difficult to draw conclusions about the TP-social process association following stress. Thus we now turn to two additional studies both conducted in the aftermath of a collectively experienced stress, thereby allowing examination of TP-social relationship associations in the context of coping with the same stressor (Table 1).

Table 1 Correlations between time perspective and social support, conflict, and undermining from three most important members of social network following recent stress as reported by students in Bay Area College Student Study

	Time 1			Time 2		
	Social support	Social conflict	Social undermining	Social support	Social conflict	Social undermining
Time 1						
Time perspective						
Past Positive	**0.33**	−0.12	−0.10	0.11	**−0.28**	**−0.27**
Past Negative	−0.17	**0.31**	**0.27**	−0.10	**0.30**	0.24
Present Hedonist	0.18	−0.00	0.03	−0.04	0.01	0.16
Present Fatalist	−0.08	0.09	−0.01	−0.24	0.25	0.15
Future	0.10	−0.00	0.20	0.16	**−0.25**	−0.12
Time 2						
Time Perspective						
Past Positive	**0.31**	−0.08	−0.02	0.22	−0.20	−0.24
Past Negative	0.07	0.12	0.05	−0.08	**0.34**	**0.33**
Present Hedonist	**0.47**	**−0.38**	−0.13	0.17	−0.10	0.00
Present Fatalist	−0.05	−0.06	−0.16	**−0.25**	**0.28**	0.24
Future	−0.01	0.15	0.28	0.19	−0.10	−0.10

Table note. Sample size varies across comparisons: T1 time perspective-T1 social N=71; T1 time perspective-T2 social N=63; T1 social-T2 time perspective N=45; T2 time perspective-T2 social N=63. Significant correlations are in **bold**

The Southern California Firestorm Study

In October 1993, the cities of Laguna Beach and Malibu, California each experienced firestorms that raged through the communities destroying hundreds of homes forcing thousands of citizens to evacuate. In the immediate aftermath of each fire, my colleague Dr. Roxane Silver and I began a study that spanned the subsequent two years and focused on identifying the early predictors of long-term adjustment following exposure to a traumatic community-based event. We previously reported that early discontinuity between past, present, and future (temporal disintegration) was associated with past (predominantly negative) TP and high psychological distress over time (Holman and Silver 1998). What we have not yet explored, however, is whether TP and social relationships work together to affect well-being over time.

Our initial assessment (36 h post fires) included early cognitive, emotional, and social responses to the fires; subsequent waves also included degree of fire exposure, generalized distress (BSI) (Derogatis and Melisaratos 1983), lifetime and recent trauma exposure, time orientation (a ZTPI-like measure that addressed past, present, and future TP), social network characteristics, and quality of social relationships (support, conflict, constraint). Table 2 presents the study's sample and response rates over time. Dropout from this study was minimal over a two year period of time (<20 %) with only 15 people leaving the study. There were no significant predictors of dropout, perhaps because the sample was small.

Table 2 Retention of 1993 Southern California firestorm sample over two-year study

	Wave 1	Wave 2	Wave 3	Wave 4	Wave 5
	36 h post-evacuation	2–4 weeks post-evacuation	6 months post-evacuation	1 year post-evacuation	2 years post-evacuation
Sample size	85	74	72	71	70
Response rate	100 %	87 %	85 %	84 %	82 %

One goal of this study was to examine the dynamic associations between TP and social relationships and their impact on adjustment in the context of coping with stress. Hence, two fundamental approaches were used. First, I examined how the quality of early social relationships (36 h to 6 months) was associated with later TP (6 months to 1 year), and whether early social processes were indirectly linked with increases in psychological distress over time (2 years) through their association with TP. Then I looked at whether early TP (2 week to 6 month) was associated with the subsequent quality of social relationships (6 month to 1 year), and whether early TP was indirectly associated with increases in psychological distress over time (2 year) through its association with subsequent social processes. In essence, the analyses were designed to examine whether one of these core psychological lenses (time, social process) had a greater influence on the other over time following stress exposure. In order to address whether one construct affects another (or vice versa) it was important that the TP, social relationship, and psychological distress measures used in these analyses were each assessed at different time points. Path models with a Sobel-Goodman test for significance of mediated indirect effects were used for these analyses. All analyses were adjusted for early post-fire psychological distress and ongoing stressors to rule out potential confounding effects of these variables.

Figure 2a presents the final path model depicting how early social support (2 weeks) and social conflict (6 months) were both indirectly associated with increases in psychological distress following the 1993 community fires through their association with past orientation (similar to ZTPI Past Negative) 1 year after the fires (Indirect effects for support on 2-year distress, 69 % of total effect, $b=-.13$, $z=-2.44$, $p=.015$; indirect effects for conflict on 2-year distress, 42 % of total effect, $b=.10$, $z=-2.36$, $p=.018$). That is, early social responses (lower social support and higher social conflict) were both significantly associated with *high* past orientation 1 year after the fires, which was, in turn, a predictor of increased distress 2 years after the fires. Similarly, Fig. 2b presents the final path model linking early social constraints (social ties did not want to hear about respondent's feelings/thoughts regarding the fires) with *low* levels of future orientation 6 months later which predicted increases in distress over the subsequent 2 years (Indirect effect for constraints on 2-year distress, 36 % of total effect, $b=.10$, $z=1.93$, $p=.053$).

Importantly, when the reverse approach was used—that is, testing whether early TP was associated with subsequent social processes that predict increases in distress—the findings were not significant (although one mediation was close with $p<.10$), suggesting that TP mediated the association between early social processes and distress, but social processes did not mediate the association between early TP

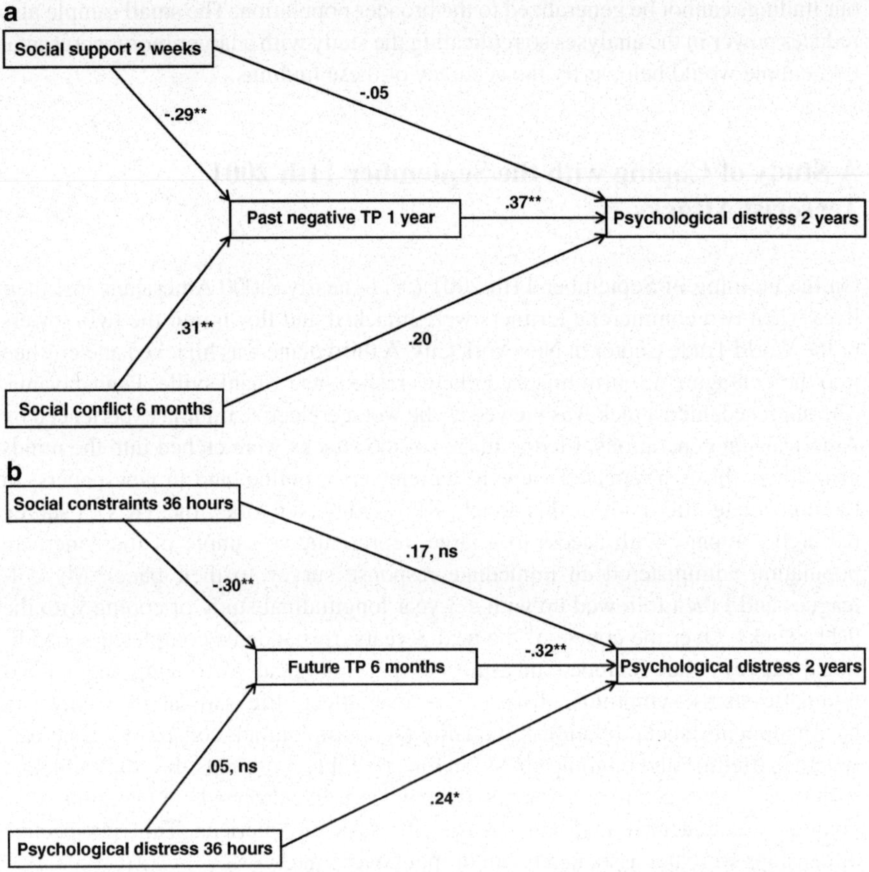

Fig. 2 (**a**) Path model showing that Past Negative TP 1 year post-fires is a mediator linking early social support (low levels at 2 weeks) and social conflict (high levels at 6 months) to psychological distress 2 years after the 1993 southern California firestorms. All analyses adjusted for early distress and ongoing stress. *$p<.05$, **$p<.01$, ***$p<.001$. (**b**) Path model showing that early social constraints on talking about fires is indirectly associated with increases in psychological distress 2 years after the 1993 southern California firestorms through Future TP as reported at 6 months post-fires. All analyses adjusted for early distress and ongoing stress. *$p<.05$, **$p<.01$, ***$p<.001$

and distress. It is important to remember that *none* of the data used in these analyses was retrospective. The entire study was conducted in real time starting 36 h after the fires, and all TP, social relationship, and distress constructs used in the analyses were temporally distinct, making this a clear test of reciprocity. Together these findings provide evidence that in the aftermath of a community-based trauma, early social responses may contribute to subsequent distress through their impact on TP, especially past and future focused TP. Moreover, past TP predicted subsequent distress independent of its associations with social processes. Nonetheless, we note that this study was conducted with a small, select group of community residents so our findings cannot be generalized to the broader population. The small sample also reduces power in the analyses so replicating the study with a larger more representative sample would help verify the accuracy of these findings.

A Study of Coping with the September 11th 2001 Terrorist Attacks

On the morning of September 11th 2001 (9/11) nearly 3,000 Americans lost their lives when two commercial airliners were hijacked and flown into the twin towers of the World Trade Center in New York City. A third plane was hijacked and crashed into the Pentagon; a fourth hijacked plane crashed near Shanksville, Pennsylvania. The unprecedented attack was viewed as the worst collective trauma experienced by Americans in generations. Media images of the attacks were etched into the minds of millions through repeated viewing on television, online, and in newspapers. In the immediate aftermath of this attack, Knowledge Networks, Inc. (KN) a survey research company with access to a large, representative sample of the American population administered an immediate response survey to their panel. My colleagues and I then followed up with a 3-year longitudinal study of coping with the 9/11 attacks. Over the course of the next 3 years, respondents completed six additional surveys that included measures of psychological well-being (e.g., posttraumatic stress symptoms, distress, positive affect, life satisfaction), physical health ailments, social relationship quality (support, conflict, constraint), time perspective, lifetime and ongoing stress, and more. Table 3 presents the study timeline with sample sizes and response rates. Respondents who dropped out over time were younger, less educated, and more likely to be African-American. Time perspective dimensions were not associated with dropout over time.

With data collected at six time points the 9/11 study allowed examination of the dynamic associations among TP and quality of social relationships over time in a large sample drawn from the American population. The focus of the analyses was to explore patterns of associations between TP and social relationships and examine how they may have affected psychological well being following collective stress. Path modeling and meditational analysis (Sobel-Goodman test for indirect effects) were used to

Table 3 Coping with the September 11th 2001 terrorist attacks study timeline, sample sizes, and response rates

	2 weeks post-9/11	2 months post-9/11**	6 months post-9/11	1 year post-9/11***	18 months post-9/11	2 years post-9/11	3 years post-9/11
Sample size	2729	933	846	2033	1666	1571	1950
Response rate*	78 %	87 %	91 %	75 %	78 %	74 %	79 %

Table note. *Response rate was calculated as number of respondents/number of available panelists who were fielded the survey. **The two month respondents were a random sample drawn from the original 2729 surveyed 2 weeks post-9/11. ***At one year post-9/11 we expanded the study to include all available panelists from the original 2729 surveyed 2 weeks post-9/11 explore the roles of early post-9/11 (2 months) social conflict, constraints, and support in relation to TP one year following the attacks, as well as the role of early TP (2 months) in relation to social conflict, constraint, and support 1 year post-9/11. Finally, analyses explored whether associations between TP and social constructs would predict increases in distress over time. All analyses were adjusted for pre-9/11 mental health, early acute stress symptoms, and ongoing stress.

Overall the findings were consistent with those of the Fire Study: early social processes were important predictors of subsequent Past Negative and Future TPs which were, in turn, associated with changes in psychological distress over time. The strongest early social predictor of TP and subsequent distress was 2-month social conflict which was associated with distress 3 years post-9/11 in part through its association with high Past Negative (Fig. 3a; indirect effect was 27 % of total effect, $b=.03$, $z=2.35$, $p<.023$) and low Future (Fig. 3b; indirect effect was 16 % of total effect, $b=.02$, $z=2.41$, $p<.016$) TPs at one year post-9/11; early social support was also indirectly associated with long-term distress through its association with Future TP 1 year post-9/11 (Fig. 3b; indirect effect was 31 % of total effect, $b=-.01$, $z=-2.21$, $p=.027$). When early 2-month TPs were examined in relation to social support, conflict, and constraint 1-year post-9/11, early Past Positive, Present Hedonist, and Future TPs were associated only with higher levels of social support one-year post-9/11. However, one-year social support was not associated with subsequent psychological distress. Early Past Negative TP was associated with one-year social conflict which partially mediated the association between early Past Negative TP and psychological distress 3 years post-9/11 (Indirect effect was 8 % of total effect, conflict $b=.01$, $z=2.64$, $p=.008$). However, both early Past Negative TP ($b=.12$, $z=6.28$, $p<.001$) and one-year social conflict ($b=.13$, $z=3.97$, $p<.001$) had substantially stronger direct associations with distress over time in this study.

In sum, although some reciprocity existed in the associations between (a) early TP and one-year social relations, and (b) early social relations and one-year TP, the pattern of findings suggests that early social conflict and support were both important predictors of subsequent TP. We note, however that although early Past Positive, Present Hedonist, and Future TPs were linked with later social support, only early Past Negative TP indirectly contributed to distress over time through its association with later social conflict.

The final set of analyses examined whether early social conflict—the strongest, most consistent early predictor of later Past Negative TP and distress—contributed to a cyclical negative spiral in which social conflict predicted increases in Past Negative TP over time which contributed to increases in social conflict over time that ultimately lead to increases in psychological distress. Not only was there evidence that this pattern of inter-relationships exists (Fig. 3c), but subsequent testing confirmed that social conflict two months post-9/11 was *indirectly* associated with higher social conflict one year post-9/11 in part *through* high Past Negative TP 6 months post-9/11 (Indirect effect was 7 % of total effect, $b=.03$, $z=2.45$, $p=.01$). Similarly, Past Negative TP at six months was *indirectly* associated with Past Negative TP at two years in part *through* high social conflict experienced one year post-9/11 (Indirect effect was 5 % of total effect, $b=.03$, $z=2.96$, $p=.003$). Finally,

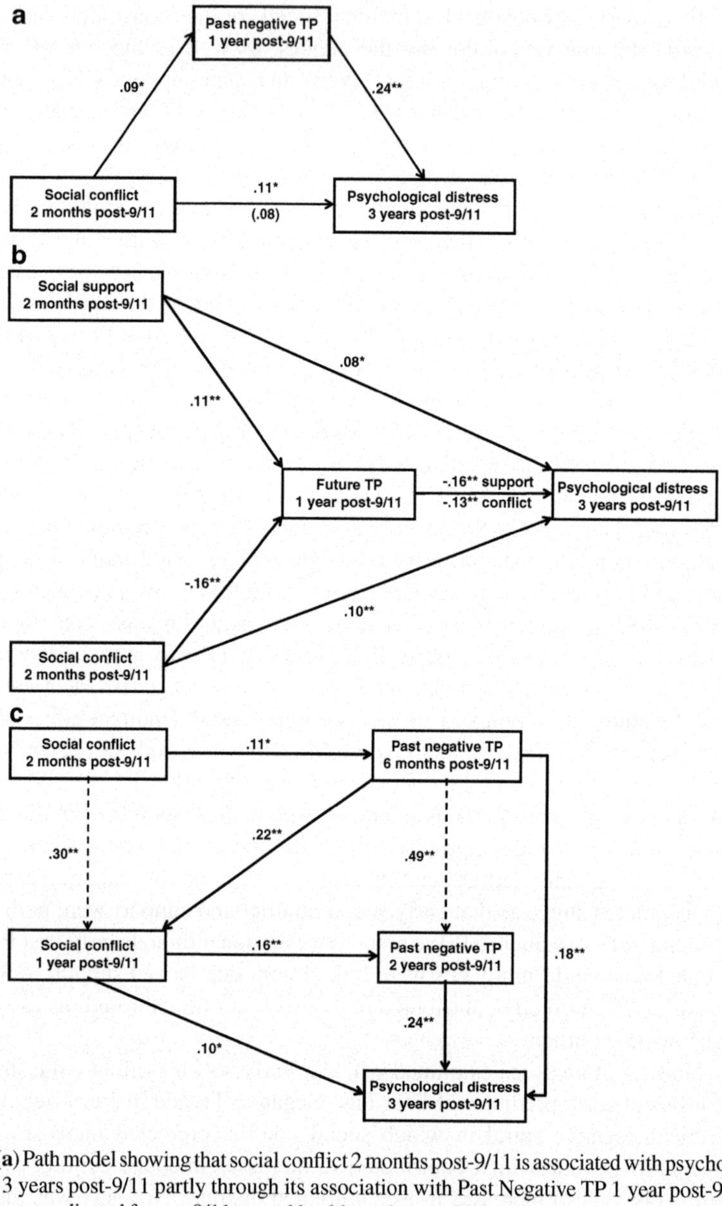

Fig. 3 (**a**) Path model showing that social conflict 2 months post-9/11 is associated with psychological distress 3 years post-9/11 partly through its association with Past Negative TP 1 year post-9/11. All analyses were adjusted for pre-9/11 mental health, early post-9/11 acute stress response, and ongoing stress. *$p<.05$, **$p<.01$, ***$p<.001$. (**b**) The quality of early post-9/11 social relationships was indirectly associated with psychological distress 3 years post-9/11 through Future TP 1 year post-9/11. All analyses were adjusted for pre-9/11 mental health, early post-9/11 acute stress response, and ongoing stress. *$p<.05$, **$p<.01$, ***$p<.001$. (**c**) The quality of early social relationships was associated with a negative downward spiral with Past Negative TP that increased distress over 3 years post-9/11. All analyses were adjusted for pre-9/11 mental health, early post-9/11 acute stress response, and ongoing stress. *$p<.05$, **$p<.01$, ***$p<.001$

Table 4 Correlations between time perspective two-months post-9/11 and the quality of social relationships one-year post-9/11

Two months post-9/11	One year post-9/11		
Time perspective	Social support	Social conflict	Social constraints
Past Positive	**0.15**	–0.04	0.01
Past Negative	–0.04	**0.17**	**0.13**
Present Hedonist	**0.07**	**–0.10**	–0.04
Future	**0.14**	**–0.09**	–0.03

Table 5 Correlations between the quality of social relations two months post-9/11 and time perspective one-year post-9/11

One year post-9/11	Two months post-9/11		
Time perspective	Social support	Social conflict	Social constraints
Past Positive	**0.12**	**–0.09**	–0.04
Past Negative	–0.04	**0.09**	**0.09**
Present Hedonist	**0.06**	–0.04	0.02
Future	**0.12**	**–0.12**	**–0.11**

Table note. Sample size varies slightly within groups: Table 4 sample includes N = 1036–1077, Table 5 includes N = 906-959. Significant correlations are in **bold**

although social conflict one year post-9/11 was directly associated with increases in distress 3 years after the attacks, it was also *indirectly* associated with distress *through* higher Past Negative TP two years post-9/11 (Indirect effect was 30 % of total effect, b = .03, z = 2.90, p = .003). It is important to note that an attempt was made to test whether Past Negative TP at two months could initiate a similar downward spiral through social conflict at six months, Past Negative TP at one year, and social conflict at two years. This approach did not work—social conflict at six months was not associated with increases in Past Negative TP one year post-9/11. A similar attempt was made to identify an upward positive spiral through which early social support contributed to higher Past Positive or Future TPs which in turn contributed to higher social support and ultimately dampened distress. Again, the data did not support this model as neither social support nor Past Positive TP were predictors of distress over time (Tables 4 and 5).

Discussion

Three independent studies provide evidence for the interdependence between TP and the quality of social relationships that may affect the degree to which we feel distressed in both everyday lives as well as in the context of coping with stress. As time perceptions and social relationships are both (a) central to how we make sense of the world around us and (b) influenced by negative life events, their interdependent roles in shaping our adaptation to stress makes intuitive sense. Unfortunately it has received too little attention in the stress and coping literature.

Importantly, the findings described in this chapter are consistent with earlier work suggesting that negative social interactions have a stronger impact on well-being than do positive ones (Rook 1984)—that is, unpleasant interactions, especially social conflict with important social network members following stress, may have enduring effects on TP. By feeding into a Past Negative TP, social conflict creates conditions for an imbalance between Past-Present-Future TPs that further contributes to desynchronized interpersonal relations (Melges 1982) and distress. In so doing, they may trigger a snowball effect of negativity where one's TP and social relations both spiral out of control.

At the same time, the Bay Area Undergraduate Study offered preliminary evidence for a "positive spiral" such that supportive relationships contributed to both higher Past Positive and Future TPs as well as greater future support and lower distress in everyday life. In other words, the interdependence of TP and social relationships and its impact on psychological functioning was not limited to the aftermath of stressful encounters.

However, none of the studies included pre-event assessments of TP. This is a very important consideration as we do not know how much pre-event TP may already have affected the quality of social interactions, especially those experienced after stress. Clearly the presence of a negative downward spiral identified in the 9/11 study suggests the need for obtaining pre-event TP assessments if we are to understand fully how TP and social relations work together both generally and following trauma to affect long-term well-being. Similarly, the general pattern of associations—Past Positive, Present Hedonist, and Future TPs being more closely associated with social support, whereas Past Negative TP being associated only with social conflict raises the possibility that dispositional optimism or pessimism may be driving these associations. In order to tease this apart, future research should include pre-event assessments of these personal qualities as well. That said, we did control for pre-9/11 mental health (measured *before* 9/11) and early post-9/11 acute stress symptoms, both of which could serve as a proxy for a pessimistic world view, making this alternative explanation less plausible for the 9/11 findings. Nonetheless, we did not have an equivalent proxy for optimism, so the "positive spiral" model remains to be confirmed in studies that include measures of optimism and have more than two time points.

Given that extremely stressful events often elicit a shift to the present, it was somewhat surprising that although present TPs were individually correlated with post-stress social relations (e.g., Table 1), these associations were neither consistent across time points or studies, nor robust in controlled analyses over time. That is, present TPs do not appear to affect the quality of post-stress social relationships and predict distress over time. Under the assumption that stress makes emotion regulation a priority and constrains TP (present focused with less attention to future), SST would predict that respondents would report less strain and more satisfaction in social relationships (Lang and Carstensen 2002)—this pattern did not consistently emerge across these three studies. In fact, Past and Future TPs had the strongest, most consistent associations with both social ties and psychological distress across all studies in the analyses over time. We recognize however, that the ZTPI does not measure the depth of TP (e.g., profiles of high vs. low in Present and Future TPs respectively). Future research needs to consider how different profiles of Past, Present, Future TP may impact responses to trauma as well as the social relationships that may affect well-being.

This pattern of findings suggests important directions for future research. First, in-depth exploration of cognitive/social processes that feed into Past Negative or Future TPs to identify targets for clinical interventions would be useful. For example, early interventions aimed at helping trauma survivors rebuild TP balance with continuity between Past-Present-Future TP can prevent them from getting stuck in the past or losing track of their future (see Zimbardo et al. 2012). Helping people develop techniques to reframe or cope with social conflict so that it doesn't simply reinforce negative world views might also be appropriate. Finally, understanding exactly how TP and social relationships play off of one another in the context of coping with stress could open avenues for TP/social relationship-focused interventions that help survivors regain TP balance or deal more effectively with people in their social networks.

At the same time, we need to address the role of a Future Negative TP—a dimension not included in the ZTPI that may also impact social relationships and well-being following stress (Carelli et al. 2011). A growing body of research demonstrates the potential health impacts of worrying and perseverative cognition (Brosschot et al. 2006; Holman and Silver 2005; Kubzansky et al. 1997), both reflecting cognitive engagement with a negative future. Given that there are many ways to engage the past (e.g., ruminating, reminiscing) and the future (e.g., planning, projecting), examining how these TPs manifest is essential to understanding how they may affect well-being over time (Atance and O'Neill 2001). Placing TP in a broader sociocultural and developmental context is also essential for understanding its meaning and impact on individuals (Atance and O'Neill 2001). For example, adolescents living in a war-zone will likely have a vastly different understanding of what "future" means than their counterparts living in relative peace (Lavi and Solomon 2005). The former may have future thoughts related to simple survival (food, shelter), whereas the latter may focus on making more abstract, distal decisions about their lives (career, family).

Finally, given the apparent benefits of maintaining a balanced TP (BTP) for well-being (Boniwell et al. 2010; Zhang et al. 2012), it seems all TP dimensions have a role to play in sustaining us. But the question remains, how do we find the right balance? Does the right balance always include moderately high Past Positive, Present Hedonist, and Future TP with relatively low Past Negative and Present Fatalist TPs (Boniwell and Zimbardo 2004)? The question arises because it has been argued that being able to shift one's TP focus is important for adaptation (Holman and Zimbardo 2009; P. G. Zimbardo and Boyd 1999). Yet an underlying assumption of the BTP definition is that one must maintain moderately high Past Positive, Present Hedonist, and Future TPs with lower Past Negative and Present fatalists scores. Does that mean there is a critical cut off point making BTP a fixed phenomenon with a static measurement (Drake et al. 2008)? Or are there optimal BTPs that vary according to one's life circumstances? For example, could there be some dynamic process by which high Past Negative TP drives people forward because they embrace a positive Future TP? Such a scenario seems well within the realm of possibility for those individuals who stubbornly refuse to let themselves be overcome by misfortune. Indeed, one could argue that one face of resilience is just that—unwillingness to succumb to persistent, powerful Past Negative forces combined with the determination and desire to create a positive future. Or, consider someone with a strong Past Positive TP who becomes overwhelmed with pain, suffering, and sadness in the present, but somehow falls back on that past to stay afloat until the present is more tolerable. Given the evolutionary value of negative emotions for learning to survive and feel appreciation, it seems possible that there may be different profiles of TPs occurring in diverse life circumstances that include moderately high levels of Past Negative or Present Fatalist TP.

Conclusion

Stress and trauma are ubiquitous. Indeed, it seems nary a day goes by without hearing of another mass murder, devastating earthquake, or war-related atrocity. As we face these experiences, how we perceive the passage of time and relate to people in our social networks will likely have a profound impact on our ability to cope. Yet we do not often recognize the subtle shifts in our TP that may affect, or result from, our social encounters. To the extent that social relationships and TP work interdependently to affect how we adapt to life's challenges it would behoove us to carefully examine the pathways linking them with psychological well-being across the lifespan. In so doing we can identify critical developmental implications that inform innovative clinical applications and help people stay grounded in the past, keenly aware of the present, and motivated toward the future despite the challenges they may face.

Acknowledgements I would like to acknowledge my collaborators for each of the studies reported herein. Dr. Philip G. Zimbardo worked closely with me on the Bay Area College Student study; Dr. Roxane C. Silver provided mentorship and support for the 1993 Southern California Fire Study (my dissertation research); and Drs. Roxane C. Silver, Michael Poulin, Danny McIntosh, Virginia Gil-Rivas, and Judith Andersen, comprise the team that conducted the 9/11 study. The Southern California Fire Study and the 9/11 study were both supported by grants provided to me and Dr. Silver by the National Science Foundation and the Josiah Macy Jr. Foundation.

References

Abbey, A., Abramis, D. J., & Caplan, R. D. (1985). Effects of different sources of social support and social-conflict on emotional well-being. *Basic and Applied Social Psychology, 6*(2), 111–129.

American Psychiatric Association. (2000). *Diagnostic and statistical manual* (Vol. 4). Washington, DC: American Psychiatric Association.

Atance, C. M., & O'Neill, D. K. (2001). Episodic future thinking. *Trends in Cognitive Sciences, 5*(12), 533–539.
Baumeister, R. F., & Leary, M. R. (1995). The need to belong – Desire for interpersonal attachments as a fundamental human-motivation. *Psychological Bulletin, 117*(3), 497–529.
Boniwell, I., & Zimbardo, P. (2004). Balancing one's time perspective in pursuit of optimal functioning. In P. Linley & S. Joseph (Eds.), *Positive psychology in practice*. Hoboken: Wiley.
Boniwell, I., Osin, E., Linley, P. A., & Ivanchenko, G. V. (2010). A question of balance: Time perspective and wellbeing in British and Russian samples. *The Journal of Positive Psychology, 5*(1), 24–40.
Brosschot, J. F., Gerin, W., & Thayer, J. F. (2006). The perseverative cognition hypothesis: A review of worry, prolonged stress-related physiological activation, and health. [Review]. *Journal of Psychosomatic Research, 60*(2), 113–124. doi:10.1016/j.jpsychores.2005.06.074.
Carelli, M. G., Wiberg, B., & Wiberg, M. (2011). Development and construct validation of the Swedish Zimbardo Time Perspective Inventory. *European Journal of Psychological Assessment, 27*(4), 220.
Carstensen, L. L., Isaacowitz, D. M., & Charles, S. T. (1999). Taking time seriously – A theory of socioemotional selectivity. *American Psychologist, 54*(3), 165–181.
Derogatis, L. R., & Melisaratos, N. (1983). The Brief Symptom Inventory: An introductory report. *Psychological Medicine, 13*, 595–605.
DeWall, C. N., Visser, P. S., & Levitan, L. C. (2006). Openness to attitude change as a function of temporal perspective. *Personality and Social Psychology Bulletin, 32*(8), 1010–1023. doi:10.1177/0146167206288009.
Drake, L., Duncan, E., Sutherland, F., Abernethy, C., & Henry, C. (2008). Time perspective and correlates of wellbeing. *Time and Society, 17*(1), 47–61.
Goldberg, J., & Maslach, C. (1996). *Understanding time: Connections between the past and future*. Paper presented at the Western Psychological Association, San Jose, CA.
Holman, E. A., & Silver, R. C. (1998). Getting "stuck" in the past: Temporal orientation and coping with trauma. *Journal of Personality and Social Psychology, 74*(5), 1146–1163.
Holman, E. A., & Silver, R. C. (2005). Future-oriented thinking and adjustment in a nationwide longitudinal study following the September 11th terrorist attacks. *Motivation and Emotion, 29*(4), 389–410. doi:10.1007/s11031-006-9018-9.
Holman, E. A., & Zimbardo, P. (2009). The social language of time: The time perspective-social network connection. *Basic and Applied Social Psychology, 31*(2), 136–147.
Kubzansky, L. D., Kawachi, I., Spiro, A., 3rd, Weiss, S. T., Vokonas, P. S., & Sparrow, D. (1997). Is worrying bad for your heart? A prospective study of worry and coronary heart disease in the Normative Aging Study. *Circulation, 95*(4), 818–824.
Lang, F. R., & Carstensen, L. L. (2002). Time counts: Future time perspective, goals, and social relationships. *Psychology and Aging, 17*(1), 125–139.
Lavi, T., & Solomon, Z. (2005). Palestinian youth of the Intifada: PTSD and future orientation. *Journal of the American Academy of Child and Adolescent Psychiatry, 44*(11), 1176–1183. doi:10.1097/01.chi.0000177325.47629.4c.
Melges, F. (1982). *Time and the inner future: A temporal approach to psychiatric disorders*. New York: Wiley.
Norbeck, J. S., Lindsey, A. M., & Carrieri, V. L. (1981). The development of an instrument to measure social support. *Nurs Research, 30*(5), 264–269.
Robins, L. N., Helzer, J. E., Croughan, J., & Ratcliff, K. S. (1981). National Institute of Mental Health Diagnostic Interview Schedule: Its history, characteristics, and validity. *Archives of General Psychiatry, 38*(4), 381–389.
Rook, K. S. (1984). The negative side of social interaction: Impact on psychological well-being. *Journal of Personality and Social Psychology, 46*(5), 1097–1108.
Tait, R., & Silver, R. C. (1989). Coming to terms with major negative life events. In J. Uleman & J. Bargh (Eds.), *Unintended thought* (pp. 351–382). New York: Guilford.

Terr, L. C. (1983). Time sense following psychic trauma: A clinical study of ten adults and twenty children. *American Journal of Orthopsychiatry, 53*(2), 244–261.

Trope, Y., & Liberman, N. (2003). Temporal construal. *Psychological Review, 110*(3), 403–421. doi:10.1037/0033-295x.110.3.403.

Twenge, J. M., Catanese, K. R., & Baumeister, R. F. (2003). Social exclusion and the deconstructed state: Time perception, meaninglessness, lethargy, lack of emotion, and self-awareness. *Journal of Personality and Social Psychology, 85*(3), 409–423.

Zhang, J. W., Howell, R. T., & Stolarski, M. (2012). Comparing three methods to measure a balanced time perspective: The relationship between a balanced time perspective and subjective well-being. *Journal of Happiness Studies*. doi:10.1007/s10902-012-9322-x.

Zimbardo, P. G., & Boyd, J. N. (1999). Putting time in perspective: A valid, reliable individual-differences metric. *Journal of Personality and Social Psychology, 77*(6), 1271–1288.

Zimbardo, P., & Boyd, J. (2009). *The Time Paradox: Using the new psychology of time to your advantage*. New York: Free Press.

Zimbardo, P., Sword, R. M., & Sword, R. K. M. (2012). *Time cure: Overcoming PTSD with the new psychology of time perspective therapy*. San Francisco: Jossey-Bass.

Time Perspective and Positive Aging

Pio Enrico Ricci Bitti, Manuela Zambianchi, and Joanna Bitner

Positive aging (or successful aging) has seen a growing interest in the field of psychogerontology research, due to the substantial changes that have occurred to the population pyramid. In developed countries, we are witnessing a progressive expansion of the elderly age group, due to an increased life-expectancy that now exceeds 80 years for women and is nearly the same for men (Eurostat 2012). A similar change brings about many challenges, including the pressing need to understand how to promote positive aging to the widest possible number of people.

Within the debate on the concept of "positive aging" itself and on the individual, psychosocial and contextual factors that could help one to reach it, time perspective is seen as a relevant factor that underlies many domains of human functioning. This chapter consists of four sections the first one focuses on the main contemporary theoretical models on positive aging that include the temporal dimension as a central feature or resource for aging well; the second one addresses the relevance of time dimensions for adopting a healthy lifestyle, while the third section considers the relevance of time perspective for well-being; the phenomenon of resilience, still to be studied in the older age, concludes the chapter. Indeed, the few available studies show the crucial role played by time in exceptional functioning late in life.

Theoretical Models of Successful Aging

The Socio-emotional Selectivity Theory: the relevance of perceived future time extension for social goals and social network.

P.E. Ricci Bitti (✉) • M. Zambianchi
Psychology Department, University of Bologna, Bologna, Italy
e-mail: pioenrico.riccibitti@unibo.it

J. Bitner
Institute of Psychology, Kasimierz Wielki University in Bydgoszcz, Bydgoszcz, Poland

M. Stolarski et al. (eds.), *Time Perspective Theory; Review, Research and Application: Essays in Honor of Philip G. Zimbardo*, DOI 10.1007/978-3-319-07368-2_28,

Developed by Carstensen et al. (1999), it is a life-cycle theory of social motivation, where the perception of future time plays a central role for the assignment of priorities to achieve social objectives, for preferences about social partners and for the extension of relational networks. It is based on three fundamental theoretical assumptions:

- social interaction is central to survival from a phylogenetic and ontogenetic human perspective;
- human beings are fundamentally agentic (active protagonist in determining and shaping his/her life through the constructive management of internal and external resources) and engage in kinds of behaviour that are driven by the mental anticipation of the realisation of important goals (objectives)
- since individuals are simultaneously committed to multiple objectives, their careful selection is a precursor of action and decision.

The socio-emotional selectivity theory maintains that the perception of future time affects the evaluation processes preceding the selection of these social objectives. It also suggests that the evaluations of individuals on the extent of their future time have a relevant impact on their emotional experience. The socio-emotional selectivity theory focuses on two different types of social objectives: the first includes expansive goals, such as acquiring knowledge or making new social contacts; the second includes goals related to feelings, such as emotional states or the perception of being needed by others. When time is perceived as open-ended (typically in the youth), expansive goals are pursued; on the contrary, when time is perceived as limited, emotionally meaningful objectives are preferred.

Social preferences are also influenced by the perception of future time: when the future is perceived as open, individuals like to meet new social partners (Lang and Carstensen 2002), while when future time is perceived as limited, individuals show preference for emotionally close social partners, who are likely to confirm their status, world vision and values. The progressive restriction of the social world of older people leads to a substantial change in their emotional feelings; they try to optimise and search for social experiences that lead to positive emotional experiences, pruning the peripheral ties, thus reducing the number of contacts, and focusing on closer friends and family.

The Proactivity Model of successful aging: time perspective as an inner resource.

This model, elaborated by Kahana and Kahana (2003) turns the perspective that characterised the theorisation of gerontology around, hypothesising that also in the late phase of life the individual maintains an agentic disposition towards his/her life context, trying to actively modify it, instead of adapting to it. Kahana and Kahana (2003) adopt a longitudinal, life-span perspective on successful aging, delineating the principal historical, contextual and individual mechanisms and processes that lead, in the long run, to positive or negative outcomes. Kahana and Kahana claim that there are two main processes available to older people to reach and maintain a high quality of life, in spite of declines and losses: the corrective adaptive behaviour and the preventive adaptive behaviour. Preventive behaviour is set in motion to reduce the risk of deleterious or critical events (eg. chronic illness, financial seatbacks, etc.) and preserve (or improve) physical, personal and social resources. Corrective behaviour is aimed, on the contrary, at managing critical ongoing events and at reducing their impact. Together, the two kinds of behaviour are viewed as proactive adaptations and defined as "the engine that drives successful aging" (Kahana et al. 2012, p. 439). These proactive adaptations are not set in motion by chance, but are preceded by motivational antecedents that can be connected to external resources and inner resources (Kahana et al. 2005). Among the inner resources we can find self-esteem, constructive coping strategies, altruism and future time orientation. Future time orientation positively influences the use of proactive adaptations (eg. active health promotion, helping others, the use of emergent technologies, such as Internet, the active modification of the life context) and directly affect perceived quality of life, the experience of positive emotions, the maintenance of valued activity and social relationships; according to Kahana and Kahana's perspective, all these factors are the core of successful aging.

The Life-Span Perspective on successful aging: primary control as a "future-centred strategy" for the optimisation of resources.

Schultz and Heckhausen (1996) claim that successful aging must be considered as a successful development and a positive adaptation to environmental circumstances and contexts, throughout all life cycles, rather than restricting it to the last decades of life. Their theoretical model is based on four general principles that regulate development during the life-span. The first principle concerns the actualisation of the individual's potential outcomes, which will only be achieved if he/she has had access to different environments and opportunities through which to understand his/her unique characteristics, talents, and in which to realise them. The second principle refers to the process of selection of life goals in order to best allocate the resources, invoking the processes of Selection, Optimisation and Compensation previously proposed by Baltes and Baltes (1990) as the basis of human development. The third principle refers to the use of constructive coping styles and compensation processes in respect to critical events and declines, while the fourth principle refers to the need to recognise the increasing specialisation of one's life-path.

The model is based on the construct of "control" that is considered the factor leading and characterising human development from infancy to old age; the underlying assumption is that humans desire to produce events or situations through which they may be able to modify the environment. The intentional actions set in motion by individuals refer to the broad category of *primary control*, through which they attempt to provoke effects in their life-context, while *secondary control* attempts to achieve changes in the inner world of the individual. Throughout life, primary and secondary controls work together to optimise development; primary control, defined as the most powerful force of development, is strictly interwoven with motivation and is guided by selection processes. Schultz & Heckhausen hypothesise that successful aging includes the development and maintenance of primary control during the course of life. Primary control, which could be compared to the proactive strategies described by Kahana and Kahana (2003), contains a future-oriented temporal quality, due to the selective activation of motivating goals. The authors indeed stress the hypothesis that long-term primary control potentials are linked to the possession of consistent resources that enable individuals to successfully engage in the environment; kinds of behaviour that maximise longevity and physical functioning potentials should receive high priority throughout life and this assumption highlights the relevance of future-orientated temporality for the adoption and maintenance of a healthy life-style (see below).

Healthy Life-Style and Time Perspective in Old Age

The debate on the relevance of time perspective on health in old age has received an important contribution by Rakowski (1986), according to whom health, illness and time perception are closely interrelated dimensions and may become increasingly integrated with age, so that health status can be considered as a "personal characteristic" that has its continuity in time.

Stressing that future temporal extension and the ability to schedule preventive behaviour can vary greatly from individual to individual, Rakowski suggested six points that represent challenges for older people; they are strictly related to the relationships between time and health in old age:

- Anticipating the trajectory of diseases in the coming months;
- Retaining the belief that one possesses one's own potential of future planning;
- Maintaining a continuity between past, present and future linked to one's identity and self-image;
- Assessing the possible future course of prescribed therapies;
- Setting short-term and long-term priorities for coping efforts;
- Adapting to future uncertainties.

Rakowski underlines the crucial importance of time perception and especially of future time for the maintenance of health throughout life and for the prevention of diseases and declines in old age, indicating that the time horizon should be considered an essential variable in adopting risk behaviours or, vice versa, in the active promotion of health behaviour.

A study carried out by Hamilton et al. (2003) analysed the relationships between time perspective and health promotion behaviour in a group of patients with a heart disease, who were attending a rehabilitation course. They assessed the relationships between time perspective (ZTPI, Zimbardo and Boyd 1999) and the presence of a healthy lifestyle, which included feeling responsible for one's own health, maintaining regular physical activity, adopting a balanced diet, the ability to handle stress, and cultivating close relationships, along with a sense of direction and purpose in life. Future time does not predict healthy behaviours, but only exerts a modest influence on the sense of responsibility for health. The close relationships between a Past-Positive and a Present-Hedonistic on one hand and the safeguard of health on the other, appears to support the hypothesis of the relevance of a balanced time perspective (Boniwell and Zimbardo 2004) for one's own health and its disappearance in the case of traumatic events such as stroke. Future time breaks down in favour of the present time, where it is possible to set important relational objectives and the past, which is the place of construction of experiences and biographical identity.

Referring to assumptions formulated by Bandura (1997) about the relevance of future orientation in determining behaviour, Kahana et al. (2001) investigated the role played by Future time perspective on physical activity in older people through a longitudinal design. The results confirm that older people who are more future-oriented keep up physical activities and non-competitive sports, such as walking, swimming, cycling, attending gymnastic courses at gym.

The positive role of future-oriented time perspectives in health protective behaviour was also confirmed by Adams and Nettle (2009) in a longitudinal study aimed at investigating the influence of individual and demographic factors on the quality of life of older people (ELSA, English Longitudinal Survey of Aging). This study assessed whether the extension of time devoted to expenses and family financial planning is associated with quitting smoking. Participants were split into those with a short Future time perspective (few weeks and months) and those who showed a long–term Future time perspective (5 and 10 years); they were evaluated three times, with an interval of 2 years. In the initial evaluation, those who planned short-range time were more likely to be smokers, compared to older people who were planning along more extended period of time. In line with this trend, long term financial planning was associated with an increased likelihood of quitting smoking in the following 4 years.

Referring to socio-emotional selectivity theory (Carstensen et al. 1999, 2006). Ziegelmann et al. (2006), highlighting the importance of perceived self-efficacy on risk perception and the formation of intentions, have investigated the role of Future time perspective (as the residual life-expectancy) in a study with a group of people aged between 18 and 80 years. They were selected at the end of a course of orthopedic rehabilitation and contacted again respectively 6 months and 12 months later for follow-up. The results confirm that the intention to perform recommended post-rehabilitation physical activity was linked to the perceived future extension: those who have limited life expectancy are driven by positive expectations, but less motivated to achieve strategic goals to ensure a better future, as to adopt a stable healthy behaviour. The group (to which belong the older people) who perceived a more limited future has less intentions to plan activities prescribed by doctors at the end of the rehabilitation programme and has carried out less physical activity in previous months, as emerged during the last follow-up.

A study on social representation of health and aging among older people (Zambianchi and Ricci Bitti 2010) evidenced that old people possess a complex and integrate representation of aging, defined as a period of life where it is possible to make future plans, to know new things and to continue to grow. This results indicate that for older people this stage of life is characterised by a complex time perspective, were both past and future represent two crucial temporal dimensions for aging well. The study also evidenced that those who perceived old age as a complex and rich stage of life open to future projects and, at the same time, enriched by Past Positive experiences possess a conception of health as a condition characterised by a biological, psychological and social well-being and by the availability of effective resources and skills in restoring, maintaining or improving well-being.

The role of future time perspective in predicting longevity was explored in a longitudinal study (Fry and Debats 2011) that involved an initial sample of 440 old people. Together with cognitive belief systems in a just world (Feather 1991) and future self-continuity perspectives (a dimension that assesses how much individuals perceive similarity between the present and future selves 15 years from now), future time perspective predicted a higher longevity. The authors postulate that the subjective sense of time plays an essential role in human motivation, so that incorporating an expansive time horizon influences individuals to pay greater attention in the time left to make decisions concerning a healthier future life, maximising attempts to preserve and protect future personal health and survival.

Time Perspective and Well-Being in Old Age

The concept of well-being has received increasing attention in recent decades from psychological research. Initially linked to the definition of *quality of life* (Camfield and Skevington 2008) originated from a sociological perspective and primarily related to material and objective life conditions of individuals, it has gradually moved towards the concept of optimal functioning and the subjective overall evaluation of life given by individuals. The study of well-being and optimal functioning gave rise to the movement of Positive Psychology (Seligman and Csikszentmihalyi 2000) which, turning the traditional line of inquiry centred on the treatment of dysfunctional conditions and illness around, emphasises the role of individual resources and potentials. The research on well-being has seen the emergence of two distinct theoretical approaches, respectively defined as *hedonic* (or *subjective well-being*) and *eudaimonic* (or *psychological well-being*) (Waterman 1993); the former based on the subjective evaluation of the emotional experiences that converges in the concept of "life satisfaction" and the latter on the definition of well-being as resulting in the development and actualisation of individual potentials within society.

A third dimension, which represents a crucial factor on the individual's positive functioning is *social well-being,* namely the perceived quality of social relationships within the communities and the society and his/her functioning within them (Keyes 1998; Mc. Millan and Chavis 1986). Psychological and social well-being have been considered by several authors as fundamental outcomes of positive aging (see par. 1) and their possible relationships with the time perspective of older people have been studied.

The current research in well-being and quality of life in older people does not provide unequivocal findings that specify the criteria for the well-being of older people. Some studies show that, in older people the satisfaction and well-being levels depend on their social activity (Diener et al. 2005) as well as, besides social commitment, their intellectual activity (Pintera 2008). The research results also show that the older people's place of residence (in care homes or with their own families) has an influential impact on the assessment of the quality of one's own life as well as on the fulfilment level of social needs (Okla 2006). Research shows that intentional social activity brought about as a part of care home residency is unquestionably beneficial; however, the entertainment does not need to be social to increase life satisfaction level. Sherer's research (1996) shows that providing computers for both residents of a care home as well as its daytime patients has a positive influence on their self-esteem and life satisfaction.

Among many concepts of quality of life, there is a consistent split between objective and subjective indicators (Sęk 2004). Subjective indicators of the quality of life are connected with, among others, a value system and individually defined meaning of life and life satisfaction. Research on the importance of values in the life of ageing people shows that religious values become more and more essential with age than edonistic values (Morcinek and Ignasiak 2009). Meaningful life feeling, seen as a fairly stable trait, is an important prerequisite for emotional balance and life satisfaction according to Wolicki (quoted by Popielski 1987). It is also stated that a meaningful life feeling is an important indicator of adaptation to reality, while life goals and the perception of time are factors related to the type of perceived meaning. Thus, it has been shown that people with a positive attitude towards life have a longer and balanced perspective of time (Zimbardo and Boyd 2008). Rakowski and Clark (1985) show that older people positively oriented towards the future have a higher life satisfaction level. Future time perspective is positively correlated with socio-economic status, while a lower status (e.g. in care homes) is concurrent with lower willingness to design the future and influences the reduction of Future time perspective (Freize et al. 1980).

Zambianchi and Ricci Bitti (2011) examined the relationship between social well-being and time perspective (ZTPI, Zimbardo and Boyd 1999) in a group of 138 older adults. Their results confirm the relevance of time perspective on the perceived overall social well-being. While Past-Negative and Present-Fatalistic perspectives exert a negative influence on it, the future time dimension shows a positive influence. Moreover, Present-Fatalistic and Past-Negative are negatively correlated with social acceptance, social contribution and social actualisation, three sub-dimensions of social well-being that respectively indicate the trust in others, the belief in one's own capacity to express potentials and talents within the society, and a positive belief towards social evolution. The Future time perspective, on the contrary, is positively associated with social actualisation and social integration: those, among older people, who are more "future-centred" have a more optimistic belief about the development and evolution of society and are more integrated in their local community, two aspects that are seen as protective and promotional of overall health during old age because they facilitate active social participation.

Bitner (2012) studied the relationship between life satisfaction (the Satisfaction with Life Scale – SWLS), as defined by Diener et al. (1985), and time perspective (the Zimbardo Time Perspective Inventory, ZTPI and the Trascendental Future Time Perspective Inventory, TFTPI – Zimbardo and Boyd 2008) as part of a research project concerning the subjective conditions of the quality of life during ageing. The research involved 445 people aged 65–96 (241 women and 204 men), of which 225 were residents of a care home and 220 were living with their own families, without cognitive deficits preventing the cognitive functioning necessary to take part in the interview. All of the older people who took part in the research received social support from their own families or institutions and reported higher life satisfaction levels than people without such care.

The results confirm the value of some of the parameters of time perspective (TP) for the subjective perception of life satisfaction in older people – depending on their place of residence (care homes or own families): people living with their own families experience higher life satisfaction levels than people living in a care homes. Overall, the subjective feeling of life satisfaction increases with age, reaching its peak in the 80–85 range. In the female group, values related to a transcendental future perspective, as well as present fatalism and future perspective, also increase with age. Older men, as years go by, think more about the future and less about their negative past. Positive past perspective is prevalent in people aged 76–85. Older people living in a care home, aged 77–82, are the most transcendental. Well-being is mainly correlated with a positive past perspective and inversely with a negative future perspective and present fatalism. Life satisfaction of older people living in a care home is only related to thinking positively about the past and hedonistically about the present, both among women and men. The well-being of people living with their own families is more influenced by the TP: they are more positively future-oriented and hedonistically present-oriented, while correlations with a negative past and present fatalism are inverse.

However, it is important to point out that subjects living with their own families present a positive relation between Future TP and happiness, whereas the experience of care home does not imply that development of future plans results in higher well-being; on the other hand Positive Past seems to influence the well-being of people living in a care home. In conclusion it seems that those who live with their own families derive joy from future planning whereas the residents in care homes are seeking their well being from their positive past experiences.

Kahana et al. (2012), according to their proactivity model of successful aging (see par. 1), examined the role of internal and external resources in the maintenance of psychological well-being and social activities among older adults. They took into account the previous health and social stress exposure and controlled factors like gender, education and age and their role on psychological well-being and social activities. Internal resources, like active and religious coping, and external resources, like available social support, were hypothesised to exert both direct and indirect influence on the psychological well-being and social activities. Their indirect influence would be achieved through proactive adaptations, among which planning for the future was considered.

The results confirm the relevance of proactive adaptations: general planning for the future and marshalling support were shown to be the strongest predictors of lack of depressive symptoms (the index of psychological well-being considered by authors) and social activities. These findings highlight the value of future-oriented planning behaviour in promoting successful aging; in this perspective, the future-oriented time perspective, assuming it is stable over time, may serve as a dispositional, inner resource in late life (Kahana et al. 2005).

Referring to the socio emotional selectivity theory and its postulated relevance of perceived future time extension for social adjustment across the life-span, Coudin and Lima (2011) investigated, in a large sample of old people from 23 European countries, whether the congruency between perceived future extension and social goals is related to subjective well-being. The congruent profile included individuals with open-ended Future time perspective and positive values in the goal index (prevalence of social acceptance and autonomy) and individuals with limited Future time perspective with negative values in the goal index (prevalence of emotional regulation and generativity, here defined as the amount of enjoyable time spent with immediate family). The incongruent profile included open ended Future time perspective and negative values in the goal index and limited Future time perspective associated with positive values in the goal index. Results show that for those with an open-ended Future time perspective, the congruency of goals leads to a higher level of subjective well-being, while for those with a future-limited time perspective the incongruity between time perception and goals is related to higher subjective well-being. These counterintuitive results are discussed by the authors assuming that goals such as having positive and active social relationships and being free to decide how to live life and thinking about creative new ideas are basic needs at all stages of life, and not only in the younger age.

As most researches on well-being and temporal organisation have been carried out in youth, adulthood and in first old age, Palgi and Shmotkin (2010) have investigated the level of life satisfaction, depression, physical health and autonomy in daily life in relation to the "temporal trajectories of life" in a sample of people aged between 85 and 106 years. They defined temporal trajectories as "a personally constructed configuration of subjective well-being composed of self-evaluations, that the person attributes to his or her past, present and anticipated future, and that represent a certain direction along the life course" (p. 578). They identified four principal temporal trajectories:

- the equilibrated trajectory, characterised by satisfaction for past, present and anticipated future;
- the descending trajectory, characterised by satisfaction for past, middle level of satisfaction for present and low satisfaction for the anticipated future;
- the unreported trajectory, characterised by no evaluation of satisfaction for any of time dimensions;
- the no-future trajectory, characterised by evaluation of satisfaction for the past and the present but not for the anticipated future.

The results indicate that the equilibrated trajectory, where the past, the present and the future (as harmonic integration between time dimensions, that could be compared to the construct of balanced time perspective of Boniwell and Zimbardo 2004) are simultaneously and positively visualised, is associated with higher level of functioning and satisfaction in this stage of life. On the contrary, the descending and no-future trajectories are characterised by a medium level of overall functioning and satisfaction, while the unreported trajectory is linked to the worse level of overall functioning.

According to Frankl (quoted by Klamut 2010), time perception can substantially influence the adaptation to old age, while the end-of-life perspective becomes a factor increasing the relevance of life experiences. A perspective of time perception driven by a transcendental future is related to a given person's religion, spirituality and their belief in life after death; (Zimbardo and Boyd 2009). Belief in a transcendental future among CH residents can lessen the severity of their life conditions, socio-economic status and current unequal treatment (Zimbardo and Boyd 2009)

The Phenomenon of Resilience in Old Age and Its *Temporal Qualities*

The concept of psychological resilience was originally developed in the field of developmental psychopathology in childhood and adolescence (Garmezy 1991; Masten and Obradovic 2006). The term *resilience* describes the fact that certain children do not become socially disfunctional despite growing up in very hard socioeconomic conditions. Garmezy defined resilience as "the capacity to recover and maintain adaptive behaviour that may follow an initial withdrawal or incapacity upon the beginning of a stressful event" (Garmezy 1991, p. 549). The concept of psychological resilience identifies two types of phenomena:

1. the maintenance of normal development despite risks and impairments;
2. the recovery of normal functioning after a traumatic experience.

Until now, the research on aging processes has seldom addressed the issue of how to define resilience in old age and what processes, conditions and resources can support it.

Staudinger et al. (2000) hypothesised that psychological resilience, related to the self and to personality, characterises the phenomenon of aging, despite the increasing risk of losses and decline. Aging satisfaction and a lower perception of depressivity are core dimensions of resilience in old age. The model they tested includes several risk factors, such as a low number of years of education, a low income, a number of diagnoses and self-related protective processes, such as coping styles, goal systems, emotions and the experience of time. The potential protective value of the experience of time was confirmed: an orientation towards the future and optimism positively predict aging satisfaction. Moreover, a strong orientation towards the future negatively influences aging satisfaction only among those who are socio-economically disadvantaged, perhaps due to the fact they cannot realise projects and goals because of their low financial conditions.

The role of the time perspective in the phenomenon of resilience is addressed by Smotkin (2003) within a study on Holocaust survivors; he claims that time perspective (Zimbardo and Boyd 1999) is important for understanding processes of coping, well-being and aging, confirming that there is both clinical and empirical evidence suggesting incongruities in the time perspective of trauma survivors and Holocaust survivors in particular. These difficulties may be expressed in either avoidance or over-emphasis on one's past history, a failure to integrate the traumatic experience with the subsequent disruption in the sense of life continuity. Shmotkin and Barilan (2002) studied medical records and interview data of 38 Holocaust survivors. The results showed two distinct factors through which the survivors related themselves to their Holocaust experience. According to the first factor, labelled Holocaust-as Present, the trauma is conceived as actually continuing in present life: this time orientation towards the Holocaust is positively correlated with mental symptoms and a number of medical diagnoses. In contrast, according to the second factor, labelled Holocaust-as Past, the trauma is conceived as a demarcated past event that ended a long time ago. This involved a relative freedom from the intrusion of traumatic memories and related emotional remnants into the present life. The Holocaust-as Past factor is associated with fewer mental symptoms and a lower number of medical diagnoses. A central aspect of this resilience, concluded the authors, is related to the ability of many survivors to formulate new meanings in life.

Conclusions

The importance of the time perspective in positive or successful aging is confirmed by several studies: time perspective and positive aging, however, show a very complex relationship. Within studies on well-being, seen in either its individual or social qualities, the presence of an harmonic integration between past, present and future time dimensions is crucial.

The older people who can look at the past as life experiences and knowledge that constitute the basis of a positive identity and that give a "positive frame of mind", to the present as a time where it is possible to have enriching and rewarding relationships, and to the future as being open to life-projects, will tend to perceive a higher level of overall well-being. Emerging data seem to endorse a complex perspective on positive aging, both regarding its outcome and the processes that lead to it, challenging those perspectives (such as the socio-emotional selectivity theory), that don't take into account the relevance of time dimensions other than the future, and other needs, such as a social network and social goals (e.g., knowledge and self-fulfilment), which have both been confirmed, by several studies, to be relevant across the entire life-span.

Future time perspective seems to be rather crucial for the promotion of a healthy lifestyle and the reduction of risk behaviour. A future-oriented time perspective is a precondition for long-term planning, for maintaining constant physical activity or other kinds of behaviour, such as adherence to medical prescriptions and adopting a healthy diet. Understanding how time perspective can be included in preventive and training programmes for older people is becoming crucial to help them take actions aimed at preventing the decline of health and their overall efficiency, thereby reducing the risk of disability (see Boniwell in this volume), as indeed evidenced by the studies of Kahana et al. (2001) and Ziegelman et al. (2006), time perspective influences the maintenance of positive healthy behaviours.

Future studies will also investigate the role of time perspective in exceptional positive functioning despite strong adversities; the phenomenon of resilience in old age, and the factors capable of promoting it, represent a further frontier of knowledge, which will surely increase the theoretical and practical responses to the contemporary challenge of successful aging.

References

Adams, J., & Nettle, D. (2009). Time Perspective, personality and smoking, body mass and physical activity: An empirical study. *British Journal of Health Psychology, 14*, 83–105.

Baltes, P. B., & Baltes, M. (1990). Theoretical propositions of life-span developmental psychology: On the dynamics between growth and decline. *Developmental Psychology, 5*, 611–626.

Bandura, A. (1997). *Self-efficacy: The exercise of control*. New York: W.H. Freeman & Company.

Bitner, J. (2012). *Podmiotowe uwarunkowania jakości życia w starości: znaczenie perspektywy czasowej*. [Subjective conditions for the quality of life of older people: value of time perspective]. Unpublished research report, Faculty of Psychology, University of Warsaw.

Boniwell, I., & Zimbardo, P. G. (2004). Balancing one's time perspective in pursuit optimal functioning. In P. A. Linley & S. Joseph (Eds.), *Positive psychology in practice* (pp. 165–178). Hoboken: Wiley.

Camfield, L., & Skevington, S. M. (2008). On subjective well-being and quality of life. *Journal of Health Psychology, 6*, 764–775.

Carstensen, L. (2006). The influence of a sense of time on human development. *Science, 312*, 1913–1915.

Carstensen, L. L., Isaacowitz, D. H., & Charles, S. T. (1999). Taking time seriously: A theory of socioemotional selectivity. *American Psychologist, 54*, 165–181.

Coudin, G., & Lima, M. L. (2011). Being well as time goes by: Future time perspective and well-being. *International Journal of Psychology and Psychological Therapy, 2*, 219–232.

Diener, E., Emmons, R. A., Larson, R. J., & Griffin, S. (1985). The satisfaction with life scale. *Journal of Personality Assessment, 49*, 71–75.

Diener, E., King, L., & Lyubomirsky, S. (2005). The benefits of frequent positive affect: Does happiness lead to success? *Psychological Bulletin, 136*(6), 803–855.

Eurostat. (2012). *Population structure and ageing*, in http://epp.eurostat.ec.europa.eu

Feather, N. T. (1991). Human values, global self-esteem, and belief in a just world. *Journal of Personality, 1*, 83–107.

Freize, E., Gorman, B., & Wessman, A. (1980). Temporal span delay of gratification socio-economic status. *Journal of Genetic Psychology, 137*, 247–255.

Fry, P. S., & Debats, D. L. (2011). Cognitive beliefs and future time perspective: Predictors of mortality and longevity. *Journal of Aging Research, 1*, 2–13.

Garmezy, N. (1991). Resilience in children's adaptation to negative live events and stressed environments. *Pediatric Annals, 20*(9), 459–466.

Hamilton, J. M., Kives, K. D., Micevski, V., & Grace, L. (2003). Time perspective and health-promoting behavior in a cardiac rehabilitation population. *Behavioral Medicine, 28*, 131–139.

Kahana, E., & Kahana, B. (2003). Contextualizing successful aging: New directions in an age-old search. In R. Settersen Jr. (Ed.), *Invitation to the life course* (pp. 225–255). Amitivylle: Baywood.

Kahana, E., Lawrence, R. H., Kahana, B., Kercher, K., Wisniewski, M. A., Stoller, E., Tobin, J. D., & Stange, K. (2001). Long-term impact of preventive proactivity on quality of life in the old-old. *Psychosomatic Medicine, 64*, 383–394.

Kahana, E., Kahana, B., & Zjiang, J. (2005). Motivational antecedents of preventive proactivity in late life: Linking future orientation and exercise. *Motivation and Emotion, 29*, 443–464.
Kahana, E., Kelley-More, J., & Kahana, B. (2012). Proactive aging: A longitudinal study of stress, agency, and well-being in late life. *Aging and Mental Health, 4*, 438–451.
Keyes, C. L. M. (1998). Social well-being. *Social Psychology Quarterly, 2*, 121–140.
Klamut, R. (2010). *Kwestionariusz Postaw Życiowych KPŻ. Podręcznik.* [Conduct of life questionnaire. Manual]. Warsaw: Psychological Test Workshop, Polish Psychological Society.
Lang, F. R., & Carstensen, L. L. (2002). Time counts: Future time perspective, goals, and social relationships. *Psychology and Aging, 1*, 125–139.
Masten, A. S., & Obradovic', J. (2006). Competence and resilience in development. *Annals of New York Academy of Sciences, 1094*, 13–27.
Mc Millan, D. W., & Chavis, D. M. (1986). Sense of community: A definition and theory. *Journal of Community Psychology, 14*, 6–23.
Morcinek, U., & Ignasiak, A. (2009). Hierarchia wartości człowieka w obliczu starości. [Hierarchy of human values in the face of old age]. In T. Ziółkowska & L. Konopska (Eds.), *W kręgu niepełnosprawności – teoretyczne i praktyczne aspekty poszukiwań w pedagogice specjalnej* (pp. 129–140). Szczecin: University of Szczecin.
Okla, W. (2006). Psychospołeczne uwarunkowania jakości życia osób starszych w rodzinach własnych i w domach opieki społecznej. [Psychosocial factors of the quality of life of older people living with their families and in care homes]. In S. Steuden & M. Marczuk (Eds.), *Starzenie się a satysfakcja z życia* (pp. 29–38). Lublin: Wydawnictwo KUL.
Palgi, Y., & Shmotkin, D. (2010). The predicament of time near the end of life: Time perspective trajectories of life satisfaction among the old-old. *Aging and Mental Health, 5*, 577–586.
Pintera, J. (2008). *Rodzaj aktywnosci i temperament a posiom inteligencji akrystalizowanej i zadowolenie z zycia w akresie pòznej dorosloscі* [Type of activity and temper in relation with the level of crystalized intelligence and life satisfaction in late adulthood]. Unpublished thesis, Faculty of Psychology, University of Warsaw, Warsaw.
Popielski, K. (Ed.). (1987). *Człowiek – pytanie otwarte. [Human – an open question]*. Lublin: Redakcja Wydawnictw KUL.
Rakowski, W. (1986). Future time perspective: Applications to the health context of later adulthood. *American Behavioural Scientist, 29*, 730–745.
Rakowski, W., & Clark, N. (1985). Future outlook, caregiving and carereceiving in the family context. *The Gerontologist, 25*, 618–623.
Schultz, R., & Heckhausen, J. (1996). A life span model of successful aging. *American Psychologist, 7*, 702–714.
Sęk, H. (Ed.). (2004). *Społeczna psychologia kliniczna. [Social clinical psychology]*. Warsaw: Polish Scientific Publishers PWN.
Seligman, M., & Csikszentmihalyi, M. (2000). Positive psychology. An introduction. *American Psychologist, 1*, 5–14.
Sherer, M. (1996). The impact of using personal computers on the lives of nursing home residents. *Physical and Occupational Therapy in Geriatrics, 14*, 13–31.
Shmotkin, D., & Barilan, Y. M. (2002). Expressions of Holocaust experience and their relationship to mental symptoms and physical morbidity among Holocaust survivors patients. *Journal of Behavioral Medicine, 25*, 115–134.
Smotkin, D. (2003). Vulnerability and resilience intertwined: A review of research on Holocaust survivors. In R. Jacoby & G. Keinan (Eds.), *Between stress and hope: From a disease-centered to a health –centered perspective* (pp. 213–233). Westport: Praeger.
Staudinger, U. M., Freund, A. M., Linden, M., & Maas, I. (2000). Self, personality and life regulation: Facets of psychological resilience in old age. In P. B. Baltes & K. U. Mayer (Eds.), *The Berlin aging study: Aging from 70 to 100* (pp. 302–328). Cambridge: Cambridge University Press.
Waterman, A. S. (1993). Two conceptions of happiness: Contrasts of personal expressiveness (eudaimonia) and hedonic enjoyment. *Journal of Personality and Social Psychology, 64*, 678–691.

Zambianchi, M., & Ricci Bitti, P. E. (2010). Rappresentazioni sociali della salute e dell'invecchiamento in un gruppo di anziani [Social representations of health and aging among the elderly]. *Psicologia della Salute, 2*, 95–110.

Zambianchi, M., & Ricci Bitti, P. E. (2011). Benessere sociale e prospettiva temporale in età anziana [Social wellbeing and time perspective in old age]. *Ricerche di Psicologia, 2*, 221–242.

Ziegelmann, J. P., Lippke, S., & Schwarzer, R. (2006). Subjective residual life expectancy in health self-regulation. *Journal of Gerontology: Psychological Science, 61 B*, 195–201.

Zimbardo, P. G., & Boyd, J. N. (1999). Putting time in perspective: A valid, reliable, individual differences metric. *Journal of Personality and Social Psychology, 6*, 1271–1288.

Zimbardo, P. G., & Boyd, J. N. (2008). *The time paradox*. New York: Free Press.

Time Perspective Coaching

Ilona Boniwell and Evgeny Osin

The centrality of time in our lives cannot be underestimated, and as many coaches would not dispute, the number of clients presenting for coaching or therapy with one or several temporal-related problems is on the rise. Issues range from not meeting deadlines, never getting on top of the to-do-list or email inbox, living things up until the last minute, through to realising that one has forgotten the birthday of his wife for the third year in a row, being too easily distracted by a more interesting task, or not quite knowing where the exit from a rat-race is.

This is precisely why time management is one of the most prolific self-help topics on offer. The term produces over a 100,000 book matches in amazon.com at a click of a button. Surely, there is nothing out there that has not been said already, so why do we need to add the time perspective into the story?

Let us first briefly consider the history and science behind time management. The term had first appeared in literature in the early 1930s, and was primarily applied to those in middle and upper-management positions in private companies. Larsson and Sanne (2005), who set themselves a task to content-analyse the advice of major self-help books on avoiding time shortage, identified six core categories of time management strategies: streamlining tasks (finding how to do the same task using less time), buying household services, minding one's basic needs (including food, exercise, time for hobbies), setting limits in relation to others (learning to say no, sharing household responsibilities with family members), setting limits to time-consuming aspirations (effectively, lowering aspirations instead of aiming for the best possible option), and using effective change methods.

Although time-management programmes are widespread and popular (e.g. Lakein 1973), the evaluation of them has been extremely limited and has rarely

I. Boniwell (✉)
Positran and Department of Psychology, Anglia Ruskin University, Paris, France
e-mail: i.boniwell@gmail.com

E. Osin
Department of Psychology, National Research University Higher
School of Economics, Moscow, Russia

M. Stolarski et al. (eds.), *Time Perspective Theory; Review, Research and Application: Essays in Honor of Philip G. Zimbardo*, DOI 10.1007/978-3-319-07368-2_29,

looked at the effects of such training on actual time-management behaviours (Claessens 2004). The only systematic review of time management literature to date has identified a total of 32 empirical studies on time management conducted between 1982 and 2004 (Claessens et al. 2007). The review demonstrates that although time management behaviours relate positively to perceived control of time, job satisfaction, and health, and negatively to stress, their relationship to performance at work and in the academic domain is not clear. Time management training seems to enhance time management skills, but this does not automatically transfer to better accomplishment. The majority of studies utilised self-reports and few have addressed the question of improvements in objective outcomes (Hanel 1982; Hall and Hursch 1982; Bost 1984). Those that did have found that time management training has little or no effect on time management behaviours, job satisfaction or performance (Macan 1994, 1996; Macan et al. 1990). These are astonishing findings, taking into account the financial and otherwise resources invested by companies into time management training.

This brief introduction raises two major questions. First of all, given the widespread use and acceptance of the value of time management behaviours, how is it possible that such a modest amount of empirical research has been conducted? Secondly, if we are to take these findings seriously, how come that time management training has such limited impact?

One possible explanation for the failure of time management training to produce desired results may be attributed to basing it on the so-called "objective paradigm of time" and thus focusing on the wrong thing – behaviour rather than psychology of time, and on efficiency rather than overall balance and satisfaction. Another possibility is that time management advocates very generalised strategies that frequently follow a "one size fits all" principle, despite most new research pointing towards developing interventions based on an understanding of an individual's specific needs (Lyubomirsky 2008). This is precisely why time perspective-based temporal coaching may offer us a unique opportunity of developing personalised interventions for the complexity of individual profiles brought about by completion of the Zimbardo Time Perspective Inventory (ZTPI, Zimbardo and Boyd 1999). Assuming a shared knowledge of the time perspective (TP) dimensions and corresponding measures, the chapter will proceed to examine how time perspective issues may be raised in coaching, focusing on the interventions and questions targeting specific TP dimensions.

Getting Started with TP Coaching

So how can the concept of TP be consciously and usefully applied in the consulting room? The first step, of course, is suggesting to the client to explore the concept together, if the coach feels it may be of relevance. Assuming the client is interested, the coach can invite him/her to discover what their time perspective profile may look like, using Zimbardo Time Perspective Inventory (ZTPI)

(Zimbardo and Boyd 1999). ZTPI is available for free on the Time Paradox website on its own[1] or as part of more comprehensive commercial diagnostics tools for coaches and clients, such as the Time Intelligence Report,[2] which also measures 10 other dimensions of the way respondent structures time and provides a range of suggestions on improving personal time management.

In some situations the coach may choose to use observation and/or questioning to gain insight into the client's TP. For instance, what stories is a client telling and re-telling him/herself and how often? What is the tone of those stories – positive, neutral or negative? How often does the client find him/herself thinking about the past? If yes, what kinds of memories come to mind (past TP, negative or positive)? Given a choice between going to a party tonight or completing an important project, what is the likely response (potentially showing the difference between the Present Positive TP and Future TP)? How far in the future does the client project their hopes and aspirations (Future TP)? What does the client feel they need to stop, start and continue in their daily routine to achieve the goals they hope to achieve?

If the client makes a choice to complete the on-line ZTPI, it may be useful to ask him or her to print the results out and then consider the results together during the next coaching session, as experience shows that many clients do not easily understand the test results and may require some help in evaluating this information. Unless the coach has existing psychometric training, which would allow him or her to interpret the questionnaire results in more depth, the basic conversation about the results is often limited to:

(a) Seeing if the client's results on each of the TP dimensions are higher or lower than the 50th percentile, the 16th/84th percentiles, and 2nd/98th percentiles? It is important to explain to the client that the absolute values are not important in comparison to the relative values, and that being in the top percentile on one of the "negative" dimensions is not the same as a similar position on one of the "positive" ones.
(b) Comparing the client's profile with the so-called "ideal time perspective" profile, discussing some research findings underlying the ideal profile (see the section on the balanced time perspective) and exploring together to what extent the ideal profile appears relevant to the client (we should not necessarily assume that it always would).

Essentially, with the exception of individuals who have had prior psychometric training, the role of the coach is not so much to communicate and explain the ZTPI results to the client, but rather to accompany the client in trying to make sense of their own results, using emerging reactions as triggers for deepening the coaching conversation. It may also happen that the client would disagree with the outcomes of the test. This may be due to a full list of extraneous factors, such as English as a second language, completing the test too fast, or without paying much attention to the questions. On the other hand, disagreeing with the results may indicate the lack

[1] http://www.thetimeparadox.com/zimbardo-time-perspective-inventory/

[2] http://www.timeintelligence.co.uk/

of awareness or acceptance of the reality on behalf of the client. In either of these cases, however, the most helpful posture of the coach would be to explore both the reaction of the client, as well as their current vision of themselves, probing this vision as appropriate.

The identification of the client's TP profile could initiate further coaching work around: raising awareness of some unproductive responses associated with habitual temporal orientations; devising strategies to develop under-used temporal zones; finding the links and connections between past, present and future temporal zones in order to develop continuity in the client's life narrative; questioning the dominance of the Future TP in Western societies and evaluating an impact that this social belief has on the individual life of the client (Boniwell 2005). The subsequent sections of the chapter will consider these avenues in further detail, taking each TP dimension in turn, suggesting some interventions and questions, and finally terminating with tools and questions for increasing the balanced TP.

Coaching Around the Past-Negative TP

As we know, the Past-Negative TP, characterised by items such as "*Painful past experiences keep being replayed in my mind*", reflects a generally negative, pessimistic and aversive attitude towards the past, which may be based on actual traumatic life events or a negative reconstruction of past occurrences. If a client exhibits a strong Past-Negative perspective and his or her coach does not have a background in counselling or psychotherapy, this might be a strong indicator for referring this client to a therapist, as the issues that may arise are likely to be outside of the scope of a coach's expertise.

Alternatively, if it is decided to continue coaching, three evidence-based interventions may be suitable for decreasing the Past-Negative TP: expressive writing, forgiveness exercises and positive portfolio. Let us consider these one by one.

The originator of the *expressive writing* Professor James Pennebaker (1997, 2004), has shown that writing can organise thoughts and emotions and help find meaning in tragic experiences, with depression, anxiety and rumination decreasing dramatically after a series of corresponding exercises. If one has experienced a particular adversity, the coach may suggest that over the next few days the client tries writing about their deepest emotions and thoughts that influenced their life the most. In this writing, the client can really let go and explore the event and how it has affected him or her. This event might be explored in the context of their childhood, child–parent relationships, people they have loved or even their career. They should write for a minimum of 20 min over four consecutive days (although they may choose write for longer and over a longer period of time). However, if the tragedy is too raw, it is usually best to wait until one is emotionally ready to take such a step.

Confucius once said: "Those who cannot forgive break the bridge over which they themselves must pass." Usually we think of *forgiveness* in terms of the victim altruistically excusing the wrongdoer, whose conscience is then eased. From this traditional perspective, the wrongdoer benefits but the victim gains nothing. But what if we take the perspective that forgiveness is something that one can primarily do for themselves? Researchers are beginning to examine the nature of forgiveness and evidence is showing that forgiveness is better for your well-being than going through life harbouring grudges and contemplating revenge (Witvliet et al. 2001). Forgiveness reduces anger, hostility, depression, anxiety, and negative emotions. In addition, forgiving people are more likely to be happier, more agreeable, and more serene. Forgiveness is also linked to physical health benefits such as a reduction in blood pressure levels and it may aid in cardiovascular recovery from stress (Friedberg et al. 2007). On the other hand, nursing grudges or dwelling on revenge not only prevents you moving on, it also prompts higher levels of anger and sadness and a significantly higher heart rate and blood pressure. Research has also shown that forgiveness can be taught, and therefore, relatively easily integrated into coaching sessions. Clients can be encouraged to read about various public figures who have practised forgiveness, such as Nelson Mandela or Mahatma Gandhi, imagining forgiving the wrongdoer or practising empathising in their daily life – avoiding jumping to conclusions if someone does something they don't understand well. A very powerful exercise involves writing a forgiveness letter to a person they believe had wronged them, being specific about the hurt, how this made them feel and what they have learnt from the experience (McCullough and Witvliet 2002). Once the letter has been written, it can be read out and discussed within a coaching session. There is little evidence that actually sending the letter is helpful and may make things worse.

Using the metaphor of the artist's portfolio, Fredrickson (2009) recommends creating a personal *positive portfolio*, unique for each individual and derived from their previous personal experience of positive emotions. A positive portfolio is a collection of texts, poetry, quotes, images, drawings, photographs, music or objects, all that can remind the client of a positive emotion they would like to focus on. This portfolio may or may not include work-related activities (this would partially depend on the coaching context - life or executive coaching). It is simply a personal collection of reminders of what triggers different positive emotions, such as joy for this person. Positive emotions could range from serenity, inspiration, awe, joy, love, gratitude, security, safety, pride, empowerment, to ebullience, etc. The portfolio can be created for one or several of these emotions, and can be utilised during the moments of depression or sadness to remind oneself of the good times in life.

The coach can use the following general questions guidelines for each of the emotions:

- Consider your life as a whole and think about (one of the positive emotions here). Think about the times you felt it clearly and deeply. What were the triggers of those nourishing states?
- When was the last time you felt this emotion?
- Where were you?

- What were you doing?
- What was happening?
- What objects or mementos would remind you of this emotion?
- How could you assemble them together?
- What could you do right now to cultivate this feeling?

Fredrickson (2009) suggests further questions that can be posed to tap into particular emotions, for example (see her book for more excellent ideas):

- When have things truly gone your way, perhaps even better than you expected? (joy)
- When do you feel the urge to replay a kindness? What inspires you to get creative about giving back? (gratitude)
- When have you felt fully at peace and serene, truly content with where and who you are? (serenity)
- When have you felt intensely open and alive, as though your own inner horizons were expanding before your eyes? (interest)
- What do you notice first when you enter a bookstore or browse through your favourite magazines? (curiosity)
- When faced with uncertainty, when have you feared the worst by still somehow believed that things could change for the good? (hope)
- What makes you hold your head high and stand up tall? What makes you want to share your good news with others? (pride)
- What makes you feel silly and fun-loving? (amusement)
- When have you come across true human excellence or virtue? (inspiration)
- When have you felt part of something much larger than yourself? (awe)
- When have you felt close, safe, and secure within your relationship, trusting? (love)

Apart from traumatic experiences that come from outside, another component of Past-Negative time perspective is regret that is usually associated with one's own actions, such as having made a mistake or missed a good opportunity. When a person is caught up in regret, he or she is unable to let go, to forgive oneself for what is seen as having made a mistake from the perspective of the present situation. When the tendency to blame oneself is particularly strong, the client may need to be referred to a therapist. A coach may help the client to turn the painful experience of regret into a learning experience by reflecting together on the following questions:

- Was it possible to recognize that the choice you made was wrong at the moment you were making it? Was there a valid reason for making the choice you made? (forgiving oneself)
- Is there something you can learn from this experience? What advice would you give to a person who finds him/herself in the same situation? (learning from experience)
- If you would ever encounter a similar situation in the future, how would you recognize it and what would you do?

Coaching Interventions Around the Past-Positive TP

The past TP is associated with focus on family, tradition, history and continuity of self over time. The Past-Positive TP reflects a warm, pleasurable, though often sentimental view of one's past, with an emphasis on maintaining relationships with family and friends. The Past-Positive scale contains items such as: *Happy memories of good times spring readily to mind* and *I enjoy stories about how things used to be in the "good old times."* The Past-Positive TP facilitates interaction in the course of meaningful activity, enables long-lasting social ties, contributes to creating a strong sense of community and increases well-being. In fact, it has the strongest association with well-being than all other individual TPs, making it an extremely important vehicle for the development of well-being (Boniwell et al. 2010). Clients low on this variable are frequently over-focused on the future, and/or present, and may need help to reconnect with their past (if they desire to do so, of course).

The last intervention introduced in the previous session (positive portfolio) would also serve as a good vehicle for the development of the Past-Positive TP. However, further work can be done to enhance so-called *positive reminiscence*.

Research has considered whether all remembering is good, whether we can identify better or worse ways to remember. For example, should one consider why and how a positive experience had occurred or just let their memory run wild? One study asked its participants to set aside 10 min twice a day for a week to engage with their positive memories. In one condition they were asked to reflect on one of their memories by allowing the associated images to come to mind. The other, memorabilia, group was asked to focus on an object associated with their good memories. Unsurprisingly, both of these groups had an increase in their positive feelings. Saying that, those asked to simply imagine their memories had seen their memories more vividly and experienced more positive emotions (Bryant et al. 2005). Similarly, Sonia Lyubomirsky's studies (2008) show that analysing one's past does little to enhance happiness, whilst replaying or reliving positive life events, as though rewinding a videotape, enhances joy. In coaching sessions, positive reminiscence can be facilitated by asking questions such as:

- What are some of the things from your past that bring a smile on your face?
- Breaking your past into life stages (pre-school, primary school, teenage years, youth, etc), what are the most memorable positive experiences that come to your mind?
- How would you connect the dots of your life, in the words of Steve Jobs? What is the positive meaning of the events and choices of your past that didn't make sense at the time, but somehow make perfect sense now?

Probably the most powerful of all coaching techniques, different variants of *what went well* exercise have been investigated by several researchers, always with substantial results (Seligman et al. 2005; Sheldon and Lyubomirsky 2004). This exercise prompts one to focus on the positive things of their recent past. It has been found to lastingly increase happiness and decrease depressive symptoms for up to 6 months. The instructions are fairly straightforward and should be given a week ahead of the next coaching session. For the duration of 1 week, the client is asked to look back at their day just before going to bed and to find three things that went well for them during the day. They need to write them down and reflect on why did the good thing happen, who or what can they be grateful for this (their own role, as well as contribution made by other people). The results can then be discussed with the coach a week later.

Ultimately, gratitude is an imperative component for well-being, which forces people to step back and reflect upon what and whom they have in their life, as well as counteract complacency and 'taken-for-grantedness'. One of the most powerful (albeit fleeting) positive impacts on well-being is achieved through *the gratitude visit* (Seligman et al. 2005). The gratitude visit requires the client to write a letter to someone they never properly thanked. Then they can either read the letter out loud in person to this individual or send the letter through the mail (though the 1st format is ideal). Even more interesting is that this exercise works even when they don't send the letter (Lyubomirsky et al. 2006), and it is easy to see how such an exercise can be integrated into a coaching session (i.e. the letter can first be read out loud and discussed with the coach).

An essential aspect of the Past-Positive TP is one's connection with people from their past, with family, with traditions, with their community, so many of the coaching interventions can be directed towards these issues, ranging from creating *a family tree,* helping a client to embark on creating a *birthdays calendar* (people low on the Past-Positive TP are usually the ones that forget everyone's birthdays) or encouraging them to participate in *community projects or events*. These developments can be facilitated by questions such as:

- Tell me about your earliest memory of your best friend?
- Who are the people from your past with whom you would like to reconnect? How would you like to proceed?
- How do you feel about traditions? Do you prefer to engage with existing traditions (which ones and why?) or create your own ones (how would you go about that?)?
- What part of your neighbourhood environment you connect with the most? Why?

Coaching Interventions Around Present-Fatalistic TP

The Present-Fatalistic TP is characterised by helplessness, hopelessness and a belief that spiritual, governmental or other outside forces control one's life. This TP orientation is expressed by statements including: *It doesn't make sense to worry about the future, since there is nothing that I can do about it anyway* and *Fate determines much in my life*. Needless to say, this TP is negatively associated with well-being, and should be decreased whenever possible (Boniwell et al. 2010). We suggest that the coaching interventions around the Present-Fatalistic TP should be focused on the reduction of passive activities, such as watching TV, and on developing autonomy and responsibility.

Evidence suggests that people with the Present-Fatalistic TP are more likely to spend their time engaging in time-wasting unproductive activities such as television watching. Having time to spare is associated with paradoxical findings. Even though people are often desperate for more free time, they sometimes do not know what to do with it when they get it. For example, unemployment is often associated with a significant decrease in well-being, mainly through loss of income and structure to the day (Jahoda 1981; Bond and Feather 1988), and few unemployed people find their leisure time very satisfying. As time perspective is likely to be affected by situational factors, we can expect that the Present-Fatalistic TP is likely to increase further during the periods of unemployment (Lewin 1942/1997).

Television viewing, despite being rated relatively low in terms of pleasure (Csikszentmihalyi 1992) is topping the list of time-wasters. Already in 1990s nearly a third of all free time (in average 3 h per day) was reported as being spent in front of the television (Tyrrell 1995). Currently, the average daily time spent in front of TV is 3 h 32 min in France, 4 h in the UK and 5 h 11 min US, accounting to 10 years of watching TV vs. 9 years of working in an average lifetime). TV viewing is associated with boredom, a low level of concentration, a low level of potency, lack of clarity of thought and lack of flow, lower flow, higher materialism, fewer social ties, lower sleep, higher fear of death, higher obesity, and increase in upwards social comparison (Desmurget 2012).

Coaching has an important role to play in identifying an challenging time spent on unproductive activities, and this role is especially relevant to clients whose present-fatalistic TP is elevated. *Reduction of TV watching* would commence with raising the client's awareness of their TV watching habits and questioning whether this time is really satisfying to them. Provided the client is motivated to moderate this habit, possible solutions could be identified through joint brainstorming, which could include:

- Not watching TV every night;
- Not switching TV on mindlessly upon arriving from work;
- Selecting the programmes one would like to watch in advance and sticking to the choices made;
- Switching the TV off immediately after the end of a watched programme, thus preventing channel-hopping;
- Taking up a new hobby to distract from habitual activities such as TV watching (same can be applied to some forms of Internet-surfing).

Developing the *capacity for choice and autonomy* is expected to be more effective than simply learning specific behaviors, as autonomy is one of the basic human psychological needs (Ryan and Deci 2000). This says a lot about how the client views the world and their role in determining the course of their life. In most cases, this is an important capacity to develop in order to succeed, as people who are high on autonomy tend to work harder and persevere longer in order to get what they want. The coaching around the issue would almost always first focus on recognising the basic fact that one always has a choice. Making no choice is actually a choice in itself, and it is, in fact, one's choice to allow other people or events decide for them. It is important to help the client to identify and challenge their self-talk, like hearing oneself saying, "I have no choice" or "There's nothing I can do". Once such self-talk is identified, the task is to step back and remind oneself that one does, in fact, have some degree of control, and it is their choice whether they exercise it or not.

Taking *responsibility* for one's time means adopting a proactive rather than reactive attitude in relation to it, preventing oneself from feeling overstressed. Atchley quotes a man in his 80s saying: "You become free of time when you realise that time is in you, not you in time" (2001, p. 168). This statement implies taking responsibility for time, rather than allowing it to run one's life. However, assuming responsibility over one's time may require a shift in one's attitudes towards responsibility in general that needs to be carefully supported. This is standard practice in some types of psychotherapy (e.g. Motivational Interviewing), but to the author's knowledge this has rarely made its way into time management programmes. The following questions can be applied to examine different life situations, helping the client to assume responsibility for the way they react to and deal with the situation:

- What happened?
- What can you learn?
- What assumptions are you making?
- How else can you think about this situation?
- What is the other person thinking, feeling, needing, and wanting?
- What is possible?
- What are you responsible for?
- What are your choices?

A fatalistic attitude may be associated with lack of meaning, when a person finds it difficult to make autonomous choices because he/she does not experience their value. The following questions could be used to facilitate the experience of meaning and help the client to make his/her activity more self-congruent:

- Why do you do this?
- Do you really like doing this? Do you do it because you experience that this is good for you?
- Do you feel like this activity is right for you? Are you happy with the way you use your time?
- Will you be happy in several years with the way you spend your time at present?
- What would be your best option, the best thing you could do in this situation? What specific steps you could take in that direction?

Coaching Interventions Around Present-Hedonistic TP

The Present-Hedonistic person lives in and for the moment, is often a pleasure seeker, enjoys high intensity activities, thrills and new sensations, and is open to adventures. He or she would score highly on items such as: *I take risks to put excitement in my life.* Children are primarily Present-Hedonistically oriented. The upside of this orientation is its correlations with the affective aspects of well-being; the downside is the lack of regard for future consequences. Coaching interventions around the Present-Hedonistic orientation might focus either on decreasing or increasing this TP, depending on the client's scores.

Decreasing the present-hedonic orientation might not be straightforward, as a client is likely to experience many rewards associated with this orientation (and often ignore the downsides). As addiction of all types (cigarettes, drugs, sex, etc) is strongly associated with this profile, at times a referral to specialist services may be necessary. Coaching interventions to *decrease* the Present-Hedonistic TP would be similar to the ones used to *increase* the Future TP, focusing on goal and principle setting, financial planning, finding a meaning in life or even identifying a higher (spiritual) calling. Some of the questions may include:

- Where do you see yourself in five years time?
- How do you plan to get there? How does your present relate to it?
- What else can you do to achieve the same satisfaction as you experience through…?

On the other end of the spectrum, coaching someone to live more in the here and now can be achieved by helping them to accept and find the enjoyment in the present, by questions such as:

- What energises you in the present?
- What gives you pleasure?
- What brings you joy? What makes you smile so broadly, that you end up with a belly-laugh?
- How can the others help you to enjoy the present?
- What activity gives you the most satisfaction?

One powerful exercise to develop the Present-Hedonistic TP is what positive psychologists call *savouring*, that brings one fully into the world of the here and now. According to Bryant and Veroff (2007, p. 2), "people have capacities to attend, appreciate and enhance the positive experiences in their lives". Savouring is about really noticing, appreciating and enhancing the positive experiences in one's life. By savouring we slow down intentionally, consciously paying attention to all our senses (touch, taste, sight, sound, smell). We stretch out the experience, and concentrate on noticing what it is about the experience that we enjoy, whether it's as simple as sipping a glass of wine, stroking the cat, or musing over the time we scored a goal for the school rugby team. Depending on the type of activity chosen, it is possible to engage physically (e.g. luxuriating in a warm bubble bath) or mentally (listening to a beautiful piece of music). Psychologists have identified several techniques that promote savouring, some of which are detailed below and can be used as savouring strategies with your clients:

- Sharing with others: seeking out others to share the experience and tell others how much one values the moment. First of all, it is nice to be with and watch loved ones enjoy themselves. Also, others may point out pleasurable aspects that

one may have not noticed and we may become more playful in the presence of others. A desire to share the pleasure makes us more attentive to all the pleasurable details of the experience. This is probably the single best way to savour pleasure.
- Memory-building: taking mental photographs of the event to reminisce about it later.
- Self-congratulation: not being afraid of pride and acknowledging the present achievement.
- Sharpening perceptions: focusing on certain elements of an immediate experience and blocking out others.
- Absorption: letting oneself get totally immersed and trying not to think, but just sense.

Savouring is not exactly the same as mindfulness because it does not imply openness to all inner and outer stimuli, and focuses solely on those generating positive affect. However, practicing *mindfulness* can also be considered a positive intervention that can be used to enhance the Present-Hedonistic orientation.

Quality of life therapy (Frisch 1998, 2006; Frisch et al. 2005) outlines the *playlist* intervention that can be employed towards the same outcome. Adults aren't really good 'players'. We tend to leave imagination and the fun stuff to children. However, recreational activities are essential ways to relax, have fun, forget worries, be creative and learn something new. These activities can renew and refresh us so that we perform better in our work and relationships. We spend too little time "playing" in our lives, despite playing being the heart of the present moment. Therefore, in this exercise a coachee is asked to list the activities that they might enjoy as a recreational outlet. Ideas on the Playlist can include visiting one's favorite (or new) sections of a book, video, or music store; playing cards or board games, singing, dancing, going to the museum or the botanical garden, visiting a neighbor, sightseeing in the city, going to an antique sale, doing woodwork, hiking, bird watching, people watching, bowling, reading do-it-yourself materials, baking, scrap booking, looking at pictures, cuddling and many others. Coaching may be used to both help generate ideas for activities, as well as making sure the playlist is put into practice.

Coaching Interventions Around Future TP

The Future time perspective is associated with delay of gratification, ability to postpone immediate pleasures for the sake of pursuing important goals. In this sense, Future and Present-Hedonistic TP are, to a certain extent, mutually exclusive (Boniwell et al. 2010), and excessive emphasis on future goals may prevent a person from enjoying the present. Future TP involves active goal-setting and prioritizing, development of action plans and implementation of these plans in a step-by-step manner. There is a wide range of coaching interventions aimed at development of these skills. However, this capacity is based on personality characteristics, such as perseverance, self-discipline, and self-regulation (impulse control), which the client needs to have or develop in order to make the new skills work.

Commitment to future plans, however, can be associated with anxiety and time pressure, or with frustration because of inability to cope with uncertainty and unexpected challenges. In cases when a person exhibits tendency to choose goals that are not self-congruent (not aligned with true values or priorities), commitment to those goals may lead to burnout (Längle 2003). Therefore, the assumption that promoting the Future TP is beneficial by default may not be true for every client, and sometimes interventions that reduce, rather than foster Future TP need to be considered. In order to help client develop and maintain a positive Future TP, it is important to ensure that the future goals chosen are in line with the client's true aspirations and life priorities, and that they are realistic, given both the client's life circumstances and personality resources.

The first step towards developing the Future TP is therefore a clarification or discovery of one's life priorities. This vision is needed in order to formulate meaningful personal goals. One possible intervention that can facilitate this process is *future best self*, or *best possible selves diary* (Lyubomirsky 2008). The client is asked to consider a desired future image of him/herself, imagining that everything has gone the way they hoped for, that they have achieved what they aimed for, and that their best potentials have come to be realised. The client is asked to write about this vision in a diary regularly, vividly imagining him/herself in the best possible future, for several weeks. Another intervention that facilitates the discovery of life priorities is based on Alfred Adler's method of discovery of personal goals and includes a series of questions that can be reflected upon in sequence:

- What are your primary life priorities, that are most important to you in your life?
- If your situation was ideal and if you could do whatever you want, how would you prefer to spend the next three years?
- Imagine that you found out you had only one year to live, starting from today. How would you spend this time and what would you do?
- Based on your answer to the previous questions, how would you formulate your life priorities?

Similar exercises that help the client to discover their life priorities are *funeral service* and *epitaph* (Frisch 2006). The client is asked to imagine what they would want to be said about them in their eulogy or in a speech at their funeral service. What would they want to be written on their tombstone? These exercises help the client to formulate and visualize what they would like to leave behind, their possibility of making a unique and personal contribution to the world which provides a personally meaningful context for formulating specific goals. In case the client has difficulties with confronting the theme of death, a less radical approach is asking them to imagine being 90, sitting in a rocking chair and remembering their life. What would they want to remember in order to experience fulfillment from a life well-lived? What would they be happy to be remembered for by others?

The second step towards fostering the Future TP is developing a habit to formulate attainable goals and make specific, realistic short-term plans coordinated with life priorities. If the coach needs to explore the client's experience of planning, the following questions may be useful:

- What is your experience of planning?
- What happened the last time you planned?
- What would happen if you planned?
- What would you advise your children about planning?

These questions help to reveal and work through the possible negative experiences associated with planning, such as sticking to plans that are too rigid, inability to cope with future anxiety that can paralyze, or unexpected stressful circumstances that can drive one out of one's way. Making and successfully carrying out future plans requires personality resources that can be developed within coaching by using evidence-based interventions. An example of such resource is existential courage, or hardiness (Maddi 2013). As part of the hardiness training, situational reconstruction is used to help client focus on stressful circumstances and to find ways towards transformational coping or compensation of the effects of stressors by means of taking a wider perspective, developing specific action plans and becoming more sensitive to positive feedback from one's actions.

If difficulties in planning and carrying out plans are not associated with deeper problems, the client may simply need instrumental skills that facilitate carrying out plans. Coach may need to help the client in formulating implementation intentions (e.g., 'Tomorrow I will have my first cigarette no sooner than 2 p.m.') instead of goal intentions ('I want to give up smoking tomorrow') (Gollwitzer 1999), and to use time management interventions that facilitate prioritizing and setting aside time to work on goals perceived as important, but not urgent. Achieving goals and carrying out future plans also requires self-regulation and impulse control. These instrumental qualities can be developed by performing any activity diligently and regularly. For instance, regular exercise does not only contribute to well-being and self-esteem by improving health and physical appearance (Penedo and Dahn 2005), but also builds up a general capacity for self-regulation as a psychological resource (Muraven et al. 1999; Oaten and Cheng 2006).

Excessive commitment to future goals, however, could also be an issue. Freedman and Edwards' (1988) experimental findings of an inverted-U relationship between time pressure and performance offer an explanation as to why pressure may become counterproductive beyond a certain point. So whilst being busy is positive and can be encouraged, an external viewpoint is often necessary to help recognise the point when time pressure enters a dangerous range, impeding performance and well-being. The client may become caught up in a vicious circle, whereby time pressure leads to decreased performance and more tasks accumulating, leading to increased time pressure.

Interventions can be used to help reduce time pressure, such as *worry reduction*. This exercise became popular as part of Quality of Life Therapy (Frisch 2006). This intervention is useful for those who find that they may be spending too much time on worrying. We cannot will ourselves not to worry, so it can easily become an unproductive pattern. Habitual worriers may find relief if they allocate a limited period (e.g. a quarter or half-an-hour) every day for worrying that is to occur at the same time and in the same place, and postpone any worrying until then.

Another possible consequence of the vicious circle of time pressure is guilt, which may accumulate in some clients who find themselves increasingly unable to carry out all their plans and tasks. Guilt may lead to depression, undermining self-esteem and self-confidence. If this is an issue, the coach may suggest that client tries to break the vicious circle by taking some time off in order to do absolutely nothing and restore their resources by participating only in activities experienced as enjoyable. This pause may help the client to rediscover their priorities and realign their everyday activities with what it really important. Reflective questions can help to focus on the present:

- What is it about the present that does not serve the future?
- What is so uncomfortable about the present for you?
- What is currently missing/absent in your life? What are you missing out on?
- Imagine you have achieved all your goals… What then?
- What if all your plans failed?
- Is there something you might be trying to run away from?
- What if the unexpected happened?
- What if today was your last day, what would you do today?

Coaching Interventions for Balanced TP

Each of the TP factors may have some personal value, but when they come to be an excessive orientation that excludes or minimizes the others, then they may become dysfunctional. There are costs and sacrifices associated with emphasising any of the individual time perspectives, whether the focus is on achievement-oriented, "workaholic" Future TP, on hedonistic present, or on nostalgic past (which is an infrequent TP in the modern society). This is where the ideal of a *Balanced Time Perspective* comes into play (Boniwell and Zimbardo 2004). It is proposed as a more positive alternative to living life as a slave to any particular temporal bias. "In an optimally balanced time perspective, the past, present and future components blend and flexibly engage, depending on a situation's demands and our needs and values" (Zimbardo 2002, p. 62).

What does it mean to have a balanced TP? People with a balanced time perspective are capable of operating within a temporal mode appropriate to the situation they find themselves in. So when they spend time with their families and friends they are fully with them and value the opportunity to connect. When they take a day off work, they get involved in recreation rather than feel guilty about the work they haven't done. However, when working and studying they approach it from the perspective of the future and work more productively. Flexibility and "switch-ability" are essential components of a balanced TP.

Are people with a balanced TP likely to be happier than the rest of us? Until very recently, there was no consistent empirical data to support this claim. The associations between time perspective and well-being differ strongly across studies; however, recent research has shown that integral profiles of time perspective are more strongly associated with happiness and well-being than individual dimensions (Boniwell et al. 2010; Stolarski et al. in this volume). The happiest people are those with a balanced time perspective (those who are able to balance the present-day enjoyment with sacrificing their time to long-term goals). Balanced time perspective is further associated with more beneficial time use.

Coaching for balanced time perspective may begin with reviewing the clients' TP profile and discovering specific aspects of TP that need to be worked on. The first possible strategy is to use interventions that give the client tools and help develop skills specific to each of the TP dimensions (examples were reviewed above). The second strategy is to help the client develop cognitive flexibility in shifting between the past, present and future mindsets. The aim is to enable the client to stay focused on one temporal dimension when this is what is needed, and to "switch off" and change their mindset when appropriate. In order to be able to make this choice, the client needs to be aware and mindful of his/her needs and priorities, as well as of the possibilities and limitations of the situation.

This can be achieved by using interventions that draw on meditation techniques. Mindfulness, otherwise defined as a receptive attention to, and awareness of, present events and experience (Brown and Ryan 2003), is one of the major topic researched in positive psychology. Mindfulness meditation is a practice that has been around for many thousands of years, is a common element of Eastern religions, and is typically associated with Buddhism (Kabat-Zinn 2005; Neale 2006). It entails the skills of paying attention purposefully, in the present moment and without judgement. This builds up the capacity to be simultaneously aware of different aspects of one's subjective experience and integrate them non-judgmentally. As a result, clients can gain a better awareness of their experience and life as a whole, as well as become more aware of every specific situation with its possibilities and limitations; thus, they can become more present in life by making more sound decisions that integrate situational and personal context (see Neale 2006, for a review of different mindfulness meditation models).

Mindfulness is not a single skill, and there is a wide range of meditation techniques that are appropriate to develop its different components. Traditional mindfulness training begins with development of attentional stability and receptive awareness, which are subsequently applied to observation of different aspects of experience: body and physical sensations, mental states, and mind objects. As a result, there emerges the effortless insight of non-attached self that allows one to choose a so-called "middle way" (Goleman 1988). Attentional stability and receptive awareness form the basis for cognitive flexibility, which refers to the mental ability to adjust thinking or attention by consciously managing one's awareness and attentional focus. One possible way to achieve it is by using the traditional focus phrase methodology (Kabat-Zinn 2005). For instance, focusing on the phrase "I feel the air flowing in and out of my nose" can turn one's attention toward the sensory experience in the present moment, whereas focusing on the phrase "I am ready to experience the feelings in my heart" facilitates non-judgmental attention towards emotional experience.

Time perspective is essentially a subjective tendency to focus on specific aspects of experience (memories, plans, pleasant feeling). Ill-balanced time perspective is inability to be flexible, becoming too attached to or too caught up in one experiential focus, so that time becomes one's master. Mindfulness meditation interventions promote flexible self-regulation and can empower clients who want to become the masters of their minds, gaining a more balanced time perspective. Asking the client the following questions can help:

- What are you experiencing right now?
- Why are you experiencing this feeling?
- What does this feeling tell you about what's really important to you in your life?
- What do you really want to do right now, in this situation?
- Given your overall experience of yourself as a person, what is the best thing you could do now? What is the best way that you could choose for today?
- How can you make good use of your past experiences in what I want to achieve?
- What is the best way for you to allocate your time today?

By reflecting on these questions regularly, the client can gain a better integration of his/her past, present, and future into a meaningful and congruent whole, so it is important to encourage the client to ask themselves these questions outside of the coaching sessions as well

Conclusion

In conclusion, we have reviewed several methods, including both evidence-based interventions and questions, that can be employed in coaching sessions to address and improve different forms of imbalance in clients' time perspective. There are sufficient theoretical grounds to assume that personalising TP interventions to suit the client's existing profile would further address their problems with time management behaviors, however, further research is needed to make this assumption a certainty. In the meanwhile, we believe that taking even baby steps towards developing a more balanced TP is already a valuable goal in itself.

Acknowledgments Support from the Basic Research Program of the National Research University Higher School of Economics is gratefully acknowledged by the second author (EO).

References

Atchley, R. C. (2001). The influence of spiritual beliefs and practices on the relation between time and aging. In S. H. McFadden & R. C. Atchley (Eds.), *Aging and the meaning of time: A multidisciplinary exploration* (pp. 157–170). New York: Springer.

Bond, M. J., & Feather, N. T. (1988). Some correlates of structure and purpose in the use of time. *Journal of Personality and Social Psychology, 55*(2), 321–329.

Boniwell, I. (2005). Beyond time management: How the latest research on time perspective and perceived time use can assist clients with time-related concerns. *International Journal of Evidence Based Coaching and Mentoring, 3*(2), 61–74.
Boniwell, I., & Zimbardo, P. (2004). Balancing time perspective in pursuit of optimal functioning. In P. A. Linley & S. Joseph (Eds.), *Positive psychology in practice* (pp. 165–179). Hoboken: Wiley.
Boniwell, I., Osin, E., Linley, P. A., & Ivanchenko, G. (2010). A question of balance: Examining relationships between time perspective and measures of well-being in the British and Russian student samples. *Journal of Positive Psychology, 5*(1), 24–40.
Bost, J. M. (1984). Retaining students on academic probation: Effects of time management peer counseling on students' grades. *Journal of Learning Skills, 3*, 38–43.
Brown, K., & Ryan, R. (2003). The benefits of being present: Mindfulness and its role in psychological well-being. *Journal of Personality and Social Psychology, 84*, 822–848.
Bryant, F. B., & Veroff, J. (2007). *Savouring: A new model of positive experiences*. Mahwah, NJ: Lawrence Erlbaum Associates.
Bryant, F. B., Smart, C. M., & King, S. P. (2005). Using the past to enhance the presence: Boosting happiness through positive reminiscence. *Journal of Happiness Studies, 6*, 227–260.
Claessens, B. J. C. (2004). *Perceived control of time: Time management and personal effectiveness at work.* Unpublished PhD dissertation, Technisce Universiteit Eindhoven, Netherlands.
Claessens, B. J. C., van Eerde, W., Rutte, C. G., & Roe, R. A. (2007). A review of the time management literature. *Personnel Review, 36*(2), 255–276.
Csikszentmihalyi, M. (1992). *Flow: The psychology of happiness*. London: Rider.
Desmurget, M. (2012). *TV Lobotomie*. Paris: Max Milo Éditions.
Freedman, J. L., & Edwards, D. R. (1988). Time pressure, task performance, and enjoyment. In J. E. McGrath (Ed.), *The social psychology of time: New perspectives* (pp. 113–133). Thousand Oaks: Sage.
Fredrickson, B. (2009). *Positivity: Top-notch research reveals the 3-to-1 ratio that will change your life*. New York: Random House.
Friedberg, J. P., Suchday, S., & Shelov, D. V. (2007). The impact of forgiveness on cardiovascular reactivity and recovery. *International Journal of Psychophysiology, 65*(2), 87–94.
Frisch, M. B. (1998). Quality of life therapy and assessment in health care. *Clinical Psychology: Science and Practice, 5*(1), 19–40.
Frisch, M. B. (2006). *Quality of life therapy: Applying a life satisfaction approach to positive psychology and cognitive therapy*. Hoboken, NJ: Wiley.
Frisch, M. B., Clark, M. P., Rouse, S. V., Rudd, M. D., Paweleck, J. K., Greenstone, A., et al. (2005). Predictive and treatment validity of life satisfaction and the Quality of Life Inventory. *Assessment, 12*(1), 66–78.
Goleman, D. (1988). *The meditative mind.* Los Angeles: J.P. Tarcher.
Gollwitzer, P. M. (1999). Implementation intentions: Strong effects of simple plans. *American Psychologist, 54*, 493–503.
Hall, B. L., & Hursch, D. E. (1982). An evaluation of the effects of a time management training program on work efficiency. *Journal of Organizational Behaviour Management, 3*, 73–96.
Hanel, F. J. (1982). Field testing the effectiveness of a self-instruction time management manual with managerial staff in an institutional setting. *Dissertation Abstracts International, 42(8-B)*, 3400.
Jahoda, M. (1981). Work, employment, and unemployment: Values, theories, and approaches in social research. *American Psychologist, 36*(2), 184–191.
Kabat-Zinn, J. (2005). *Wherever you go, there you are: Mindfulness meditation in everyday life*. New York, NY: Hyperion Books.
Lakein, A. (1973). *How to get control of your time and your life*. New York: Signet.
Längle, A. (2003). Burnout–Existential meaning and possibilities of prevention. *European Psychotherapy, 4*(1), 107–121.
Larsson, J., & Sanne, C. (2005). Self-help books on avoiding time shortage. *Time and Society, 14*, 213–230.

Lewin, K. (1942/1997). Time perspective and morale. In K. Lewin (Ed.), *Resolving social conflicts and field theory in social science* (pp. 80–93). Washington, DC: APA.

Lyubomirsky, S. (2008). *The how of happiness: A practical guide to getting the life you want.* London: Sphere.

Lyubomirsky, S., Sousa, L., & Dickerhoof, R. (2006). The costs and benefits of writing, talking, and thinking about life's triumphs and defeats. *Journal of Personality and Social Psychology, 90*(4), 692.

Macan, T. H. (1994). Time management: Test of a process model. *Journal of Applied Psychology, 79*, 381–391.

Macan, T. H. (1996). Time-management training: Effects on time behaviors, attitudes, and job performance. *Journal of Psychology, 130*, 229–237.

Macan, T. H., Shahani, C., Dipboye, R. L., & Phillips, A. P. (1990). College students' time management: Correlations with academic performance and stress. *Journal of Educational Psychology, 82*, 760–768.

Maddi, S. R. (2013). *Hardiness: Turning stressful circumstances into resilient growth.* Dordrecht: Springer.

McCullough, M. E., & Witvliet, C. V. (2002). The psychology of forgiveness. In C. R. Snyder & S. J. Lopez (Eds.), *Handbook of positive psychology* (pp. 446–458). New York: Oxford University Press.

Muraven, M., Baumeister, R. F., & Tice, D. M. (1999). Longitudinal improvement of self-regulation through practice: Building self-control strength through repeated exercise. *The Journal of Social Psychology, 139*(4), 446–457.

Neale, M. I. (2006). *Mindfulness meditation: An integration of perspectives from Buddhism, science, and clinical psychology.* Unpublished doctoral thesis, California Institute of Integral Studies, San-Francisco.

Oaten, M., & Cheng, K. (2006). Longitudinal gains in self-regulation from regular physical exercise. *British Journal of Health Psychology, 11*(4), 717–733.

Penedo, F. J., & Dahn, J. R. (2005). Exercise and well-being: A review of mental and physical health benefits associated with physical activity. *Current Opinion in Psychiatry, 18*(2), 189.

Pennebaker, J. W. (1997). Writing about emotional experiences as a therapeutic process. *Psychological Science, 8*(3), 162–166.

Pennebaker, J. W. (2004). Expressive writing and the regulation of emotion over time. *Psychophysiology, 41*, S23–S23.

Ryan, R. M., & Deci, E. L. (2000). Self-determination theory and the facilitation of intrinsic motivation, and well-being. *American Psychologist, 55*, 68–78.

Seligman, M. E. P., Steen, T., Park, N., & Peterson, P. (2005). Positive psychology progress, empirical validation of interventions. *American Psychologist, 60*(5), 410–421.

Sheldon, K. M., & Lyubomirsky, S. (2004). Achieving sustainable new happiness: Prospects, practices, and prescriptions. In P. A. Linley & S. Joseph (Eds.), *Positive psychology in practice* (pp. 127–145). Hoboken: Wiley.

Tyrrell, B. (1995). Time in our lives: Facts and analysis on the 90s. *Demos, 5*, 23–25.

Witvliet, C. V., Ludwig, T. E., & Vander Laan, K. L. (2001). Granting forgiveness or harboring grudges: Implications for emotion, physiology, and health. *Psychological Science, 12*(2), 117–123.

Zimbardo, P. G. (2002). Just think about it: Time to take our time. *Psychology Today, 35*, 62.

Zimbardo, P. G., & Boyd, J. N. (1999). Putting time in perspective: A valid, reliable individual-differences metric. *Journal of Personality and Social Psychology, 77*, 1271–1288. doi:10.1037/0022-3514.77.6.1271.

Friend or Foe? Escape from Death, or Death as an Escape?

Wessel van Beek and Ksenia Chistopolskaya

General Introduction

Time is limited for all of us, but some people chose to end their own lives by committing suicide. How can something so horrible, our own death, become an ultimate choice for some people? Human beings are the only species that can think about their eventual death. And this awareness of one's mortality is something that people have to deal with. On the other hand, humans are most likely the only species capable of deliberately taking one's own life by committing suicide.[1]

Every year about one million people commit suicide worldwide, possibly growing towards one suicide per every 20 s in the year 2020 (Bertolote and Fleischmann 2002). This reflects a worldwide increase in suicide rates, and suicide is among the three leading causes of death among those aged 15–44 (male and female). The World Health Organization defines suicide as "the result of an act, deliberately initiated and performed by a person in the full knowledge or expectation of its fatal outcome" (Murthy 2001, p. 37). This is in our opinion only part of the truth, because suicide is not always, or maybe hardly ever, the outcome of a conscious and deliberate process. Most people commit suicide under the influence of alcohol, drugs, or medication, and in almost every case the suicidal patient is suffering from a comorbid psychiatric disorder (O'Connor et al. 2011). As we will discuss in this chapter, suicide is much more complicated behavior. First, people need to overcome their death anxiety to take such a step. Negate one's intrinsic tendency to survive, and mentally create personal approval: it is

[1] Some animals seem to be aware of their upcoming death, for instance elephants. Claims that animals commit suicide have not been acknowledged (the lemmings story is made up).

W. van Beek (✉)
GGZ Veenendaal, Veenendaal, The Netherlands
e-mail: wessel.van.beek@gmail.com

K. Chistopolskaya
Moscow Research Institute of Psychiatry, Moscow, Russia

M. Stolarski et al. (eds.), *Time Perspective Theory; Review, Research and Application: Essays in Honor of Philip G. Zimbardo*, DOI 10.1007/978-3-319-07368-2_30,

the right thing to do. This is, in most of the cases, a process over time. People learn to tolerate suicide as the only way out (Shneidman 1996).

In this chapter we discuss how people deal with the knowledge that they are going to die, and why some people decide to choose death themselves. We relate this to Time Perspective Theory, and provide some guidance on how to integrate this in treatment.

Escape from Death, or Death as an Escape?

Escape from Death

Psychiatrist Robert Lifton was convinced that the feeling of immortality is universal and gives people self-continuity, as it is "humanity's symbolization of ties with both biological fellows and history, past and future" (Lifton 1977, p. 277). He wrote that the loss of immortality, or impaired death imagery, is characterized by (1) death anxiety (manifested in war neurosis, guilt over survival); (2) psychic numbing (the constant restriction of life because of the fear of death, "If I feel nothing, then death doesn't exist," a shrinking of the ego, and a diminished capacity for experience); (3) suspicion of counterfeit nurturance ("If death exists, then life is counterfeit").

Cultural anthropologist Ernest Becker (1924–1974) needed the construct of death for his model of a moral society (Becker 1968). At first he stated that death is the ultimate evil and that humans are the only animals that await their death. People build their individual symbolic projects (*causa sui*) because symbols are infinite and body is finite and reminds of death. People sacrifice their physical existence in exchange for symbolic immortality (Becker 1973). Becker agreed with Zilboorg that the fear of death is always present in our mental functioning. This fear is an expression of the instinct for self-preservation, which functions as a constant drive to maintain life and to master the dangers that threaten life: "Such constant expenditure of psychological energy on the business of preserving life would be impossible if the fear of death were not as constant. The very term 'self-preservation' implies an effort against some force of disintegration; the affective aspect of this is fear, fear of death" (Zilboorg 1943, p. 467).

Becker was highly censorious of the feeling of immortality. Lifton (1977) considered it obligatory and healthy, but Becker pointed out many of its morbid weaknesses. He warned that the pursuit of immortality—or *causa sui* (self-esteem)—may lead to tragedies and injustices, that people have to live with a constant feeling of the frailty of their being, in permanent awe of creation.

The ideas of Becker are continued in Terror Management Theory, proposed in 1986 by Greenberg, Pyszczynski, and Solomon. They state that most of human behavior can be understood as an attempt to achieve *psychological equanimity* in the face of mortality. People gain this equanimity through culture, which raises them above other animals (Goldenberg et al. 2001). The cultural anxiety buffer consists of (a) belief in one's cultural worldview and (b) self-esteem, which is derived from living up to the standards of that worldview (Pyszczynski et al. 2004). In defence of their feelings of personal value and their worldviews people are prone to risk their lives (for example, to drive recklessly), to have negative feelings toward opponents, to prefer authoritarian leaders, to demand tough sentencing for relatively minor faults and crimes (Harmon-Jones et al. 1996; Hirschberger 2006).

But other defences have less negative effects. First, there are attachment relationships: people choose them and as a result give up their worldviews and self-esteem. Such a compromise has its emotional price: the choice is accompanied by a reduced feeling of pride and an intensification of guilt and shame (Mikulincer et al. 2003). Second, there is nostalgia. Sedikides and colleagues (Sedikides et al. 2008; Wildschut et al. 2006) defined nostalgia as a self-relevant, primarily positive emotion with some 'bittersweet' elements. People recall their loved and close ones, social contexts as a whole, places, objects, events. The authors prove that nostalgia repairs discontinuity of the self, binds the past and the present. Their studies show that people restore their individual and collective selves by reminiscing about their past when they lack resources to deal with the situation in the present.

A few years later Wong formulated the Meaning Management Theory, in which attitudes toward life and death are connected like communicating vessels (2007). He believes that people who fear death and try to avoid any reminders of it in their daily life are extremely attached to life. People who are in difficult life circumstances or who are terminally ill accept death as an escape and even welcome it, or death just seems more attractive to them than life. Wong proposes that the most 'healthy' and benign death attitude is neutral, when one sees death as a natural and unavoidable phenomenon.

Death as an Escape

Traditionally the act of committing suicide is regarded as a mental illness, or as a side effect of it. This is an overly simplistic view of complex human behavior. As we discussed in the prior paragraph, all people have to deal with the awareness of eventual death, and this knowledge is likely to be associated with the unique human capacity to end one's life. But under what circumstances would a person commit suicide? Over the years several psychological theories of suicide and suicidal behavior have been published (for an overview see Rudd et al. 2009). The renowned suicidologist Shneidman (1985) introduced the term 'egression', as one of the ten commonalities of suicide. Suicide as an act of intended escape. This has become one of the most influential perspectives in both research and practice: suicide as an escape from unbearable life (e.g. Baumeister 1990; Williams 1997). The subjective perception that self-chosen death brings relief, and ends a situation that is experienced as unbearable. This 'subjective perception' implies that emotional and cognitive aspects influence the judgment of life to be unliveable. In this paragraph we have a closer look at how this judgment takes place, and how it is related to Time Perspective Theory.

One core element in suicidal thinking is hopelessness, a component of Beck's theory of depression. According to Beck's classic model (1967) three variables constitute the negative triad of depression: hopelessness, self-esteem, and a negative perception of the environment. Hopelessness is considered to be the best predictor or indicator of the risk of suicidal behaviour (Vinas et al. 2002). Research has shown that hopelessness in suicidal people can be further operationalized as a decrease in positive future thinking, but not an increased anticipation of unpleasant events (MacLeod et al. 1993, 1998). We know from our own research (Van Beek et al. submitted) that suicidal people are not only less able to generate positive future ideas, but they also tend to overproduce negative thoughts about the present.

Apparently, future thinking plays an important role in suicidality, but how does that help us to understand why hopeless people would commit suicide? What makes hopelessness, or an inability to imagine positive future scenarios, so unliveable? One possible starting point can be found in discrepancy theory. According to discrepancy theory people are motivated to reach a condition where their self-concept matches their personally relevant internalized values (Higgins 1987), by a process that is generally described as self-regulation. People construct self-guides (wishes and oughts), which, when elicited, stimulate the individual to retrieve autobiographical material. The actual:ought discrepancy leads to a negative evaluation of oneself, and likely the retrieval of negative memories (Strauman 1996). When people form the idea that they cannot live up to their own personal standards, or the ones of significant others, they may become hopeless. Research stresses the significance of feeling hopeless about ever achieving important personal ideals in suicidal ideation (Chatard and Selimbegoviç 2011; Cornette et al. 2009). This prediction, partly based upon the retrieved negative memories, may lead to an unbearable ought:future discrepancy. The inability to envision a future in which this ought Self—future Self mismatch will be resolved, is likely to be influenced by personal tendencies to be oriented on the Past Negative, in terms of Time Perspective.

In order to examine the role of Time Perspective in suicidality, we investigated a group of 195 depressed psychiatric patients, referred to us because they reported suicidal thoughts. The Table shows the outcome of our hierarchical cluster analyses. The most interesting is the second cluster, which consists of severely depressed patients, who report significantly more negative symptoms and distress, and who are highly suicidal. The group is characterized by high Past Negative, low Past Positive, high Present Fatalistic, and low Future scores. They also reported to be hedonistic in the Present, most likely as a means to escape their daily suffering (engaging in self-soothing behavior, like alcoholism) (Table 1).

This seems to reflect the group of patients who are too overwhelmed by their negative memories, depressed feelings, and inability to foresee positive future. This group can no longer cling onto, or escape to, the Positive Past.

The first cluster consists of people who are suicidal, but who have a higher Past Positive score, and higher Future scores than the people in the second cluster. This appears to reflect a subgroup of suicidal patients who cling onto the good memories, and are still able to foresee positive future scenarios. This is comparable to the findings in our Russian sample (paragraph 3.b).

Table 1 Cluster mean scores of time perspective, depression and quality of life; hierarchical cluster analyses

	Cluster			
	1	2	3	4
	$n=48$	$n=42$	$n=92$	$n=13$
	Suicidal/ future	Suicidal/ depressed	Less suicidal/ here and now	Not suicidal/ future
Past Negative	3.76	4.33***	3.57	2.48***
Past Positive	2.18***	1.69***	3.21	3.43**
Present Fatalistic	3.11	3.72***	3.34	2.38***
Present Hedonistic	2.61***	3.37*	3.38**	3.07
Future	3.41**	2.77**	3.00	3.74***
Suicidal ideation	12.15	12.98	6.83***	1.38 a)***
Depression	35.43	41.10***	27.82*	15.77***
Symptoms and distress	106.25	113.38**	100.69	75.77***

Note. a) only 1 participant scored > 0 on the SSI in this cluster
*$p<.05$, **$p<.01$, ***: $p<.001$

Suicide and Time Perspective (Time Lost and Found)

Objectives of Research

JUAN I have a stratagem, Holy Father, to outwit their cannon.
ALEXANDER Would you be so good as to share it with us?
JUAN Indeed. Just give me some time with my condottieri.
ALEXANDER *Time is what we do not have!* The barbarians are approaching!
Rome has been sacked twice in her past.
We would spare her a third such indignity.
The Borgias

The above-mentioned dialogue from the T.V. series 'The Borgias' gives us an example of how people deal with the threat of death. There is some rumination and a feeling of urgency and scarce resources. Let us imagine that the condottieri are the time perspectives themselves, the psychological constructs which when being balanced coincide with the feeling of well-being (Boniwell and Zimbardo 2004; Drake et al. 2008). But in the state of panic, with a discontinuity created by an unbearable situation and the suicidal attempt, there is no place for equanimity and the mind gives way for a band-aid approach, when each time perspective solves its own function, exerts its own defence.

We hypothesized that suicide attempt serves as a strong mortality salience, from which people need to defend themselves. The impact of this salience corresponds with the suicidal intent and the suicidal experience. It further influences the pattern of defences, which comply with the defences, found in Terror Management Theory.

Russian Findings

A total of 336 young people (ranging in age from 18 to 25) participated in the study. In the control group there were undergraduate students (n=156). The experimental group (n=180) consisted of patients in the department of toxicology at the N. V. Sklifosovsky Research Institute of Emergency Medicine. All of them had recently (in the past 2 to 14 days) tried to poison themselves. Thirty-seven had made two or more suicide attempts, 103 had made one attempt, and 40 denied recent suicidal thoughts and actions (they explained the acts as 'accidents', 'mistakes' or that they 'just wanted to frighten somebody', regardless of the severity of the medical consequences).

Suicidals were significantly higher on Past Negative and Present Fatalistic and lower on Hardiness than the control group. The study has also shown that cultural defences—literal immortality (religion, belief in an afterlife) (Dechesne et al. 2003; Wong 2007) and rationalization (neutral acceptance of death as a natural phenomenon) (Wong 2007)—don't work for suicidal people: they also scored lower on them than the control sample. They are highly emotional about death and their attitude is mostly characterised by the *fear of death*, which serves as a defence against suicidal behaviour, but at the same time, being a painful experience, in its turn calls for a defence.

Feelings of *nostalgia*, warm remembrances of one's childhood (Past Positive), allow one to cope with the task the best, but the group with the *denial of the attempt*, which exerts this defence most prominently, plunges into illusions and denies reality. The *Future*, the ability to work for some far-reaching goals, the formation of one's *causa sui* project, as Becker would put it, is a more fragile defence, and it leaves one in the group with *one attempt* with the awareness of one's finitude (high fear of *consequences of death for body*). A *positive attitude toward death*, as Ambrumova has put it (Ambrumova and Kalashnikova 1998), is seen in people with *several suicide attempts*—as their established style of coping with the fear of death. They fear only of *oblivion,* of being forgotten by significant others. Notably, these suicidals combine the fear of death with Past Positive, Present Hedonistic, and Future time perspectives, which usually give an appreciation for life, but they score equally low on them. Escape Acceptance lets them build an alternative worldview, which is desirable, but non-existent. It is another type of flight from reality.

Implications

It is known that the risk of suicide is higher in those who have got more suicidal attempts in the past and high in suicide ideation. Our research has shown that those people exert escape acceptance of death and detachment from everything positive in life (score low on hardiness, Past Positive, Present Hedonistic and Future). Their social and psychological situation is so bad that the only thing they fear is oblivion.

Another group of suicidal patients is characterised by low psychological well-being. They try to fall back on future, be efficient in daily life, but this defence is weak and leaves place for negative time perspective, which is linked with aversion of physicality.

The third group of suicidals is unlikely to be seen in therapy, as those people deny having a problem. They rely on nostalgia, Past Positive time perspective, as if making a step back and trying to solve their situation with different resources. It is unknown how do they cope in the long run. Probably they become more desperate or maybe this defence actually helps them. We only know that it hides part of the truth from them and still leaves them with the fear of death.

We believe that for the healthy functioning people who feel suicidal have to lose their fear of death as a defence, to find neutral acceptance of death, without overloading death with extra-meaning. They need to start breathing freely again, come to terms with their negative time perspectives and feel themselves "immortal" again (in terms of Lifton).

Dutch Findings

We did two studies in which we investigated the role of time perspective in suicidality. In our first study we examined 76 individuals, patients in treatment (n=32), and participants currently not in treatment (n=44). We found that higher levels of suicidality are associated with higher Past Negative, lower Past Positive, higher Present Fatalistic, and lower Future scores. Most subscales of the ZTPI correlated high with the scales of two other important instruments used in mental health care research (NEO-PI II and the SIPP), but the Future scale of the ZTPI appears to measure a distinct and unique characteristic. This is important, because in this study low Future scores were related to higher levels of suicidality.

In our second study we looked at differences between suicidal (n=105) and non-suicidal depressed (n=94) patients. The findings were almost similar to the first study: suicidal patients were less oriented on Past Positive, more on Past Negative, more on Present Fatalistic, but this time we found no significant differences on the Future scale between suicidal and non-suicidal patients.

Our hypothesis is that within the depressed patients group, most participants have an anxious and worrisome outlook on the future. The Future scale of the ZTPI might not differentiate enough in severity, and it does not distinguish positive and negative ideas about the future. Further research on the role of positive and negative aspects of the future in clinical psychology is needed.

Suicidal Process: To Be or Not to Be

Suicidality is a process over time, with or without an eventual suicide attempt as the outcome. Whereas patients are afraid to die in the beginning of this process, death anxiety loses its defensive value when feelings of hopelessness are not alleviated during this process. The future loses its hope-giving capacity. Not only the present is unliveable, but the current suffering will continue in the future. During this development over time death, normally experienced as aversive, gradually changes to ambivalence about dying. People get detached from the positive past, present, and future. They lose the connection with others, but also with their own life story and their own uniqueness: the threat of further deterioration of the Self. Many hopeless patients attempt to escape their situation, either by taking alcohol or drugs, by escaping in numbness, passivity, and isolation, in which depression might be a protective mechanism against suicide. But when no other escape routes are available, a suicide attempt might become the only available option to stop the psychic pain. We know from research that most patients were ambivalent about their intention to die from a suicide attempt. The majority of patients who attempted suicide report they needed to escape the unliveable moment. Possibly, various fears encourage some of these attempters to re-attach to their former lives and relationships. But others are unable to do so, they further withdraw from their personal place in this world. Those patients create a mental reality in which death is acceptable, because they are no longer part of a larger whole, like a relationship, family, or community.

Friend or Foe, or Time Found?

Time is precious for most of us. We are aware that we have a limited amount of it, before we eventually have to die. But for some human beings, particularly depressed, hopeless, and suicidal people, there is too much time. Their time perspectives are blurred or, probably more precisely, bound. Used not for the purposes of well-being, but as band-aids for the fears and wishes of death. Zimbardo and Boyd (2008) write about suicide as avoiding the future, time has become a burden to someone who no longer wants to endure the suffering (p. 222). The future (the causa sui project, the wishes of perfection) corresponds to the strongest fears of death, when the smallest mistake becomes a problem, which is difficult to overcome. Past Positive becomes characteristic for some the suicidals, who feel the need to cling to the close ones, but it also provides an opportunity for the illusion that there wasn't any suicide attempt. It may hurt when being remembered in reality it was a suicide attempt. Bound by the fear and avoidance of death Past Positive shuts people out from the present and the future. Probably only those who had several suicidal attempts understand the need for balance, but they are too negative about their lives to make changes straight after the suicidal attempt. Death is probably not a friend nor a foe, but a highly emotional expected event which leaves people in confusion. It is our task to untangle those emotions and let people see what they can do.

This leads to the conclusion that Time Perspective Theory also should have an important role in the treatment of suicidal patients. The distinct role of future thinking provides an opportunity for clinicians. Fostering realistic hope, embracing positive memories, and stimulating constructive, goal-oriented behaviour in the present, may lead to a decrease in the need to escape.

Further research could focus on the different aspects of suicidality. Suicidality is a multifaceted, multidimensional and complex phenomenon and we need to know more about the commonalities and differences when it comes to time perspective. Can Past Negative be disseminated, to further understand its importance in suicidality? Maybe it is helpful to discriminate a Positive and Negative Future, and Transcendental Future, as has been suggested in different chapters in this book. (see chapters "Broadening the TP Profile: Future Negative Time Perspective" by Carelli et al., this volume, and "Time Perspective and Transcendental Future Thinking" by van Beek and Kairys, this volume).

References

Ambrumova, A. G., & Kalashnikova, O. E. (1998). Kliniko-psihologicheskie aspekty samoubijstva [Clinical and psychological aspects of suicide]. *Socialnaya i klinicheskaya psihiatriya [Social and Clinical Psychiatry], 8*(4), 65–77.

Baumeister, R. F. (1990). Suicide as escape from self. *Psychological Review, 97*(1), 90–113.

Beck, A. T. (1967). *Depression: Clinical, experimental, and theoretical aspects*. New York: Harper & Row.

Becker, E. (1968). *The structure of evil: An essay on the unification of the science of man*. New York: Braziller.

Becker, E. (1973). *The denial of death*. New York: Free Press.

Beek, W. van, Beekman, A. T. F., & Kerkhof, A. J. F. M. (submitted). Past, present and future fluency in depressed suicidal and non-suicidal patients. Manuscript submitted for publication.

Bertolote, J. M., & Fleischmann, A. (2002). Suicide and psychiatric diagnosis: A worldwide perspective. *World Psychiatry, 1*(3), 181–185.

Boniwell, I., & Zimbardo, P. (2004). Balancing one's time perspective in pursuit of optimal functioning. In P. A. Linley & S. Joseph (Eds.), *Positive psychology in practice* (pp. 165–178). Hoboken: Wiley.

Chatard, A., & Selimbegović, L. (2011). When self-destructive thoughts flash through the mind: Failure to meet standards affects the accessibility of suicide-related thoughts. *Journal of Personality and Social Psychology, 100*, 587–605.

Cornette, M. M., Strauman, T. J., Abramson, L. Y., & Busch, A. M. (2009). Self-discrepancy and suicidal ideation. *Cognition and Emotion, 23*, 504–527.

Dechesne, M., Pyszczynski, T., Arndt, J., Ransom, S., Sheldon, K., van Knippenberg, A., & Janssen, J. (2003). Literal and symbolic immortality: The effect of evidence of literal immortality on self-esteem striving in response to mortality salience. *Journal of Personality and Social Psychology, 84*(4), 722–737.

Drake, L., Duncan, E., Sutherland, F., Abernethy, C., & Henry, C. (2008). Time perspective and correlates of wellbeing. *Time and Society, 17*(1), 47–61.

Goldenberg, J. M., Pyszczynski, T., Greenberg, J., Solomon, S., Kluck, B., & Cornwell, R. (2001). I am not an animal: Mortality salience, disgust and the denial of human creatureliness. *Journal of Experimental Psychology, 130*(3), 427–435.

Greenberg, J., Pyszczynski, T., & Solomon, S. (1986). The causes and consequences of a need for self-esteem: A terror management theory. In R. F. Baumeister (Ed.), *Public self and private self* (pp. 189–212). New York: Springer.

Harmon-Jones, E., Greenberg, J., Solomon, S., & Simon, L. (1996). The effects of mortality salience on intergroup bias between minimal groups. *European Journal of Social Psychology, 25*, 781–785.

Higgins, E. T. (1987). Self-discrepancy: A theory relating self and affect. *Psychological Review, 94*, 319–340.

Hirschberger, G. (2006). Terror management and attributions of blame to innocent victims: Reconciling compassionate and defensive responses. *Journal of Personality and Social Psychology, 91*(5), 832–844.
Lifton, R. (1977). The sense of immortality: On death and the continuity of life. In H. Feifel (Ed.), *New meanings of death* (pp. 273–290). New York: McGraw-Hill.
MacLeod, A. K., Rose, G. S., & Williams, M. G. (1993). Components of hopelessness about the future in parasuicide. *Cognitive Therapy and Research, 5*, 441–455.
MacLeod, A. K., Tata, P., Evans, K., Tyrer, P., Schmidt, U., Davidson, K., Thornton, S., & Catalan, J. (1998). Recovery of positive future thinking within a high-risk parasuicide group: Results from a pilot randomized controlled trial. *British Journal of Clinical Psychology, 37*, 371–379.
Mikulincer, M., Florian, V., & Hirschberger, G. (2003). The existential function of close relationships: Introducing death into the science of love. *Personality and Social Psychology Review, 7*, 20–40.
Murthy, R. S. (Ed.). (2001). *The World health report 2001: Mental health: New understanding, new hope*. Geneva: World Health Organization.
O'Connor, R. C., Platt, S., & Gordon, J. (Eds.). (2011). *International handbook of suicide prevention: Research, policy and practice*. Chichester: Wiley-Blackwell.
Pyszczynski, T., Greenberg, J., Solomon, S., Arndt, J., & Schimel, J. (2004). Why do people need self-esteem? A theoretical and empirical review. *Psychological Bulletin, 130*, 435–468.
Rudd, M., Trotter, D., & Williams, B. (2009). Psychological theories of suicidal behaviour. In D. Wasserman & C. Wasserman (Eds.), *Oxford textbook of suicidology and suicide prevention* (pp. 159–164). New York: Oxford University Press Inc.
Sedikides, C., Wildschut, T., Routledge, C., & Arndt, J. (2008). Nostalgia as enabler of self-continuity. In F. Sani (Ed.), *Self-continuity. Individual and collective perspectives* (pp. 227–239). New York: Psychology Press.
Shneidman, E. S. (1985). *Definition of suicide*. New York: Wiley.
Shneidman, E. S. (1996). *The suicidal mind*. New York: Oxford University Press.
Strauman, T. J. (1996). Stability within the self: A longitudinal study of the structural implications of self-discrepancy theory. *Journal of Personality and Social Psychology, 71*(6), 1142–1153.
Vinas, F., Canals, J., Gras, E., Ros, C., & Domenech-Llaberia, E. (2002). Psychological and family factors associated with suicidal ideation in pre-adolescents. *Spanish Journal of Psychology, 5*, 20–28.
Wildschut, T., Sedikides, C., Arndt, J., & Routledge, C. (2006). Nostalgia: Content, triggers, functions. *Journal of Personality and Social Psychology, 91*(5), 975–993.
Williams, M. (1997). *Cry of pain: Understanding suicide and self harm*. London: Penguin Books, Ltd.
Wong, P. T. (2007). Meaning management theory and death acceptance. In A. Tomer, G. T. Eliason, & P. T. Wong (Eds.), *Existential and spiritual issues in death attitudes* (pp. 65–87). New York: Erlbaum.
Zilboorg, G. (1943). Fear of death. *Psychoanalytic Quarterly, 12*, 465–475.
Zimbardo, P., & Boyd, J. (2008). *The Time Paradox: The new psychology of time that will change your life*. New York: Free Press.

Time Perspective Therapy: Transforming Zimbardo's Temporal Theory into Clinical Practice

Richard M. Sword, Rosemary K.M. Sword, and Sarah R. Brunskill

In October 2008, Dr. Philip Zimbardo was the keynote speaker at the Hawaii Psychological Association (HPA) where he introduced his intriguing new book, *The Time Paradox* (Zimbardo and Boyd 2008) and detailed Temporal Theory (TT). It became obvious to attendees Rick and Rosemary Sword, private practice clinicians on the island of Maui, Hawaii, that the concept of "Time Perspective" could have a notable effect on mental health and clinical practice. During questions and answers, a clinician in the audience asked Zimbardo how he applied TT, "I'm an academic psychologist and researcher. It's my job to point out the problems and the clinician's job to solve them…"

Time Perspective

What is one's Time Perspective (TP)? At its most basic level, it is how one views themselves, their life as a whole, and the world around them. This perspective is an ever shifting view point that affects – either positively or negatively – our daily lives. Consequently these same experiences and memories of our past can be extremely biased. Neurological research has shown that when recalling past events, the same regions in the brain are activated as when thinking about the future (Addis et al. 2009, 2007). This provides strong evidence that one's future is highly influenced by his or her past and further indicates that the can past shape one's understanding of their everyday life, which in turn, influences how they view the future. Research has shown that stress (e.g., Kuhlmann et al. 2005; Roberts 2002; Sandi

Dr. R.M. Sword (Deceased)

R.M. Sword • R.K.M. Sword (✉)
The Z Team, 30 Ahuwale Place, Makawao, 96768, HI, USA
e-mail: dr.sword@hawaiiantel.net; rosemarysword@hawaiiantel.net

S.R. Brunskill
The Z Team, Concord, CA, USA

M. Stolarski et al. (eds.), *Time Perspective Theory; Review, Research and Application: Essays in Honor of Philip G. Zimbardo*, DOI 10.1007/978-3-319-07368-2_31,

and Pinelo-Nava 2007) can influence and shape one's memory by effecting the encoding and retrieval of information (Kuhlmann et al. 2005; Sandi and Pinelo-Nava 2007). Additionally, TPs have been shown to influence both recall and one's anticipation of mood (Stolarski et al. 2013). Extensive research indicates that Past Negative, Past Positive and Present Fatalist orientations are associated with problems in mental health, for example, depression (Griffin and Wildbur 2013; Naeger 2001; Van Beek et al. 2011; Zimbardo and Boyd 1999) and anxiety (Anagnostopoulos and Griva 2011; Griffin and Wildbur 2013; Zimbardo and Boyd 1999). Those who are depressed tend to score significantly higher on Past Negative, Present Hedonism, and Present Fatalism, while scoring lower on Future and Past Positive (Zimbardo and Boyd 1999). In contrast, Future and Past Positive orientation have been associated with wellbeing (Boniwell et al. 2010; Drake et al. 2008; Naeger 2001; Zimbardo and Boyd 1999), and protective against psychopathology issues (Van Beek et al. 2011; Zimbardo et al. 2012a, b).

Time Perspective in a Health Care Setting

The concept of TP is a growing movement in the health care research. The ZTPI has been used to better understand substance use (Apostolidis et al. 2006; Keough et al. 1999; Wills et al. 2001), risky sexual behaviors (Henson et al. 2006), treatment of chronic illness, (Hamilton et al. 2003), physical activity (Hall and Fong 2003), weight management behaviors (Hall et al. 2012) poverty (Boniwell and Zimbardo 2003; Epel et al. 1999) and a patient's ability to cope with medical conditions (Livneh and Martz 2007). Unfortunately, the mental health field has been slower to adopt the idea of TPs. There are few known interventions that use the concept of time at their foundation. Currently, researchers in the Netherlands are using a TP-based therapy called Future Oriented Group Training (FOGT) with suicidal patients (Van Beek 2013). They found that FOGT had a significant effect on suicidal ideations, reported distress and on depressive symptoms. In the United Kingdom, Mindfulness Based Cognitive Therapy (MBCT; Segal et al. 2002) focuses on helping patient's interrupt incoming negative/intrusive thoughts to help prevent or manage negative thinking patterns that are linked to a downward spiral and depressive relapses (Teasdale 1988, 1997). Research on MBCT has shown to decrease depression relapse by 50 % (Teasdale et al. 2000; Ma and Teasdale 2004).

By studying Zimbardo's various TPs and the different forms of applying them, the Swords noted that the instability of Past Negative memories and/or Present Fatalistic thoughts could be balanced with Past Positive memories, healthy or selected Present Hedonism and a Future Positive TP (Zimbardo et al. 2012a, b; Sword et al. 2012a, b, 2014a, b). Review of the thought patterns as indicated in the treatment notes of their clients suffering from PTSD (anxiety, depression and trauma) indicated that many did not consider the future, especially a positive future, at all. They were stuck in a pattern of reliving their Past Negatives over and over again to the point of being unable to enjoy them selves in the present or consider their futures. To put this into

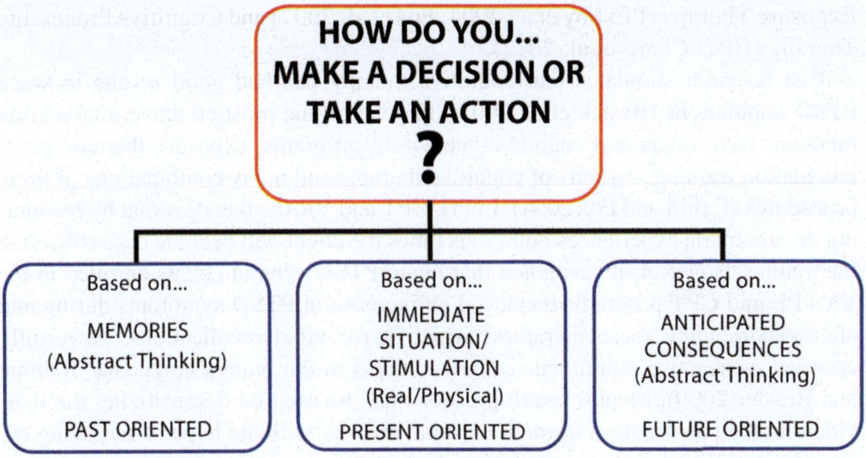

Fig. 1 Decision making typical for particular time orientations

perspective, in Fig. 1 we see *past-oriented* people make decisions based on negative or positive memories of similar situations. *Present-oriented* people take immediate action based on pleasure or avoidance, without thought for consequences. *Future-oriented* people make decisions based on a reasoned assessment of the future consequences, engaging in cost-versus-benefits reasoning.

PTSD and Other Therapies

Clinical psychology, in general, tends to focus on the past. In therapy, patients are encouraged to re-experience, articulate and integrate previous events in the hope of coping or creating a healthy understanding of them. In regard to PTSD, psychological conceptions of the problem posit that being stuck in the past is what prevents actualization in the present. In the United States of America, the majority of therapies implemented to treat PTSD - Cognitive Behavioral Therapy (CBT), Prolonged Exposure Therapy (PE), Cognitive Processing Therapy (CPT) and Virtual Reality Therapy (VR) - are used by the Veterans Administration (VA) and Department of Defense (DoD) for active duty military personnel and veterans. These therapies are based on the present and largely the past.

Cognitive Behavioral Therapy (CBT; e.g., Beck 1967; Suinn and Richardson 1971) focuses on the past trauma with the thought of reframing the past and redirect to a better present. In CBT (Beck 1967), the clinician focuses on the patient's automatic thoughts, assumptions and cognitive distortions and how they influence the patient's understanding of events. Intervention involves teaching patient's how to reinterpret their thinking and assumptions. This focus is similarly true of subsets of CBT such as exposure therapies like Prolonged

Exposure Therapy (PE; Foy et al. 2004; Foa et al. 2007) and Cognitive Processing Therapy (CPT; Chard et al. 2012).

Past research stipulates that cognitive therapy has had good results in some PTSD populations (Resick et al. 2002). In general, the most effective intervention therapies have integrated cognitive-behavioral programs, exposure therapy, stress inoculation training, variants of cognitive therapy, and many combinations of these procedures (Cahill and Foa 2004). In PE, CPT and VR the theory is that by recounting the traumatic experiences numerous times the client will become desensitized to the trauma. However, it was noted that many PTSD veteran clients enrolled in the VA's PE and CPT programs displayed an increase in PTSD symptoms during and after experiencing these therapies[1] which leave vivid recollections, powerfully encoded as negative emotional scenarios buried in the brain's amygdala (Rainnie and Ressler 2009). Mental health professionals focused on desensitizing the individual to the past traumas through multiple reviews with the hope of removing the negative emotional valence attached to the memory.

After studying TT in light of these previous therapies, it was clear that without positive reinforcement, and with little or no emphasis on a Future time perspective, it was no wonder that the PTSD sufferer could not focus on anything other than their Past Negative or their depressing Present Fatalism. It seemed logical that applying the opposite TP, (e.g., Past Positive for Past Negative and Present Hedonism for Present Fatalism), would create balance (Zimbardo et al. 2012a, b; Sword et al. 2014a, b); and emphasis on a brighter future would further assist to balance the Past Negative experiences of those suffering from chronic and severe PTSD.

Time Perspective and PTSD

Reflection on past events is often seen as the best way to understand, describe, and predict ones future. For individuals suffering from PTSD, there is a tendency to relive their past and personal traumas through trademark symptoms such as nightmares, flashbacks and invasive distressing memories of their experiences (American Psychiatric Association 2013; APA). Generally, symptoms surface within a month or two after the triggering event(s) and can persist for months, years or a lifetime. When left untreated, the patients Past Negative experiences influence their present, which can transition their present toward a negative orientation. The present becomes plagued with the hallmark PTSD symptoms, thereby creating a wary and

[1] Our review of the cognitive processing therapy studies show that a significant number of veterans drop out or fail to complete their study. No reason is given for why they failed to completed the study or why they dropped out. Statistical analyses were produced only on the program completers, which positively skewed the results. It would be instructive and responsible for these researchers to follow up with the "dropouts" to determine whether they were harmed by the process and the reason for their leaving the study.

paranoid mindset. Over time, if not corrected the overall negative disposition can carry on into the patient's future, frequently through self-fulfilling prophecy.

The consequences of living in a present negative TP fueled by PTSD are momentous. Significant research shows that impairment in relationships is greatly affected (e.g., APA 2013; Byrne and Riggs 1996; Ruscio et al. 2002; Taft et al. 2011.) Classic diagnostic symptoms such as avoiding stimuli the individual associates with the stressor (e.g., triggers) and their arousal responses (e.g., startle responses and hypervigilance) can generate debilitating fear of unfamiliar social situations causing one to live in a constant state of anxiety about the present and the perceived future. In this mindset, the past seems the best predictor of the future, and in their future it seems inevitable that they are bound to re-live their past traumas or some variation of these negative self-narratives, repeatedly.

Time Perspective Therapy

Using Zimbardo's TT as defined in *The Time Paradox* (Zimbardo and Boyd 2008) and the Zimbardo Time Perspective Inventory (ZTPI; Zimbardo and Boyd 1999), a new talk-therapy was adapted, Time Perspective Therapy (TPT), that offered a unique approach to clinical treatment (Zimbardo et al. 2012a, b; Sword et al. 2012a, b). Over the course of several months following the 2008 HPA conference, this time perspective-based therapy was applied in the Swords private practice, to better understand how it works and to improve it.

Steps of Time Perspective Therapy

As with any therapy, TPT has outlined steps to help guide the therapist and client. First, the therapist administers the ZTPI to determine the individual's TP and assesses the results for any time bias that may be associated with the reported problems. Second, once the biases have been determined, the therapist teaches the individual about TT and the importance of a balanced time perspective. TPT embraces the idea that individuals have a unique TP which can shift or alter depending on one's experiences (Sword et al. 2009, 2013; Zimbardo et al. 2012a, b). However, in times of anguish, our TP can shift for the worse. This second step is illustrated in Fig. 2 which illustrates what happens when the negatives of the past outweigh hope for a better future. The Past Negatives have been stuffed into a box that is spilling over. The bar runs out just past the balance point of the present, the past is so heavy that the future is uncertain (Zimbardo et al. 2012a, b).

As TPT progresses, several things change: (1) the negative past becomes much more manageable, (2) the timeline extends much further into the future where positive goals are beginning to balance out negative past. Through helping the individual become more aware of their overall TP and how this factors into their mental

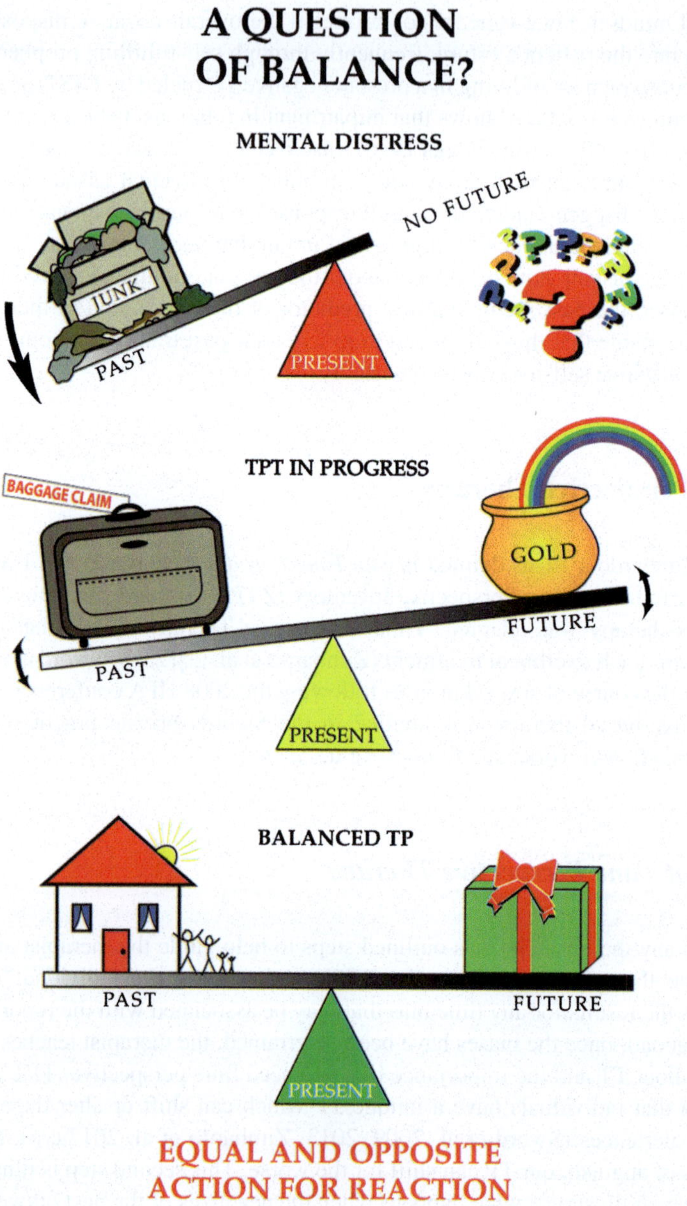

Fig. 2 Illustration of the essence of the idea of Balanced Time Perspective

health (step 3) they work to balance out their time bias (step 4). In a balanced TP, a more positive past and a positive future rest on the fulcrum of the present (see Fig. 2). Further, we see in Fig. 2 that as future goals become present realities, self-confidence and mental health improves. The positive things that happened in the past once again become more readily accessible helping Past Negatives to shrink in importance. In this highly desirable state, positive relationships and experiences of our past outweigh the negative and we look forward to the yet undisclosed gifts the future has in store for each of us (Zimbardo et al. 2012a, b).

The third component and last step of TPT is behavioral. Individuals are taught and encouraged to practice self-soothing activities. When our minds and bodies are in good working order, we automatically know when we are close to reaching our limits of stress and exhaustion and what it takes for us to recuperate. But when our minds and bodies, for whatever reason, aren't in good working order, trouble can ensue. To help with this, TPT participants are encouraged to use meditation and physical exercise (e.g., walking, yoga, dancing, or a regimented gym routine) to reintroduce these important self-soothing behaviors (Zimbardo et al. 2012a, b). Additionally, individuals are encouraged to engage in more pro-social activities and practice selected present hedonism to offset avoidance and isolation experienced when one is depressed.

Time Perspective Therapy Pilot

In January 2009, three months after implementation of TPT, Zimbardo suggested a pilot study of a select group of the Swords' PTSD veteran clients. He introduced the Swords to two graduate researchers from San Francisco State University, Anthony Ferreras and Sarah Brunskill. Over the course of several months, Ferreras, Brunskill and the Swords met together via Skype to discuss and develop a plan for the TPT pilot study that would be implemented in the summer of 2009 to determine the effects of the time based therapy on real situations.

The four year long pilot study (2009–2012) consisted of twenty-nine male United States veterans who were clients in the Sword private practice. On average, participants received 29 (about 10 sessions per year) TPT sessions during the pilot. All participants had a DMS-IV-TR (APA 2000) diagnosis of PTSD that could be linked to a traumatic event that occurred while serving in the military; however, not all were combat related. Participants represented World War II, Korean, Vietnam, Gulf and the Iraq Wars.

At the start of the pilot in June of 2009, participants were tested for self-reports of depression, anxiety and PTSD using the Burns Anxiety Inventory (BAI; Burns 1999), Burns Depression Checklist (BDC; Burns 1997, 1999, 2006), PTSD Checklist – Military Version (PCL-M; Weathers et al. 1993) and Zimbardo Time Perspective Inventory (ZTPI; Zimbardo and Boyd 1999). Participants were retested every 12 months to track their progress. Once participants exited therapy and again one year later, they were given the same measures (BAI, BDC, PCL-M and the ZTPI) to track pre-, post-treatment, one-year follow up to determine and changes while using TPT. The therapy focused on the TPT method of identifying time biases and restructuring their self-narratives to construct a more positive view of their life (Sword et al. 2014a, b; Zimbardo et al. 2012a, b). The overall goal was to decrease

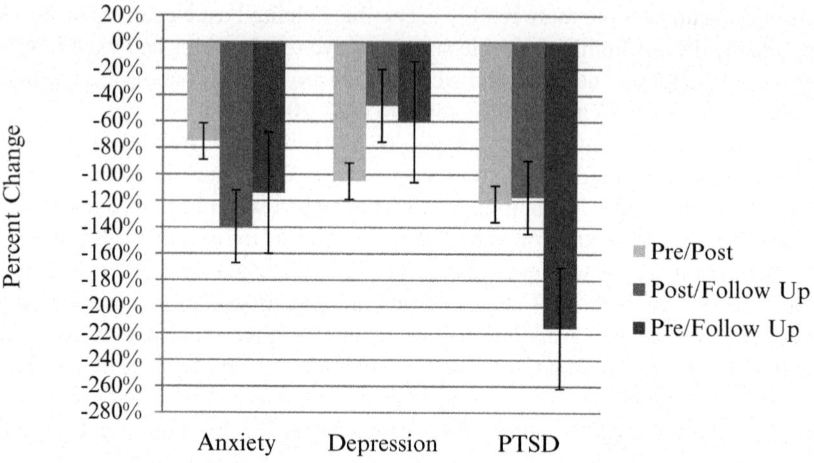

	Anxiety	Depression	PTSD
Pre/Post	-75%	-105%	-122%
Post/Follow Up	-139%	-48%	-117%
Pre/Follow Up	-114%	-60%	-216%

Fig. 3 Anxiety, depression, and PTSD percent change across times measured

reported symptoms (e.g., depression, anxiety and PTSD) by improving the participants' TP (Zimbardo et al. 2014).

When compared to their baseline, participants reported an overall reduction of symptoms for anxiety, depression, and PTSD (see Fig. 3). From their anxiety baseline, there was an overall 75 % decrease in post-treatment reports, 114 % at their one-year follow up and 139 % between post- to one-year follow up. Participant's depression baseline was compared to post scores and found a 105 % drop and an overall decrease of 60 % at one-year follow up. Additionally, depression reports continued to decrease from post-treatment to one-year follow. Lastly, PTSD baseline scores dramatically dropped when they were compared to post-treatment reports and continued to improve at the one-year follow up. Nevertheless, scores slipped from post-treatment to one-year follow up (Fig. 3; Sword et al. 2012a, b, 2014a, b).

With regards to TP, over time a significant shift of both negative and positive TP was observed that trended towards the ideal established by Zimbardo and Boyd (2008; Past Negative = 1.95, Past Positive = 4.60, Present Fatalism = 1.40, Present Hedonism = 3.90 and Future = 4.00). From pre- to post-treatment, participants reported a decrease of Past Negative, Present Fatalism, and Present Hedomism, with an increase of Past Positive and Future thoughts. As with any therapy, the scores leveled off from post-treatment to the one year follow up with Past Negative and Present Fatalism increasing, Past Positive and Future decreasing and Present Hedonism remaining the same. However, when the pre-treatment

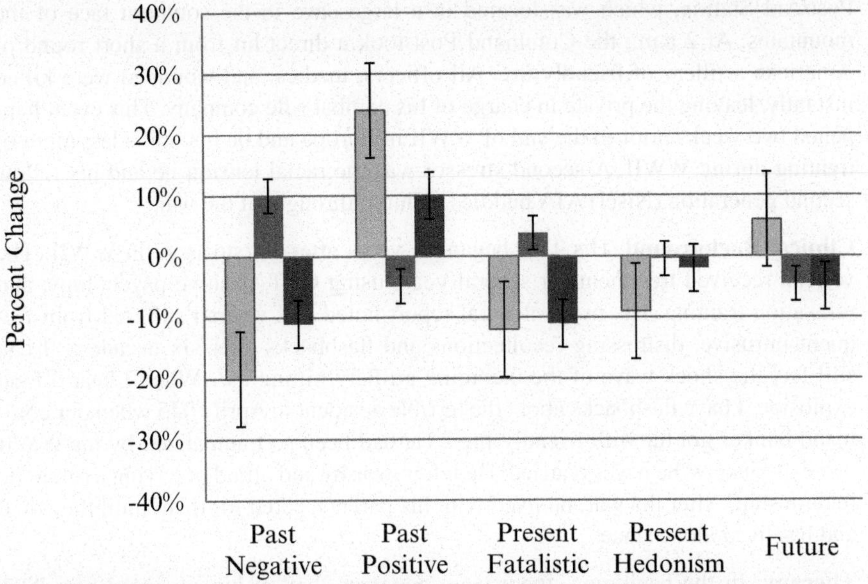

	Past Negative	Past Positive	Present Fatalistic	Present Hedonism	Future
Pre/Post	-20%	24%	-12%	-9%	6%
Post/Follow Up	10%	-5%	4%	0%	-5%
Pre/Follow Up	-11%	10%	-11%	-2%	-5%

Fig. 4 ZTPI percent change across times measured

were compared to one-year follow, patients self reported TP remained healthier than prior to starting TPT which was seen by an overall decrease in Past Negative, Present Fatalism and Present Hedonism and an increase in Past Positive. We did find an overall decline in future reports. This is explained by the higher average age ($m=62.44$) of our participants at the start of the pilot study (see Fig. 4 for percent change; Sword et al. 2012a, b, 2014a, b).

Case Study 1

Demographics. 89 year-old American of Japanese Ancestry (AJA) WWII veteran, a member of the 442nd Regimental Combat Team.

Main Military Stressors. This veteran joined the U.S. Army during WWII to prove his loyalty to the United States. Shortly after being deployed to Europe, he was sent as a rifleman replacement and singularly arrived one evening at the front on the Gothic Line (Nazi line of defense in the spring of 1944, located in the mountains bordering Southern Germany and Northern Italy). He checked into the Command

Post/Aid Station, which was located in a large cave in the southern face of the mountains. At 2 a.m., the Command Post took a direct hit from a short round of American artillery of friendly fire. All officers, medics, and wounded were killed instantly, leaving the private in charge of his combat rifle company. This event happened two weeks prior to the end of WWII in Europe and on his unit's last night of fighting during WWII. A second stressor was the racial tension he and his fellow second generation (Nisei) AJA buddies endured throughout the war.

Clinical Background. His TPT began 64 years after his stressors in WWII. The veteran received treatment for several years using CBT, positive psychology, and relaxation training. His psychological report noted this veteran suffered from frequent intrusive, distressing recollections and flashbacks after six decades: "I can still feel the shock wave of the incoming artillery hitting us…When I hear a loud explosion, I have flashbacks about the terrible accident in April 1945 when our command bunker got hit with friendly fire." He had been so traumatized by his WWII war experiences, he never married. He felt unworthy and afraid of having a romantic relationship. After the war, he lived with his parents, cared for them until they died and has lived alone since.

Therapy. In the beginning, there were concerns that, at his advanced age, TPT would not be effective; however, the client seemed to understand and relate to TPT much more readily than the previous CBT-based, cross-cultural approaches. He related to the simplicity and the positive focus of TPT. Culturally, TPT was a good fit. He quickly grasped the concept of working together and focusing on the good things that can be planned and accomplished in order to create a brighter Future. He pointed out that the pro-social group focus was in keeping with the social nature of the Japanese WWII 442nd culture, which emphasizes the goals of the group above the agenda of the individual.

TPT was explained and reviewed with him in a cross-culturally sensitive manner. The focus was on a brighter future positive TP and he was encouraged to participate in the local WWII 442nd Veterans Club social activities. It is interesting to note his social bonding with his WWII 442nd Unit was so intense that in the seventy years since the end of WWII he has not made close friends outside his elite fighting unit. Since TPT his social ties with his old military buddies are more frequent, which has invoked more upbeat memories of the past and propels him toward a higher future positive TP. However, he is being encouraged to enjoy his present TP a little more fully as ideally his present hedonism score could be higher. He feels that his life is within his control and he believes, if he tries, he can make it even better. This gives him an optimistic outlook for the future.

Results. This veteran's depression, anxiety and PTSD scores fell significantly from severe to within the normal range. His post ZTPI scoring reflected improvement; decrease in Past Negative and Present Fatalism, stabilized Past Positive and Present Hedonism and increased Future (Fig. 5).

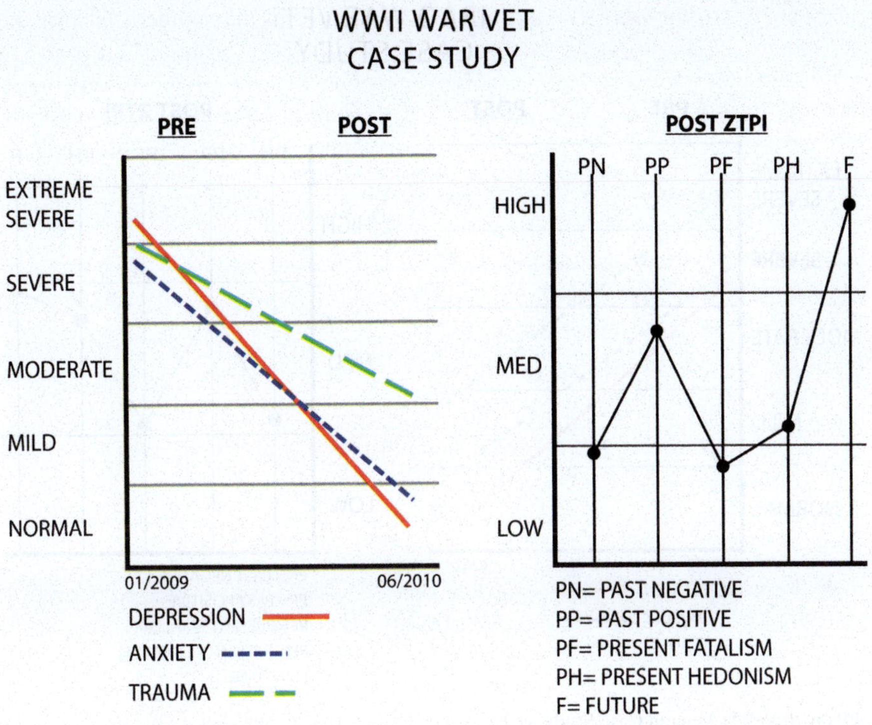

Fig. 5 WWII War Veteran Case Study TPT

Case Study 2

Demographic. 27-year-old Iraq War Veteran of Hawaiian/Japanese/Caucasian Ancestry

Main Military Stressors. At the age of 19, this veteran was deployed to Iraq and served as an escort for detainees at Abu Ghraib prison outside Baghdad. In one incident, he was escorting a detainee when another tried to escape. He chased after the escapee and head butted him with his night optical helmet. The veteran left him on the ground in the heat while he escorted the other detainee to a helicopter. By the time he returned to the downed escapee, the escapee had died. (Note: During the autopsy, it was discovered the escapee was in the final stage of a terminal illness). His second major stressor took place while he was part of the Quick Reaction Force responding to his company's convoy being hit, in which four GIs were KIA. After discovering that two of the KIAs were his cousin and his uncle, an uncontrollable rage descended upon him toward the enemy. He suffered from an all-encompassing blanket of stress in regards to his intolerance of the incompetence of officers and other troops.

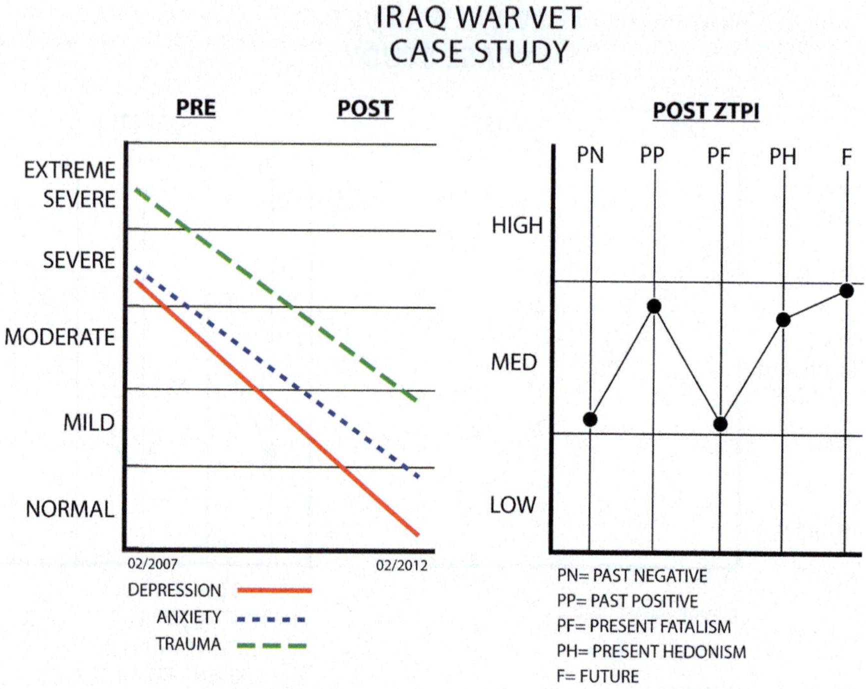

Fig. 6 Iraq War Veteran Case Study TPT

Clinical Background. He returned from Iraq and took a job in pharmaceuticals, but suffered from severe to extreme PTSD symptoms, including frequent suicidal and homicidal ideations. His concerned uncle, who worked with Rick in the National Disaster Medical System's Disaster Mortuary Operational Response Team, insisted he seek help for his chronic/severe service-connected PTSD.

Therapy. The veteran quickly grasped TT as well as TPT and became intent on making positive changes in his life. Although he was anti-social upon entering therapy, he reestablished relationships with family members he had ignored since returning from Iraq. Plans for his future were mapped and be began implementing the steps necessary to secure a productive, pro-social future. Through the course of therapy, he decided to attend a university with the academic goal of completing medical school and becoming a psychiatrist. Although he will always suffer from PTSD, his symptoms have improved significantly, and he now has goals in line for his future positive with his education, career and relationships.

Results. Clinical reports for depression, anxiety and PTSD significantly dropped for this veteran and his ZTPI score reflect these improvements; decrease in Past Negative, Present Hedonism and Present Fatalism and increased Future and Past Positive which led all scores to fall around the ideal (Fig. 6).

Other Components of TPT

Pro-social Behaviors

In the development of TPT, the importance of pro-social behaviors became a critical part of therapy, especially with veterans. The strong social bond the veterans had experienced while in the military is rarely duplicated once they become civilians (Zimbardo et al. 2014). In fact, for PTSD veterans, isolation and avoidance are the norm (Glover 1984). But just as Zimbardo emphasizes the importance of family meals together as a way of bonding in *The Time Paradox* (Zimbardo and Boyd 2008), *The Demise of Guys* (Zimbardo and Duncan 2012) and other works, the Swords also used food to bring the veterans together (Laffaye et al. 2008). Every Wednesday afternoon, veterans gather at the Swords' clinic for war trauma group sessions which includes a meal consisting of food each brings to share. Brunskill and Fererras attended two such meetings. They noted that these veterans who had once lived lives of social isolation were now commiserating, helping each other, planning community projects and competing over who brought the best, freshest food for all to enjoy. Several veterans were hunters, fishermen and farmers and took great satisfaction in providing food they had personally hunted, gathered or cultivated. One or two veterans took it upon themselves to become the grill sergeants and each week performed the duties of cooking what others had brought. After years of social isolation, with the help of TPT, these men created a brotherhood based in their common bond of service to country.

Coronary Rehabilitation

Rick was confident TPT would assist in reducing stress for cardiac patients as he had worked with Meyer Freidman, MD, founder of Type A Behavior Modification which is based on time urgency. TPT was adapted for behavioral medical use for the Maui Memorial Medical Center's cardiac rehabilitation community outreach program. A six week program was created and is provided free of charge to anyone in the community with cardiac concerns interested in learning how to live a healthy life style. Attendees are educated about how to take care of their heart, learn to prepare food and eat healthily, exercise properly (e.g., dance fitness, yoga and Tai Chi), conduct cardio pulmonary resuscitation and live less stressful lives. Participants are taught about TPs and how to healthfully adapt to pre- and post-surgery difficulties

Disaster Stress Control

For two decades, Rick was a member of the U.S. Federal Government's Hawaii Disaster Medical Assistance Team and Hawaii Disaster Mortuary Operational Response Team. He insured the behavioral health of the teams and stress management. Since its development, he utilized TPT in his deployments. His results were qualified by team members during 'hot wash' debriefings following deployments and reported to command staff (Sword and Sword 2013).

Future Directions of TPT

US Department of Defense

In January 2011, Surgeon General of the Pentagon's Joint Chiefs of Staff -U.S. Department of Defense (DoD) Major General Douglas Robb, MD requested an audience with Zimbardo and the Swords to discuss if and how TPT might be implemented into the behavioral health component of the DoD's health care system. General Robb explained that the suicide rate among active military personnel as well as veterans was escalating; his primary focus was to find a way to deal with this problem. The team explained the results from the pilot study and the overall conclusion that when you balance negative TPs with a strong future, the positive focus gave veterans with chronic and severe PTSD something they had lacked, hope. The same would likely be true for active duty military personnel.

In December 2012, the team began working with US Army Lieutenant Colonel Melba Stetz who acquired the necessary funding for a TPT efficacy research study at Tripler Army Medical Center, the largest military medical facility in the Pacific. The study's focus is the use of TPT as a preventative measure for undiagnosed active duty military personnel suffering from PTSD symptoms. It includes TPT's use in individual and group sessions as well as telemedicine (Skype for participants in remote areas). The Swords trained military mental health professionals the summer of 2013; the study will commence in 2014.

Middle East Connection

Throughout the years since the inception of TPT, Phil has traveled the world, talking at international conferences, congresses, universities and symposiums about TT and TPT. At one such international congress, he met a young Iranian graduate student, Marjan Haghighatgoo. Marjan had presented the findings of her study on Iranian university students and the use of the ZTPI. Impressed with Marjan, Zimbardo volunteered to be her mentor and encouraged her TT work in addition to putting in contact with the Swords. Plans for TPT education of Iranian psychologists working with veterans in Tehran were made for early 2012. Unfortunately this humanitarian visit was scrapped due to political concerns brought about by The Arab Spring. They continue to help Marjan as they can (e.g., providing a step-by-step TPT process guidebook) with her work at the Iranian VA with not only veterans but also the women and children affected by wars in Iran.

Future Endeavors

The Time Cure was published in October 2012 (Zimbardo et al. 2012a, b) and unveiled during Zimbardo and the Swords' presentation at HPA Conference in Honolulu, Hawaii (Zimbardo et al. 2012a, b) and elaborated on in their talk during the August 2013 American Psychological Association Conference in Orlando, Florida (Zimbardo et al. 2013). Currently, Zimbardo and the Swords are in negotiations for a two book deal regarding other TPT applications such as depression, anxiety, stress, family and couples counseling, as well as time perspective and sexuality. The team continues to work towards the development of The Time Perspective Therapy Institute where in-person as well as virtual trainings will be offered to all interested therapist TPT sessions will be possible for all.

Conclusion

By using *The Time Paradox* (Zimbardo and Boyd 2008) and ZTPI (Zimbardo and Boyd 1999), the Swords were able to adapt TT into a new treatment, TPT. With an approach aimed at changing the patient's thought process and view of the world, TPT has seen positive results. This led us to argue that time-orientation is a vital component in treatment and is worthy of further exploration as an alternative therapy and extension of CBT. By identifying the client's TP, clinicians were able to assist clients by restructuring their views about the past, present and future as well as impart a self-sustaining, long-lasting way of thinking to gain a more balanced overall TP. Through balancing an individual's time orientation, vital tools can be implemented in their daily life for both the short- and long-term gains. It is understood that TPT may not the right fit for every person or problem, but all indications are it is a promising new tool for the mental field.

References

Addis, D. R., Wong, A. T., & Schacter, D. L. (2007). Remembering the past and imagining the future: Common and distinct neural substrates during event construction and elaboration. *Neuropsychologia, 45*(7), 1363.

Addis, D. R., Pan, L., Vu, M. A., Laiser, N., & Schacter, D. L. (2009). Constructive episodic simulation of the future and the past: Distinct subsystems of a core brain network mediate imagining and remembering. *Neuropsychologia, 47*(11), 2222–2238.

American Psychiatric Association. (2000). *Diagnostic and statistical manual of mental disorders* (4th ed., Text Revision). Washington, DC; Author.

American Psychiatric Association. (2013). *Diagnostic and statistical manual of mental disorders* (5th ed.). Washington, DC: Author.

Anagnostopoulos, F., & Griva, F. (2011). Exploring time perspective in Greek young adults: Validation of the Zimbardo Time Perspective Inventory and relationships with mental health indicators. *Social Indicators Research, 106*(1), 41–59.

Apostolidis, T., Fieulaine, N., & Soulé, F. (2006). Future time perspective as predictor of cannabis use: Exploring the role of substance perception among French adolescents. *Addictive Behaviors, 31*(12), 2339–2343.

Beck, A. T. (1967). *Depression: Clinical, experimental, and theoretical aspects*. New York, NY: Harper and Row. Republished as: Beck, A. T. (1970). *Depression: Causes and treatment.* Philadelphia, PA: University of Pennsylvania Press.

Boniwell, I., & Zimbardo, P. (2003). Time to find the right balance. *The Psychologist.*

Boniwell, I., Osin, E., Linley, P. A., & Ivanchenko, G. V. (2010). A question of balance: Time perspective and well-being in British and Russian samples. *The Journal of Positive Psychology, 5*(1), 24–40.

Burns, D. D. (1997, 2006). Therapist's toolkit: 1997 upgrade; 2006 upgrade. Los Altos Hills: Author.

Burns, D. D. (1999). *Therapist's toolkit*. Palo Alto: D. D. Burns.

Byrne, C. A., & Riggs, D. S. (1996). The cycle of trauma: Relationship aggression in male Vietnam veterans with symptoms of posttraumatic stress disorder. *Violence and Victims, 11*(3), 213–225.

Cahill, S. P., & Foa, E. B. (2004). A glass half empty or half full? Where we are and directions for future research in the treatment of PTSD. In S. Taylor (Ed.), *Advances in the treatment of post-traumatic stress disorder: Cognitive– behavioral perspectives* (pp. 267–313). New York: Springer.

Chard, K. M., Ricksecker, E. G., Healy, E. T., Karlin, B. E., & Resick, P. A. (2012). Dissemination and experience with cognitive processing therapy. *Journal of Rehabilitation Research and Development, 49*(5), 667–678.

Drake, L., Duncan, E., Sutherland, F., Abernethy, C., & Colette, H. (2008). Time perspective and correlates of wellbeing. *Time and Society, 17*(1), 47–61.

Epel, E. S., Bandura, A., & Zimbardo, P. G. (1999). Escaping homelessness: The influences of self-efficacy and Time Perspective on coping with homelessness. *Journal of Applied Social Psychology, 29*(3), 575–596.

Foa, E. B., Hembree, E. A., & Rothbaum, B. O. (2007). *Prolonged exposure therapy for PTSD: Emotional processing of traumatic experiences, therapist guide*. New York: Oxford University Press.

Foy, D. W., Glynn, S. M., Shnurr, P. P., Jankowski, M. K., Wattenberg, M. S., Weiss, D. S., Marmar, C. R., & Gusman, F. D. (2004). Group therapy. In E. B. Foa, T. M. Keane, & M. J. Friedman (Eds.), *Effective treatments for PTSD*. New York: Guilford Press.

Glover, H. (1984). Themes of mistrust and the posttraumatic stress disorder in Vietnam veterans. *American Journal of Psychotherapy, 38*(3), 445–452.

Griffin, E., & Wildbur, D. (2013). Effects of Time-Perspective on the Well-being, Success and Mental Health of Undergraduate Students.

Hall, P. A., & Fong, G. T. (2003). The effects of a brief time perspective intervention for increasing physical activity among young adults. *Psychology and Health, 18*(6), 685–706.

Hall, P. A., Fong, G. T., & Cheng, A. Y. (2012). Time perspective and weight management behaviors in newly diagnosed Type 2 diabetes: A mediational analysis. *Journal of Behavioral Medicine, 35*(6), 569–580.

Hamilton, J. M., Kives, K. D., Micevski, V., & Grace, S. L. (2003). Time perspective and health-promoting behavior in a cardiac rehabilitation population. *Behavioral Medicine, 28*(4), 132–139.

Henson, J. M., Carey, M. P., Carey, K. B., & Maisto, S. A. (2006). Associations among health behaviors and time perspective in young adults: Model testing with boot-strapping replication. *Journal of Behavioral Medicine, 29*(2), 127–137.

Keough, K. A., Zimbardo, P. G., & Boyd, J. N. (1999). Who's smoking, drinking, and using drugs? Time perspective as a predictor of substance use. *Basic and Applied Social Psychology, 21*(2), 149–164.

Kuhlmann, S., Piel, M., & Wolf, O. T. (2005). Impaired memory retrieval after psychosocial stress in healthy young men. *The Journal of Neuroscience, 25*(11), 2977–2982.

Laffaye, C., Cavella, S., Drescher, K., & Rosen, C. (2008). Relationships among PTSD symptoms, social support, and support source in veterans with chronic PTSD. *Journal of Traumatic Stress, 21*, 394–401.

Livneh, H., & Martz, E. (2007). Reactions to diabetes and their relationship to time orientation. *International Journal of Rehabilitation Research, 30*(2), 127–136.

Ma, S. H., & Teasdale, J. D. (2004). Mindfulness-based cognitive therapy for depression: Replication and exploration of differential relapse prevention effects. *Journal of Consulting and Clinical Psychology, 72*(1), 31–40.

Naeger, M. (2001). *Temporal perspectives, dispositional styles, and subjective well being*. Masters thesis, Western Kentucky University, Masters theses & specialist projects, paper 690.

Rainnie, D., & Ressler, K. (2009). Physiology of the amygdala: Implications for PTSD. In J. E. LeDoux, T. Keane, & P. Shiromani (Eds.), *Post- traumatic stress disorder: Basic science and clinical practice* (pp. 39–78). Totowa: Humana Press.

Resick, P. A., Nishith, P., Weaver, T. L., Astin, M. C., & Feuer, C. A. (2002). A comparison of cognitive-processing therapy with prolonged exposure and a waiting condition for the treatment of chronic post traumatic stress disorder in female rape victims. *Journal of Consulting and Clinical Psychology, 70*, 867–879.

Roberts, P. (2002). Vulnerability to false memory: The effects of stress, imagery, trait anxiety, and depression. *Current Psychology, 21*(3), 240–252.

Ruscio, A. M., Weathers, F. W., King, L. A., & King, D. W. (2002). Male war-zone veterans' perceived relationships with their children: The importance of emotional numbing. *Journal of Traumatic Stress, 15*(5), 351–357.

Sandi, C., & Pinelo-Nava, M. T. (2007). Stress and memory: Behavioral effects and neurobiological mechanisms. *Neural Plasticity*. Segal, Z. V., & Williams, J. M. G. (2012). *Mindfulness-based cognitive therapy for depression*. Guilford Press.

Segal, Z., Williams, M., & Teasdale, J. (2002). *Mindfulness-based cognitive therapy for depression: A new approach to preventing relapse*. New York: Guilford Press.

Stolarski, M., Matthews, G., Postek, S., Zimbardo, P. G., & Bitner, J. (2013). How we feel is a matter of time: Relationships between time perspectives and mood. *Journal of Happiness Studies*, 1–19. doi:10.1007/s10902-013-9450-y.

Suinn, R., & Richardson, F. (1971). Anxiety management training: A non-specific behavior therapy program for anxiety control. *Behavior Therapy, 2*, 498–510.

Sword, R. M., & Sword, R. K. M. (2013, August). *Time perspective therapy: From theory to clinical trauma conversion therapy—Temporal rebalancing past downers into future uppers*. Paper presented at the annual meeting of the American Psychological Association, Honolulu.

Sword, R. M., Sword, R. K. M., & Zimbardo, P. (2013, August). *Time perspective therapy: New and effective cure for PTSD in vets and civilians*. Paper presented at the annual meeting of the American Psychological Association, Honolulu.

Sword, R. M., Sword, R. K. M., Brunskill, S. R., Ferreras, A. C., Calleon, K., & DePont, K. (2009). *Zimbardo's temporal theory: An emerging therapy for PTSD vets*. Paper presented at the Hawaiian Psychological Association.

Sword, R. M., Sword, R. K. M., Zimbardo, P., & Brunskill, S. R. (2012a, September). *Time Perspective Therapy: An interactive therapy that lasts*. Paper presented at the International Time Perspective Conference, Portugal.

Sword, R. M., Sword, R. K. M., Zimbardo, P., & Brunskill, S. R. (2012b, April). *Time Perspective Therapy: From theory to clinical practice*. Paper presented at the annual meeting of the Western Psychological Association, San Francisco.

Sword, R. M., Sword, R. K. M., Brunskill, S. R., & Zimbardo, P. G. (2014a). Time perspective therapy: A new time-based metaphor therapy for PTSD. *Journal of Loss and Trauma*, (accepted).

Sword, R. M., Sword, R. K. M., Brunskill, S. R., Ferreras, A. C., & Zimbardo, P. (2014b). Time perspective therapy: Time perspective therapy pilot study. *Journal of Professional Psychology*. Submitted and under review.

Taft, C. T., Watkins, L. E., Stafford, J., Street, A. E., & Monson, C. M. (2011). Posttraumatic stress disorder and intimate relationship problems: A meta-analysis. *Journal of Consulting and Clinical Psychology, 79*(1), 22.

Teasdale, J. D. (1988). Cognitive vulnerability to persistent depression. *Cognition and Emotion, 2*, 247–274.

Teasdale, J. D. (1997). The relationship between cognition and emotion: The mind-in-place in mood disorders. In D. M. Clark & C. G. Fairburn (Eds.), *Science and practice of cognitive behaviour therapy* (pp. 67–93). New York: Oxford University Press.

Teasdale, J. D., Segal, Z. V., Williams, J. M. G., Ridgeway, V. A., Soulsby, J. M., & Lau, M. A. (2000). Prevention of relapse/recurrence in major depression by mindfulness-based cognitive therapy. *Journal of Consulting and Clinical Psychology, 68*(4), 615.

Van Beek, W. (2013). Future thinking in suicidal patients: Development and evaluation of a future oriented group training in a randomized controlled trial.

Van Beek, W., Berghuis, H., Kerkhof, A., & Beekman, A. (2011). Time perspective, personality and psychopathology: Zimbardo's time perspective inventory in psychiatry. *Time and Society, 20*(3), 364–374.

Weathers, F. W., Litz, B. T., Herman, D. S., Huska, J. A., & Keane, T. M. (1993). The PTSD checklist (PCL): Reliability, validity, and diagnostic utility. In *Proceedings of the Annual Meeting of the International Society for Traumatic Stress Studies*, San Antonio, TX.

Wills, T. A., Sandy, J. M., & Yaeger, A. M. (2001). Time perspective and early-onset substance use: A model based on stress–coping theory. *Psychology of Addictive Behaviors, 15*(2), 118.

Zimbardo, P. G., & Boyd, J. N. (1999). Putting time in perspective: A valid, reliable individual-differences metric. *Journal of Personality and Social Psychology, 77*(6), 1271–1288.

Zimbardo, P. G., & Boyd, J. N. (2008). *The Time Paradox: The new psychology of time that will change your life*. New York: The Free Press, Simon & Schuster.

Zimbardo, P. G., & Duncan, N. (2012). *The demise of guys: Why boys are struggling and what we can do about it* (TED ebooks). New York: TED Conferences.

Zimbardo, P. G., Sword, R. M., & Sword, R. K. (2012a). *The time cure: Overcoming PTSD with the new psychology of time perspective therapy*. San Francisco: Jossey-Bass.

Zimbardo, P. G., Sword, R. M., & Sword, R. K. M. (2012b, October). *Time Perspective Therapy: From theory to clinical practice*. Paper presented at the Hawaiian Psychological Association Conference, Hawaii.

Zimbardo, P. G., Sword, R. M., & Sword, R. K. M. (2013, August). *Time Perspective Therapy: New and effective cure for PTSD in vets and civilians*. Paper presented at the American Psychological Association Conference, Florida.

Zimbardo, P., Ferreras, A. C., & Brunskill, S. R. (2014). Social intensity syndrome: Why men prefer males to females. *Psychology of Men and Masculinity*. Submitted and under review.

The Uncharted Territory: Time Perspective Research Meets Clinical Practice. Temporal Focus in Psychotherapy Across Adulthood and Old Age

Elena Kazakina

Overview

The goal of this chapter is to demonstrate how time perspective research can inform clinical practice and how, reciprocally, clinical practice can contribute to further research. I will highlight some aspects of the interaction between research and practice (dissemination of knowledge; converting biography into theory, self-reflection) and point out the role of Philip Zimbardo in promoting time studies in mainstream psychology. In my own work, during the last 15 years I have been applying time perspective-focused psychotherapy to clinical practice with adults ranging in age from early 20s to late 90s. My approach is based on the multidimensional study of time perspective and concepts of temporal balance and time continuity elaborated in my doctoral dissertation (Kazakina 1999). My clinical work was enriched by the construct of balanced time perspective derived from the research of Philip Zimbardo and colleagues. Further in this chapter I demonstrate how the temporal focus of clinical strategies can be combined with other psychotherapy approaches (cognitive, behavioral, psychodynamic, and existential) to enhance the effectiveness of treatment. I review two clinical cases, pointing out the reduction of symptoms and increase in positive functioning associated with self-actualization, interpersonal effectiveness, and well-being. The chapter also focuses on the empirical and theoretical implications of clinical practice as well as points out some clinically relevant time studies. I introduce the notion of optimal time perspective, useful in my clinical work, and suggest a redefinition of the concept of Time Competence (Shostrom 1968). Further development of time-perspective focused clinical practice is examined in the conclusion.

E. Kazakina (✉)
Independent Private Practice, East Brunswick, NJ, USA
e-mail: ekazakina@comcast.net

M. Stolarski et al. (eds.), *Time Perspective Theory; Review, Research and Application: Essays in Honor of Philip G. Zimbardo*, DOI 10.1007/978-3-319-07368-2_32,

Crossroads: Research, Practice, Biography

The theory and research always aim at enriching practice. However, this task, demanding for any field of knowledge, can be particularly challenging for the newly unified domain of time perspective. First, this research has to overcome its former "disjointed" and "noncumulative" nature (Zimbardo and Boyd 1999, p. 1272). Second, the relevance of time perspective studies to practice, and more specifically to the practice of psychotherapy has to be ensured and enhanced. This is a challenging task because mainstream psychologists are largely unaware of "this intriguing, seemingly central aspect of human functioning." (Zimbardo and Boyd 1999, p. 1272).

The growing movement towards evidence-based practice in modern counseling and psychotherapy aims at the "the integration of best available research with clinical expertise in the context of patient characteristics, culture and preferences" (American Psychological Association 2006, p. 273). To reach this goal, practitioners have to avoid "reckless extrapolation of research from the lab to the consulting room…" (Norcross et al. 2008, p. xiii), while not overlooking or even disregarding existing scholarly empirical findings. However, prior to choosing the best available time perspective research, clinicians have to become aware that this research does exist and can contribute to their work with patients. Therefore dissemination of knowledge obtained in time perspective studies among practitioners takes a more central role. No one may give a better example of this professional competency than Philip Zimbardo. Zimbardo with his colleague John Boyd developed theory and instrument (Zimbardo and Boyd 1999) that inspired a solid body of research (Paixao et al. 2012). Zimbardo also promoted the understanding of the concept of balanced time perspective and its connections with optimal human functioning in his publications and talks for the psychology community at large (e.g., Boniwell and Zimbardo 2004; Chamberlin 2008). His books "Time Paradox" (Zimbardo and Boyd 2008) and most recent "Time Cure" (Zimbardo et al. 2012) bring time perspective research and theory closer to practice, capturing interest of both the general public and professional audience.

However, dissemination of knowledge is a two-way street on which clinicians share the road. Clinical work is viewed (Goldfried 2000) as providing the *context of discovery* (emphasis added) which helps to formulate meaningful research questions and to garner clinical hypotheses that later can be studied under rigorous research conditions (p. 21). I suggest that clinicians utilizing time perspective-focused approach recognize the value of their clinical discoveries, register benefits and challenges in applying research findings and disseminate this knowledge within the clinical and research community. I hope this chapter will be a step in that direction.

Another task essential for both scientists and clinicians is objective and subjective observation including empathic observation and self-examination (Stricker and Trierweiler 1995). Here I would like to illuminate the importance of self-examination in regard to evolution of one's interest in psychology of time and also in the current status and the evolution of one's own time perspective. As clinicians, we bring our views of past, present and future into the therapy setting and they affect every phase of treatment.

Scientist-practitioner's temporal sensibility and temporal sensitivity – from my point of view – have to address the following issues: How was the interest in time research and practice developed? What in one's intellectual and experiential history instigated interest and sensitivity to the psychology of time? How biography can be converted into theory (Ash 1992), creating the context of discovery for research and clinical practice? How does individual experience shape our time perspective outlook and research interests? What do we bring into the consultation room, what are our own biases and preferences in perception of past, present and future?

How does one's biography become a catalyst of temporal sensitivity? Zimbardo (Zimbardo and Boyd 1999, 2008) shared with us several experiences that shaped his deep interest in time, such as being sick for a long time as a child and growing up poor among intensely present and past-oriented childhood family members. The latter propelled his almost rebellious emphasis on future orientation, facilitated by his dedicated elementary school teachers. The profound changes in time perspective of the participants of his dramatic Stanford Prison Experiment further deepened his fascination with time.

My observation is that an individual's emotional struggle to cope with disruptions or contradictions in surrounding reality can become *a powerful catalyst of temporal sensitivities*. It was remarkable for me to discover that two important figures in psychology of time and temporal theory, French psychiatrist, Eugene Minkowski, the author of fundamental volume "Lived time" (1933/1970) and Kurt Lewin, founder of American social psychology, emigrated from their native countries following the persecution of Jews. Minkowski left czarist Russia early in the 1900s and Lewin escaped Nazi Germany in 1933. Both were decorated World War I veterans fighting on the opposite sides... Less well-known among TP research community is Hans Loewald (1906–1993), one of the major psychoanalytic thinkers who highlighted the centrality of temporal dimension in human life and psychoanalysis (Loewald 1962/1980a, 1972/1980b). His life was marked by a life saving move to the U.S. from Europe in 1940. To what extent personal transitions affect intellectual biography sparking one's interest in temporal phenomena?

My own experience of emigration from the former Soviet Union to the U.S. in 1989 and multiple cultural adjustments that followed compelled me to understand how people perceive time, the time of their lives. The captivating personal puzzle translated later into a research question for my doctoral dissertation was whether positive functioning was compatible with holding on to all three time orientations, past, present and future, rather than sacrificing one for another, with future orientation predominating over the temporal perspective, as American culture seemed to require. Could continuity or connections among personal past, present and future help in navigating life changes? Is it possible to retain one's past while moving towards the promising future? It was difficult to find the answers in the literature: the studies of the future rarely informed how their participants viewed their present or past. The reminiscences research by and large remained isolated from the investigation of the present and future in the same groups of participants (see review in Kazakina 1999).

I believed that in order to obtain a deep and comprehensive understanding of individuals' time perspective all three time frames, past, present and future, had to be represented in the same research studies. It was my conviction that the respect to all three temporal regions in the American culture and society might enhance the depth and meaning of American cultural and public life, which seems focused primarily on the future with its cultural value of progress and achievement (Gorman and Wessman 1977; Kastenbaum 1964).

In retrospect, it appears that it was my biography and desire to retain the best of my personal and cultural past while intensely focusing on the present and moving towards an uncertain but exciting future that were shaping my thinking at the time. It was striking to find out from Philip Zimbardo's talk about history of the ZTPI development (Zimbardo 2012) that the creation of the past orientation scale was influenced by the comments of the foreign students, his study participants. They pointed to the absence of questions about the past in the initial version of his questionnaire that focused on the differences between present and future oriented individuals (Gonzalez and Zimbardo 1985; Zimbardo and Boyd 1999).

Perhaps, these young people wanted to honor or recognize their past along with their present and future, sharing with me similar temporal sensibility. That is how my biography was converted into theory explaining the personal aspect of my commitment to each temporal orientation, past, present, and future, to be given a full representation in the individuals' experience of time.

Theoretical and Empirical Foundation of the Temporal Focus of My Clinical Practice

Central concepts, variables and findings of my dissertation research: Time perspective of older adults: Relationships to attachment style, psychological well-being and psychological distress (Kazakina 1999).[1]

The theory and findings of my study completed in the late 90s laid the foundation of the time perspective focus in counseling and psychotherapy that I have been applying for 15 years. What did I take from this work into my clinical practice?

Theoretical Background

One of the study's major theoretical concepts is the concept of temporal integration. The human capacity to extend beyond the present moment, making connections among past, present and future, is viewed as a special "time-binding" quality of the

[1] I would like to thank my dissertation advisor, Dr. Elizabeth Midlarsky for her thoughtful guidance and insightful suggestion to examine the relationship between temporal phenomena and attachment style (capacity for trusting and enduring relationship), an essential but then rarely investigated aspect of functioning in late life.

human mind, or temporal integration, necessary for successful adaptation (Hearnshaw 1956; Melges 1982). Particularly relevant to the temporal focus of my clinical interventions is Lewin's (1942/1997) strong emphasis that psychological past and psychological future are *simultaneous* and *interdependent* parts of the psychological field existing at a given time (p. 208). The distinction of temporal regions in the time perspective and their coexistence and inner correlation provide a comprehensive view of the nature of personal experience of time. Thus, the psychological present is conceptualized as a "mixture" of past events (recollections of the past), responses to present events (experience in the present), and anticipations of future events (Block 1990; Doob 1971).

However, research frequently reduced time perspective to a single time orientation (e.g., future), or to a single temporal dimension (e.g., extension – projection into the future or past) (see review in Kazakina 1999). My study investigated all three time orientations in one population and along multiple dimensions. Each time orientation was examined along the dimensions of density, emotional valence, and extension (i.e., number of experiences, thoughts and feelings allocated to each temporal frame, their emotional tone, and length of period over which they are projected into the past or future). In addition, my study distinguished two rarely examined variables – temporal continuity (ability to see past, present and future as meaningfully connected) and temporal balance (relative equilibrium of thoughts and feelings allocated to each temporal region). Both variables characterized time perspective as a whole, expressing interconnectedness and coexistence of the three temporal regions.

Traditionally, a dominant focus on futurity was regarded as an indicator of adaptation and mental health (Kahana and Kahana 1983; Schonfield 1973; Seginer 2009; Vilhauer et al. 2012). By contrast, my study emphasized the importance of balanced temporal orientations for psychological health based on the concepts of "open mind" (Rokeach 1960), "healthy" time line (Rappaport 1990), "time competence" (Shostrom 1968), and "openness" of an individual to past, present and future (Nuttin 1985; Rappaport 1990).

The basic hypothesis (by and large confirmed) was that the balance of time orientations and their interconnectedness (concepts of temporal balance and temporal continuity), as well as their disruptions, could be more essential and perhaps sophisticated indicators and predictors of positive and negative aspects of individual functioning than time-related phenomena associated with only one particular time frame, such as positive or negative future outlook.

Zimbardo and Boyd's seminal publication (1999) offered the concept and measure of time perspective including all three temporal frames and generated a solid body of research around the world. However, time studies combining all three time referents, past, present, and future, remain infrequent (Webster 2011), and particularly rare in the samples of older adults (Desmyter and De Raedt 2012; Kazakina 2012, 2013; Webster and Ma 2013). TP research often continues to focus on one temporal region, as it is done for example in a comprehensive volume by Seginer (2009) "Future orientation" as well as in many studies presented at the ITPC12 (Paixao et al. 2012).

It is fascinating to see that the emphasis on the future prevalent in research has been carried over into the time-oriented psychotherapy both in the earlier approaches (Melges 1982; Rappaport 1990) and recent nascent time perspective therapy developments such as future directed therapy for major depressive disorder (Vilhauer and Deepika 2012), and future oriented group training for suicidal patients (van Beek et al. 2009).

Major Findings

(Findings most relevant to my clinical work are presented here).[2]

My study documented that older adults who were securely attached (those with close and trusting interpersonal connections) had the more balanced time orientations and experienced a greater sense of connection among personal past, present, and future.

The strongest predictor of life satisfaction was positive present attitude, followed by positive past attitude (Kazakina 1999, p. 210; p. 213). Important correlates of psychological distress were negative feelings about the present and an imbalance of positive experiences, thoughts and feelings across time regions – past, present, and future.

It should be noted that only one type of temporal balance contributed to psychological distress as well as attachment security: the balance of positive experiences, thoughts and feelings across time regions (positive emotional valence measure derived from Time Reference Inventory) (Roos and Albers 1965).

In addition, my empirical findings pointed out connections among rarely examined phenomena: secure attachment (capacity for close, enduring relationships), balance and continuity of time perspective, and level of educational attainment. Individuals with secure attachment style of relationships had a greater balance of positive aspects of past, present and future and greater ability to see them in a meaningful continuity. Also, more educated participants in this study demonstrated higher time continuity – greater ability to use one's past in understanding the present and planning for the future (Shostrom 1968). This finding resonates with most recent research on connections of balanced TP with emotional intelligence (Stolarski et al. 2011) and wisdom (Webster et al. 2012).

The Notions of Balanced Temporality and Optimal Time Perspective

Balanced temporality was initially defined as a relatively balanced combination of past, present and future orientations in the individual's time perspective that was distinguished as an essential part of the subjective experience of time (Kazakina 1999).

[2] Please see Kazakina (1999) for the full discussion of limitations of the study and findings. The brief description of study design, variables and measures can be found in Kazakina (2013).

My approach was based on the conceptualization of the balance of temporal orientations necessary for temporal integration and psychological health (Rappaport 1990; Shostrom 1968).

Later I extended this concept to include those aspects of time perspective that were found in my research to be the most relevant temporal correlates of positive functioning in late life. These "healthy" time perspective variables involved a specific type of temporal balance – a balance of positive experiences, thoughts and feelings that older adults referred to their past, present and future. Other essential dimension included temporal continuity – a sense of connection among past, present and future. Other "healthy" temporal elements included positive feelings about the present, followed by positive feelings about the past; positive future was found to be a part of this formulation but its role in late life had to be clarified further due to inconsistent findings. I suggested that these aspects of temporal experience needed to be evaluated and enhanced in counseling and psychotherapy.[3]

In my study balance and continuity of past, present and future were found to be independent from each other, presenting two distinct manifestations of temporal integration. New operational definitions of these variables as well as age groups other than older adults should be included in further research to collaborate this finding. However, I believe that theoretically these concepts should be looked at as distinct. It is beyond the scope of this chapter to elaborate on the clarification of the related constructs – balanced time perspective (Zimbardo and Boyd 1999, 2008), temporal expansion (Webster 2011; Webster and Ma 2013), and temporal holism (Sirois 2012). These constructs and their relevant measures seem to reflect both balance and continuity in individual's experience of past, present, and future.

Further development of the notion of balanced temporality incorporated Zimbardo and Boyd's (1999) dynamic understanding of "balanced time perspective" associated with positive functioning. This balance was viewed not only as a state but also as an *ongoing process of balancing* (emphasis added) (Boniwell and Zimbardo 2004). The key part of this process is the flexible switching of temporal frames among past, future and present, depending on situational demands and personal resources to avoid temporal bias (overuse or underuse of any particular time orientation) (Zimbardo and Boyd 1999, p. 1272).

Most recently, I have developed a clinically useful notion of the "Optimal Time Perspective" (OTP). It includes balance of time orientations, subjective sense of their connections, temporal flexibility – ability to switch from one temporal frame to another depending on situational demands (Zimbardo and Boyd 1999), and also if necessary – an adaptive over-focus on a specific time region or regions. OTP allows for an adaptive limited engagement with one (or two) particular time zone, past, present or future unless it becomes a rigid defense or as Zimbardo and Boyd (1999) described it as *habitual* over-focus or temporal bias. This adaptive or coping over-focus seems to help individuals to navigate through traumatic, transitional or demanding experiences (e.g., grief and mourning; emigration, meeting deadlines, etc.).(see, for example, Turnip 2012).

---

[3] A careful consideration is given to the generalizability of results obtained in the older sample (65+) to the middle-aged and younger individuals (21+).

Time Perspective Psychotherapy

Time perspective therapy from my point of view is psychotherapy in which temporal focus – awareness of psychological concepts of past, present and future, and their interaction – underlies clinical interventions. I view temporal flexibility – ability to switch from one temporal frame to another not only as a goal for the patient to acquire but also as a tool for the clinician to use. Keeping in mind a patient's past, present and future while moving swiftly to the time orientation in need of immediate attention, and choosing the most appropriate clinical intervention, is at the core of my time perspective focused therapeutic approach.

My clinical work incorporated a conceptual framework of time competence and self-actualization (Maslow 1970; Shostrom 1968). It was also informed by Temporally Oriented Psychotherapy (Rappaport 1990) and later by the seminal contribution of Philip Zimbardo and colleagues to time perspective theory and research (Zimbardo and Boyd 1999, 2008; Boniwell and Zimbardo 2004).

The notions of balanced temporality and optimal time perspective help me to do assessment and formulate treatment goals. "If psychotherapy may be considered to be a process of value re-orientation for the patient, a significant step can be made in helping the client to realize the proper balance between past, present, and future orientations." (Shostrom 1968, p. 19). However, I specify that this temporal balance is in fact a balance of the positive elements of past, present, and future in individual's experience of time (Kazakina 1999, 2013).

It is also important to emphasize that in the course of treatment I use temporal balance "as a yardstick of health in trying to ascertain the relative progress of a given patient" (Rappaport 1990, p. 189). I also review "the status" of my patients' sense of meaningful continuity among their past, present and future as treatment unfolds.

My strong suggestion is that the first step for clinicians has to include evaluation of their own cultural and personal values about the concepts of past, present and future. Are there any implicit "favorites" or, as Gorman and Wessman (1977) noted, "good guys versus bad guys?" Thomas Jefferson wrote once that he liked dreams of the future more than the memories of the past. This view may have been forever embedded in American cultural tradition. However, the basic attitude that followed from my study was based on respect for each temporal region and the enhancement of its balanced participation in an individual's functioning.

Another important step is to gain awareness of how we view the temporality of adults of different age – young, middle-aged and older adults. Are there any stereotypes about the experience of time in old age, such as "the elderly live only by their memories" or "old people have no future"? Do we have any preconceptions about younger people that their past is insignificant or it is good for them to only live for the future?

A multidimensional approach to time perspective applied in my study (Kazakina 1999) has become a part of my clinical work, both in the evaluation phase and as treatment unfolds. It means that I have to understand how patients think and feel about each period of their lives–past, present, and future–and about their connections or disconnections. To what extent is each time period full or empty? What is the emotional tone associated with different aspects of each temporal frame? How far in both directions–past and future–can a person see? What is the relative importance of past, present, and future for each individual? Can patients find positive experiences in each temporal region in a relatively even fashion? If past, present, and future are split or disconnected, if one temporal zone "outweighs" another, is it an adaptive transient state or a potential temporal bias? If one temporal period is excluded from an individual's perspective, this may be a signal for a careful exploration of a personal coping style and also a sign of a possible problem that needs to be addressed in psychotherapy.

"Problems" in time perspective based on my clinical experience could be triggered by various developmental and transitional issues of younger, middle and late adulthood. Among them stands out achieving and re-establishing ego identity based on what an individual was, has come to be and promises to be in the future (Erikson 1985). Transitional issues characterized by change may include relocation, sudden illness, change of jobs or residence, wedding, pregnancy, divorce, and among older adults, retirement, declining health and widowhood.

Clinical Theoretical Perspectives

Temporal focus of my clinical work is implemented within the context of my psychotherapy approach, which is informed by several theoretical perspectives. Theoretical framework of enhancing actualizing tendency of an individual (Maslow 1970) (humanistic/positive psychology) also includes psychodynamic, cognitive-behavioral and existential perspectives. The elements of these diverse schools of psychotherapy constitute one combined approach to my clinical work.

Psychodynamic perspective emphasizes the role of unconscious motivation and defense mechanisms. (See Shedler's (2010) well-written presentation of theory and efficacy of psychodynamic psychotherapy). I became particularly affiliated with the psychoanalytic self psychology developed by Heinz Kohut (1971, 1984). It expands clinician's empathic ability focusing on "how to be with a patient" rather than "what to do with a patient." This becomes a core of what I call the empathic present of therapy sessions. Empathic bond established in sessions as well as an understanding of patients' experience effectively conveyed to them eventually helps to strengthen the self as independent center of initiative and the organizing center of skills and talents of personality (Kohut 1971).

Cognitive-behavioral aspects of my work involve examining patients' automatic thoughts, schemata (core beliefs), and cognitive distortions; using relaxation techniques as well as cognitive and behavioral rehearsals (Dobson 2010). Based on existential perspective associated with Victor Frankl (1976), I address an individual's search for meaning which is identified as a primary motivational force in a human being (Frankl 1976).

Clinical Case: Creating Positive Past to Alleviate Negative Experience in the Present[4]

Mr. Michael Jones (not his real name), is a 45 year old Caucasian man, gainfully employed professional, happily married with two children. He reported recurrent depressive episodes and anxiety, easily succumbing to the emotion of disappointment in the search of greater fulfillment of his ambitions unrelated to his occupation. Focus on his past helped him gain insight in the siblings' rivalry, and desire to distinguish himself in the area where he could avoid competition with his older powerful brother. Finding a more realistic path to assert his unmet needs for recognition became one of the longer-term treatment goals. Our sessions addressed the development of Michael's interests and abilities across time periods with the emphasis on the future.

The short-term goal of treatment was to help the patient regulate his mood in the present alleviating his chronic dysphoria. Michael was capable of experiencing positive emotions but unlike negative ones, they were extremely short-lived. Commonly my temporal intervention would be to activate Positive Past (ZTPI, Zimbardo and Boyd 1999) in order to search and accumulate positive images that can be used for enhancing positive present or positive future. However, this patient reported immense difficulty looking for good memories: he was immediately overtaken by powerful negative feelings associated with his past. Instead a very specific temporal intervention has been developed in our close collaboration during therapy session.

Michael was instructed to detect his positive experiences in the present as they were happening, being mindful of his positive affect. He would turn to these images (e.g., playing with his children, intimate moments with wife, early morning run) of his purposefully constructed recent positive past at the first signals of distress.

Obtaining sense of mastery in coping with disturbing symptoms is one of the key interventions for anxiety reduction (Dobson 2010). Sense of mastery also became a necessary component for Michael's confidence building and enhancing his sense of self.

Clinical Case: Obtaining Balance and Continuity of Time Perspective

Ms. Lillian Jacksons is a 71-year-old Caucasian female, divorced, with no children, retired college professor. She initially came for treatment to help her cope with transitional and adjustment issues following her retirement and move from another state. Therapy sessions brought out her interests in arts that she was never able to pursue; as a young adult she dreamt of having an art gallery. Her volunteer work in the local Arts Center which she became engaged with in the course of treatment gave her a strong sense of meaning connecting her past and present together. She became more optimistic about her future at a new place: her new friends, relatively

[4] ***Clinical Cases*:** patients' names and background details are changed to protect confidentiality.

stable health, developing her talent representing artists to the bigger art galleries. It seemed that after a period of disruption she was helped to regain a sense of balance and continuity between her past, present and future.

However, Lillian's present unexpectedly turned into turmoil. She became romantically interested in one of the artists, who participated in the exhibit she helped to organize. Mr. Robert Williams (not his real name) was 10 years younger and recently separated from his wife. Lillian's long dormant sexuality was re-awakened as well as her feelings of abandonment and loss associated with her earlier experiences of love.

Several important things happened in treatment. While providing an empathic therapy present in which patient could freely express her passionate longings, I had to re-evaluate my own preconception of sexuality and the prospect of extra-marital affair – not uncommon topics in therapy – but taking place in later life and with full messiness of "a younger love affair". Rarely themes of love and sexuality are considered in the context of old age in research and psychotherapy (Hillman 2012).

Therapy sessions helped Lillian explore and sort out powerful feelings that she experienced in the present. For the first time in two decades she felt fully alive, but overcome with intolerable jealousy that seemed to outweigh the moments of tenderness and thoughtfulness in her new relationship. Lillian was also preoccupied with the potential destructiveness that a possible affair may bring into her life. Therapy sessions switched focus from patient's past to her present and future. Cognitive approach helped patient identify her thoughts that triggered her jealousy. For example, while waiting longer for Robert's telephone call – being in the near Future temporal frame – her internal monologue would be: "He had a car accident; He is with another woman, younger and prettier; He will never call me again, he does not love me anymore." "I am writing a negative script again," she would comment, learning to register and then stop her catastrophic and self-deprecating thoughts.

Psychodynamic interventions exploring patient's associations to her experience "of being unlovable" took us to her distant past producing her important insight: "Robert is my mother!" Indeed, my patient's earlier childhood memories of trying to gain love from her distant and unpredictable mother pointed out her "transference reaction". Patient realized that some of her communications with Robert in the present (e.g., her multiple telephone calls, anger outbursts) reflected her extreme childhood neediness interfering with their emerging closeness. She learnt to recognize the intrusion of unwelcome elements from the past into her adult present. It enhanced her motivation to change her maladaptive behaviors not only in relationship with Robert but with other important people in her life as well.

Attachment problems in early childhood may have contributed to my patient negative sense of self as well as her lifelong difficulty to form trustful and close romantic relationships. Quality of mothering was highlighted as a possible common root for the empirical findings between time perspective variables and attachment security among older adults (Kazakina 1999, 2013). Her impatience, in contrast with her overall rational and mature presentation, pointed to her distorted experience of duration, usually strongly affected by emotional distress (Fraisse 1975).

In the process of therapy she learned to cope with anxiety and bouts of acute loneliness when her love object was unavailable or his reassurances were delayed,

"It will pass. I am drawing on imagination of good times and memory of good times. I know it will pass." This statement reflects the patient's mastering of the temporal strategy proved to be effective in my clinical work. This strategy includes eliciting positive aspects of one's past and creating new appealing or comforting images extending them in one's future. It also involves training the temporal flexibility – the patient's ability to switch from one time frame to another and to travel fluidly across temporal regions. This intervention capitalizes on the patient's growing sense of self, and in fact, reveals the building blocks of such temporal phenomena as trust and hope.

However, Lillian's difficulties were dramatically exacerbated by Robert's own way of relating to his past, present and future. "He is unpredictable" "He is in the now". He does not have memory!" He could forget about an important studio visit for any number of reasons: being carried away by his work process, an exciting discussion with fellow artists, or a festive gathering. He could spend hours on the phone with my patient but may forget to call her as promised to follow up on their romantic or business arrangement. By and large, her boyfriend exhibited what Zimbardo and Boyd (1999) described as hedonistic present. Lillian like some of my other patients was more receptive to psychological educational information about problems with time perspective when it was introduced as explanation of their significant others' behavior rather than their own.

The treatment of this patient is still in progress. Lillian continues to struggle with recurrent although less frequent and severe bouts of anxiety and depressed mood. She remains conflicted about her current romantic involvement, but begins to consider the possibility of joining the internet dating service to find a more suitable partner. However, future is no longer dismal without Robert in her life. She became able to access to her distant past gaining insight in the impact of her attachment insecurity on her present interpersonal struggle. Her temporal flexibility – ability to switch from one temporal frame to another – improved. She also learned to recognize an imbalance in time perspective (over-focus on the present) in people she loved. She is ready to carry on the positive aspects of her exciting yet stressful present, re-awakened femininity, art business skills, improved interpersonal effectiveness and overall enhanced sense of self from present to the future.

Thus my patient's improvement in psychotherapy is associated with her obtaining temporal characteristics that I link with a notion of optimal time perspective: balance and connections of positive aspects of past, present and future as well as flexible travel across time regions (Webster 2013). This allows her to be fully engaged with life that presents one of the key features of successful aging (Rowe and Kahn 1998).

Recommendations for Further Research and Clinical Practice

Theoretical and empirical clarification of several related concepts are necessary.

It seems that the concept of balanced time perspective and Zimbardo Time Perspective Inventory (Zimbardo and Boyd 1999) contain two characteristics: balance and connectedness of time regions. BTPS developed by Webster (2011) and its variable Time Expansion also seem to reflect both of these characteristics. The Zimbardo's idea about holistic present (Zimbardo and Boyd 2008), which awaits investigation, appears to resonate with a notion of temporal holism (Sirois 2012). Temporal holism points out the dimension of connectedness of time present and future illuminating the role of the reinforced present that contains past and future. Webster's approach overtly eliminates clinically invaluable concept of the present but focuses to a large degree on the connections of present to past and future. Theoretical and empirical distinction of temporal balance and temporal continuity is very important because of their high relevance to clinical practice.

In this regard it can be of interest to see further TP research that provides data on theoretical and empirical investigation of the "Optimal Time Perspective" (OTP) that I suggested in this chapter. I included in this notion: balance of time orientations, subjective sense of their connections, temporal flexibility – ability to switch from one temporal frame to another depending on situational demands (Zimbardo and Boyd 1999), and also – an adaptive time limited over-focus on a specific time region or regions.

I believe that the concept of Optimal Time Perspective has a potential to include new interesting aspects of individuals' relations to their past, present and future as TP research continues. For example, a concept of transcendental future (Zimbardo and Boyd 1999, 2008), particularly resonating with my patients facing issues of mortality and mourning has already been an object of investigation (Kairys et al. 2012); a concept of the prenatal past has been offered for consideration by Wessel van Beek (2012) and seems very promising both theoretically and clinically. Also a valuable focus on the interconnections of reminiscences and anticipations of the future (Webster 2013) may allow to empirically approach the concept of temporal integration testing its adaptive outcomes as well as further develop temporal aspect of clinical interventions.

The Concept of "Time Competence" Redefined

"Time Competence" – one of the two major scales in the POI, questionnaire determining personality level of self-actualization (Shostrom 1968). The concept had been originally developed by Everett Shostrom under the impact of Abraham Maslow's theory of self-actualizing personality. The essence of "a Time Competent orientation" according to Shostrom (1968) was represented in the POI statement: "For me, past, present and future is in meaningful continuity" (p. 19). In my study (Kazakina 1999, 2013) Time Competence scale was used as a measure of temporal continuity. However, Shostrom's conceptualization of Time Competence also included ideas of balance (over-focus on time region versus more competent balanced orientation to past, present and future).

It seems that the concept of "Time Competence" is not sufficiently utilized or in Maslow's terms – "actualized." I suggest that it may be revisited and extended because the very wording of it -"time competence" – may allow to highlight mastery over time related phenomena. Optimal time perspective as it is suggested in this chapter is definitely a component of overall time competence. Additionally, time competence could include understanding of time perspective of our significant others, family members, co-workers, friends. Further, time competence can embrace managing cultural differences in time perspectives. It may involve increased awareness of our beliefs and attitudes to both "lived" time and used time as they are operating in the society we live in (Levine 1997).

Time management efficiency can also be viewed as a part of time competence. It seems promising to follow Boniwell's (2005) approach in considering the problems with time use as connected with imbalances in time perspective. The constant feeling of lack of time, or failure to be on time can for some individuals reach a point of disturbing symptoms that are brought in therapy session. In this case these troubling concerns can be considered in the context of their time perspective profile, which may reveal problems such as over-dominant future or over-dominant Present Hedonistic orientations.

Another manifestation of time competence may be seen in managing effectively our biologically based preferences for morning-evening functioning, defined as chronotypes, Their correlations with personality and time perspective measures established in recent TP studies (Milfont and Schwarzenthal 2014; Stolarski et al. 2013) present exciting discoveries that carry most promising clinical relevance. What is behind my patient's difficulty to keep her appointments on time? Is it a failure in executive functions such as planning? Or her difficulty to terminate pleasurable experience in the present? Or avoidance of interpersonal difficulties? Fear of future success or failure that her scheduled activities can bring? Or her life long struggle with early morning rising?

Here the practice illuminates a question for further research: to provide more data on the connections between temporal phenomena of different levels: Time perspective, time use, as well as morning-evening biologically based preferences. It is interesting that in mid 90s when I worked on my dissertation research, it was critical for me to conceptually and empirically distinguish time perspective from other temporal phenomena, such as chronological time, time perception and time management. Remarkably, time research has reached another stage that is reflected in one of the symposia at ICTP2012 titled "From time perception to time perspective: connecting different levels in the study of temporal processes" (Vasquez and Maiche 2012, p. 82).

A good initial step in this direction, from my point of view, has been made in regard to the study of a disturbing symptom of procrastination (Sirois and Pychyl 2012a). The efforts of different scholars (Engberding et al. 2012; Sirois and Pychyl 2012b) presented at ICTP12 allow clinicians to better understand the temporal aspects of this phenomenon and find out about initial attempts to develop clinical interventions "to manage this form of temporal self-regulation failure" (Sirois and Pychyl 2012b, p. 92).

The efficacy of time perspective psychotherapy will probably become a task for the research as TP informed clinical work accumulates more data.

Further Development of TP Focused Clinical Practice

TP clinicians are a very small but growing group of practitioners interested in applying temporal focus and TP interventions in their clinical practice. I believe that ongoing consultations with each other and communications with the TP research community are paramount. Conferences, workshops and publications are among our traditional venues. However, creating an ongoing web seminar on TP psychotherapy can be considered as well.

Some of the topics can include:

(a) In-depth case discussions (identifying cases that require temporal focus, treatment planning, integration with various treatment modalities and theoretical perspectives, e.g., cognitive-behavioral, psychodynamic).
(b) Development of effective time perspective focused clinical interventions.
(c) Keeping up with most current research; examining challenges and benefits in the application of theory and empirical findings into clinical practice.
(d) Finally, dissemination of TP focused psychotherapy in the larger clinical community.

References

APA Task Force on Evidence-Based Practice. (2006). Evidence-based practice in psychology. *American Psychologist, 61*, 271–285.

Ash, M. G. (1992). Cultural context and scientific change in psychology. *American Psychologist, 47*, 198–207.

Block, R. A. (1990). Introduction. In R. A. Block (Ed.), *Cognitive models of psychological time* (pp. xiii–xix). Hillsdale: Erlbaum.

Boniwell, I. (2005). Beyond time management: how the latest research on time perspective and perceived time use can assist clients with time-related concerns. *International Journal of Evidence Based Coaching and Mentoring, 3*(2), 61–74.

Boniwell, I., & Zimbardo, P. G. (2004). Balancing time perspective in pursuit of optimal functioning. In P. A. Liney & S. Joseph (Eds.), *Positive psychology in practice* (pp. 165–178). Hoboken: Wiley.

Chamberlin, J. (2008). The time of our lives. *Monitor on Psychology, 39*(9), 20–21.

Desmyter, F., & De Raedt, R. (2012). The relationship between time perspective and subjective well-being of older adults. *Psychologica Belgica, 52*(1), 19–38.

Dobson, K. S. (Ed.). (2010). *Handbook of cognitive-behavioral therapies* (3rd ed.). New York: The Guilford Press.

Doob, L. W. (1971). *Patterning of time*. New Haven: Yale University Press.

Engberding, M., Hocker, A., Haferkamp, R., Krumm, K, & Rist, F. (2012). Focused clinical treatment of procrastination by means of working time-restriction. In M. P. Paixao, V. E. C. Ortuno, P. Cordeiro, & R. David (Eds.), *First international conference on time perspective: Converging paths in psychology time theory and research. book of abstracts* (p. 94). Portugal: University of Coimbra.

Erikson, E. H. (1985). *Childhood and society* (35th ed.). New York: Norton.

Fraisse, P. (1975). *The psychology of time* (J. Leith, Trans.). Westport, CT: Greenwood Press. (Reprinted from the edition published 1963, New York: Harper & Row)

Frankl, V. E. (1976). *Man's search for meaning: An introduction to logotherapy*. (I. Lasch, Trans.). New York: Pocket Books.

Goldfried, M. R. (2000). Reflections of a scientist practitioner. In S. Soldz & L. McCullough (Eds.), *Reconciling empirical knowledge and clinical experience* (pp. 17–32). Washington, DC: American Psychological Association.

Gonzalez, A., & Zimbardo, P. G. (1985). Time in perspective. *Psychology Today, 19*, 21–26.

Gorman, B. S., & Wessman, A. E. (1977). Images, values, and concepts of time in psychological research. In B. S. Gorman & A. E. Wessman (Eds.), *The personal experience of time* (pp. 217–263). New York: Plenum Press.

Hearnshaw, L. S. (1956). Temporal integration and behavior. *Bulletin of the British Psychological Society, 30*, 1–20.

Hillman, J. L. (2012). *Sexuality and aging: Clinical Perspectives*. New York: Springer.

Kahana, E., & Kahana, B. (1983). Environmental continuity, futurity and adaptation of the aged. In G. D. Rowles & R. J. Ohta (Eds.), *Aging and milieu* (pp. 205–228). New York: Academic.

Kairys, A., van Beek, W., & Zimbardo, P. G. (2012). Transcendental future time perspective: How life after death motivates us? In M. P. Paixao et al. (Eds.), *First international conference on time perspective: Converging paths in psychology time theory and research. Book of abstracts* (p. 87). Portugal: University of Coimbra.

Kastenbaum, R. (1964). The crisis of explanation. In R. Kastenbaum (Ed.), *New thoughts of old age* (pp. 316–323). New York: Springer.

Kazakina, E. (1999). *Time perspective of older adults: Relationships to attachment style, psychological well-being and psychological distress*. Unpublished doctoral dissertation, Columbia University.

Kazakina, E. (2012). Time perspective of older adults: Research and clinical practice. In M. P. Paixao et al. (Eds.), *First international conference on time perspective: Converging paths in psychology time theory and research. Book of abstracts* (p. 78). Portugal: University of Coimbra.

Kazakina, E. (2013). Time perspective of older adults: Research and clinical practice. In *International studies in time perspective*. Impresa da Universidade de Coimbra.

Kohut, H. (1971). *The analysis of the self*. New York: International Universities Press.

Kohut, H. (1984). *How does analysis cure?* Chicago: The University of Chicago Press.

Levine, R. (1997). *A geography of time*. New York: Basic Books.

Lewin, K. (1943/1997). Defining the "field at a given time." In D. Cartwright (Ed.), *Field theory in social science. Selected theoretical papers. In Resolving social conflicts. Field theory in social science*. (pp. 200–211). Washington, DC: American Psychological Association (Original work published 1943).

Loewald, H. W. (1980a). Superego and time. In H. W. Loewald (Ed.), *Papers on psychoanalysis* (pp. 43–52). New Haven, CT: Yale University Press. (Reprinted from *International Journal of Psycho-Analysis*, 1962, 43)

Loewald, H. W. (1980b). The experience of time. In H. W. Loewald (Ed.), *Papers on psychoanalysis* (138–147). New Haven, CT: Yale University Press. (Reprinted from *The Psychoanalytic Study of the Child*, 1972, 27)

Maslow, A. H. (1970). *Motivation and personality* (2nd ed.). New York: Harper & Row.

Melges, F. T. (1982). *Time and the inner future*. New York: Wiley.

Milfont, T. L., & Schwarzenthal, M. (2014). Explaining why lars future are future oriented and owls are present-oriented: Self-control mediates the chronotype-time perspective relationships. *Chronobiology International, 31*(4), 581–588. New York: Informa Healthcare ISSN 0742–0528.

Minkowski, E. (1970). *Lived time* (N. Metzel, Trans.). Evanston, IL: Northwestern University Press. (Original work published 1933)

Norcross, J. C., Hogan, T. P., & Koocher, G. P. (2008). *Clinician's guide to evidence- based practice*. New York: Oxford University Press.

Nuttin, J. (1985). *Future time perspective and motivation*. Hillsdale: Lawrence Erlbaum.

Paixao, M. P., Ortuno, V. E. C., Cordeiro, P., & David, R. (Eds.). (2012). First *international conference on time perspective: Converging paths in psychology time theory and research. Book of abstracts*. Portugal: University of Coimbra.

Rappaport, H. (1990). *Marking time*. New York: Simon and Shuster.

Rokeach, M. (1960). *The open and closed mind*. New York: Basic Books.

Roos, P., & Albers, R. (1965). Performance of alcoholics and normals on a measure of temporal orientation. *Journal of Clinical Psychology, 21*(1), 34–36.

Row, J., & Kahn, R. L. (1998). *Successful aging*. New York: Pantheon Books.

Schonfield, D. (1973). Future commitments and successful aging. *Journal of Gerontology, 28*, 189–196.

Seginer, R. (2009). *Future orientation*. New York: Springer.

Shedler, J. (2010). The efficacy of psychodynamic psychotherapy. *American Psychologist, 65*, 98–109.

Shostrom, E. L. (1968). *EITS manual for the personal orientation inventory*. Educational and Industrial Testing Service.

Sirois, F. (2012). What was, is, and will be: temporal holism, well-being, and the pursuit of goals. In M. P. Paixao et al. (Eds.), *First international conference on time perspective: Converging paths in psychology time theory and research. Book of abstracts* (p. 72). Portugal: University of Coimbra.

Sirois, F., & Pychyl, T. (2012a). Procrastination and the priority of short-term mood regulation: Consequences for future self. *Social and Personality Psychology Compass*, 1–13. Blackwell Publishing. doi:10.1111/spc3.12011

Sirois, F., & Pychyl, T. (2012b). Procrastination and perception of time: Implications for theory and practice. In M. P. Paixao et al. (Eds.), *First international conference on time perspective: Converging paths in psychology time theory and research. Book of abstracts* (p. 92). Portugal: University of Coimbra.

Stolarski, M., Bitner, J., & Zimbardo, P. G. (2011). Time perspective, emotional intelligence and discounting of delayed awards. *Time and Society, 20*(3), 346–363.

Stolarski, M., Ledzinska, M., & Matthews, G. (2013). Morning is tomorrow, evening is today: Relationships between chronotype and time perspective. *Biological Rhythm Research, 44*(2), 181–196.

Stricker, G., & Trierweiler, S. J. (1995). The local clinical scientist: A bridge between science and practice. *American Psychologist, 50*, 995–1002.

Turnip, S. S. (2012). Time dominance and relatedness as protective factors against mental health problems among internally displaced adolescents in Ambon Indonesia. In M. P. Paixao et al. (Eds.), *First international conference on time perspective: Converging paths in psychology time theory and research. Book of abstracts* (p. 62). Portugal: University of Coimbra.

van Beek, W. (2012). What was, what is, and what will be: Temporal thinking in suicidal individuals and how to change it in therapy. In M. P. Paixao et al. (Eds.), *First international conference on time perspective: Converging paths in psychology time theory and research. Book of abstracts* (p. 49). Portugal: University of Coimbra.

van Beek, W., Kerkhof, A., & Beekman, A. (2009). Future oriented group training for suicidal patients: a randomized clinical trial. *BMC Psychiatry,* 9(65). doi:10.1186/1471-244X-9-65

Vasquez, A., & Maiche, A. (2012). From time perception to time perspective: Connecting different levels in the study of temporal processes. In M. P. Paixao et al. (Eds.), *First international conference on time perspective: Converging paths in psychology time theory and research. Book of abstracts* (p. 82). Portugal: University of Coimbra.

Vilhauer, J. S., & Deepika, C. (2012). Future directed therapy for the treatment of major depressive disorder. In M. P. Paixao et al. (Eds.), *First international conference on time perspective: Converging paths in psychology time theory and research. Book of abstracts* (p. 79). Portugal: University of Coimbra.

Vilhauer, J. S., Young, S., Kealoha, C., Borrman, J., IsHak, W. W., Rapaport, M. H., et al. (2012). Treating major depression by creating positive expectations for the future: A pilot study for the effectiveness of future directed therapy (FDT) on symptoms severity and quality of life. *CNS Neuroscience and Therapeutics, 18*(2), 102–109. doi:10.1111/j 1755-5949.2011.00235.x.

Webster, J. D. (2011). A new measure of time perspective: Initial psychometric findings for the balanced time perspective scale (BTPS). *Canadian Journal of Behavioral Science, 43*(2), 11–118. doi:10.1037/a0022801.

Webster, J. W. (2013). Is it time to reminiscence about the future? *The International Journal of Reminiscence and Life Review, 1*(1), 51–54.

Webster, J. W., & Ma, X. (2013). A balanced time perspective in adulthood: Well-being and developmental effects. *Canadian Journal on Aging, 32*(4), 433–442.

Webster, J. D., Westerhof, G., & Bohlmeijer, E. (2012). Is balanced time perspective wise? In M. P. Paixao et al. (Eds.), *First international conference on time perspective: Converging paths in psychology time theory and research. Book of abstracts* (p. 81). Portugal: University of Coimbra.

Zimbardo, P. G. (2012, September). Time perspective network history and goals. Presentation at the *Time perspective network meeting* conducted at the first international conference on time perspective: Converging paths in psychology time theory and research. Portugal: University of Coimbra.

Zimbardo, P. G., & Boyd, J. N. (1999). Putting time in perspective: A valid, reliable individual-differences metric. *Journal of Personality and Social Psychology, 77*, 1271–1288.

Zimbardo, P. G., & Boyd, J. N. (2008). *The time paradox*. New York: Free Press.

Zimbardo, P. G., Sword, R. M., & Sword, R. K. M. (2012). *Time cure: Overcoming PTSD with new psychology of time perspective therapy*. San Francisco: Jossey-Bass a Wiley Imprint.

Afterword

My Perspective on This Gift of Time

By the time a man arrives at the over-ripe age of 80, he has received many gifts on each of those previous annual celebrations of his survival mission through life. With increasing age, just making it to the next marker is a reason to be joyful, yet increasingly cautious about making plans for an ever more uncertain future. But of all the gifts I have ever been given, the one I will treasure most, is this one, this book, this sharing of friendship and camaraderie, and even love, with my colleagues around the world and at home. It is a rare and wonderful honor to have so many scholars dedicate to me their special contributions to this remarkable volume of the wisdom of Time Perspective. It is also a testimonial to what is best in cross-cultural psychology with its three editors—Maciej Stolarski, Nicolas Fieulaine and Wessel van Beek—from three European nations, integrating the ideas of an amazing gathering of researchers, theorists and practitioners from many nations around the world. Their overview chapter is brilliant in distilling key concepts in the genesis of time perspective theory, research and applications, along with a concise thumbnail description of the key features of the contributions in each of the five areas around which they have organized this unique volume.

With their contributions presented here, each one has given me a most precious gift, the gift of time, or more precisely the gift of imaginative and important research on the psychology of time perspective. I am happy to share my personal and professional joy with the readers of this volume, whom I hope have been well informed, even entertained, by the writings of ***103 authors, from 27 different nations, across six continents, in these 32 chapters.*** Before reflecting back on my reactions to the ideas presented in some of them, I want to detour and go way back in time to my first involvement, or entanglement, with this topic of time psychology.

It all began in my childhood, growing up in poverty in the inner city of the South Bronx, New York, from a family with a Sicilian heritage. My father, George Zimbardo, was a brilliant man, although uneducated, whom I witnessed doing

M. Stolarski et al. (eds.), *Time Perspective Theory; Review, Research and Application: Essays in Honor of Philip G. Zimbardo*, DOI 10.1007/978-3-319-07368-2,

amazing feats of mechanical and musical genius. He could play all stringed instruments without lessons, by ear and improvise any thing he heard. He built one of the first television sets in 1947 from a wiring diagram, the year after TV was invented! Again, he did so without any formal training in electronics.

My admiration, however, did not extend to the rest of his non-creative life style, which was focused around personal pleasure pursuits, in what now would be termed the Present Hedonistic life style that he created. He was often unemployed—it was the time of the Big Depression in the 1930s—but never seemed to be concerned about it, although my mother did, since she had to feed our family of six.

It was obvious to me that the only way out of our poverty was through hard work. That meant becoming educated, graduating from schools and eventually college and then getting a good paying job. So even as a pre-teenager, my eye was on planning for tomorrow, not living for today. That meant developing a focus on the future, with clear plans for how to get from the terrible present to ultimately achieving those positive future goals.

With much hard work, but without much family support, I managed to realize that goal of becoming extremely well educated, very future oriented, and financially successful. Of course, in the bargain, I did forfeit enjoying many of the pleasures of the moment that come packaged with a hedonistic life style.

However, upon further reflection, this personal experience seemed not idiosyncratic of just me, but typical of many people around the world. How was it that someone developed a temporal focus on the past, or the present, or the future? Once they did so, what were the consequences of living in a particular time zone rather than another one?

These generic questions encouraged me to begin a systematic program of research at Stanford University, to explore unanswered questions about the nature of psychological time. First, as I am reminded here in the foreword by Christina Maslach, the earliest work we did (in 1971) was on varying the time concept of tempo, as well as using hypnosis to manipulate time zones, by putting future-oriented students into a present-focused mind set and then observing the range of dramatic consequences. However, the key to future research involved something that was alien to my training as an experimental social psychologist, namely developing a scale that could be used to systematically differentiate and profile individual differences in time perspective in order to more precisely identify some of its causes, and correlates, and consequences. After many years of trial and error, we succeeded in realizing that goal and published in 1999 our seminal article on that scale and its associated research—as described in John Boyd's initial chapter in this volume. Since then, an enormous amount of research erupted in academic, clinical, and business settings around the world to understand the hows and whys of time perspective, some of which you have read here.

Our initial scale of 56 items that identified five different time factors, as well as a sixth factor (transcendental future) in an associated scale, has been reduced to 36-items that are universal across two dozen nations, as can be seen in the cross-cultural research article just published by our Z-Time Team, headed by Anna Sircova (*Sage Open,* Jan-March, 2014). Nicolas Fieulaine has developed a useful

15-item short form. I am also currently in the process of developing another time perspective factor—that of the Holistic Expanded Present—as in Zen mediation—with Rose McDermott and Zara Zimbardo.

After more than four decades of being immersed in this domain of human nature, I have come to believe that time perspective is a most fundamental aspect of human nature, even foundational to much of our motivations, judgments, decisions and actions—both mundane ones and our grandly significant ones. Time Perspective is precious in our personal life and essential in our business life. The concept of time is one of the most basic, yet rather curious aspects in human thought.

We often think about time as if it were a commodity, a thing, and a resource that we say can be saved, can be wasted, can be spent, and can be misused. And of course, in our current time-pressured cultures around the world, time is our most precious asset, or which we want more of, can't have enough of, and resent anything that makes us lose some of it—such as the burden of waiting for anything not instantaneously available to us.

In most cultures, we have proverbs or sayings in which time is central, such as "a stitch in time will save nine" (saving many later stitches if done correctly and soon enough the first time). We also say "a bird in the hand is worth two in the bush," meaning take what is available in the present rather than plan for something that might be better in the future—but not certain. At the same time, we also acknowledge "haste makes waste," so slow down and do it right the first time. In addition, there are an endless number of songs that feature basic time themes, such as: "As Time Goes By; Your Time Is Now; I Didn't Know What Time It Was; Time After Time," and many others. Interesting to me is discovering that in Bali, Indonesia, the word for time translates into "rubber time," meaning that time is stretched to fit human affairs. 'People time' is modified to accommodate the irregular timing of daily religious and artistic events. This seems to be the opposite of time concepts in most Western cultures where human affairs are compressed to fit the fleeting time that presses us, and that now crunches us into an ever more narrow time zone.

Although I know many of the contributors here personally and have heard them present earlier versions of their ideas, it was a refreshing experience to reconnect with each and all of them here as they put forward their best organized work within special contexts created by our three editors.

We began with fascinating ideas about how to balance TP to make it optimally functional, then we journeyed into the life of time after death, we saw links to personality and to learning, as well as discovering that what had always seemed only positive about being future oriented, can have a negative side of worry and anxiety about not being able to meet the demands of one's to do list.

Next up were a group of authors who took us wide and deep, to evolutionary perspectives, broad cross-cultural vistas, and important links to poverty and social insecurity (reminding me again of my early life condition).

We were then treated to a journey into the core of basic psychology where we learned about links of TP to affect, cognition, and motivation. They revealed how these basic processes form the foundations of human action—for better or for worse, for richer or for poorer, for success or for failure.

Then, what is rare in most academic treatises on research and theory, came two final sections on practical applications of TP to everyday life and also to problematic life experiences. First, we discovered links to health improvement, well- being enhancement, better financial decisions, effective persuasion approaches, and grounding pro-environmental attitudes in TP frameworks.

This volume ended with a powerhouse section on clinical applications—from reduction of stress, promotion of positive aging, more effective life coaching, and new conceptions of some psychopathological challenges, such as a new treatment for the previously intractable post-traumatic stress disorder (PTSD), in evidence-based new Time Therapy on which I have been fortunate to work with my Hawaiian colleagues, Richard and Rosemary Sword. Wow! What a tasty treat from beginning to end.

I wish to end this brief final section with the declaration of my new mission life, as a **Time Maker**: Encouraging everyone to learn how to practice MAKING TIME work for themselves, rather than work against them. What time?

MAKING TIME FOR FAMILY, MAKING TIME FOR FRIENDS, MAKING TIME FOR FUN, MAKING TIME FOR NATURE, MAKING TIME FOR SPIRITUALITY, MAKING TIME FOR CULTURE, AND ESPECIALLY MAKING TIME FOR MORE ROMANCE IN OUR LIVES.

And now a tender farewell, until we meet next time around,

CIAO!

Appendix

Table S1 Nomological network summary of the five scales of the Zimbardo Time Perspective Inventory

ZTPI scale	Related variables	Country	Reference
Past-Negative			
Positive relations	Anxiety	USA/Greece/Russia/ France	Zimbardo and Boyd (1999), Anagnostopoulos and Griva (2012), Sircova et al. (2008), Fieulaine et al. (2006)
	Aggression	USA/Greece/Russia	Zimbardo and Boyd (1999), Anagnostopoulos and Griva (2012), Sircova et al. (2008)
	Suicidal ideation	Italy/Netherlands	Laghi et al. (2009), van Beek et al. (2011)
	Depression	USA/Russia/ Netherlands/ Sweden/France	Zimbardo and Boyd (1999), Sircova et al. (2008), van Beek et al. (2011), Carelli and Wiberg (2012), Fieulaine et al. (2006)
	Childhood stresses and Ambivalent-Anxious attachment to family	USA	Thornhill et al. (2007)
	Physical activity	Canada	Hamilton et al. (2003)
	Use of approaches that search for meaning in study	Australia	Horstmanshof and Zimitat (2004)
	Being a pathological gambler or psychiatric patient	Canada	Hodgins and Engel (2002)

(continued)

M. Stolarski et al. (eds.), *Time Perspective Theory; Review, Research and Application: Essays in Honor of Philip G. Zimbardo*, DOI 10.1007/978-3-319-07368-2,

ZTPI scale	Related variables	Country	Reference
	Being female	Brazil	Milfont et al. (2008)
	Being older	Lithuania	Kairys (2010)
	Being 50 year older female	Russia	Sircova and Mitina (2008)
	Gambling	USA	McKillop et al. (2006)
	Depression in adolescent cancer	USA	Bitsko et al. (2008)
	External control, neuroticism, pessimism	USA	Shipp et al. (2009)
	Conflict with members of social network	USA	Holman and Zimbardo (2009)
	Cooperation in Prisoner's dilemma	USA	Thoms (2004)
	Search for meaning in life (MLQ)	USA	Steger et al. (2008)
	Being homeless	England	Pluck et al. (2008)
	Frequency of future self thought	USA	McElwee and Haugh 2009
	Proneness to mania (Hypomanic Personality Scale)	USA	Gruber et al. (2012)
	Higher chance of reporting severe personality problems	Netherlands	van Beek et al. (2011)
	Binge eating and drinking	Italy	Laghi et al. (2012)
	Negative affect, depressive feelings in older adults	Belgium	Desmyter and De Raedt (2012)
	Socioeconomic deprivation	France	Fieulaine et al. (2006), Merson and Perriot (2011)
	Lower education level, unemployment, lack of family relations, not in couple	France	Fieulaine et al. (2006)
	Diffused Ego Identity Status	Italy	Laghi et al. (2013)
	Problematic Internet Use	Italy	Chittaro and Vianello (2013)
Negative relations	Students' satisfaction with their university experience	Australia	Horstmanshof and Zimitat (2004)
	Mindfulness, Happiness	Scotland	Drake et al. (2008)
	Right wing authoritarianism, conservatism; Secure attachment to family	USA	Thornhill and Fincher (2007)

(continued)

ZTPI scale	Related variables	Country	Reference
	Happiness and quality of life in adolescent cancer	USA	Bitsko et al. (2008)
	Life satisfaction, optimism, conscientiousness, extraversion, agreeableness, risk-taking	USA	Shipp et al. (2009)
	Present and Future satisfaction in life, affective balance, Self-actualisation	UK	Boniwell et al. (2010)
	Satisfaction with life, happiness, purpose in life, self-efficacy, optimism	Russia	Boniwell et al. (2010)
	Positive relations with others, autonomy, environmental mastery, personal growth, purpose in life, self-acceptance (Scales of Psychological Well-Being); Dispositional hardiness, tolerance for ambiguity, satisfaction with life, Self-actualization	Russia	Sircova and Mitina (2008)
	Meaning in life (MLQ)	USA	Steger et al. (2008)
	Support from members of social network	USA	Holman and Zimbardo (2009)
	Conscientiousness, risk-taking	Russia	Sircova et al. (2008)
	Patience	USA	Schnitker and Emmons (2007)
	Being female	USA	Ely and Mercurio (2010)
	Clarity of future self thought	USA	McElwee and Haugh (2009)
	Emotional intelligence	Poland	Stolarski et al. (2011)
	Positive affect, satisfaction with life in older adults	Belgium/France	Desmyter and De Raedt (2012), Gana et al. (2012)
	Self-esteem, optimism, proactive coping	Greece	Anagnostopoulos and Griva (2012)
Past-Positive			
Positive relations	Self-esteem	USA, Greece	Zimbardo and Boyd (1999), Anagnostopoulos and Griva 2012

(continued)

ZTPI scale	Related variables	Country	Reference
	Health responsibility, nutrition, and spiritual growth	Canada	Hamilton et al. (2003)
	Wristwatch use	USA	Zimbardo and Boyd (1999)
	Use of approaches that search for both meaning and reproduction in study	Australia	Horstmanshof and Zimitat (2004)
	Being a pathological gambler or psychiatric patient	Canada	Hodgins and Engel (2002)
	Secure attachment to family, right wing authoritarianism	USA	Thornhill and Fincher (2007)
	Pro-environmental attitudes	Brazil	Milfont and Gouveia (2006)
	Concern about the correct time	Brazil	Milfont et al. (2008)
	Being male	Lithuania	Linauskaité and Kairys (2009)
	Being female	Australia/Lithuania/USA	Horstmanshof and Zimitat (2004), Kairys (2010), Zimbardo and Boyd (1999), Ely and Mercurio (2010)
	Arousal procrastination	USA, Spain	Ferrari and Diaz-Morales (2007)
	Life satisfaction, internal control, optimism, conscientiousness, agreeableness, extraversion	USA	Shipp et al. (2009)
	Larger Social network, length of relationships, Support from members of social network	USA	Holman and Zimbardo (2009)
	Present and future satisfaction in life, affective balance, Self-actualisation	UK	Boniwell et al. (2010)
	Satisfaction with life in older adults	Belgium	Desmyter and De Raedt (2012)
	Satisfaction with life, happiness, purpose in life, self-efficacy, optimism	Russia	Boniwell et al. (2010)

(continued)

ZTPI scale	Related variables	Country	Reference
	Positive relations with others, environmental mastery, personal growth, purpose in life, self-acceptance (Scales of Psychological Well-Being); Dispositional hardiness, satisfaction with life, Self-actualization	Russia	Sircova and Mitina (2008)
	Patience	USA	Schnitker and Emmons (2007)
	Strong predictor of many aspects of autobiographical memory; tendency to talk about the past. Relationship between TP and autobiographical memory are independent of personality traits	USA	Ely and Mercurio (2010)
	ADHD status	Sweden	Carelli and Wiberg (2011)
	Being older	Lithuania/Brazil/USA	Kairys (2010), Milfont et al. (2008), Shores and Scott (2007)
	Emotional intelligence	Poland	Stolarski et al. (2011)
	Less personality problems	Netherlands	van Beek et al. (2011)
	Empathy	Russia	Sircova et al. (2008)
	Higher level of education, higher income; seeking physical fitness, spiritual benefits, family togetherness, learning during recreation	USA	Shores and Scott (2007)
	Clarity and frequency of future self thought	USA	McElwee and Haugh (2009)
	Seeing life as meaningful	UK	Routledge et al. (2008)
	Fear of death	Russia	Chistopolskaya and Enikolopov (2012)
Negative relations	Depression, and anxiety	USA/Greece/Sweden	Zimbardo and Boyd (1999), Anagnostopoulos and Griva (2012), Carelli and Wiberg (2012)

(continued)

ZTPI scale	Related variables	Country	Reference
	Anxiety	USA/Greece	Zimbardo and Boyd (1999), Anagnostopoulos and Griva (2012)
	Aggression	USA	Zimbardo and Boyd (1999)
	Ambivalent-Anxious and avoidant attachment to family, childhood stresses	USA	Thornhill and Fincher (2007)
	Neuroticism, chance (locus of control)	USA	Shipp et al. (2009)
	Treatment optimism in drug treatment patients	Switzerland	Klingemann (2001)
	Conflict with members of social network	USA	Holman and Zimbardo (2009)
	Meaning in life (MLQ)	USA	Steger et al. (2008)
	Being homeless	England	Pluck et al. (2008)
	Being older	Greece	Anagnostopoulos and Griva (2012)
Present-Fatalistic			
Positive relations	Depression	USA/Greece/Sweden	Zimbardo and Boyd (1999), Anagnostopoulos and Griva (2012), Carelli and Wiberg (2012)
	Anxiety	USA/Greece/Russia	Zimbardo and Boyd (1999), Anagnostopoulos and Griva (2012), Sircova et al. (2008)
	Aggression	USA	Zimbardo and Boyd (1999)
	Physical activity	Canada	Hamilton et al. (2003)
	Being a pathological gambler or psychiatric patient	Canada	Hodgins and Engel (2002)
	Suicidal ideation	Italy/Netherlands	Laghi et al. (2009), van Beek et al. (2011)
	Tobacco, alcohol and drug use,	USA	Daugherty and Brase (2010)
	Being male	Lithuania/USA	Linauskaitė and Kairys (2009), Mello and Worrell (2006)
	Being female	Italy/Lithuania/Brazil/Russia	D'Alession et al. 2003, Kairys (2010), Rego-Leite (2008), Sircova and Mitina (2008)
	Diffuse-avoidant style of identity formation	Belgium	Luyckx et al. (2010)

(continued)

ZTPI scale	Related variables	Country	Reference
	Search for meaning in life (MLQ)	USA	Steger et al. (2008)
	Being older	Italy/Lithuania/ Brazil/Russia	D'Alession et al. (2003), Kairys (2010), Milfont et al. (2008) Sircova and Mitina (2008)
	Impulsivity	USA	MacKillop et al. (2006)
	External control, neuroticism, pessimism	USA	Shipp et al. (2009)
	Avoidant procrastination	USA, Spain	Ferrari and Diaz-Morales (2007), Diaz-Morales et al. (2008)
	Neuroticism	Netherlands	van Beek et al. (2011)
	Alcohol consumption	Brazil	Milfont et al. (2008)
	Depression, anxiety, aggression, low self-esteem	Russia	Sircova et al. (2008)
	Proneness to mania (Hypomanic Personality Scale)	USA	Gruber et al. (2012)
	Health destructive behaviours (regular smokers, less seatbelt use)	USA	Henson et al. (2006)
	Depressive feelings in older adults	Belgium	Desmyter and De Raedt (2012)
	Time-moving representation of time	UK	Richmond et al. (2012)
	Socioeconomic deprivation	France	Fieulaine et al. (2006), Merson and Perriot (2011)
	Lower education level	France	Fieulaine et al. (2006)
	Non-planning	USA	Baumann and Odum (2012)
	Impulsive buying tendency	Korea	Lee and Song (2011)
Negative relations	Consideration of future consequences	USA	Zimbardo and Boyd (1999)
	Health concerns	USA	Daugherty and Brase (2010)
	Students' satisfaction with their university experience, and the use of approaches that search for meaning in study	Australia	Horstmanshof and Zimitat (2004)
	Life satisfaction, internal control, optimism, conscientiousness, agreeableness	USA	Shipp et al. (2009)

(continued)

ZTPI scale	Related variables	Country	Reference
	Extraversion, conscientiousness	Netherlands	van Beek et al. (2011)
	Seat belt use, condom use, birth control	USA	Henson et al. (2005)
	Pro-environmental behaviour and attitudes	Mexico/Brazil	Corral-Verdugo et al. (2006), Milfont and Gouveia (2006)
	Quality of life in HIV	France	Préau et al. (2007)
	Education degree	USA	Guthrie et al. (2009)
	Commitment and information-oriented style in identity formation	Belgium	Luyckx et al. 2010
	eating breakfast, using safety belts	USA	Daugherty and Brase (2010)
	Satisfaction with life, happiness, purpose in life, self-efficacy, optimism	Russia	Boniwell et al. (2010)
	Retirement planning (financial)	Australia	Petkoska and Earl (2009)
	Conscientiousness	Russia	Sircova et al. (2008)
	Positive relations with others, autonomy, environmental mastery, personal growth, purpose in life, self-acceptance (Scales of Psychological Well-Being);	Russia	Sircova and Mitina (2008)
	Dispositional hardiness, tolerance for ambiguity, satisfaction with life, Self-actualization		
	Patience	USA	Schnitker and Emmons (2007)
	Emotional intelligence	Poland	Stolarski et al. (2011)
	Academic orientation, meaningful approach	Australia	Horstmanshof and Zimitat (2007)
	Clarity of future self thought	USA	McElwee and Haugh (2009)
	Intention-behavior consistency (intention of purchasing understated)	USA	Van Ittersum (2011)

(continued)

ZTPI scale	Related variables	Country	Reference
	Self-esteem, optimism, proactive coping	Greece	Anagnostopoulos and Griva (2012)
	Academic achievement	USA	Mello and Worrell (2006)
	Intention to have unprotected sex	Greece & UK	Protogerou and Turner-Cobb (2011)
Present-Hedonistic			
Positive relations	Ego undercontrol, novelty, and sensation seeking	USA	Zimbardo and Boyd (1999)
	Desire for control	France	Fieulaine and Martinez (2010)
	Health responsibility and interpersonal relations	Canada	Hamilton et al. (2003)
	Tobacco, alcohol and drug use, exercise	USA	Daugherty and Brase (2010)
	Life satisfaction, risk-taking (JPI-R), optimism, extraversion, openness; locus of control – chance	USA	Shipp et al. (2009)
	Curiosity and exploration	USA	Kashdan et al. (2004)
	Substance use	USA, France	Keough et al. (1999), Henson et al. (2005), Fieulaine and Martinez (2010, 2012), Cheong et al. (2014)
	Condom use and birth control	USA	Henson et al. (2005)
	Risky driving	USA	Zimbardo et al. (1997)
	Being a pathological gambler	Canada	Hodgins and Engel (2002)
	Being younger	Italy/Australia/ Lithuania/USA/ Russia	D'Alession et al. (2003), Horstmanshof and Zimitat (2004), Kairys 2010, Keough et al. (1999), Zimbardo et al. (1997), Sircova and Mitina (2008)
	Present and future satisfaction in life, affective balance, Self-actualisation	UK	Boniwell et al. (2010)
	Happiness, self-efficacy, optimism	Russia	Boniwell et al. (2010)

(continued)

ZTPI scale	Related variables	Country	Reference
	Being male	Italy/Australia/USA/ Lithuania	D'Alessio et al. (2003), Horstmanshof and Zimitat (2004), Keough et al. (1999), Zimbardo et al. (1997), Linauskaitė and Kairys (2009)
	Gambling	USA	MacKillop et al. (2006)
	Impulsivity	USA, Russia	MacKillop et al. (2006), Sircova et al. (2008)
	Procrastination	USA, Spain	Ferrari and Diaz-Morales (2007), Diaz-Morales et al. (2008)
	Quality of life in HIV	France	Préau et al. (2007)
	Diffuse-avoidant style of identity formation	Belgium	Luyckx et al. (2010)
	Retirement planning (interpersonal/ leisure)	Australia	Petkoska and Earl (2009)
	Risk taking, empathy	Russia	Sircova et al. (2008)
	Positive relations with others, personal growth, (Scales of Psychological Well-Being); tolerance for ambiguity, satisfaction with life, Self-actualization	Russia	Sircova and Mitina (2008)
	Alcohol related problems, blood alcohol concentration, heavy drinking days, high number of drinks per week	USA	Carey et al. (2007)
	Patience	USA	Schnitker and Emmons (2007)
	Emotional intelligence	Poland	Stolarski et al. (2011)
	Being an older adolescent	USA	Mello and Worrell (2006)
	Being older; Opportunity for risk taking during recreation	USA	Shores and Scott (2007)

(continued)

ZTPI scale	Related variables	Country	Reference
	Alcohol, tobacco, drug, seat belt use, number of sex partners (but no condom use), exercise; increased risky health behaviours; stronger predictor for females; A much stronger predictor of health behaviours than Future TP	USA	Henson et al. (2006)
	Longer time spent eating, watching TV or passing time	USA	Epel et al. (1999)
	Re-experiencing remembered events and pre-experiencing future events ; Mental time travels	USA	Arnold et al. (2011)
	Proneness to mania (Hypomanic Personality Scale)	USA	Gruber et al. (2012)
	Positive affect in older adults	Belgium	Desmyter and De Raedt (2012)
	Eveningness	Poland	Stolarski et al. (2013)
	Time moving representation of time	UK	Richmond et al. (2012)
	Motor impulsiveness (restlessness)	USA	Baumann and Odum (2012)
	Impulsive buying tendency	Korea	Lee and Song (2011)
Negative relations	Preference for consistency, religiosity, and wristwatch use	USA	Zimbardo and Boyd (1999)
	Eating breakfast, safety belt use	USA	Daugherty and Brase (2010)
	Intentions to participate in Diabetes screening; socio-economic status	UK	Crockett et al. (2009)

(continued)

ZTPI scale	Related variables	Country	Reference
	Education degree	USA	Guthrie et al. (2009)
	Conscientiousness, neuroticism	USA	Shipp et al. (2009)
	Treatment optimism in drug treatment patients	Switzerland	Klingemann (2001)
	Pro-environmental behaviours	Mexico	Corral-Verdugo et al. (2006)
	Regular screenings for breast cancer	Italy	Guarino et al. (1999)
	Hours spent preparing, academic application, academic orientation	Australia	Horstmanshof and Zimitat (2007)
	Clarity of future self thought	USA	McElwee and Haugh (2009)
	Practicing safe sex	USA	Rothspan and Read (1996)
	Being older	Greece	Anagnostopoulos and Griva (2012)
	Intention-behavior consistency (intention of purchasing overstated)	USA	Van Ittersum (2011)
	Using risk reduction initiative in rural substance users living with AIDS	USA	Tucker et al. (2012)
Future			
Positive relations	Conscientiousness, preference for consistency, consideration of future consequences, and self-report hours spent studying per week	USA	Zimbardo and Boyd (1999)
	Avoidant attachment to family	USA	Thornhill and Fincher (2007)
	Internal control	USA	Shipp et al. (2009)
	Curiosity and exploration	USA	Kashdan et al. (2004)
	Conscientiousness	Lithuania/USA/Russia/UK	Kairys (2010), Shipp et al. (2009), Sircova et al. (2008), Adams and Nettle (2009)
	Support from members of social network	USA	Holman and Zimbardo (2009)

(continued)

ZTPI scale	Related variables	Country	Reference
	Health responsibility	Canada	Hamilton et al. (2003)
	Perceived control, positive well-being, adaptive (behavioural, cognitive, and distract) coping, positive affective symptomatology, and resistance efficacy		Wills et al. (2001)
	Satisfaction with life, purpose in life, optimism	Russia	Boniwell et al. (2010)
	Students' satisfaction with their university experience, and the use of approaches that search for both meaning and reproduction in study	Australia	Horstmanshof and Zimitat (2004)
	Concern for own health	Brazil/Israel	Milfont et al. (2008), Carmi (2012)
	Quality of life in HIV	France	Préau et al. (2007)
	Pro-environmental behaviour and attitudes	Mexico/Brazil	Corral-Verdugo et al. (2006), Milfont and Gouveia (2006)
	Initiating alliance in Prisoner's dilemma	USA	Thoms 2004
	Being male	Lithuania	Linauskaité and Kairys (2009)
	Being female	Lithuania/USA/ Latvia/Brazil/ France	Kairys (2010), Keough et al. (1999), Zimbardo and Boyd (1999), Zimbardo et al. (1997), Kolesovs (2002, 2004), Rego-Leite (2008), Ely and Mercurio (2010), Harber et al. (2003); Apostolidis et al. (2006a)
	Being female between 40–60 years old	Russia	Sircova and Mitina (2008)
	Being younger	Canada	Hamilton et al. (2003)
	Exercise	USA	Henson et al. (2005), Guthrie et al. (2013)
	Condom use		Henson et al. (2005)
	Maternal Foetal attachment	USA	Levine-Kornfield (2010)

(continued)

ZTPI scale	Related variables	Country	Reference
	Treatment optimism in drug treatment patients	Switzerland	Klingemann (2001)
	Moderates intention-quitting behaviour; significant relation between planning to quit smoking and actual behaviour	Norway	Kovač and Rise (2007)
	Exercise, eating breakfast, safety belt, expected life longevity	USA	Daugherty and Brase (2010)
	Commitment and information-oriented style in identity formation	Belgium	Luyckx et al. (2010)
	Being older	Lithuania/Russia/USA	Kairys (2010), Sircova and Mitina (2008), Holman and Silver (2005)
	Environmental mastery, purpose in life (Scales of Psychological Well-Being);	Russia	Sircova and Mitina (2008)
	Dispositional hardiness, satisfaction with life,		
	Patience	USA	Schnitker and Emmons (2007)
	Increased protective and decreased risky health behaviours (less drinking, drug use, smoking, more exercise, safe sex behaviors)	USA	Henson et al. (2006)
	Influences nature and valence of post-traumatic reactions (positively related with acknowledgement and adjustment)	USA	Martz and Livneh (2007)
	Emotional intelligence	Poland	Stolarski et al. (2011)
	Academic achievement	USA/Fiji/Australia	Mello and Worrell (2006), Phan (2009), Horstmanshof and Zimitat (2007)

(continued)

ZTPI scale	Related variables	Country	Reference
	Important factor mediating student's engagement with their university studies, leading to completing the higher education	Australia	Horstmanshof and Zimitat (2007)
	Hours spent preparing, academic application, academic orientation, meaningful approach, reproductive approach	Australia	Horstmanshof and Zimitat (2007)
	Higher level of education, higher income	USA	Shores and Scott (2007), Holman and Silver (2005); Epel et al. (1999), Vinkers et al. (2012)
	Seeking physical fitness, family togetherness, learning during recreation	USA	Shores and Scott (2007)
	Robust predictor of many aspects of autobiographical memory.	USA	Ely and Mercurio (2010)
	Relationship between TP and autobiographical memory are independent of personality traits		
	Active coping in the first few weeks following 9/11; lower levels of psychological distress and higher positive affect	USA	Holman and Silver (2005)
	Clarity and frequency of future self thought	USA	McElwee and Haugh (2009)
	Sign-ups for the experiment participation, reliable participation in the longitudinal research	USA	Harber et al. (2003)

(continued)

ZTPI scale	Related variables	Country	Reference
	Intention-behavior consistency	USA	Van Ittersum (2011)
	Re-experiencing remembered events and pre-experiencing future events; Mental time travels	USA	Arnold et al. (2011)
	Proactive coping	Greece/The Netherlands	Anagnostopoulos and Griva (2012), Vinkers et al. (2012)
	Smoking	USA	Guthrie et al. (2013)
	Positive affect in older adults	Belgium	Desmyter and De Raedt (2012)
	Morningness	Poland	Stolarski et al. (2013)
	Ego-moving representation of time	UK	Richmond et al. (2012)
	Performance in creative imagination for distant future thinking	Taiwan	Chiu (2012)
	Regulatory focus (prevention and promotion)	The Netherlands	Vinkers et al. (2012)
	Continued completion of a self-management intervention for weight control	The Netherlands	Vinkers et al. (2012)
	Increased money management	USA	Donnelly et al. (2012)
	Increased medication adherence	USA	Sansbury et al. (2014)
	Self-reported cervical cancer screening	USA	Roncancio et al. (2013)
	Achieved and foreclosed Ego Identity Status	Italy	Laghi et al. (2013)
	Cognitive performance in processing of chronologically presented events	Germany	Nowack et al. (2013)
Negative relations	Novelty and sensation seeking, anxiety, and depression	USA	Zimbardo and Boyd (1999)
	Anxiety, and depression	Russia	Sircova et al. (2008)
	Ambivalent-Anxious attachment to family; social dominance	USA	Thornhill and Fincher (2007)

(continued)

ZTPI scale	Related variables	Country	Reference
	Substance use	USA, France	Keough et al. (1999), Henson et al. (2005), Fieulaine and Martinez (2010, 2012)
	Risky driving	USA	Zimbardo et al. (1997)
	Diffuse-avoidant style in identity formation	Belgium	Luyckx et al. (2010)
	Procrastination	USA, Spain	Ferrari and Diaz-Morales (2007), Diaz-Morales et al. (2008)
	Gambling	USA	MacKillop et al. (2006)
	Impulsivity	USA/ Russia	MacKillop et al. (2006), Sircova et al. (2008)
	Number of sexual partners and relations	USA	Henson et al. (2005)
	External control, risk-taking (JPI-R)	USA	Shipp et al. (2009)
	Smoking	UK	Adams and Nettle (2009)
	Tobacco use, Drug use, Socio-sexual orientation,	USA	Daugherty and Brase (2010)
	Alcohol consumption	Brazil, USA	Milfont et al. (2008), Henson et al. (2005)
	Cannabis use and perception as a drug	France	Apostolidis et al. (2006a, b)
	Living within 25–100 mile radius of the WTC (World Trade Center); being widowed	USA	Holman and Silver (2005)
	Proneness to mania (Hypomanic Personality Scale)	USA	Gruber et al. (2012)
	Longer homelessness duration, longer time spent watching TV or passing time	USA	Epel et al. (1999)
	Binge eating and drinking	Italy	Laghi et al. (2012)
	Socioeconomic deprivation	France	Merson and Perriot (2011)
	Motor impulsiveness (restlessness)	USA	Baumann and Odum (2012)
	willingness to sacrifice for the sake of the environment	Israel	Carmi (2012)
BTP			
	Emotional intelligence	Poland	Stolarski et al. (2011)
	Patience construct	USA	Schnitker and Emmons (2007)

(continued)

ZTPI scale	Related variables	Country	Reference
	Deviation from BTP – predictor of the tendency to delay gratification	Poland	Stolarski et al. (2011)
	Satisfaction with life	USA/Russia	Shipp et al. (2009), Sircova and Mitina (2008), Zhang et al. (2012)
	Quality of life construct	France	Préau et al. (2007)
	Purpose in Life (Ryff); Hardiness (Maddi)	Russia	Sircova and Mitina (2008)
	Subjective happiness, mindfulness	UK, USA	Drake et al. (2008), Zhang et al. (2012)
	Well-being	UK/Russia/USA	Boniwell et al. (2010), Zhang et al. (2012)
Issues	Insensitivity of the measure to distinguish between groups of (1) pathological gamblers, (2) potential pathological gamblers and (3) non-pathological gamblers	USA	MacKillop et al. (2006)
	EFA and CFA proposes 6 factors – two for future (positive and negative)	USA	Mello and Worrell (2006)
	In general population samples ZTPI is less reliable, but more readable; 6 factor structure was emerging; ZTPI-R (9 items) was developed	UK	Crocket et al. (2009)
	Classifying students on the basis of studying expectancies (beliefs about the long-term gain inherent in studying) rather than FTP criteria was a stronger predictor of drinking habits and problems (similar to MacKillop – low sensitivity)	USA	Levy and Earleywine (2004)

Originally presented as a supplementary material in Sircova, van de Vijver, Osin, Milfont, Fieulaine, Kislali-Erginbilgic, Zimbardo & 50 members of the International Network on Time Perspective, 2014

References

Adams, J., & Nettle, D. (2009). Time perspective, personality and smoking, body mass, and physical activity: An empirical study. *British Journal of Health Psychology, 14*, 83–105. doi:10.1348/135910708X299664.

Anagnostopoulos, F., & Griva, F. (2012). Exploring time perspective in Greek young adults: Validation of the Zimbardo Time Perspective Inventory and relationships with mental health indicators. *Social Indicators Research, 106*(1), 41–59. doi:10.1007/s11205-011-9792-y.

Apostolidis, T., Fieulaine, N., & Soulé, F. (2006a). Future time perspective as predictor of cannabis use: Exploring the role of substance perception among French adolescents. *Addictive Behaviors, 31*(12), 2339–2343. doi:10.1016/j.addbeh.2006.03.008.

Apostolidis, T., Fieulaine, N., Rolland, G., & Simonin, L. (2006b). Cannabis use, time perspective and risk perceptions: Evidence of a moderating effect. *Psychology and Health, 21*, 571–592.

Arnold, K. M., McDermott, K. B., & Szpunar, K. K. (2011). Individual differences in time perspective predict autonoetic experience. *Consciousness and Cognition, 20*, 712–719. doi:10.1016/j.concog.2011.03.006.

Baumann, A. A., & Odum, A. L. (2012). Impulsivity, risk taking, and timing. *Behavioural Processes, 90*, 408–414.

Bitsko, M. J., Stern, M., Dillon, R., Russell, E. C., & Laver, J. (2008). Happiness and time perspective as potential mediators of quality of life and depression in adolescent cancer. *Pediatric Blood and Cancer, 50*(3), 613–619.

Boniwell, I., Osin, E., Linley, P. A., & Ivanchenko, G. (2010). A question of balance: Time perspective and well-being in British and Russian samples. *Journal of Positive Psychology, 5*, 24–40.

Carelli, M. G., & Wiberg, B. (2011). Time out of mind: Temporal perspective in adults with ADHD. Prepublished April, 13, 2011, *Journal of Attention Disorders.* doi:10.1177/1087054711398861

Carelli, M. G., & Wiberg, B. (2012). Time out of mind: Temporal perspective in adults with ADHD. *Journal of Attention Disorders, 16*(6), 460–466.

Carey, K. B., Henson, J. M., Carey, M. P., & Maisto, S. A. (2007). Which heavy drinking college students benefit from a brief motivational intervention? *Journal of Consulting and Clinical Psychology, 75*(4), 663–669. doi:10.1037/0022-006X.75.4.663.

Carmi, N. (2012). Caring about tomorrow: Future orientation, environmental attitudes and behaviors. *Environmental Education Research*. doi:10.1080/13504622.2012.700697.

Cheong, J., Tucker, J. A., Simpson, C. A., & Chandler, S. D. (2014). Time horizons and substance use among African American youths living in disadvantaged urban areas. *Addictive Behaviors*. doi:10.1016/j.addbeh.2013.12.016.

Chistopolskaya, K. A., & Enikolopov, S. N. (2012). Terror management after a recent suicide attempt. *Psychology in Russia: State of the Art, 5*, 142–156.

Chittaro, L., & Vianello, A. (2013). Time perspective as a predictor of problematic Internet use: A study of Facebook users. *Personality and Individual Differences, 55*(8), 989–993.

Chiu, F.-C. (2012). Fit between future thinking and future orientation on creative imagination. *Thinking Skills and Creativity, 7*, 234–244.

Corral-Verdugo, V., Fraijo-Sing, B., & Pinheiro, J. Q. (2006). Sustainable behavior and time perspective: Present, past, and future orientations and their relationship with water conservation behavior. *Interamerican Journal of Psychology, 40*(2), 139–147.

Crockett, R. A., Weinman, J., Hankins, M., & Marteau, T. (2009). Time orientation and health-related behaviour: Measurement in general population samples. *Psychology & Health, 24*(3), 333–350.

D'Alessio, M., Guarino, A., De Pascalis, V., & Zimbardo, P. G. (2003). Testing Zimbardo's Stanford Time Perspective Inventory (STPI)-Short Form. *Time and Society, 12*(2–3), 333–347.

Daugherty, J. R., & Brase, G. L. (2010). Taking time to be healthy: Predicting health behaviors with delay discounting and time perspective. *Personality and Individual Differences, 48*, 202–207.

Desmyter, F., & De Raedt, R. (2012). The relationship between time perspective and subjective well-being of older adults. *Psychologica Belgica, 52*(1), 19–38.

Díaz-Morales, J. F., Ferrari, J. R., & Cohen, J. R. (2008). Indecision and avoidant procrastination: The role of morningness—eveningness and time perspective in chronic delay lifestyles. *The Journal of General Psychology, 135*(3), 228–240.

Donnelly, G., Iyer, R., & Howell, R. T. (2012). The Big Five personality traits, material values, and financial well-being of self-described money managers. *Journal of Economic Psychology, 33*(6), 1129–1142. doi:10.1016/j.joep.2012.08.001.

Drake, L., Duncan, E., Sutherland, F., Abernethy, C., & Henry, C. (2008). Time perspective and correlates of wellbeing. *Time and Society, 17*(1), 47–61.

Ely, R., & Mercurio, A. (2010). Time perspective and autobiographical memory: Individual and gender differences in experiencing time and remembering the past. *Time and Society, 20*, 375–400. doi:10.1177/0961463X10366081.

Epel, E. S., Bandura, A., & Zimbardo, P. G. (1999). Escaping homelessness: The influences of self-efficacy and time perspective on coping with homelessness. *Journal of Applied Social Psychology, 29*(3), 575–596. doi:10.1111/j.1559-1816.1999.tb01402.x.

Ferrari, J. R., & Diaz-Morales, J. (2007). Procrastination: Different time orientations reflect different motives. *Journal of Research in Personality, 41*(3), 707–714. doi:10.1016/j.jrp.2006.06.006.

Fieulaine, N., & Martinez, F. (2010). Time under control: Time perspective and desire for control in substance use. *Addictive Behaviors, 35*, 799–802. doi:10.1016/j.addbeh.2010.03.022.

Fieulaine, N., & Martinez, F. (2012). About the fuels of self-regulation: Time perspective and desire for control in adolescents substance use. In V. Barkoukis (Ed.), *The psychology of self-regulation* (pp. 83–102). New York: Nova.

Fieulaine, N., Apostolidis, T., & Olivetto, F. (2006). Précarité et troubles psychologiques: l'effet médiateur de la perspective temporelle [Time perspective and psychological distress: the mediating role of time perspective]. *Les Cahiers Internationaux de Psychologie Sociale, 72*, 51–64.

Gana, K., Klein, V., Saada, Y., & Trouillet, R. (2012). Relationship between time perspective and life satisfaction among older adults: Test of mediating effect of self-efficacy. *European Review of Applied Psychology*. doi:10.1016/j.erap.2012.07.001.

Gruber, J., Cunningham, W., Kirkland, T., & Hay, A. (2012). Feeling stuck in the present? Mania proneness and history associated with present-oriented time perspective. *Emotion, 12*(1), 13–17.

Guarino, A., De Pascalis, V., & Di Chiacchio, C. (1999). Breast cancer prevention, time perspective, and trait anxiety. *Unpublished manuscript,* University of Rome.

Guthrie, L. C., Butler, S. C., & Ward, M. M. (2009). Time perspective and socioeconomic status: A link to socioeconomic disparities in health? *Social Science and Medicine, 68*(12), 2145–2151.

Guthrie, L. C., Lessl, K., Ochi, O., & Ward, M. M. (2013). Time perspective and smoking, obesity, and exercise in a community sample. *American Journal of Health Behavior, 37*(2), 171–180.

Hamilton, J., Kives, K., Micevski, V., & Grace, S. (2003). Time perspective and health promoting behavior in a cardiac rehabilitation population. *Behavioral Medicine, 28*, 132–139.

Harber, K. D., Zimbardo, P. G., & Boyd, J. N. (2003). Participant self-selection biases as a function of individual differences in time perspective. *Basic and Applied Social Psychology, 25*(3), 255–264. doi:10.1207/S15324834BASP2503_08.

Henson, J. M., Carey, M. P., Carey, K. B., & Maisto, S. A. (2005). Associations among health behaviors and time perspective in young adults: Model testing with boot-strapping replication. *Journal of Behavioral Medicine, 29*, 127–137.

Henson, J. M., Carey, M. P., Carey, K. B., & Maisto, S. A. (2006). Associations among health behaviors and time perspective in young adults: Model testing with boot-strapping replication. *Journal of Behavioral Medicine, 29*(2), 127–137. doi:10.1007/s10865-005-9027-2.

Hodgins, D., & Engel, A. (2002). Future time perspective in pathological gambling. *Journal of Nervous and Mental Disease, 190*(11), 775–780.

Holman, A. E., & Silver, R. C. (2005). Future-oriented thinking and adjustment in a nationwide longitudinal study following the September 11th terrorist attacks. *Motivation and Emotion, 29*(4), 389–410. doi:10.1007/s11031-006-9018-9.

Holman, E. A., & Zimbardo, P. G. (2009). The social language of time: The time perspective–social network connection. *Basic and Applied Social Psychology, 31*, 136–147. doi:10.1080/01973530902880415.

Horstmanshof, L., & Zimitat, C. (2004, July). *Time for persistence*. Paper presented at the 8th Pacific Rim First Year in Higher Education Conference, Melbourne, Australia.

Horstmanshof, L., & Zimitat, C. (2007). Future time orientation predicts academic engagement among first-year university students. *British Journal of Educational Psychology, 77*(3), 703–718. doi:10.1348/000709906X160778.

Kairys, A. (2010). *Time Perspective: Its link to personality traits, age and gender.* Unpublished doctoral thesis, Vilnius University, Lithuania.

Kashdan, T. B., Rose, P., & Fincham, F. D. (2004). Curiosity and exploration: Facilitating positive subjective experiences and personal growth opportunities. *Journal of Personality Assessment, 82*, 291–305.

Kati Nowack, K., Milfont, T. L., & van der Meer, E. (2013). Future versus present: Time perspective and pupillary response in a relatedness judgment task investigating temporal event knowledge. *International Journal of Psychophysiology, 87*(2), 173–182. doi:10.1016/j.ijpsycho.2012.12.006.

Keough, K. A., Zimbardo, P. G., & Boyd, J. N. (1999). Who's smoking, drinking, and using drugs? Time perspective as a predictor of substance use. *Basic and Applied Social Psychology, 21*(2), 149–164.

Klingemann, H. (2001). The Time Game: Temporal perspectives of patients and staff in alcohol and drug treatment. *Time and Society, 10*(2–3), 303–328.

Kolesovs, A. (2002). The relation between time perspective and locus of control in high school students. *Baltic Journal of Psychology, 3*(2), 7–19.

Koļesovs, A. (2004). Gender differences in time perspective of high school students in Latvia. *Comparison of State and Trait Anxiety of Latvians and Russians Residing in Latvia, 5*(1), 14.

Kovač, V. B., & Rise, J. (2007). The relation between past behavior, intention, planning, and quitting smoking: The moderating effect of future orientation. *Journal of Applied Biobehavioral Research, 12*(2), 82–100. doi:10.1111/j.1751-9861.2007.00015.x.

Laghi, F., Baiocco, R., D'Alessio, M., & Gurrieri, G. (2009). Suicidal ideation and time perspective in high school students. *European Psychiatry, 24*, 41–46.

Laghi, F., Liga, F., Baumgartner, E., & Baiocco, R. (2012). Time perspective and psychosocial positive functioning among Italian adolescents who binge eat and drink. *Adolescence, 35*(5), 1277–1284.

Laghi, F., Baiocco, R., Liga, F., Guarino, A., & Baumgartner, E. (2013). Identity status differences among Italian adolescents: Associations with time perspective. *Children and Youth Services Review, 35*(3), 482–487.

Lee, S., & Song, E. (2011). Influences of time perspective on impulsive purchase tendency. *Journal of Global Scholars of Marketing Science, 21*(4), 210–217.

Levine-Kornfield, S. (2010). *Maternal-Fetal attachment, temporal orientation and locus of control: Implications for prenatal care behaviors and HIV risk reduction during pregnancy.* Unpublished Doctoral thesis, Drexel University, USA.

Levy, B., & Earleywine, M. (2004). Discriminating reinforcement expectancies for studying from future time perspective in the prediction of drinking problems. *Addictive Behaviors, 29*(1), 181–190. doi:10.1016/S0306-4603(03)00073-X.

Liniauskaitė, A., & Kairys, A. (2009). The lithuanian version of the Zimbardo time perspective inventory. *Psichologija, 40*, 66–87.

Luyckx, K., Lens, W., Smits, I., & Goossens, L. (2010). Time perspective and identity formation: Short-term longitudinal dynamics in college students. *International Journal of Behavioral Development, 34*(3), 238–247.

MacKillop, J., Anderson, E. J., Castelda, B. A., Mattson, R. E., & Donovick, P. J. (2006). Divergent validity of measures of cognitive distortions, impulsivity, and time perspective in pathological gambling. *Journal of Gambling Studies, 22*(3), 339–354. doi:10.1007/s10899-006-9021-9.

Martz, E., & Livneh, H. (2007). Do posttraumatic reactions predict future time perspective among people with insulin-dependent diabetes mellitus? *Rehabilitation Counseling Bulletin, 50*(2), 87–98. doi:10.1177/00343552070500020701.

McElwee, R. O.'. B., & Haugh, J. A. (2009). Thinking clearly versus frequently about the future self: Exploring this distinction and its relation to possible selves. *Self and Identity, 9*(3), 298–321. doi:10.1080/15298860903054290.

Mello, Z. R., & Worrell, F. C. (2006). The relationship of time perspective to age, gender, and academic achievement among academically talented adolescents. *Journal for the Education of the Gifted, 29*(3), 271–289.

Merson, F., & Perriot, J. (2011). Précarité sociale et perception du temps, impact sur le sevrage tabagique [Social deprivation and time perception, the impact on smoking cessation]. *Santé Publique, 23*(5), 359–370.

Milfont, T. L., & Gouveia, V. V. (2006). Time perspective and values: An exploratory study of their relations to environmental attitudes. *Journal of Environmental Psychology, 26*(1), 72–82. doi:10.1016/j.jenvp.2006.03.001.

Milfont, T. L., Andrade, T. L., Belo, R. P., & Pessoa, V. S. (2008). Testing Zimbardo time perspective inventory in a Brazilian sample. *Interamerican Journal of Psychology, 42*, 49–58.

Nowack, K., Milfont, T. L., & van der Meer, E. (2013). Future versus present: Time perspective and pupillary response in a relatedness judgment task investigating temporal event knowledge. *International Journal of Psychophysiology, 87*, 173–182.

Petkoska, J., & Earl, J. K. (2009). Understanding the influence of demographic and psychological variables on retirement planning. *Psychology and Ageing, 24*(1), 245–251.

Phan, H. P. (2009). Amalgamation of future time orientation, epistemological beliefs, achievement goals and study strategies: Empirical evidence established. *British Journal of Educational Psychology, 79*, 155–173. doi:10.1348/000709908X306864.

Pluck, G., Lee, K. H., Lauder, H. E., Fox, J. M., Spence, S. A., & Parks, R. W. (2008). Time perspective, depression, and substance misuse among the homeless. *The Journal of Psychology, 142*(2), 159–168.

Préau, M., Apostolidis, T., Francois, C., Raffi, F., & Spire, B. (2007). Time perspective and quality of life among HIV-infected patients in the context of HAART. *AIDS Care, 19*(4), 449–458. doi:10.1080/09540120601017464.

Protogerou, C., & Turner-Cobb, J. (2011). Predictors of non-condom use intentions by university students in Britain and Greece: The impact of attitudes, time perspective, relationship status, and habit. *Journal of Child & Adolescent Mental Health, 23*(2), 91–106.

Rego-Leite, U. (2008). Estudo de validaçao do inventario de perspectiva de tempo de Zimbardo (Brazilian – Validation study of the Zimbardo Time Perpective Inventory). *Avaliaçao Psicologica, 7*(3), 301–320.

Richmond, J., Clare Wilson, J., & Zinken, J. (2012). A feeling for the future: How does agency in time metaphors relate to feelings? *European Journal of Social Psychology*. doi:10.1002/ejsp.1906.

Roncancio, A. M., Ward, K. K., & Fernandez, M. E. (2013). The influence of time perspective on cervical cancer screening among Latinas in the United States. *Journal of health psychology*. doi:10.1177/1359105313495073.

Rothspan, S., & Read, S. J. (1996). Present versus future time perspective and HIV risk among heterosexual college students. *Health Psychology, 15*(2), 131–134. doi:10.1037/0278-6133.15.2.131.

Routledge, C., Arndt, J., Sedikides, C., & Wildschut, T. (2008). A blast from the past: The terror management function of nostalgia. *Journal of Experimental Social Psychology, 44*, 132–140. doi:10.1016/j.jesp.2006.11.001.

Sansbury, B., Dasgupta, A., Guthrie, L., & Ward, M. (2014). Time perspective and medication adherence among individuals with hypertension or diabetes mellitus. *Patient Education and Counseling*, e-first. doi.org/10.1016/j.pec.2013.12.016.

Schnitker, S. A., & Emmons, R. A. (2007). Patience as a virtue: Religious and psychological perspectives. *Research in the Social Scientific Study of Religion, 18*, 177–207. doi:10.1163/ej.9789004158511.i-301.69.

Shipp, A. J., Edwards, J. R., & Lambert, L. S. (2009). Conceptualization and measurement of temporal focus: The subjective experience of the past, present, and future. *Organizational Behavior and Human Decision Processes, 110*, 1–22.

Shores, K., & Scott, D. (2007). The relationship of individual time perspective and recreation experience preferences. *Journal of Leisure Research, 39*(1), 28–59.

Sircova, A., & Mitina, O. V. (2008). Age dynamics of time orientations [in Russian]. *Voprosi Psikhologii, 2*, 41–55.

Sircova, A., Mitina, O. V., Boyd, J. N., Davydova, I. S., Zimbardo, P. G., Nepryakho, T. L., Nikitina, E. A., Semenova, N. S., Fieulaine, N., & Yasnaya, V. A. (2007). Phenomenon of time perspective in different cultures (based on research materials using ZTPI) [in Russian]. *International Journal of Cultural-Historical Psychology, 4*, 19–31.

Sircova, A., Sokolova, E. T., & Mitina, O. V. (2008). Adaptation of Zimbardo time perspective inventory [in Russian]. *Psikhologichesky Journal, 29*(3), 101–109.

Steger, M. F., Kashdan, T. B., Sullivan, B. A., & Lorentz, D. (2008). Understanding the search for meaning in life: Personality, cognitive style, and the dynamic between seeking and experiencing meaning. *Journal of Personality, 76*, 199–228. doi:10.1111/j.1467-6494.2007.00484.x.

Stolarski, M., Bitner, J., & Zimbardo, P. G. (2011). Time perspective, emotional intelligence and discounting of delayed awards. *Time and Society, 20*, 346–363. doi:10.1177/0961463X11414296.

Stolarski, M., Ledzinska, M., & Matthews, G. (2013). Morning is tomorrow, evening is today: Relationships between chronotype and time perspective. *Biological Rythm Research, 44*(2), 181–196.

Thoms, P. (2004). *Driven by time: Time orientation and leadership*. Westport/London: Praeger.

Thornhill, R., & Fincher, C. L. (2007). What is the relevance of attachment and life history to political values? *Evolution and Human Behavior, 28*, 215–222.

Tucker, J. A., Blum, E. R., Xie, L., Roth, D. L., & Simpson, C. A. (2012). Interactive voice response self-monitoring to assess risk behaviors in rural substance users living with HIV/AIDS. *AIDS Behavior, 16*(2), 432–440.

van Beek, W., Berghuis, H., Kerkhof, A., & Beekman, A. (2011). Time perspective, personality and psychopathology: Zimbardo's time perspective inventory in psychiatry. *Time and Society, 20*, 364–374. doi:10.1177/0961463X10373960.

Van Ittersum, K. (2011). The effect of decision maker's time perspective on intention-behavior consistency. doi:10.1007/s11002-011-9152-3.

Van Ittersum, K. (2012). The effect of decision maker's time perspective on intention-behavior consistency. *Marketing Letters, 23*(1), 263–277.

Vinkers, C. D. W., Adriaanse, M. A., & De Ridder, D. T. D. (2012). In it for the long haul: Characteristics of early and late drop out in a self-management intervention for weight control. *Journal of Behavioral Medicine*. doi:10.1007/s10865-012-9446-9.

Wills, T. A., Sandy, J. M., & Yaeger, A. M. (2001). Time perspective and early-onset substance use: a model based on stress-coping theory. *Psychology of Addictive Behaviors, 15*(2), 118–125.

Zhang, J.W., Howell, R.T., & Stolarski, M. (2012). Comparing three methods to measure a balanced time perspective: The relationship between a balanced time perspective and subjective well-being. *Journal of Happiness Studies*, 1–16. doi:10.1007/s10902-012-9322-x

Zimbardo, P. G., & Boyd, J. N. (1999). Putting time in perspective: A valid, reliable individual-differences metric. *Journal of Personality and Social Psychology, 77*(6), 1271–1288.

Zimbardo, P., Keough, K., & Boyd, J. (1997). Present time perspective as a predictor of risky driving. *Personality and Individual Differences, 23*, 1007–1023. doi:10.1016/S0191-8869(97)00113-X.

Index

M. Stolarski et al. (eds.), *Time Perspective Theory; Review, Research and Application: Essays in Honor of Philip G. Zimbardo*, DOI 10.1007/978-3-319-07368-2,

The manufacturer's authorised representative in the EU is Springer Nature Customer Service Centre GmbH, Europaplatz 3, 69115 Heidelberg, Germany. If you have any concerns regarding our products, please contact ProductSafety@springernature.com

Printed and bound by CPI Group (UK) Ltd, Croydon, CR0 4YY
30/09/2026
02225593-0016